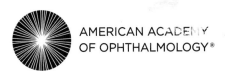

AMERICAN ACADEMY
OF OPHTHALMOLOGY®

External Disease and Cornea

Last major revision 2017–2018

2018–2019
BCSC
Basic and Clinical
Science Course™

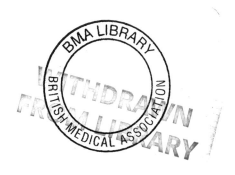
Protecting Sight. Empowering Lives.®

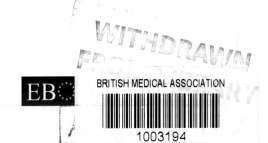

The American Academy of Ophthalmology is accredited by the Accreditation Council for Continuing Medical Education (ACCME) to provide continuing medical education for physicians.

The American Academy of Ophthalmology designates this enduring material for a maximum of 15 *AMA PRA Category 1 Credits*™. Physicians should claim only the credit commensurate with the extent of their participation in the activity.

CME expiration date: June 1, 2020. *AMA PRA Category 1 Credits*™ may be claimed only once between June 1, 2017, and the expiration date.

BCSC® volumes are designed to increase the physician's ophthalmic knowledge through study and review. Users of this activity are encouraged to read the text and then answer the study questions provided at the back of the book.

To claim *AMA PRA Category 1 Credits*™ upon completion of this activity, learners must demonstrate appropriate knowledge and participation in the activity by taking the posttest for Section 8 and achieving a score of 80% or higher. For further details, please see the instructions for requesting CME credit at the back of the book.

Cover image: From BCSC Section 12, *Retina and Vitreous.* End-stage chorioretinal atrophy in pathologic myopia. *(Courtesy of Richard F. Spaide, MD.)*

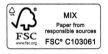

MIX
Paper from
responsible sources
FSC
www.fsc.org   FSC® C103061

Basic and Clinical Science Course

Louis B. Cantor, MD, Indianapolis, Indiana, *Senior Secretary for Clinical Education*

Christopher J. Rapuano, MD, Philadelphia, Pennsylvania, *Secretary for Lifelong Learning and Assessment*

George A. Cioffi, MD, New York, New York, *BCSC Course Chair*

Section 8

Faculty

Robert W. Weisenthal, MD, *Chair,* De Witt, New York
Mary K. Daly, MD, Lexington, Massachusetts
Denise de Freitas, MD, São Paulo, Brazil
Robert S. Feder, MD, Chicago, Illinois
Stephen E. Orlin, MD, Philadelphia, Pennsylvania
Elmer Y. Tu, MD, Chicago, Illinois
Woodford S. Van Meter, MD, Lexington, Kentucky
David D. Verdier, MD, Grand Rapids, Michigan

The Academy wishes to acknowledge the *Cornea Society* for recommending faculty members to the BCSC Section 8 committee.

The Academy also wishes to acknowledge the following committees for review of this edition:

Committee on Aging: Rahul T. Pandit, MD, Houston, Texas

Vision Rehabilitation Committee: John D. Shepherd, MD, Omaha, Nebraska

Practicing Ophthalmologists Advisory Committee for Education: Dasa V. Gangadhar, MD, *Primary Reviewer,* Wichita, Kansas; Edward K. Isbey III, MD, *Chair,* Asheville, North Carolina; Alice Bashinsky, MD, Asheville, North Carolina; David Browning, MD, PhD, Charlotte, North Carolina; Bradley D. Fouraker, MD, Tampa, Florida; Steven J. Grosser, MD, Golden Valley, Minnesota; Stephen R. Klapper, MD, Carmel, Indiana; James A. Savage, MD, Memphis, Tennessee; Michelle S. Ying, MD, Ladson, South Carolina

European Board of Ophthalmology: Joseph Colin, MD, PhD, *EBO Chair,* Bordeaux, France; Marie-José Tassignon, MD, PhD, FEBO, *EBO Liaison,* Antwerp, Belgium; Massimo Busin, MD, Forlì, Italy; Béatrice Cochener-Lamard, MD, PhD, Brest, France; Sheraz M. Daya, MD, London, England, United Kingdom; Günther Grabner, MD, Salzburg, Austria; Rudy M.M.A. Nuijts, MD, PhD, Maastricht, the Netherlands

Financial Disclosures

Academy staff members who contributed to the development of this product state that within the 12 months prior to their contributions to this CME activity and for the duration of development, they have had no financial interest in or other relationship with any entity discussed in this course that produces, markets, resells, or distributes ophthalmic health care goods or services consumed by or used in patients, or with any competing commercial product or service.

The authors and reviewers state that within the 12 months prior to their contributions to this CME activity and for the duration of development, they have had the following financial relationships:*

Dr Browning: Aerpio Therapeutics (S), Alcon (S), Alimera Sciences (C), Genentech (S), Novartis Pharmaceuticals (S), Ohr Pharmaceutical (S), Pfizer (S), Regeneron Pharmaceuticals (S)

Dr Busin: Moria (L, P)

Dr Cochener-Lamard: Alcon (L), Bausch + Lomb (L), Laboratoires Théa (C), Novagali-Santen (C), PhysIOL (L), ReVision Optics, Inc (L)

Dr Colin: Abbott Medical Optics (C), Addition Technology, Inc (C), Alcon (C)

Dr Daya: Bausch + Lomb (C, L), PhysIOL (C), STAAR Surgical (C), Technolas Perfect Vision GmbH (C, L), Zeiss Acri.Tec (C)

Dr Fouraker: Addition Technology (C, L), Alcon (C, L), KeraVision (C, L), OASIS Medical (C, L)

Dr Grabner: Abbott Medical Optics (C, L, S), AcuFocus Inc (L, S), Polytech (C)

Dr Grosser: Ivantis (O)

Dr Isbey: Alcon (S), Allscripts (C), Bausch + Lomb (S), Medflow (C), Oculos Clinical Research (S)

Dr Nuijts: Alcon (L, S), ASICO (P), Bausch + Lomb (C), SensoMotoric Instruments (C, L)

Dr Savage: Allergan (L)

Dr Tassignon: Morcher GmbH (P)

Dr Tu: Eye Bank Association of America (S), Seattle Genetics (C)

The other authors and reviewers state that within the 12 months prior to their contributions to this CME activity and for the duration of development, they have had no financial interest in or other relationship with any entity discussed in this course that produces, markets, resells, or distributes ophthalmic health care goods or services consumed by or used in patients, or with any competing commercial product or service.

*C = consultant fees, paid advisory boards, or fees for attending a meeting; L = lecture fees (honoraria), travel fees, or reimbursements when speaking at the invitation of a commercial sponsor; O = equity ownership/stock options of publicly or privately traded firms (excluding mutual funds) with manufacturers of commercial ophthalmic products or commercial ophthalmic services; P = patents and/or royalties that might be viewed as creating a potential conflict of interest; S = grant support for the past year (all sources) and all sources used for a specific talk or manuscript with no time limitation

Recent Past Faculty

Natalie A. Afshari, MD

Charles S. Bouchard, MD

Kathryn A. Colby, MD, PhD

David S. Rootman, MD

In addition, the Academy gratefully acknowledges the contributions of numerous past faculty and advisory committee members who have played an important role in the development of previous editions of the Basic and Clinical Science Course.

American Academy of Ophthalmology Staff

Dale E. Fajardo, EdD, MBA, *Vice President, Education*

Beth Wilson, *Director, Continuing Professional Development*

Ann McGuire, *Acquisitions and Development Manager*

Stephanie Tanaka, *Publications Manager*

D. Jean Ray, *Production Manager*

Beth Collins, *Medical Editor*

Naomi Ruiz, *Publications Specialist*

American Academy of Ophthalmology
655 Beach Street
Box 7424
San Francisco, CA 94120-7424

Contents

6 Clinical Approach to Depositions and Degenerations of the Conjunctiva, Cornea, and Sclera 111

7 Corneal Dystrophies and Ectasias 133

8 Systemic Disorders With Corneal and Other Anterior Segment Manifestations 173

11   Diagnosis and Management of Immune-Related Disorders of the External Eye 285

General Introduction

The Basic and Clinical Science Course (BCSC) is designed to meet the needs of residents and practitioners for a comprehensive yet concise curriculum of the field of ophthalmology. The BCSC has developed from its original brief outline format, which relied heavily on outside readings, to a more convenient and educationally useful self-contained text. The Academy updates and revises the course annually, with the goals of integrating the basic science and clinical practice of ophthalmology and of keeping ophthalmologists current with new developments in the various subspecialties.

The BCSC incorporates the effort and expertise of more than 90 ophthalmologists, organized into 13 Section faculties, working with Academy editorial staff. In addition, the course continues to benefit from many lasting contributions made by the faculties of previous editions. Members of the Academy Practicing Ophthalmologists Advisory Committee for Education, Committee on Aging, and Vision Rehabilitation Committee review every volume before major revisions. Members of the European Board of Ophthalmology, organized into Section faculties, also review each volume before major revisions, focusing primarily on differences between American and European ophthalmology practice.

Organization of the Course

The Basic and Clinical Science Course comprises 13 volumes, incorporating fundamental ophthalmic knowledge, subspecialty areas, and special topics:

1 Update on General Medicine
2 Fundamentals and Principles of Ophthalmology
3 Clinical Optics
4 Ophthalmic Pathology and Intraocular Tumors
5 Neuro-Ophthalmology
6 Pediatric Ophthalmology and Strabismus
7 Orbit, Eyelids, and Lacrimal System
8 External Disease and Cornea
9 Intraocular Inflammation and Uveitis
10 Glaucoma
11 Lens and Cataract
12 Retina and Vitreous
13 Refractive Surgery

In addition, a comprehensive Master Index allows the reader to easily locate subjects throughout the entire series.

References

Readers who wish to explore specific topics in greater detail may consult the references cited within each chapter and listed in the Basic Texts section at the back of the book.

These references are intended to be selective rather than exhaustive, chosen by the BCSC faculty as being important, current, and readily available to residents and practitioners.

Multimedia

This edition of Section 8, *External Disease and Cornea,* includes videos related to topics covered in the book. The videos were selected by members of the BCSC faculty and are available to readers of the print and electronic versions of Section 8 (www.aao.org/bcscvideo _section08). Mobile-device users can scan the QR code below (a QR-code reader must already be installed on the device) to access the video content.

Self-Assessment and CME Credit

Each volume of the BCSC is designed as an independent study activity for ophthalmology residents and practitioners. The learning objectives for this volume are given on page 1. The text, illustrations, and references provide the information necessary to achieve the objectives; the study questions allow readers to test their understanding of the material and their mastery of the objectives. Physicians who wish to claim CME credit for this educational activity may do so by following the instructions given at the end of the book.

This Section of the BCSC has been approved by the American Board of Ophthalmology as a Maintenance of Certification Part II self-assessment and CME activity.

Conclusion

The Basic and Clinical Science Course has expanded greatly over the years, with the addition of much new text, numerous illustrations, and video content. Recent editions have sought to place a greater emphasis on clinical applicability while maintaining a solid foundation in basic science. As with any educational program, it reflects the experience of its authors. As its faculties change and medicine progresses, new viewpoints emerge on controversial subjects and techniques. Not all alternate approaches can be included in this series; as with any educational endeavor, the learner should seek additional sources, including Academy Preferred Practice Pattern Guidelines.

The BCSC faculty and staff continually strive to improve the educational usefulness of the course; you, the reader, can contribute to this ongoing process. If you have any suggestions or questions about the series, please do not hesitate to contact the faculty or the editors.

The authors, editors, and reviewers hope that your study of the BCSC will be of lasting value and that each Section will serve as a practical resource for quality patient care.

Objectives

Upon completion of BCSC Section 8, *External Disease and Cornea,* the reader should be able to

- describe the anatomy of the external eye and cornea

- describe the techniques used for systematic evaluation of the cornea, including tests for assessing corneal topography, tensile strength, and endothelial function

- identify the distinctive clinical signs of specific diseases of the ocular surface

- identify the two most common underlying causes of dry eye

- identify and differentiate the corneal dystrophies

- select the appropriate management of the corneal dystrophies

- recognize common corneal manifestations of systemic disease

- outline an approach to the evaluation, diagnosis, and management of immune-related and neoplastic disorders of the external eye and anterior segment

- describe the indications for and techniques of surgical procedures used in the management of corneal disease, trauma, and refractive error

- discuss common surgical interventions for ocular surface disorders such as pterygium and corneal melts

- explain the role of full-thickness and lamellar transplantation in the treatment of corneal disease

CHAPTER 1

Structure and Function of the External Eye and Cornea

Highlights

- Diseases of the external eye and cornea include a wide range of conditions affecting the eyelids, sclera, and ocular surface (cornea, conjunctiva, and limbus). The external eye has both anatomical and immunologic defense mechanisms that protect the eye against infection and other ocular conditions.
- Current corneal disease classifications and evolving corneal grafting techniques make knowledge of corneal anatomy of the utmost clinical and surgical importance.
- The total dioptric power of a normal human eye is 58.60 diopters (D), to which the cornea contributes 74%.

Eyelids

The functions of the eyelid are protection of the eye, distribution of tears, mechanical cleaning of the ocular surface, regulation of light exposure for the eye, and partial production of the tear film. The eyelid is composed of skin, subcutaneous connective tissue, fibrous tissue (tarsus), muscle, and mucous membrane (palpebral conjunctiva). The eyelid skin varies in thickness, from 0.5 mm at the eyelid margin to 1 mm at the orbital rim. Except for fine vellus hairs, the eyelashes (cilia) are the only hairs of the eyelids and are twice as numerous along the upper eyelid compared with the lower margin. Eyelashes are replaced every 3–5 months and usually regrow in 2 weeks when cut and within 2 months if epilated. They catch small particles and also work as sensors to stimulate reflex eyelid closure. Blinking stimulates the lacrimal pump to release tears, which are then spread across the cornea, flushing foreign material. Most individuals blink an average of 10–15 times per minute at rest, 20 times per minute or more during a conversation, and as few as 5 times per minute when concentrating (eg, reading). Blink frequency has also been shown to change in different positions of gaze. The orbicularis oculi muscle, which is innervated by cranial nerve (CN) VII, closes the upper and lower eyelids (Fig 1-1). The levator palpebrae muscle, innervated by CN III, inserts into the tarsal plate and skin and elevates the upper eyelid. The Müller muscle, innervated by sympathetic nerves, increases the width of the palpebral fissure.

The epidermis of the eyelids abruptly changes from keratinized to nonkeratinized stratified squamous epithelium at the mucocutaneous junction of the eyelid margin, along

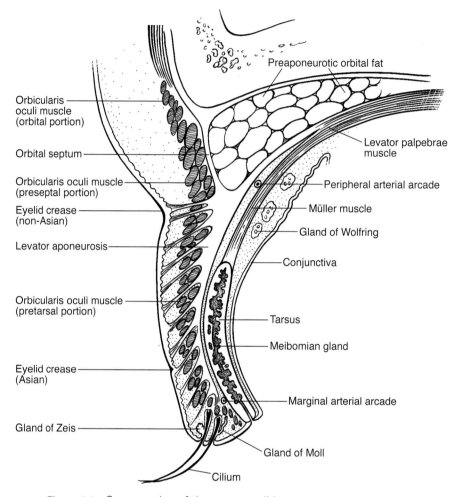

Figure 1-1 Cross section of the upper eyelid. *(Illustration by Christine Gralapp.)*

the row of *meibomian gland* orifices. Holocrine sebaceous glands and eccrine sweat glands are present in the eyelid skin. Near the eyelid margin are apocrine sweat glands (the *glands of Moll*) and numerous modified sebaceous glands (the *glands of Zeis*).

See BCSC Section 2, *Fundamentals and Principles of Ophthalmology*, and Section 7, *Orbit, Eyelids, and Lacrimal System*, for additional discussion of eyelid anatomy.

Argilés M, Cardona G, Pérez-Cabré E, Rodríguez M. Blink rate and incomplete blinks in six different controlled hard-copy and electronic reading conditions. *Invest Ophthalmol Vis Sci.* 2015;56(11):6679–6685.

Lin LK, Gokoffski KK. Eyelids and the corneal surface. In: Mannis MJ, Holland EJ, eds. *Cornea.* Vol 1. 4th ed. Philadelphia: Elsevier; 2017:40–45.

Lacrimal Functional Unit

The lacrimal functional unit (LFU; Fig 1-2) is a highly complex apparatus comprising the lacrimal glands, ocular surface, and eyelids, as well as the sensory and motor nerves that

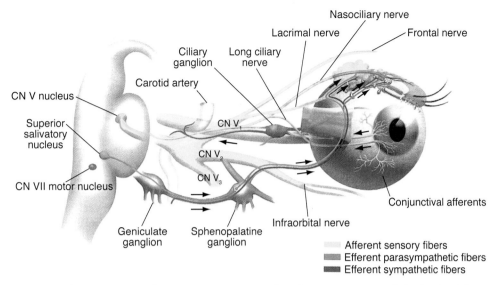

Figure 1-2 The sensory and motor nerves connecting the components of the lacrimal functional unit. CN = cranial nerve. *(Modified with permission from Pflugfelder SC, Beuerman RW, Stern ME, eds. Dry Eye and Ocular Surface Disorders. New York: Marcel Dekker; 2004.)*

connect these components. The LFU is responsible for the regulation, production, and health of the tear film. The LFU responds to environmental, endocrinologic, and cortical influences. Its overall functions are to preserve the following:

- integrity of the tear film (by carrying out lubricating, antimicrobial, and nutritional roles)
- health of the ocular surface (by maintaining corneal transparency and the surface stem cell population)
- the quality of the image projected onto the retina

The afferent component of the LFU is mediated through ocular surface and trigeminal nociceptors, which synapse in the brainstem with autonomic and motor (efferent) nerves. The autonomic nerve fibers innervate the meibomian glands, conjunctival goblet cells, and lacrimal glands. The motor nerve fibers innervate the orbicularis muscle to initiate blinking. During blinking, the meibomian glands express lipid, and the tears are replenished from the inferior tear meniscus and spread across the cornea while excess tears are directed into the lacrimal puncta.

Pflugfelder SC, Beuerman RW, Stern ME, eds. *Dry Eye and Ocular Surface Disorders.* Boca Raton, FL: CRC Press/Taylor & Francis; 2004.

Tear Film

Our understanding of the structure and composition of the tear film has gradually evolved. The tear film was formerly described as a structure composed of 3 layers: lipid (expressed from the meibomian glands), aqueous (expressed from the lacrimal gland), and mucin (produced primarily by goblet cells). It is now thought of as a uniform gel consisting of

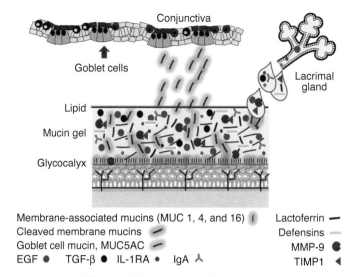

Figure 1-3 Components of the tear film—produced by the lacrimal glands, conjunctival goblet cells, and surface epithelium—lubricate (mucins), heal (epidermal growth factor [EGF]), and protect the cornea from infection (lactoferrin, defensins, immunoglobulin A [IgA]). When the tear film is inflamed, it produces interleukin-1 receptor antagonist (IL-1RA), transforming growth factor β (TGF-β), and tissue inhibitor of matrix metalloproteinase 1 (TIMP 1). MMP-9 = matrix metalloproteinase 9. *(Modified with permission from Pflugfelder SC. Tear dysfunction and the cornea: LXVIII Edward Jackson Memorial Lecture.* Am J Ophthalmol. *2011;152(6):902.)*

soluble mucus, which is secreted by conjunctival goblet cells, mixed with fluids and proteins secreted by the lacrimal glands (Fig 1-3).

The air–tear film interface at the surface of the cornea constitutes the primary refractive element of the eye. The tear film is primarily responsible for maintaining a smooth optical surface between blinks. It also serves as a medium to remove irritants and pathogens and contains a variety of elements that control the normal ocular flora. Further, tears dilute toxins and allergens and allow for the diffusion of oxygen and other nutrients. Maintenance of the tear film is thus critical to normal corneal function.

Pflugfelder SC. Tear dysfunction and the cornea: LXVIII Edward Jackson Memorial Lecture. *Am J Ophthalmol.* 2011;152(6):900–909.

Conjunctiva

The conjunctiva can be broadly divided as follows: bulbar (covers the eyeball), forniceal (covers the superior and inferior fornices), and palpebral, or tarsal (starts at the mucocutaneous junction of the eyelid and covers the inner eyelid). The *caruncle*—a fleshy, ovoid modified mass approximately 5 mm high and 3 mm wide, containing the lacus lacrimalis—is attached to the inferomedial side of the plica semilunaris and bears goblet cells and lacrimal tissue, as well as hairs, sebaceous glands, and sweat glands. The *plica semilunaris* is a crescent-shaped vertical fold at the medial angle of the eye. The *palpebral,* or *tarsal, conjunctiva* is tightly adherent to the underlying tarsus. The *bulbar conjunctiva* is loosely attached to the Tenon capsule, and both insert into the limbus.

The cell morphology of the conjunctival epithelium varies from stratified cuboidal over the tarsus and columnar in the fornices to squamous on the globe. Goblet cells account for up to 10% of basal cells of the conjunctival epithelium and are most numerous in the tarsal conjunctiva, the inferonasal bulbar conjunctiva, and in the area of the plica semilunaris.

The *substantia propria* of the conjunctiva consists of loose connective tissue. Conjunctiva-associated lymphoid tissue (CALT), which consists of lymphocytes and other leukocytes, is present, especially in the fornices. Lymphocytes interact with mucosal epithelial cells through reciprocal regulatory signals mediated by growth factors, cytokines, and neuropeptides.

The palpebral conjunctiva shares its blood supply with the eyelids. The bulbar conjunctiva is supplied by the anterior ciliary arteries, which arise from muscular branches of the ophthalmic artery. These capillaries are fenestrated and leak fluid, producing chemosis (conjunctival swelling), as a response to allergies or other inflammatory events.

Cornea

The cornea is a transparent, avascular tissue that consists of 5 layers (Fig 1-4): epithelium, Bowman, stroma, Descemet membrane, and endothelium; these are discussed in the following subsections.

In adults, the cornea measures 11–12 mm horizontally and 10–11 mm vertically. It is approximately 500–600 μm thick at its center and gradually increases in thickness toward the periphery. The cornea is aspheric, although the central portion of the anterior corneal

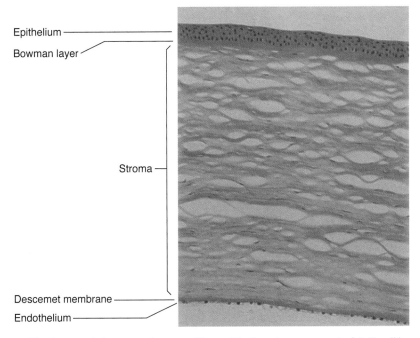

Figure 1-4 The layers of the normal cornea. The epithelium is composed of 4–6 cell layers, but it can increase in thickness to maintain a smooth surface (hematoxylin-eosin, ×32).

surface is often described as a spherocylindrical convex mirror. The general refractive index of the cornea is 1.376. The average radius of curvature of the anterior central cornea is 7.8 mm, which would produce a dioptric power of 43.25 D for the front surface of the cornea, using the keratometer calibration index of 1.3375. The total dioptric power of a normal human eye is 58.60 D, to which the cornea contributes 74%. The cornea is also the major source of astigmatism in the human optical system. For further discussion of corneal optics, see Evaluation of Corneal Curvature in Chapter 2.

For its nutrition, the cornea depends on diffusion of glucose from the aqueous humor and of oxygen through the tear film. In addition, the peripheral cornea is supplied with oxygen from the limbal circulation.

The density of nerve endings in the cornea is among the highest in the body, and the sensitivity of the cornea is 100 times that of the conjunctiva. Sensory nerve fibers extend from the long ciliary nerves and form a subepithelial plexus.

Corneal Epithelium

The corneal epithelium is composed of 4–6 layers, which include 1–2 layers of superficial squamous cells, 2–3 layers of broad wing cells, and an innermost layer of columnar basal cells. It is 40–50 μm thick (see Fig 1-4; also see the Pachymetry section in Chapter 2). The epithelium and tear film form an optically smooth surface. Tight junctions between superficial epithelial cells prevent penetration of tear fluid into the stroma. Continuous proliferation of limbal stem cells gives rise to the other layers, which subsequently differentiate into superficial cells. With maturation, these differentiated cells become coated with microvilli on their outermost surface and then desquamate into the tears. The process of differentiation takes approximately 7–14 days. Basal epithelial cells secrete a continuous, 50-nm-thick basement membrane, which is composed of type IV collagen, laminin, and other proteins. Corneal clarity depends on the tight packing of epithelial cells, which results in a layer with a nearly uniform refractive index and minimal light scattering.

Bowman Layer

The Bowman layer lies anterior to the corneal stroma. Previously considered a membrane, the Bowman layer is rather the acellular condensate of the most anterior portion of the stroma (see Fig 1-4). This layer is 15 μm thick and helps maintain the shape of the cornea. When disrupted, it will not regenerate.

Corneal Stroma

The corneal stroma makes up roughly 90% of the total corneal thickness (see Fig 1-4). The regular arrangement of stromal cells (keratocytes), fibers, and extracellular matrix is necessary for a clear cornea. Keratocytes vary in size and density throughout the stroma and form a 3-dimensional network throughout the cornea. They are flattened fibroblasts, located between the stromal collagen lamellae (Fig 1-5), and they continually digest and manufacture stromal molecules. Keratocyte density declines with age, by 0.9% per year for

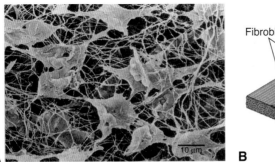
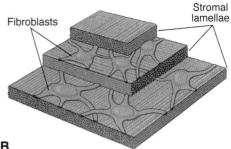

Figure 1-5 Keratocytes **(A)** are flattened fibroblasts **(B)** situated between the stromal collagen lamellae. *(Reproduced with permission from Oyster CW. The Human Eye: Structure and Function. Sunderland, MA: Sinauer Associates; 1999:331.)*

anterior density and by 0.3% per year for posterior density. It can also decline with refractive laser surgery and may not be completely restored.

The corneal stroma is composed of an extracellular matrix formed of collagens and proteoglycans. Type I and type V fibrillar collagens are intertwined with filaments of type VI collagen. The major corneal proteoglycans are decorin (associated with dermatan sulfate) and lumican (associated with keratan sulfate).

Corneal transparency depends on maintaining the water content of the corneal stroma at 78%. Corneal hydration is largely controlled by intact epithelial and endothelial barriers and the functioning of the endothelial pump, which is linked to an ion-transport system controlled by temperature-dependent enzymes such as Na^+,K^+-ATPase. In addition, negatively charged stromal glycosaminoglycans tend to repel each other, producing a *swelling pressure (SP)*. Because the intraocular pressure (IOP) tends to compress the cornea, the overall imbibition pressure of the corneal stroma is given as IOP – SP. The total transendothelial osmotic force is calculated by adding the imbibition pressure and the various electrolyte gradients produced by the endothelial transport channels. Corneal hydration varies from anterior to posterior and increases closer to the endothelium.

Schlötzer-Schrehardt U, Bachmann BO, Tourtas T, et al. Ultrastructure of the posterior corneal stroma. *Ophthalmology.* 2015;122(4):693–699.

Descemet Membrane

The Descemet membrane is the basement membrane of the corneal endothelium (see Fig 1-4). It is 3 μm at birth and increases in size, to 10–12 μm in adulthood, as the endothelium gradually lays down a posterior amorphous, nonbanded zone. Though controversial, a novel layer in the posterior part of the cornea (pre-Descemet layer or Dua's layer) has been reported. This layer may be important during deep anterior lamellar keratoplasty. The *Schwalbe line* is a gonioscopic landmark that defines the end of the Descemet membrane and the beginning of the trabecular meshwork.

Dua HS, Faraj LA, Said DG, Gray T, Lowe J. Human corneal anatomy redefined: a novel pre-Descemet's layer (Dua's layer). *Ophthalmology.* 2013;120(9):1778–1785.

Corneal Endothelium

Corneal endothelial cells lie on the posterior surface of the cornea, composing a mono-layer of closely interdigitated cells arranged in a mosaic pattern of mostly hexagonal shapes (see Fig 1-4). Human endothelial cells do not proliferate in vivo, but they can divide in cell culture. If cell loss occurs, especially as a result of trauma or surgery, the defective area is covered via enlargement and spread of residual cells or perhaps peripheral stem cells. These cell findings can be observed by specular microscopy as polymegethism (variability in cell size) and polymorphism (variability in cell shape). Cell density varies over the endothelial surface; normally, the concentration is highest in the periphery. Central endothelial cell density decreases with age at an average rate of approximately 0.6%/year, diminishing from a count of about 3400 cells/mm^2 at age 15 years to about 2300 cells/mm^2 at age 85 years. The normal central endothelial cell count is between 2000 and 3000 cells/mm^2. It has been observed that eyes with an endothelial cell count below 500 cells/mm^2 may be at risk for development of corneal edema. The endothelium maintains corneal transparency by controlling corneal hydration and maintaining stromal deturgescence through its functions as a barrier to the aqueous humor and as a metabolic pump that moves ions, and draws water osmotically, from the stroma into the aqueous humor. The barrier and pump functions of the endothelium can be measured clinically by fluorophotometry and pachymetry. The endothelium must also be permeable to nutrients and other molecules from the aqueous humor. Increased permeability and insufficient pump sites occur with reduced endothelial cell density, although the cell density at which clinically evident edema occurs is not an absolute.

For more detailed information on the histology and physiology of the cornea, see BCSC Section 2, *Fundamentals and Principles of Ophthalmology,* Chapter 8.

Bourne WM. Biology of the corneal endothelium in health and disease. *Eye (Lond).* 2003; 17(8):912–918.

DelMonte DW, Kim T. Anatomy and physiology of the cornea. *J Cataract Refract Surg.* 2011; 37(3):588–598.

Gambato C, Longhin E, Catania AG, Lazzarini D, Parrozzani R, Midena E. Aging and corneal layers: an in vivo corneal confocal microscopy study. *Graefes Arch Clin Exp Ophthalmol.* 2015;253(2):267–275.

Nishida T, Saika S, Morishige N. Cornea and sclera: anatomy and physiology. In: Mannis MJ, Holland EJ, eds. *Cornea.* Vol 1. 4th ed. Philadelphia: Elsevier; 2017:1–22.

Whikehart DR, Parikh CH, Vaughn AV, Mishler K, Edelhauser HF. Evidence suggesting the existence of stem cells for the human corneal endothelium. *Mol Vis.* 2005;11:816–824.

Limbus

The limbus is the transition zone between transparent cornea and opaque sclera. This area harbors corneal epithelial stem cells, which are responsible for the normal homeostasis and wound repair of the corneal epithelium. The *palisades of Vogt,* which are concentrated in the superior and inferior limbus, are thought to be the site of the limbal stem cells' niche and can be observed biomicroscopically as radially oriented fibrovascular ridges concentrated along the corneoscleral limbus (Fig 1-6). The posterior limbus appears to be

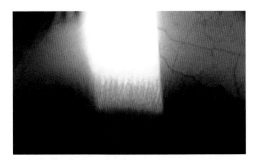

Figure 1-6 Slit-lamp photograph showing the corneoscleral limbus with radially oriented fibrovascular ridges (palisades of Vogt). *(Courtesy of Cornea Service, Paulista School of Medicine, Federal University of São Paulo.)*

responsible for stem cell maintenance, while the function of the anterior limbus may be to prompt regeneration of corneal epithelium. Renewal occurs from basal cells, with centripetal migration of stem cells from the periphery. This is known as the *XYZ hypothesis*, where *X* represents proliferation and stratification of limbal basal cells; *Y*, centripetal migration of basal cells; and *Z*, desquamation of superficial cells. The health of the cornea depends on the sum of X and Y being equal to Z. Damage to epithelial stem cells impairs long-term regeneration of corneal epithelial cells. Damage to the limbus leads to loss of the barrier that prevents invasion of the conjunctiva and neovascularization of the ocular surface.

Singh V, Shukla S, Ramachandran C, et al. Science and art of cell-based ocular surface regeneration. *Int Rev Cell Mol Biol.* 2015;319:45–106.

Yoon JJ, Ismail S, Sherwin T. Limbal stem cells: central concepts of corneal epithelial homeostasis. *World J Stem Cells.* 2014;6(4):391–403.

Defense Mechanisms of the External Eye and Cornea

The external eye and cornea comprise complexly integrated tissues that, along with the tear film, help protect the eye against infection. For an in-depth discussion of the various features of the innate and adaptive arms of the immune system, see BCSC Section 9, *Intraocular Inflammation and Uveitis.* BCSC Section 2, *Fundamentals and Principles of Ophthalmology,* discusses the biochemistry, metabolism, and immunology of the tear film and cornea in detail.

Components of the ocular adnexa—periorbital area, eyelids and lashes, lacrimal and meibomian glands—play different but important roles in the production, spread, and drainage of the tear film. As discussed earlier, the tear film serves as a protective layer, washing away irritants and pathogens and diluting toxins and allergens. Each functional blink promotes tear turnover. Tears are secreted from the lacrimal gland and spread across the cornea while excess tears are directed into the lacrimal puncta; all of these actions reduce the contact time of microbes and irritants with the ocular surface.

Immunoregulation of the ocular surface occurs through tolerance and regulation of the innate and adaptive arms of the ocular immune response (Fig 1-7). The normal tear film contains components of the complement cascade, proteins, growth factors, and an array of cytokines. Cytokines such as interleukin-1 and tumor necrosis factor α are

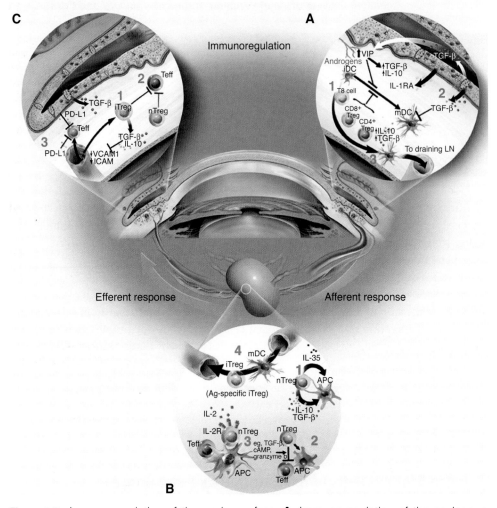

Figure 1-7 Immunoregulation of the ocular surface. **A,** Immunoregulation of the ocular surface: The ocular surface tissues contain a variety of soluble and cellular factors to reduce inflammation-induced pathology in the lacrimal functional unit. Those implicated in immunoregulation within the ocular surface tissues include the following: (1) Natural regulatory T cells (nTreg cells) (eg, CD4+, CD8+, and natural killer T cells), which include many of the conjunctival intraepithelial lymphocytes, are thought to dampen or inhibit the inflammatory/autoimmune response on the ocular surface. (2) The anti-inflammatory cytokine transforming growth factor β (TGF-β) is present on the ocular surface and has profound suppressive effects on resident dendritic cell (DC) maturation in the cornea; proliferation, differentiation, and survival of autoreactive T cells; and Treg cell differentiation and maintenance. The activity of the potent acute-response, proinflammatory cytokine interleukin-1 (IL-1) is modulated by the IL-1 receptor antagonist (IL-1RA), which is expressed and secreted by corneal and conjunctival epithelial cells. Vasoactive intestinal peptide (VIP) also seems to be protective; VIP secreted by sensory nerve endings in the cornea increases production of TGF-β and IL-10 and inhibits expression of the proinflammatory cytokines and chemokines, IL-1β, tumor necrosis factor α, interferon-γ, and chemokine (C-X-C motif) ligand 2. Hormones are also implicated in curbing inflammation and maintaining homeostasis. In addition, the corneal epithelium expresses vascular endothelial growth factor (VEGF) receptor-1 to sequester VEGF and reduce neovascularization. (3) Antigen-presenting cells (APCs) bearing self-antigen derived at the ocular surface may migrate to the regional lymph nodes to induce antigen-specific Treg cells (iTreg cells). **B,** Immunoregulation in the lymphoid organs: nTreg cells may exert their immunosuppressive function through (1) release of soluble factors (eg, TGF-β, IL-10);

(Continued)

Figure 1-7 *(continued)* (2) cell–cell contact, which disables pathogenic effector T cells (Teff cells) and/or APCs; and/or (3) competition for soluble factors (eg, IL-2). (4) iTreg cells may use similar mechanisms to inhibit cells bearing or responding to autoantigens. It is possible that these Treg-dependent mechanisms may also function within the ocular surface tissues. **C,** Other peripheral immunoregulatory mechanisms: additional mechanisms also limit access and effector function of autoreactive T cells within the ocular surface tissues: (1) TGF-β and (2) nTreg and iTreg cells are thought to suppress infiltrating autoreactive lymphocytes, and (3) low-level expression of integrins in endothelial cells of the healthy ocular surface, coupled with expression of the programmed death ligand-1 (PD-L1), negatively regulates activated T cells within the ocular surface tissues. *(Modified with permission from Stern ME, Schaumburg CS, Dana R, Calonge M, Niederkorn JY, Pflugfelder SC. Autoimmunity at the ocular surface: pathogenesis and regulation.* Mucosal Immunol. *2010;3(5):425–442.)*

significantly upregulated in a variety of corneal inflammatory diseases, such as corneal graft rejection and dry eye disease. Similarly, increased expression of growth factors, prostaglandins, neuropeptides, and proteases has been observed in a wide array of immune disorders of the ocular surface.

The normal, uninflamed conjunctiva contains polymorphonuclear leukocytes (neutrophils), lymphocytes (including regulatory T cells [Treg cells], which dampen the immune response), macrophages, plasma cells, and mast cells. The conjunctival stroma has an endowment of dendritic antigen-presenting cells (APCs). The conjunctival epithelium contains a special subpopulation of dendritic APCs known as *Langerhans cells*, which are capable of both uptake of antigens and priming (sensitizing) of naive (antigen-inexperienced) T lymphocytes. Hence, these dendritic cells serve as the sentinel cells of the immune system of the ocular surface. In addition to containing immune cells, the conjunctiva has a plentiful supply of blood vessels and lymphatic vessels, which facilitate the trafficking of immune cells and antigens to the draining lymph nodes, where the adaptive immune response is generated. This occurs through the recruitment of Treg cells, which return to the ocular surface to modulate and suppress the local immune response.

The normal, uninflamed cornea, like the conjunctiva, is also endowed with dendritic cells. Like those in the conjunctiva, the dendritic APCs in the corneal epithelium are Langerhans cells. They are located primarily in the corneal periphery and limbus (Fig 1-8).

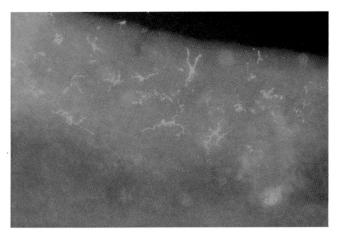

Figure 1-8 Langerhans cells. This micrograph shows the predominance of major histocompatibility complex class II⁺ Langerhans cells in the limbus of the uninflamed eye. *(Courtesy of the laboratory of M. Reza Dana, MD.)*

These APCs are in an activated, mature state (expressing class II major histocompatibility complex [MHC] antigens and costimulatory molecules) and hence are capable of efficiently stimulating T cells. In addition to these dendritic cells, small numbers of lymphocytes are present in the peripheral epithelium and anterior stroma of the cornea. A highly regulated process, mediated by vascular endothelial adhesion molecules and cytokines, controls the recruitment of the various leukocyte subsets from the intravascular compartment into the limbal matrix. Immune responses are also mediated by Treg cells in the regional lymph nodes and perhaps at the local level as well. See also Chapter 11 on corneal graft rejection.

Ecoiffier T, Yuen D, Chen L. Differential distribution of blood and lymphatic vessels in the murine cornea. *Invest Ophthalmol Vis Sci.* 2010;51(5):2436–2440.

Niederkorn JY. Cornea: window to ocular immunology. *Curr Immunol Rev.* 2011;7(3): 328–335.

Stern ME, Schaumburg CS, Dana R, Calonge M, Niederkorn JY, Pflugfelder SC. Autoimmunity at the ocular surface: pathogenesis and regulation. *Mucosal Immunol.* 2010; 3(5):425–442.

CHAPTER 2

Examination Techniques for the External Eye and Cornea

Highlights

- Placement of a hard contact lens on an irregular cornea provides a smooth anterior surface, helping the clinician to determine the contribution of the surface irregularity to vision loss.
- Evaluation of the mires projected onto the cornea during keratometry and Placido disk–based topography can help distinguish irregular astigmatism (distorted mires) due to ocular surface irregularity from regular corneal astigmatism (clear but oval mires).
- Corneal topography and tomography can give the clinician accurate data on corneal power, elevation, and thickness that are useful in diagnosis and surgical planning.

Direct Visualization

Slit-Lamp Biomicroscopy

The slit lamp is a fundamental and invaluable tool in the ophthalmologist's armamentarium. Mastery of the slit-lamp examination is critical in categorizing corneal pathology and formulating a diagnostic (Fig 2-1) and therapeutic plan.

The slit-lamp biomicroscope has 2 rotating arms—one for the slit illuminator and the other for the biomicroscope—mounted on a common axis. The illumination unit is essentially a projector with a light beam that is adjustable in width, height, direction, intensity, and color. The biomicroscope is a binocular Galilean telescope that offers a choice of magnifications. The illumination and microscope arms are parfocal, arranged so that both focus on the same spot, with the slit beam centered on the field of view. This setup provides direct illumination, and purposeful shifting of alignment allows for indirect illumination.

Four reflections of light can be seen when the eye is examined with the slit lamp. These reflections are known as Purkinje images or reflexes, named after the Czech anatomist Jan Evangelista Purkyně. The first Purkinje image is reflection off the surface of the cornea. The second is from the inner surface of the cornea. The third and fourth are from the anterior and posterior surfaces of the lens, respectively.

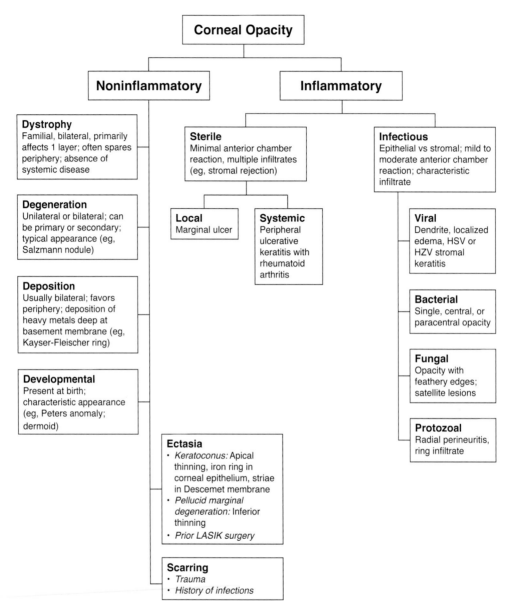

Figure 2-1 Flowchart for diagnosis of corneal opacity. HSV = herpes simplex virus; HZV = herpes zoster virus.

The slit lamp allows clinicians to examine the eye in a variety of ways, as described in the discussions that follow.

Direct illumination methods

Diffuse illumination With diffuse illumination, the light beam is broadened, reduced in intensity, and directed at the eye from an oblique angle. Swinging the illuminator arm to produce highlights and shadows can enhance the visibility of raised lesions of the ocular surface and iris (Fig 2-2).

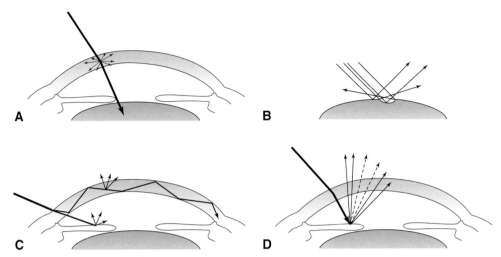

Figure 2-2 Diagram of how light rays interact with the eye in slit-lamp biomicroscopic examination. **A,** Direct illumination. **B,** Specular reflection. **C,** Sclerotic scatter. **D,** Retroillumination. *(From Tasman W, Jaeger AE, eds. The slit lamp: history, principles, and practice. In: Duane's Clinical Ophthalmology. Philadelphia: Lippincott; 1995–1999:33. Redrawn by Cyndie C. H. Wooley.)*

Focal illumination With focal illumination, the light and the microscope are focused on the same spot, and the slit aperture is adjusted from wide to narrow. Broad-beam illumination, which uses a beam width of about 3 mm, is optimal for visualizing eyelid lesions as well as the corneal opacities seen in dystrophies or scarring. Slit-beam illumination, which uses a beam width of about 1 mm or less, gives an optical section of the cornea (Fig 2-3); this section is essential for evaluation of corneal thinning, edema, stromal infiltrates, and endothelial abnormalities. The examiner can use a very narrow slit beam to help identify differences in refractive index between transparent structures as light rays pass through the cornea, anterior chamber, and lens. The examiner can also reduce the height of a narrow beam to determine the presence and amount of cell and flare in the anterior chamber.

Specular reflection Specular reflections are normal light reflexes bouncing off a surface (see Fig 2-2B). An example is the bright round or oval spot seen reflected from the ocular surface in a typical flash photograph of an eye. These mirror images of the light source can be annoying, and it is tempting to ignore them during slit-lamp examination. However, the clarity and sharpness of these reflections from the tear film give clues to the condition of the underlying tissue.

A faint reflection also comes from the posterior corneal surface. The examiner can enhance this specular reflection by placing a light beam at an appropriate angle, revealing the corneal endothelium. Following are the steps for examining the corneal endothelium with specular reflection:

1. Begin by setting the slit-beam arm at an angle of 60° from the viewing arm and using a short slit or 0.2-mm spot.
2. Identify the very bright mirror image of the lightbulb's filament and the paired epithelial and endothelial Purkinje light reflexes.

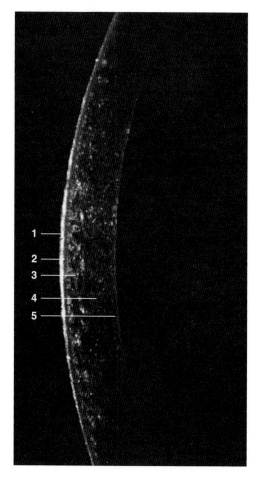

Figure 2-3 Slit section of normal cornea. *1,* Tear film. *2,* Epithelium. *3,* Anterior stroma with a high density of keratocytes. *4,* Posterior stroma with a lower density of keratocytes. *5,* Descemet membrane and endothelium. *(Reproduced with permission from Krachmer JH, Mannis MJ, Holland EJ, eds. Cornea. 2nd ed. Vol 1. Philadelphia: Elsevier/Mosby; 2005:201. © CL Mártonyi, WK Kellogg Eye Center, University of Michigan.)*

3. Superimpose the corneal endothelial light reflex onto the filament's mirror image, giving a bright glare.
4. Use the joystick to move the biomicroscope slightly forward in order to focus the endothelial reflex.

Specular reflection is monocular, and 1 eyepiece may require focusing. A setting of 25× to 40× is usually necessary to obtain a clear view of the endothelial mosaic. Cell density and morphology are noted (Fig 2-4); guttae and keratic precipitates appear as nonreflective dark areas.

Indirect illumination methods

Proximal illumination Turning a knob on the illumination arm slightly decenters the light beam from its isocentric position, causing the light beam and the microscope to be focused at different but adjacent spots. This technique, proximal illumination, highlights an existing opacity against deeper tissue layers and allows the examiner to see small irregularities that have a refractive index similar to that of their surroundings. Moving the light beam

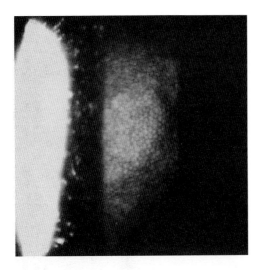

Figure 2-4 Corneal endothelium seen with specular reflection using the slit-lamp biomicroscope at 40× magnification. *(Reproduced with permission from Krachmer JH, Mannis MJ, Holland EJ, eds. Cornea. 2nd ed. Vol 1. Philadelphia: Elsevier/Mosby; 2005:208. © CL Mártonyi, WK Kellogg Eye Center, University of Michigan.)*

back and forth in small oscillations can help the examiner detect small 3-dimensional lesions, such as a corneal foreign body.

Sclerotic scatter Total internal reflection in the cornea makes possible another form of indirect illumination, sclerotic scatter. (See BCSC Section 3, *Clinical Optics,* for a discussion of total internal reflection.) Decentering the isocentric light beam so that an intense beam shines on the limbus and scatters off the sclera causes a very faint glow of the cornea (see Fig 2-2C). Reflective opacities stand out against the dark field, whereas areas of reduced light transmission in the cornea are seen as shades of gray. This technique is effective in demonstrating epithelial edema, mild stromal infiltration, nebulae, and cornea verticillata.

Retroillumination Retroillumination can be used to examine more than one area of the eye. Retroillumination from the iris is performed by displacing the beam tangentially while examining the cornea (see Fig 2-2D). Through observing the zone between the light and dark backgrounds, the examiner can detect subtle corneal abnormalities. Retroillumination from the fundus is performed by aligning the light beam nearly parallel with the examiner's visual axis and rotating the light so that it shines through the edge of the pupil. Opacities in the cornea, phakic or pseudophakic lens, or posterior capsule (Fig 2-5) are highlighted against the red reflex, and iris defects can be transilluminated.

Mártonyi CL, Maio M. Slit lamp examination and photography. In: Mannis MJ, Holland EJ, eds. *Cornea.* Vol. 1. 4th ed. Philadelphia: Elsevier; 2017:79–109.

Clinical use
The slit-lamp examination should be performed in an orderly fashion, beginning with direct illumination of the eyelids (margin, meibomian glands, and eyelashes), conjunctiva, and sclera. A broad beam illuminates the cornea and overlying tear film in the optical section. Details are examined with a narrow beam. The examiner estimates the height

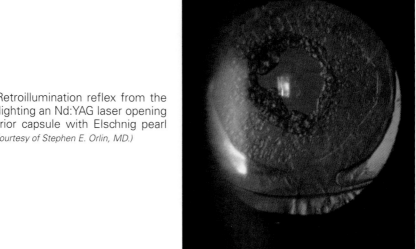

Figure 2-5 Retroillumination reflex from the fundus, highlighting an Nd:YAG laser opening in the posterior capsule with Elschnig pearl formation. *(Courtesy of Stephen E. Orlin, MD.)*

of the tear meniscus and looks for mucin cells and other debris in the tear film. Discrete lesions are measured with a slit-beam micrometer or an eyepiece reticule. All indirect illumination methods, including retroillumination, accentuate fine changes. The examiner then uses specular reflection to inspect the endothelium and has the patient shift gaze in different directions so that each corneal quadrant can be surveyed. A slit beam is used to estimate the thickness of the cornea and the depth of the anterior chamber. A short beam or spot will show flare or cells in the aqueous humor. Direct and indirect illumination and retroillumination techniques are used to identify abnormalities of the iris and lens.

With all illumination methods, the examiner actively controls the light beam to sweep across the eye, using shadows and reflections to bring out details. Having the patient blink can help the examiner distinguish ocular surface changes from tiny opacities floating in the tear film. After initial low-power screening, much of the slit-lamp examination is performed using higher magnifications.

Visualization of deeper and peripheral intraocular structures, except for the anterior vitreous humor, requires special lenses. A contact lens allows examination of the intermediate and posterior portions of the eye; its use is often combined with angled mirrors and prisms for gonioscopy and peripheral fundus examination.

Scanning

Ultrasound Biomicroscopy

High-frequency ultrasound biomicroscopy (UBM) provides high-resolution in vivo imaging of the anterior segment (Fig 2-6). Tissues visualized include the cornea, the anterior and posterior surface of the iris, the ciliary body, zonular fibers, angle structures, and the anterior lens capsule. UBM technology incorporates 50–100-MHz transducers into

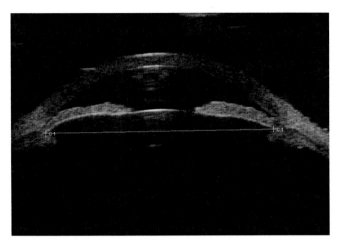

Figure 2-6 Ultrasound biomicroscopic visualization of the entire anterior segment, including structures behind the iris pigment epithelium, thereby permitting precise determination of the sulcus-to-sulcus measurements prior to implantation of a phakic refractive intraocular lens. *(Reproduced from Goins KM, Wagoner MD. Imaging the anterior segment.* Focal Points: Clinical Modules for Ophthalmologists. *San Francisco: American Academy of Ophthalmology; 2009, module 11.)*

a B-mode clinical scanner. Paradigm Medical Industries (Salt Lake City, UT) and Ophthalmic Technologies (Toronto, ON, Canada) UBM scanners utilize 50-MHz transducers and provide axial and lateral physical resolutions of 25 μm and 50 μm, respectively. UBM allows structures to be viewed through an opaque cornea and total hyphema. The scleral spur, located where the trabecular meshwork meets an interface line between the sclera and ciliary body, is a constant landmark that aids the clinician in the examination of various angle configurations.

UBM is a helpful adjunct in the assessment of ciliary body pathology, including cysts and tumors. It is also very useful in the evaluation of various angle anomalies, including angle recession, occludable angles, pupillary block, plateau iris, malignant glaucoma, and cyclodialysis clefts. In addition, clinicians can use UBM to assist with accurate placement of phakic intraocular lenses (IOLs), identify pigment dispersion syndrome, and locate IOL haptic positions and foreign bodies in the angle. Its major advantage is its ability to visualize structures behind the iris; most of its other capabilities in visualizing the anterior segment have been supplanted by anterior segment optical coherence tomography.

Goins KM, Wagoner MD. Imaging the anterior segment. *Focal Points: Clinical Modules for Ophthalmologists.* San Francisco: American Academy of Ophthalmology; 2009, module 11.

Anterior Segment Optical Coherence Tomography

Optical coherence tomography (OCT) is a noninvasive technology that produces 2-dimensional, high-resolution, and high-definition cross-sectional images of ocular tissue. These images are similar to ultrasonographic images, but they are based on the emission and reflection of light (low-coherence interferometry). The extremely fine resolution of the images (5–10 μm) allows exquisite delineation of the layers of the cornea, anterior chamber, and iris. There are 2 types of anterior segment OCT: time-domain (TD-OCT) and frequency-domain (FD-OCT). Spectral-domain OCT (SD-OCT), also called Fourier-domain OCT, is a subtype of the latter. A new, faster OCT technique that features components of both TD- and SD-OCT, called swept-source OCT, has been developed; it is being used both in the clinical setting and in real time in the operating room as an attachment to the operating microscope.

OCT scans can measure the depth, width, and angle of the anterior chamber (Fig 2-7). The corneal pachymetry feature of these devices is useful in the preoperative evaluation of patients with Fuchs endothelial corneal dystrophy. In postoperative follow-up of endothelial keratoplasty cases, the shape, thickness, and attachment of the donor lenticule can be visualized and quantified. In patients who have undergone laser in situ keratomileusis (LASIK), clinicians can use OCT to measure the thickness of the corneal flap and the residual stromal bed to determine the safety of an enhancement (re-treatment). Recent software provides information on corneal curvature and epithelial thickness that is helpful in screening refractive surgery patients. Software is also available to calculate the true corneal power, which can be used in IOL power calculation after LASIK or photorefractive keratectomy. Intraoperative OCT has also recently been developed as an adjunct in Descemet membrane endothelial keratoplasty (DMEK) to ensure correct orientation of endothelial grafts.

Dada T, Sihota R, Gadia R, Aggarwal A, Mandal S, Gupta V. Comparison of anterior segment optical coherence tomography and ultrasound biomicroscopy for assessment of the anterior segment. *J Cataract Refract Surg.* 2007;33(5):837–840.

Goins KM, Wagoner MD. Imaging the anterior segment. *Focal Points: Clinical Modules for Ophthalmologists.* San Francisco: American Academy of Ophthalmology; 2009, module 11.

Jancevski M, Foster CS. Anterior segment optical coherence tomography. *Semin Ophthalmol.* 2010;25(5–6):317–323.

Zhou SY, Wang CX, Cai XY, Huang D, Liu YZ. Optical coherence tomography and ultrasound biomicroscopy imaging of opaque corneas. *Cornea.* 2013;32(4):e25–e30.

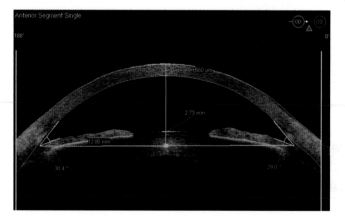

Figure 2-7 Anterior segment optical coherence tomography image of a phakic eye. The central anterior chamber depth is 2.73 mm, and there is moderate narrowing of the anterior chamber angle. *(Reproduced from Goins KM, Wagoner MD. Imaging the anterior segment.* Focal Points: Clinical Modules for Ophthalmologists. *San Francisco: American Academy of Ophthalmology; 2009, module 11.)*

Specular Microscopy

Specular microscopy (contact and noncontact techniques) provides an objective measurement of corneal endothelial cells. The following parameters can be calculated from a specular or confocal image:

- *Density.* Endothelial cell density decreases with age. The endothelial cell count normally exceeds 3500 cells/mm² in children and gradually declines with age to approximately 2000 cells/mm² in older individuals. An average value for adults is 2400 cells/mm² (with a range of 1500–3500 cells/mm²), with a mean cell size of 150–350 μm². Low cell density (ie, fewer than 1000 cells/mm²) may provide for a transparent cornea, but such corneas are at greater risk for corneal decompensation with intraocular surgery. Dark, "punched out" areas might represent cornea guttae (Fig 2-8).
- *Coefficient of variation.* The standard deviation of the mean cell area divided by the mean cell area gives the *coefficient of variation,* a unitless number that is normally less than 0.30. *Polymegethism* is increased variation in individual cell areas; it typically increases with contact lens wear. Corneas with significant polymegethism (>0.40) might not tolerate intraocular surgery.
- *Percentage of hexagonal cells.* Ideally, the percentage of cells with 6 apices is close to 100%. Lower percentages indicate a diminishing state of endothelial health. *Pleomorphism* is increased variability in cell shape. Corneas with high pleomorphism (more than 50% nonhexagonal cells) might not tolerate intraocular surgery.

American Academy of Ophthalmology. *Corneal Endothelial Photography.* Ophthalmic Technology Assessment. San Francisco: American Academy of Ophthalmology; 1996. (Reviewed for currency 2003.)

Sayegh RR, Benetz BA, Lass JH. Specular microscopy. In: Mannis MJ, Holland EJ, eds. *Cornea.* Vol. 1. 4th ed. Philadelphia: Elsevier; 2017:160–179.

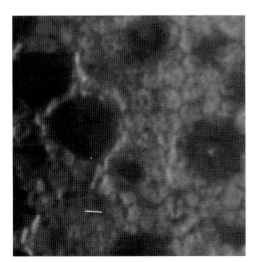

Figure 2-8 Specular microscopy showing Fuchs endothelial corneal dystrophy with guttae. *(Courtesy of John E. Sutphin, MD.)*

Confocal Microscopy

Confocal corneal microscopy is a noninvasive technique for in vivo imaging of the living cornea; it compares to in vitro histochemical analysis of the 5 layers of the cornea. The basic principle of confocal microscopy is that a single point of tissue can be illuminated by a point source of light or laser and simultaneously imaged by a camera in the same plane (ie, confocal). Because this technique involves scanning a small region of tissue with thousands of spots of light, it produces a usable field of view at a cellular level and an image of very high resolution. A number of units are available for clinical use: (1) tandem scanning, (2) scanning-slit, and (3) laser scanning confocal microscopes. The major advantage of laser scanning confocal systems is the ability to serially produce extremely thin images of the cornea. The depth of focus is 7–9 μm in tandem scanning, 26 μm in slit scanning, and 5–7 μm in laser scanning.

Confocal microscopy is useful in identifying causative organisms in cases of infectious keratitis, such as *Acanthamoeba* keratitis, fungal keratitis, microsporidiosis, and herpetic eye disease. It is also helpful in evaluating corneal nerve morphology in diabetic neurotrophic keratitis and neuropathic pain occurring in ocular surface disease and after refractive surgery (Fig 2-9); it is similarly useful in evaluating the corneal endothelial layer. In addition, confocal microscopy may help differentiate some corneal dystrophies, for example, Reis-Bücklers corneal dystrophy from Thiel-Behnke corneal dystrophy, both of which involve the Bowman layer, as well as Fuchs and posterior polymorphous dystrophies, both of which involve the corneal endothelium (see Chapter 7, Figs 7-6A and 7-7A).

Alzubaidi R, Sharif MS, Qahwaji R, Ipson S, Brahma A. In vivo confocal microscopic corneal images in health and disease with an emphasis on extracting features and visual signatures for corneal diseases: a review study. *Br J Ophthalmol.* 2016;100(1):41–55.

Petroll WM, Cavanagh HD, Jester JV. Confocal microscopy. In: Mannis MJ, Holland EJ, eds. *Cornea.* Vol. 1. 4th ed. Philadelphia: Elsevier; 2017:180–191.

Villani E, Baudouin C, Efron N, et al. In vivo confocal microscopy of the ocular surface: from bench to bedside. *Curr Eye Res.* 2014;39(3):213–231.

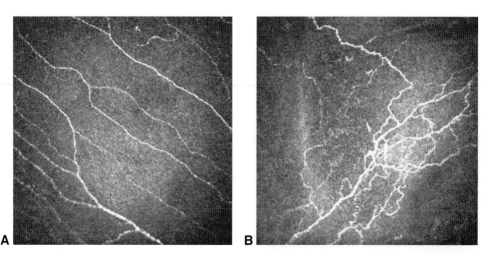

A B

Figure 2-9 Confocal microscopy of corneal nerves. **A,** Normal nerve architecture. **B,** Tortuous branching patterns. *(Courtesy of Mina Massaro-Giordano, MD.)*

Evaluation of Corneal Curvature

Zones of the Cornea

For more than 100 years, the corneal shape has been known to be aspheric. Typically, the central cornea is about 3 diopters (D) steeper than the periphery, a positive shape factor *(prolate)*. Clinically, the cornea may be divided into zones (Fig 2-10). The *central zone* is 1–3 mm in diameter and closely resembles a spherical surface. It is surrounded by the *paracentral zone,* a 3- to 4-mm "doughnut" with an outer diameter of 7–8 mm that progressively flattens from the center. Together, the paracentral and central zones constitute the *apical zone,* which is used in contact lens fitting. The central and paracentral zones are primarily responsible for the refractive power of the cornea. Adjacent to the paracentral zone is the *peripheral zone* or *transitional zone,* which has an outer diameter of approximately 11 mm. This is the area of greatest flattening and asphericity in the normal cornea. Finally, there is the limbus *(limbal zone),* where the cornea steepens prior to joining the sclera at the limbal sulcus; its outer diameter averages 12 mm.

The *optical zone* is the portion of the cornea that overlies the entrance pupil of the iris. The *corneal apex* is the point of maximum curvature, typically temporal to the center of the pupil. The *corneal vertex* is the point located at the intersection of the patient's line of fixation and the corneal surface. It is represented by the corneal light reflex when the cornea is illuminated coaxially with fixation. The corneal vertex is the center of the keratoscopic image and does not necessarily correspond to the point of maximum curvature at the corneal apex (Fig 2-11).

Shape, Curvature, and Power

Three topographic properties of the cornea are important to its optical function: the underlying *shape,* which determines its *curvature* and, hence, its refractive *power.* Shape and curvature are geometric properties of the cornea, whereas power is a functional property. Historically, power was the first parameter of the cornea to be described, and a unit

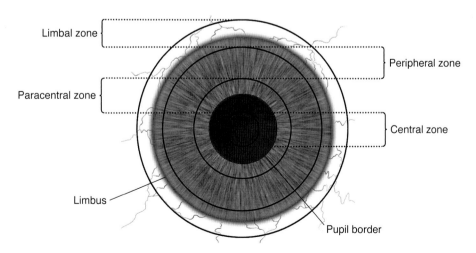

Figure 2-10 Topographic zones of the cornea. *(Illustration by Christine Gralapp.)*

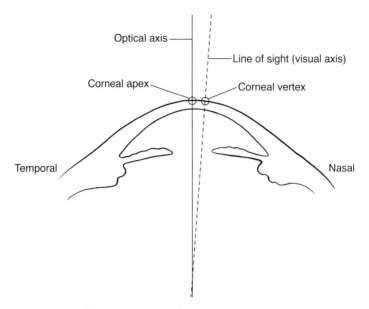

Figure 2-11 Corneal vertex and apex. *(Illustration by Christine Gralapp.)*

representing the refractive power of the central cornea, the *diopter,* was accepted as its basic unit of measurement. However, with the advent of contact lenses and refractive surgery, knowing the overall shape and the related property of curvature has become increasingly important.

The refractive power of the cornea is determined by *Snell's law,* the law of refraction. Snell's law is based on the difference between 2 refractive indices (in this case, of the cornea and of air), divided by the radius of curvature. The refractive index of air is 1.000; aqueous and tears, 1.336; and corneal stroma, 1.376. Although the air–tear film interface constitutes the primary refractive element of the eye, the difference between total corneal power calculated based on stroma alone and corneal power calculated with both stroma and tears is only –0.060, a clinically insignificant difference.

Calculating the anterior corneal power using the refractive indices overestimates the true power because it does not take into account the negative contribution of the posterior cornea. Average refractive power of the central cornea is about +43 D, which is the sum of the refractive power at the air–stroma interface of +49 D minus the endothelium–aqueous power of 6 D. For most clinical purposes, a derived corneal refractive index of 1.3375 is used in calculating central corneal power. This value was chosen to allow +45 D to equate to a 7.5-mm radius of curvature. BCSC Section 3, *Clinical Optics,* covers these topics in greater depth.

Dawson DG, Ubels JL, Edelhauser HF. Cornea and sclera. In: Alm A, Kaufman PL, eds. *Adler's Physiology of the Eye.* 11th ed. New York: Elsevier; 2011:71–130.

Keratometry

The ophthalmometer (keratometer) was invented by Hermann von Helmholtz in 1853. It empirically estimates, but does not directly measure, the central corneal power. It reads

2 points in the 2.8- to 4.0-mm zone. A simple vergence formula used in computing the corneal power in this region is then utilized to calculate the radius of curvature. Results are reported as *radius of curvature* in millimeters or *refracting power* in diopters.

The 2 basic keratometers are the Helmholtz type and the Javal-Schiøtz type. The former is more commonly used. The Helmholtz type is a 1-position device in which the image size is adjustable; the examiner aligns the "plus sign" and "minus sign" mires (Fig 2-12). The Javal-Schiøtz type is a 2-position instrument in which the object size is adjustable; the examiner aligns mires resembling a red square and a green staircase.

The manual keratometer has certain limitations. It measures only a small region of the cornea without providing information about the cornea central or peripheral to these points. Keratometry assumes that the cornea has a symmetric spherocylindrical shape with a major and minor axis separated by 90°. It also does not account for spherical aberration, and it is susceptible to focusing and misalignment errors. Finally, if the cornea is irregular, distortion of the mires reduces the accuracy of the measurement.

Despite these drawbacks, the manual keratometer provides accurate information for most patients. It is a valuable instrument in ophthalmology for measuring astigmatism. Clinically, corneal curvature data are used primarily for contact lens fitting, IOL calculations, and planning for corneal refractive surgery. However, it is not accurate for IOL power calculations in patients who have undergone previous corneal refractive surgery. It is also helpful for detecting irregular astigmatism, which is visible as distortion or irregularity in the appearance of the mires. Clinicians can also use the keratometer dynamically by comparing the measurements in primary gaze with those in upgaze. Steepening of the measurements in upgaze is an early sign of keratoconus.

Keratoscopy and Placido Disk–based Topography

The keratoscope, which is based on the original prototype invented by Antonio Plácido da Costa in 1880 (Placido disk), projects circular, concentric, illuminated mires onto the corneal surface. Unlike keratometry, which measures quantitative data and is limited to the

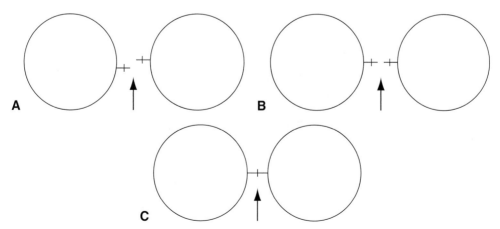

Figure 2-12 Diagrammatic representation of manual keratometry. **A,** Misalignment of the horizontal axis (plus sign). **B,** Correct alignment of the horizontal axis just before the power is corrected (horizontal dial). **C,** Alignment of axes and vertical and horizontal power.

central 4.0 mm, keratoscopy provides a qualitative evaluation of a larger surface of the cornea, based on the shape and dimension of and the distance between the projected rings. It is helpful in the detection of paracentral and peripheral disorders of corneal contour, such as keratoconus, pellucid marginal degeneration, and astigmatism following penetrating keratoplasty (Fig 2-13). In addition, distorted mires can aid clinicians in identifying surface irregularity.

Topography

Corneal topography is based on the Placido disk principle of reflecting images of multiple concentric rings onto the cornea; in corneal topography, the projected images are digitally captured and analyzed by computer software. Generally, in steeper parts of the cornea, the reflected mires appear closer together and thinner and the axis of the central mire is shorter. Conversely, along the flat axis, the mires are farther apart and thicker and the central mire is longer. Thousands of points are measured, and, using complex algorithms, the software generates color-coded maps of the topographic curvature of the cornea. These topographers assess only the anterior corneal surface and tear film.

There are 3 types of maps. The first is the *axial curvature map,* which closely approximates the power of the central 1–2 mm of the cornea but fails to describe the true shape and power of the peripheral cornea. The second is a *tangential map,* which typically shows better sensitivity to peripheral changes, with less "smoothing" of the curvature than the axial map (Fig 2-14). (In these maps, diopters are relative units of curvature and do not equate to diopters of corneal power.) A third map, the *mean curvature map,* uses an infinite number of spheres to fit the curvature. The algorithm determines a minimum- and maximum-size best-fit sphere and, from the radius of each, determines an average curvature (arithmetic mean of the principal curvatures) known as the mean curvature. These powers are then mapped using standard colors to represent diopter changes, allowing for more sensitivity to peripheral changes of curvature (Fig 2-15).

Before any topographic maps are interpreted, the color scale needs to be evaluated, because it can grossly influence the interpretation of the map. Arranging the color bar

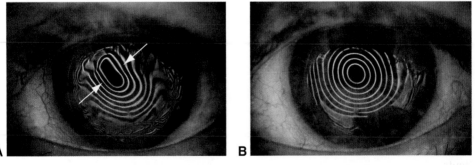

Figure 2-13 **A,** Videokeratoscopic mires are closer together in the axis of steep curvature *(arrows)* and farther apart in the flat axis in this postkeratoplasty patient. **B,** Videokeratoscopic mires round out after keratoplasty sutures are cut. *(Courtesy of Stephen E. Orlin, MD.)*

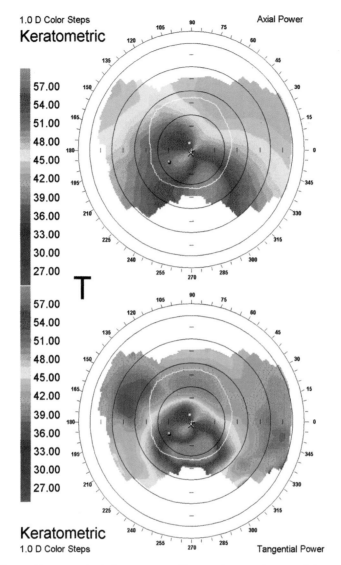

Figure 2-14 Corneal topography in keratoconus. The top image shows axial curvature; the bottom shows tangential curvature. Note that the steeper curve on the bottom is more closely aligned with the cone. *(Courtesy of John E. Sutphin, MD.)*

in 0.50-D increments may improve accuracy in interpretation of the map. Smaller increments greatly exaggerate minor or normal changes and increase sensitivity. Larger increments decrease sensitivity and can mask significant changes. The absolute scale is constant for all examinations and is useful for comparisons over time and between patients. The normalized or relative scale adjusts to the range of powers on the corneal surface and differs for each cornea. Thus, the power range and step size may be narrow or broad, thereby magnifying or minifying significant changes. Besides the limitations of the

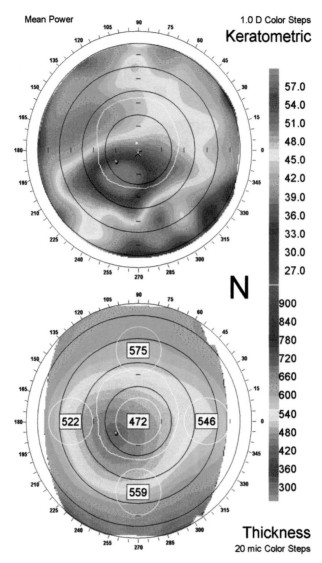

Figure 2-15 The top image shows mean curvature in keratoconus for the same patient as in Figure 2-14. The local curvature outlines the cone, as shown by the thinnest point in the pachymetry map in the bottom figure. *(Courtesy of John E. Sutphin, MD.)*

algorithms and the variations in terminology used by manufacturers, various other problems may affect the accuracy of corneal topography:

- misalignment
- limited stability (test-to-test variation)
- sensitivity to focus errors
- tear film effects
- distortions

- limited area of coverage (central and limbal)
- no standardized data maps
- colors that may be absolute or varied (normalized)

Despite these limitations, corneal topography maps allow clinicians to detect forme fruste and frank keratoconus in refractive surgery screenings and identify and predict corneal ectasia following refractive surgery. A normal astigmatic profile has a symmetric bow-tie pattern (Fig 2-16). Keratoconus can be represented by a central cone or inferotemporal steepening (Fig 2-17) (see Chapter 7 for a discussion of keratoconus). Skew deviations and asymmetric bow ties associated with focal steepening inferiorly are also suggestive of keratoconus. The ratio between the inferior and superior keratometry values can be indicative of keratoconus. The inferior–superior value (I–S value) is derived by calculating the difference between inferior and superior corneal curvature measurements at a defined set of 5 points above and below the horizontal meridian. I–S values greater than 1.4 and central corneal powers greater than 47.2 D are all suggestive of corneal ectatic disorders, but there is some overlap between normal and abnormal eyes (Table 2-1). Pellucid marginal degeneration has a characteristic "crab-claw" configuration with against-the-rule astigmatism (Fig 2-18). However, this pattern is not pathognomonic, as it can also be seen in keratoconus. Corneal topography can aid in accurately monitoring progression of these ectatic corneal diseases and in planning procedures such as corneal crosslinking. Prior refractive surgery leads to central flattening in myopic corrections and steepening in hyperopic corrections.

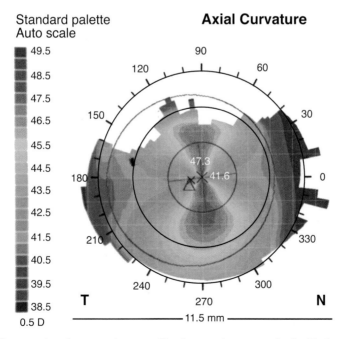

Figure 2-16 Topography of a normal cornea. The image shows regular "with-the-rule" astigmatism with a symmetric bow-tie pattern. *(Courtesy of Stephen E. Orlin, MD.)*

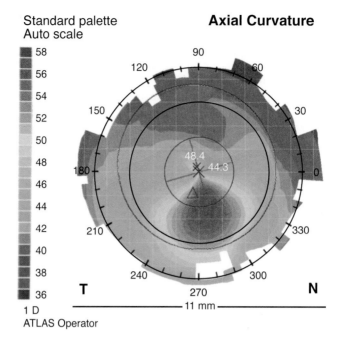

Standard palette
Auto scale

Axial Curvature

ATLAS Operator

Figure 2-17 Corneal topography in keratoconus. The image shows inferior steepening. *(Courtesy of Stephen E. Orlin, MD.)*

Table 2-1 Corneal Topography Signs Suggestive of Keratoconus or Corneal Ectasia

Axial Map Abnormalities	Elevation Map Abnormalities	Pachymetry Map Abnormalities
Central corneal power >47.2 D	Isolated islandlike or tonguelike extension on anterior or posterior surface	Thinnest location is <470 μm
I–S value >1.4 D	Elevation values >12 μm on anterior elevation map at 5 mm	Displacement of thinnest point is >500 μm from center
Skewed radial axis index >21°	Elevation values >15 μm on posterior elevation map	Pachymetry difference at thinnest point between 2 eyes is >30 μm
Corneal astigmatism (anterior or posterior) >6.0 D	—	I–S difference at the 5-mm circle is >30 μm
Against-the-rule astigmatism	—	Conelike pattern on thinnest map
I–S value at 5-mm zone >2.5 D	—	—

I–S = Inferior–superior.

Corneal mapping is useful in managing congenital and postoperative astigmatism, particularly following penetrating keratoplasty. Complex peripheral patterns may result in a refractive axis of astigmatism that is not aligned with a topographic axis.

In addition to displaying power maps, computerized topography systems may display other data: pupil size and location, indices estimating degrees of regular and irregular

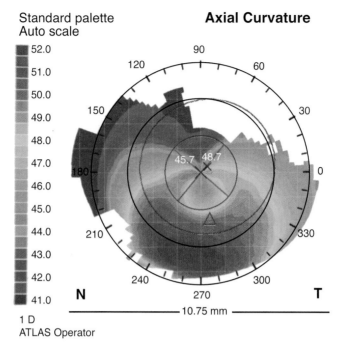

Figure 2-18 Corneal topography map showing the classic "crab-claw" configuration with inferior steepening and against-the-rule astigmatism seen in pellucid marginal degeneration. *(Courtesy of Stephen E. Orlin, MD.)*

astigmatism, estimates of the probability that the patient has keratoconus, simulated corneal curvature measurements, wavefront analysis, results of dry eye screening, meibomian gland imagery, and chord μ (angle kappa).

Angle kappa, the angle formed between the visual axis and the optical (or pupillary) axis, is particularly useful in the selection of basic or premium IOLs for cataract surgery and in detailed planning of astigmatic correction. Generally, an angle kappa less than 0.4 mm is desired. If angle kappa is greater than 0.4 mm, the clinician may choose to avoid multifocal IOLs. The ideal amount of spherical aberrations varies by individual, and appropriate IOL selection might offset these aberrations.

Corneal mapping can also be useful in the selection of lens implants for patients with previous refractive surgery who are considering cataract surgery. Hyperopic ablation induces negative spherical aberrations because the central cornea is steeper, and myopic ablation induces positive spherical aberrations because the central cornea is flattened. To avoid halos in eyes with positive aberrations, the clinician may consider an IOL with negative or zero spherical aberrations.

Tomography

Placido disk–based topography describes only the surface corneal curvature (power), whereas corneal tomography computes a 3-dimensional image of the cornea, providing details such as the anterior and posterior corneal curvature, corneal thickness, and anterior chamber depth, as well as information on the iris and lens. Various technologies, including scanning-slit and Scheimpflug imaging, are utilized to obtain these images.

Scanning-slit technology has been combined with Placido disk–based topography; this combination of technologies derives its posterior elevation map mathematically. This map may overestimate the posterior corneal curvature, however, especially in patients who have undergone LASIK procedures.

Other systems are based on the Scheimpflug principle, which is a geometric rule that describes the orientation of the plane of focus of an optical system, such as a camera, when the lens plane is not parallel to the image plane. The principle is named after Austrian army captain Theodor Scheimpflug, who used it to devise an apparatus for correcting perspective distortion in aerial photography. In Scheimpflug-based corneal tomography, a thin layer of the cornea is illuminated with the slit. Because they are not entirely transparent, the cells scatter the light, creating a sectional image. This image is photographed according to the Scheimpflug principle, resulting in an image of the illuminated plane in complete focus from the anterior surface of the cornea to the posterior surface of the crystalline lens. A number of devices have employed the Scheimpflug principle with rotational scanning, dual rotational scanning, and Placido disk–based topography.

Scheimpflug-based systems present considerable information, including anterior curvature, corneal thickness, anterior chamber depth, anterior and posterior elevation, and pupil diameter. As a result, the thickness and topography of the entire anterior and posterior surface of the cornea can be displayed (Fig 2-19). In addition, a densitometry function measures the amount of corneal or lens opacification.

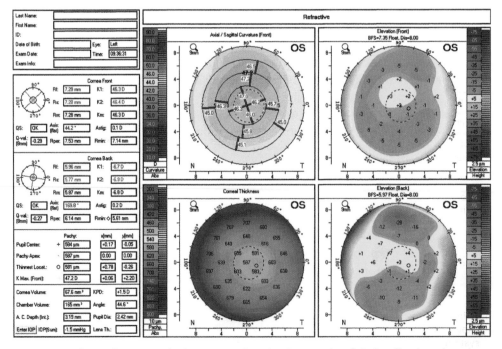

Figure 2-19 Corneal tomography image, produced using rotating Scheimpflug imaging, demonstrates normal axial curvature, corneal thickness, and anterior and posterior elevation. *(Courtesy of Stephen E. Orlin, MD.)*

Corneal tomography systems also employ keratoconus detection and classification algorithms. In keratoconus suspects, corneal tomography may provide additional useful information, as it may reveal subtle changes in the posterior corneal curvature that can precede anterior steepening. Measurements of the posterior corneal curvature and thickness provide important confirmation of thinning and steepening (Fig 2-20).

See Table 2-2 for an overview of methods and instruments used for corneal topography and tomography.

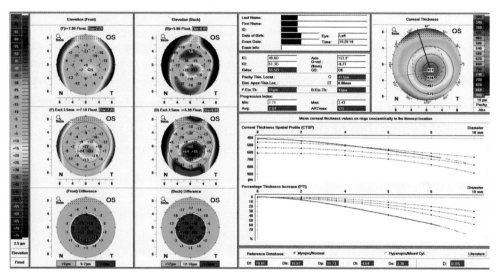

Figure 2-20 An inferior displacement and posterior elevation suggestive of keratoconus are shown in these images produced using a rotating Scheimpflug camera. *(Courtesy of Robert W. Weisenthal, MD.)*

Table 2-2 Methods and Instruments for Corneal Topography and Tomography

Method(s)	Instruments
Videokeratoscopy or Placido disk–based topography	Atlas (Carl Zeiss Meditec, Jena, Germany)
	Topographic Modeling System (TMS-5; Tomey, Nagoya, Japan)
	OPD-Scan III (Nidek, Gamagori, Japan)
Horizontal slit-scan	Orbscan IIz (Bausch + Lomb, Bridgewater, NJ, USA)
Rotating Scheimpflug imaging	Pentacam (Oculus Optikgeräte, Wetzlar, Germany)
	TMS-5 (Tomey)
	Oculyzer (WaveLight Laser Technologie AG, Erlangen, Germany)
Scheimpflug imaging with Placido disk–based topography	Galilei (Ziemer Ophthalmic Systems AG, Port, Switzerland)
	Sirius (Costruzione Strumenti Oftalmici, Florence, Italy)
Rotating optical coherence tomography integrated into the Atlas topography system	Visante (Carl Zeiss Meditec)
	SS-1000 Casia (Tomey)
Arc scanning with very-high-frequency ultrasound	Artemis II (ArcScan, Morrison, CO, USA)

Ambrósio R Jr, Belin MW. Imaging of the cornea: topography vs tomography. *J Refract Surg.* 2010;26(11):847–849.

Belin MW, Asota IM, Ambrósio R Jr, Khachikian SS. What's in a name: keratoconus, pellucid marginal degeneration, and related thinning disorders. *Am J Ophthalmol.* 2011;152(2): 157–162.

Courville CB, Klyce SD. Corneal topography. In: Foster CS, Azar DT, Dohlman CH, eds. *Smolin and Thoft's The Cornea: Scientific Foundations and Clinical Practice.* 4th ed. Philadelphia: Lippincott Williams & Wilkins; 2004:175–185.

Dharwadkar S, Nayak BK. Corneal topography and tomography. *J Clin Ophthalmol Res.* 2015; 3(1):45–62.

Kim EJ, Weikert MP, Martinez CE, Klyce SD. Keratometry and topography. In: Mannis MJ, Holland EJ, eds. *Cornea.* Vol. 1. 4th ed. Philadelphia: Elsevier; 2017:144–153.

Oliveira CM, Ribeiro C, Franco S. Corneal imaging with slit-scanning and Scheimpflug imaging techniques. *Clin Exp Optom.* 2011;94(1):33–42.

Clinical Evaluation of the Ocular Surface

Ocular Surface Staining

Fluorescein

Topical fluorescein is a nontoxic, water-soluble, synthetic organic hydroxyxanthene dye that is available in several forms: as a 0.25% solution with an anesthetic (benoxinate or proparacaine) and a preservative, as a 2% nonpreserved unit-dose eyedrop, and in impregnated paper strips. Fluorexon, a related macromolecular compound, is available as a 0.35% nonpreserved solution that does not stain most contact lenses. Staining is easily detected with a cobalt-blue filter.

Fluorescein is most commonly used for applanation tonometry and evaluation of the tear film, including filaments. *Tear breakup time (TBUT)* is measured by instilling fluorescein, asking the patient to hold the eyelids open after 1 or 2 blinks, and counting the seconds until a dry spot appears. The appearance of dry spots in less than 10 seconds is considered abnormal. TBUT is further discussed in Chapter 3. Fluorescein detects disruption of intercellular junctions and stains punctate and macroulcerative epithelial defects (positive staining), such as herpetic dendritic lesions and dysplastic epithelium. It can also highlight nonstaining lesions that project through the tear film (negative staining), as in epithelial basement membrane dystrophy and Thygeson superficial punctate keratitis. Different disease states can produce various punctate staining patterns (Fig 2-21). Fluorescein that collects in an epithelial defect will diffuse into the corneal stroma and cause a green flare in the anterior chamber. Pooling of the dye due to an indentation or thinning of the cornea must be distinguished from actual staining. This can be done by anesthetizing the eye and using a wisp of cotton from a cotton-tipped applicator to absorb the fluorescein in the area of concern. If the epithelium is intact, the dye will be removed, with no staining noted in the base. In the *dye disappearance test,* the tear meniscus is observed for the disappearance of fluorescein. Prolonged presence of the dye suggests a blockage of the drainage system.

The *Seidel test* is used to detect seepage of aqueous humor through a corneal perforation (Fig 2-22) or a conjunctival defect, such as a leaking trabeculectomy bleb. The

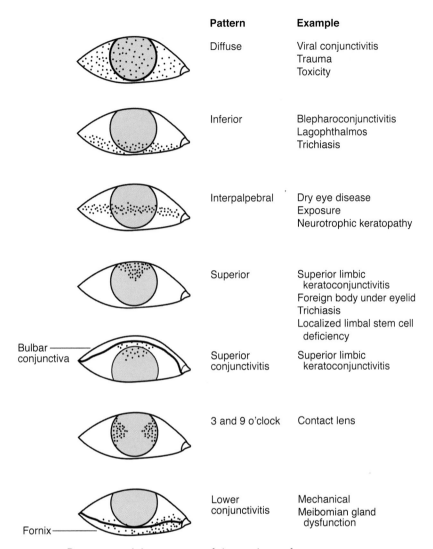

	Pattern	Example
	Diffuse	Viral conjunctivitis Trauma Toxicity
	Inferior	Blepharoconjunctivitis Lagophthalmos Trichiasis
	Interpalpebral	Dry eye disease Exposure Neurotrophic keratopathy

	Superior	Superior limbic
		  keratoconjunctivitis
		Foreign body under eyelid
		Trichiasis
		Localized limbal stem cell
		  deficiency

Bulbar conjunctiva	Superior conjunctivitis	Superior limbic keratoconjunctivitis
	3 and 9 o'clock	Contact lens
Fornix	Lower conjunctivitis	Mechanical Meibomian gland dysfunction

Figure 2-21 Punctate staining patterns of the ocular surface. *(Illustration by Joyce Zavarro.)*

examiner applies fluorescein to the site of suspected leakage using a moistened strip or concentrated drop and looks for a flow of clear fluid streaming through the orange dye under cobalt-blue light.

Rose bengal and lissamine green

Rose bengal and lissamine green (both available as a 1% solution or in impregnated strips) are other water-soluble dyes. They stain the epithelial cells of the cornea and conjunctiva when a disruption occurs in the protective mucin coating. These dyes are routinely used for evaluating tear-deficiency states and for detecting and assessing various epithelial lesions, such as evaluating the extent of corneal intraepithelial neoplasia (Fig 2-23). Rose bengal is toxic to the epithelium. Lissamine green is better tolerated and has fewer toxic effects on cultured human corneal epithelial cells.

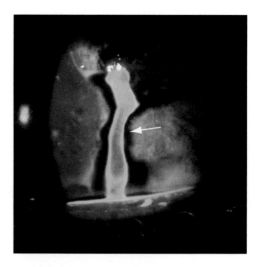

Figure 2-22 Leakage of fluid from the anterior chamber *(arrow)* following a corneal perforation, indicating a positive Seidel test result. *(Courtesy of Stephen E. Orlin, MD.)*

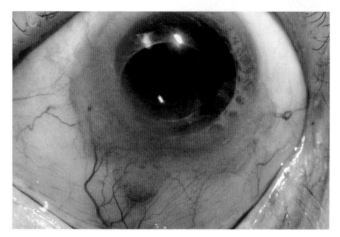

Figure 2-23 Slit-lamp photograph from a patient with conjunctival intraepithelial neoplasia shows staining with lissamine green dye. *(Courtesy of Stephen E. Orlin, MD.)*

Evaluation of Tear Production

The *basic secretion test* is performed after instillation of a topical anesthetic and light blotting of residual fluid from the inferior fornix. To minimize irritation to the cornea during the test, a thin filter-paper strip (5 mm wide, 30 mm long) is placed at the junction of the middle and lateral thirds of the lower eyelid, with 5 mm of the paper's length folded within the inferior cul-de-sac and the remaining 25 mm projecting over the lower eyelid. The test can be performed with the patient's eyes open or closed, but some recommend that the eyes be closed to eliminate blinking. Although normal tear secretion is quite variable, repeated measurements of less than 3 mm of wetting after 5 minutes, with anesthetic, are highly suggestive of aqueous tear deficiency (ATD), whereas 3–10 mm is equivocal. See Chapter 3 for a discussion of ATD.

The *Schirmer I test,* which is similar to the basic secretion test but is done without topical anesthetic, measures both basic and reflex tearing. Less than 5.5 mm of wetting after 5 minutes is diagnostic of ATD. Although this test is relatively specific, its sensitivity is poor. Using lower thresholds increases the specificity of the test but decreases its sensitivity. The *Schirmer II test,* which measures reflex secretion, is performed in a similar manner but with topical anesthetic. However, after the filter-paper strips have been inserted into the inferior fornices, a cotton-tipped applicator is used to irritate the nasal mucosa. Wetting of less than 15 mm after 2 minutes is consistent with a defect in reflex secretion. Although an isolated abnormal result for any of these tests can be misleading, serially consistent results are highly suggestive of ATD. Schirmer testing is also useful in demonstrating to patients the presence of ATD. An alternative to use of the classic Schirmer strips involves use of a cotton thread impregnated with phenol red, which allows for quicker assessment of tear secretion but has not been fully validated.

Greiner MA, Faulkner WJ, Vislisel JM, Varley GA, Goins KM. Corneal diagnostic techniques. In: Mannis MJ, Holland EJ, eds. *Cornea.* Vol. 1. 4th ed. Philadelphia: Elsevier; 2017:116–122.

Tear Film Quantitative Tests

As our understanding of the tear film has improved (see Chapter 1), commercial assays to measure its various components have been developed. The objectivity and reproducibility of many of these tests have yet to be confirmed, and the results need to be evaluated in conjunction with symptoms and other clinical findings.

Microliter samples of tears can be used to measure tear film osmolarity. Values higher than 306–308 mOsm/L are considered highly indicative of ATD. Other studies, however, have shown a lack of correlation between tear osmolarity and symptoms and objective signs of dry eye.

Lactoferrin, an iron-binding protein secreted directly by the acinar cells of the lacrimal gland, plays an important antibacterial role in the tear film. Although it does not play a role in tear production, its levels are directly correlated to aqueous production. Microassays are now available to measure levels of lactoferrin, providing an indirect measure of lacrimal gland function.

Immunoglobulin E (IgE) levels in the tear film can also be measured with microassay technology, and increased levels can help distinguish between ATD and ocular allergies. Lactoferrin and IgE biomarkers can be measured in a single commercially available test requiring only 0.5 μL of tears.

Matrix metalloproteinase 9 (MMP-9) is an inflammatory cytokine released by distressed epithelial cells. Dry eye is multifactorial and can be associated with inflammation of the ocular surface and eyelids (eg, blepharitis), which in turn can cause the release of the inflammatory marker MMP-9. Elevated values (>40 ng/mL) might indicate evaporative dry eye (see Chapter 3). However, this test is not specific for dry eyes, as high levels of MMP-9 are reported in conditions other than blepharitis, such as allergy, infection, and peripheral ulcerative keratitis.

Sjögren syndrome is commonly associated with dry eye. Early biomarkers for this autoimmune disease may support the diagnosis in patients with systemic symptoms such as dry mouth and joint pains. A proprietary biomarker test is available that may be more sensitive than other blood tests, such as SS-A and SS-B antibody and rheumatoid factor tests.

Tear Film Qualitative Tests

Meibomian gland dysfunction (MGD) is a major cause of evaporative dry eye and is discussed in Chapter 3. Slit-lamp examination of the eyelid margin and meibomian gland orifices is an important clinical tool in the evaluation of MGD, but interferometry and infrared meibography have enhanced the ability to assess meibomian gland structure and pathology (Fig 2-24). These tools allow clinicians to measure the height of the tear film meniscus and examine, with submicrometer accuracy, the thickness and structure of the lipid layer (Fig 2-25). They also allow real-time evaluation of the blink rate, the completeness of blink patterns, and TBUT (noninvasive) and provide objective recordings of meibomian gland dropout.

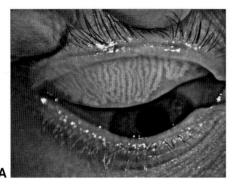
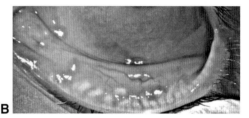

A   **B**

Figure 2-24   **A,** Upper eyelid infrared meibography image (Keratograph; Oculus, Arlington, WA) demonstrates normal meibomian gland architecture. Note the long, straight glands with very little tortuosity. **B,** Lower eyelid meibography image shows severe gland truncation and atrophy. *(Courtesy of Mina Massaro-Giordano, MD.)*

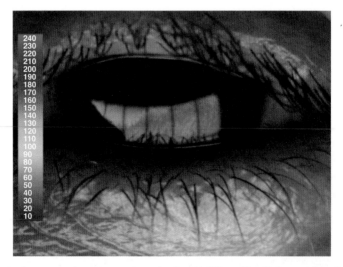

Figure 2-25   Interferometry image, produced using LipiView (TearScience, Morrisville, NC) and showing the "rainbow" pattern of the normal lipid layer in the tear film. *(Courtesy of Mina Massaro-Giordano, MD.)*

American Academy of Ophthalmology Cornea/External Disease Panel. Preferred Practice Pattern Guidelines. *Dry Eye Syndrome.* San Francisco: American Academy of Ophthalmology; 2013. Available at www.aao.org/ppp.

Bunya VY, Langelier N, Chen S, Pistilli M, Vivino FB, Massaro-Giordano G. Tear osmolarity in Sjögren syndrome. *Cornea.* 2013;3(32):922–927.

The definition and classification of dry eye disease: report of the Definition and Classification Subcommittee of the International Dry Eye WorkShop (2007). *Ocul Surf.* 2007;5(2):75–92.

Pachymetry

A corneal pachymeter measures corneal thickness, a sensitive indicator of endothelial physiology that correlates well with functional measurements. Optical pachymetry, which is performed using a special device attached to the slit-lamp biomicroscope, is somewhat imprecise and is rarely used today. Ultrasonic pachymetry, which is based on the speed of sound in the normal cornea (1640 m/sec), is both easier to perform and more accurate. The applanating tip of the pachymeter must be perpendicular to the ocular surface because errors are induced by tilting. Scanning-slit technology, Scheimpflug-based anterior segment imaging, OCT, and high-resolution ultrasonography are newer techniques that can be used to produce precise maps of the entire corneal thickness, including curvature (see Fig 2-19).

The thinnest zone of the cornea is usually about 1.5 mm temporal to the geographic center, and the cornea becomes thicker in the paracentral and peripheral zones. The average central thickness of the normal human cornea is between 540 and 550 μm. In the Ocular Hypertension Treatment Study, the average central corneal thickness was higher, at 573 ± 39 μm, but it was acknowledged that central corneal thickness was probably higher in the study population than in the general population. Corneal thickness affects the measurement of intraocular pressure (IOP), with thicker corneas producing falsely higher IOP readings and thinner corneas producing falsely lower readings. However, Liu and Roberts demonstrated that the biomechanical properties of the cornea, particularly stiffness, may have a greater impact on IOP measurement errors than does corneal thickness or corneal curvature. Adjustment for corneal biomechanical properties may lead to a more accurate measurement of the IOP. Despite these adjustments, low pachymetry measurements have been shown to be an independent risk factor for glaucoma even when the artificial lowering of IOP is accounted for.

Pachymetry can also be used to assess corneal hydration and the function of the corneal endothelium in its dual role as a barrier to aqueous humor and as a metabolic pump. When functioning normally, the endothelial pump balances the leak rate to maintain the corneal stromal water content at 78% and the central corneal thickness at about 540 μm. Acute corneal edema is often the result of an altered barrier effect of the endothelium or epithelium. Chronic corneal edema is usually caused by an inadequate endothelial pump. Early signs of corneal edema evident on slit-lamp examination include patchy or diffuse haze of the epithelium, mild stromal thickening, faint but deep stromal wrinkles (Waite-Beetham lines), Descemet membrane folds, and a patchy or diffuse posterior collagenous layer. Folds in the Descemet membrane are first seen when corneal thickness increases by

10% or more; epithelial edema occurs when corneal thickness exceeds 700 μm. Stromal edema alters corneal transparency, but vision loss is most severe when epithelial microcysts or bullae occur. A central corneal thickness greater than 640 μm, corneal thickening that is asymmetric between the 2 eyes, or a thicker central cornea compared with inferior corneal measurements within the same eye may indicate a higher risk for symptomatic corneal edema after intraocular surgery.

Brandt JD, Beiser JA, Kass MA, Gordon MO. Central corneal thickness in the Ocular Hypertension Treatment Study (OHTS). *Ophthalmology.* 2001;108(10):1779–1788.

Khaja WA, Grover S, Kelmenson AT, Ferguson LR, Sambhav K, Chalam KV. Comparison of central corneal thickness: ultrasound pachymetry versus slit-lamp optical coherence tomography, specular microscopy, and Orbscan. *Clin Ophthalmol.* 2015;12(9):1065–1070.

Liu J, Roberts CJ. Influence of corneal biomechanical properties on intraocular pressure measurement: quantitative analysis. *J Cataract Refract Surg.* 2005;31(1):146–155.

Corneal Esthesiometry

Corneal sensation is supplied by the ophthalmic division of the fifth (trigeminal) cranial nerve. Corneal esthesiometry is typically used clinically to evaluate for neurotrophic keratopathy.

In the clinical setting, an evaluation of corneal sensation is most commonly achieved with a cotton-tipped applicator. This is performed without topical anesthesia and should be done before IOP is checked. A wisp of cotton from the cotton-tipped applicator is used to compare sensation in each eye. Approaching the patient from the side and testing all 4 quadrants has the advantage of eliminating false-positive responses, which result when the patient sees the cotton-tipped applicator approaching the eye. The sensation in each location is recorded as normal, reduced, or absent.

Various quantitative methods exist, but they are typically reserved for research or complex cases. The most common quantitative method is use of the handheld (Cochet-Bonnet) esthesiometer; this is discussed in the following section. Other methods include the noncontact air-puff technique, chemical stimulation using capsaicin, and thermal stimulation with a carbon dioxide laser.

Handheld Esthesiometer

The handheld (Cochet-Bonnet) esthesiometer is a device that contains a thin, retractable nylon monofilament. Adjusting the length of the monofilament changes the pressure applied by the device. The maximum length is 60 mm, and the minimum length is 5 mm; as the length decreases, the pressure increases from a minimum of 11 mm/gm to a maximum of 200 mm/gm.

Steps for using the handheld esthesiometer are as follows:

1. Extend the filament to the full length of 60 mm.
2. Retract the filament in 5-mm increments until the patient can feel its contact.
3. Record the length. (Note: The shorter the length, the lower the sensation.)

4. Repeat steps 1–3 in the fellow cornea.
5. Repeat steps 1–4 in each quadrant: superior, temporal, inferior, and nasal.
6. Clean the filament and retract it into the device.

Greiner MA, Faulkner WJ, Vislisel JM, Varley GA, Goins KM. Corneal diagnostic techniques. In: Mannis MJ, Holland EJ, eds. *Cornea.* Vol. 1. 4th ed. Philadelphia: Elsevier; 2017:116–122.

Measurement of Corneal Biomechanics

The biomechanical properties of the cornea affect its functional responses and can have a significant impact on vision. The cornea has both elastic and viscous elements, and these play a role in conditions such as keratoconus and ectasia. *Corneal hysteresis* is defined as the difference between the pressure at which the cornea bends inward during air-jet applanation and the pressure at which it bends out again. This difference, which is measured in millimeters of mercury, gauges elasticity, a biomechanical property of the cornea. Theoretical applications of these measurements might enable detection of corneas at risk for ectasia following corneal refractive surgery.

A commercially available instrument now allows in vivo clinical testing of a cornea's direct biomechanical properties. The *corneal resistance factor (CRF)* is calculated based on a mathematical correlation between hysteresis and corneal thickness. CRF values have a normal distribution within the general population but are lower in patients who have undergone LASIK or photorefractive keratectomy or whose corneas have an inherent biomechanical weakness, like forme fruste keratoconus. These values are also lower in patients who have corneal edema secondary to Fuchs endothelial corneal dystrophy. These measurements might also increase the accuracy of IOP measurements, which are affected by corneal properties such as thickness. However, use of the device may not be particularly effective in screening refractive surgery patients for risk of keratectasia or in documenting the increased stiffness associated with corneal crosslinking, aging, and diabetes mellitus, because it measures the viscous and not the elastic properties of the cornea.

Newer technologies for evaluating corneal biomechanics integrate dynamic corneal imaging instruments using Placido disk–based technology, Scheimpflug imaging, or OCT and allow more accurate measurement of the corneal deformation produced by the collimated air puffs. These devices can differentiate the elastic biomechanical properties of normal corneas from those of ectatic corneas. They can also distinguish corneal crosslinking–treated corneas from pretreatment corneas, using variables such as the quantitative amplitude of inward deformation (greater in softer, ectatic corneas) and the area of corneal tissue experiencing inward deformation (less in softer, ectatic corneas). Using these devices, investigators have shown that corneal deformation is influenced by the IOP and corneal thickness as well as the innate elastic biomechanical properties of the cornea.

Dawson DG, Ubels JL, Edelhauser HF. Cornea and sclera. In: Alm A, Kaufman PL, eds. *Adler's Physiology of the Eye.* 11th ed. New York: Elsevier; 2011:71–130.

Piñero DP, Alcón N. In vivo characterization of corneal biomechanics. *J Cataract Refract Surg.* 2014;40(6):870–887.

CHAPTER 3

Clinical Approach to Ocular Surface Disease

Highlights

- It is helpful both diagnostically and therapeutically to divide dry eye into 2 categories, aqueous tear deficiency (ATD) and evaporative dry eye.
- Mucous discharge is common in patients with moderate to severe ATD and in patients with infectious conjunctivitis; consequently, ATD is frequently misdiagnosed as infectious conjunctivitis.
- Eyelid margin disease is commonly associated with dry eye; effective treatment of eyelid disease is therefore an important adjunct to dry eye management.

Common Clinical Findings in Ocular Surface Disease

The following sections and tables introduce and define common clinical findings of the external eye and cornea that aid in the diagnosis of ocular surface disease (Table 3-1).

Table 3-1 Common Clinical Findings of the External Eye and Cornea

Tissue	Finding	Description
Eyelid	Macule	Spot of skin color change
	Papule	Small, solid elevation of the skin
	Vesicle	Blister filled with serous fluid
	Bulla	Large blister
	Pustule	Pus-filled blister
	Keratosis	Scaling from accumulated keratinized cells
	Eczema	Scaly crust on a red base
	Erosion	Excoriated epidermal defect
	Ulcer	Epidermal erosion with deeper tissue loss
Conjunctiva	Hyperemia	Focal or diffuse dilation of the subepithelial plexus of conjunctival blood vessels, usually with increased blood flow; other changes include fusiform vascular dilations, saccular aneurysms, petechiae, and intraconjunctival hemorrhage
	Chalasis	Laxity of conjunctiva; tissue may roll up onto the eyelid margin or cover the lacrimal punctum

(Continued)

45

Table 3-1 *(continued)*

Tissue	Finding	Description
	Chemosis	Conjunctival edema caused by a transudate leaking through fenestrated conjunctival capillaries as a result of altered vascular integrity (eg, inflammation and vasomotor changes) or hemodynamic changes (eg, impaired venous drainage or intravascular hyposmolarity)
	Epiphora	Excess tears from increased lacrimation or impaired lacrimal outflow
	Mucus excess	Increased amount of mucin relative to aqueous component of tears
	Discharge	Exudate on the conjunctival surface, varying from proteinaceous (serous) to cellular (purulent)
	Papillae	Dilated, telangiectatic conjunctival blood vessels, varying from dotlike changes to enlarged tufts, surrounded by edema and a mixed inflammatory cell infiltrate
	Follicle	Focal lymphoid nodule with accessory vascularization
	Pseudomembrane	Inflammatory coagulum on the conjunctival surface that does not bleed during removal
	Membrane	Inflammatory coagulum suffusing the conjunctival epithelium that bleeds when stripped
	Granuloma	Nodule consisting of chronic inflammatory cells with fibrovascular proliferation
	Phlyctenule	Nodule consisting of chronic inflammatory cells, often at or near the limbus
	Punctate epithelial erosion	Loss of individual epithelial cells in a stippled pattern
	Epithelial defect	Focal area of epithelial loss
Sclera	Episcleritis	Focal or diffuse dilation of radial superficial episcleral vessels
	Nonnecrotizing scleritis	Dilated deep episcleral vessels with scleral edema
	Necrotizing scleritis	Area of avascular sclera
Cornea	Punctate epithelial erosion	Fine, slightly depressed stippling caused by altered or desquamated superficial epithelium
	Punctate epithelial keratitis	Swollen, slightly raised epithelial cells that can be finely scattered, coarsely grouped, or arranged in an arborescent pattern
	Epithelial edema	Swollen epithelial cells (intraepithelial edema) or intercellular vacuoles (microcystic edema)
	Bulla	Fluid pocket within or under the epithelium
	Epithelial defect	Focal area of epithelial loss, caused by trauma (abrasion) or other condition
	Dendrite	Branching linear epithelial ridge with swollen cells, terminal bulbs, and possible central ulceration
	Ulcer	Epithelial defect, stromal loss, stromal inflammation, or any combination of these changes
	Filament	Strand (filament) or clump (mucous plaque) of mucus and degenerating epithelial cells attached to an altered ocular surface
	Subepithelial infiltrate	Coin-shaped inflammatory opacity in the anterior portion of Bowman layer
	Suppurative stromal keratitis	Focal yellow-white infiltrate of neutrophils
	Nonsuppurative stromal keratitis	Focal gray-white infiltrate of lymphocytes and other mononuclear cells; also called *interstitial keratitis,* especially when accompanied by stromal neovascularization

Conjunctival Signs

Table 3-2 lists conjunctival findings, with examples of ocular and systemic conditions in which they are seen.

Papillae

Papillae are vascular changes seen most easily in the palpebral conjunctiva where fibrous septa anchor the conjunctiva to the tarsus. With progression, these dilated vessels sprout spokelike capillaries that become surrounded by edema and a mixed inflammatory cell infiltrate, producing raised elevations under the conjunctival epithelium (Fig 3-1).

A mild papillary reaction produces a smooth, velvety appearance (Fig 3-2A). Chronic or progressive changes result in enlarged vascular tufts that obscure the underlying

Table 3-2 Conjunctival Signs

Finding	Examples of Ocular or Systemic Conditions
Papillary conjunctivitis	Allergic conjunctivitis
	Bacterial conjunctivitis
Follicular conjunctivitis	Adenovirus conjunctivitis
	Herpes simplex virus conjunctivitis
	Molluscum contagiosum blepharoconjunctivitis
	Chlamydial conjunctivitis
	Drug-induced (eg, brimonidine) conjunctivitis
Conjunctival pseudomembrane or membrane	Severe viral or bacterial conjunctivitis
	Stevens-Johnson syndrome
	Chemical burn
Conjunctival granuloma	Cat-scratch disease
	Sarcoidosis
	Foreign-body reaction
Conjunctival erosion or ulceration	Stevens-Johnson syndrome
	Mucous membrane pemphigoid
	Graft-vs-host disease
	Factitious conjunctivitis
	Mechanical or chemical trauma
Conjunctival cicatrization	Stevens-Johnson syndrome
	Mucous membrane pemphigoid
	Chemical injury

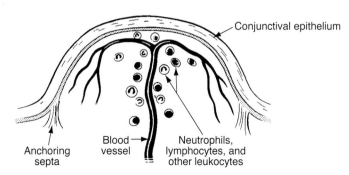

Figure 3-1 Cross-sectional diagram of a conjunctival papilla with a central vascular tuft surrounded by acute and chronic leukocytes.

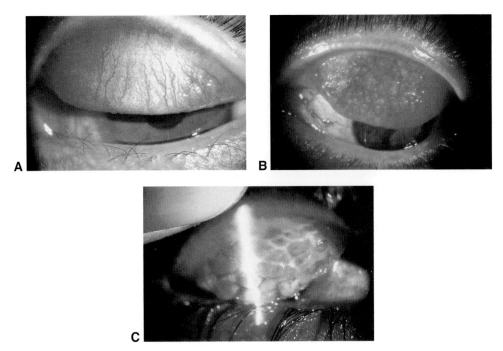

Figure 3-2 Papillary conjunctivitis. **A,** Mild papillae. **B,** Moderate papillae. **C,** Marked (giant) papillae.

blood vessels (Fig 3-2B). Connective tissue septa restrict inflammatory changes to the fibrovascular core, producing the appearance of elevated, polygonal, hyperemic mounds. Each papilla has a central red dot that represents a dilated capillary viewed end-on. Examination of the palpebral, bulbar, and forniceal conjunctivae beyond the tarsus is less helpful in revealing the nature of an inflammatory reaction, because the anchoring septa become sparser toward the fornix and permit undulation of less adherent tissue. With prolonged, recurrent, or severe conjunctival inflammation, the anchoring fibers of the tarsal conjunctiva stretch and weaken, leading to confluent papillary hypertrophy. *Giant papillae* are defined as those with a diameter greater than 0.3 mm (Fig 3-2C). The furrows between these enlarged fibrovascular structures collect mucus and purulent material. After treatment, a fibrotic subepithelial scar may be seen at the apex of the former giant papilla.

Follicles

Conjunctival lymphoid tissue is normally present within the substantia propria except in neonates, who do not have visible follicles. Conjunctival follicles are round or oval clusters of lymphocytes (Fig 3-3). Small follicles are often visible in the normal lower fornix. Clusters of enlarged, noninflamed follicles are occasionally seen in the forniceal or inferior palpebral conjunctiva of children and adolescents, a condition known as *benign lymphoid folliculosis* (Fig 3-4).

Follicular conjunctivitis is characterized by conjunctival injection and the presence of new or enlarged follicles (Fig 3-5). Vessels surround and encroach on the raised surface

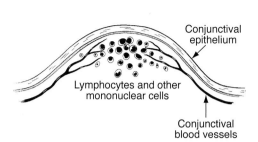

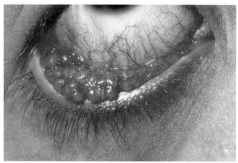

Figure 3-3 Cross-sectional diagram of a con-junctival follicle with mononuclear cells ob-scuring conjunctival blood vessels.

Figure 3-4 Benign lymphoid folliculosis. *(Courtesy of Kirk R. Wilhelmus, MD.)*

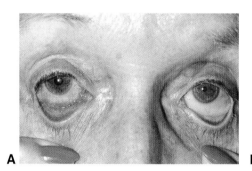

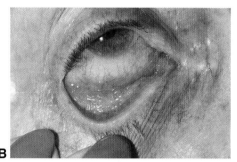

A **B**

Figure 3-5 Follicular conjunctivitis. **A,** Inflammation of the right eye from glaucoma medication. **B,** Right eye showing follicular conjunctivitis in the inferior fornix. *(Courtesy of John E. Sutphin, MD.)*

of follicles but are not prominently visible within the follicle. Follicles can be seen in the inferior and superior tarsal conjunctiva and, less often, on the bulbar or limbal conjunc-tiva. They must be differentiated from cysts produced by tubular epithelial infoldings dur-ing chronic inflammation and lymphangiectasis.

See also BCSC Section 4, *Ophthalmic Pathology and Intraocular Tumors.*

Stern G. Chronic conjunctivitis, Parts 1–2. *Focal Points: Clinical Modules for Ophthal-mologists.* San Francisco: American Academy of Ophthalmology; 2012, modules 11–12.

Corneal Signs

Corneal signs of inflammation are described in Table 3-3. The pattern of corneal inflam-mation, or *keratitis,* can be described according to the following:

- *distribution:* diffuse, focal, or multifocal
- *depth:* epithelial, subepithelial, stromal, or endothelial
- *location:* central, paracentral, or peripheral
- *shape:* dendritic, disciform, and so on

The clinician should also note any structural or physiologic changes associated with kera-titis, such as ulceration or endothelial dysfunction.

Table 3-3 Corneal Signs

Finding	Examples of Ocular Conditions
Punctate epithelial erosions	Dry eye Toxic reaction Atopic keratoconjunctivitis
Punctate epithelial keratitis	Adenovirus keratoconjunctivitis Herpes simplex virus epithelial keratitis Herpes zoster virus epithelial keratitis Thygeson superficial punctate keratitis
Stromal keratitis, suppurative	Bacterial keratitis Fungal keratitis
Stromal keratitis, nonsuppurative	Herpes simplex virus stromal keratitis Varicella-zoster virus stromal keratitis Syphilitic interstitial keratitis
Peripheral keratitis	Blepharitis-associated marginal infiltrates Peripheral ulcerative keratitis caused by connective tissue diseases Mooren ulcer

Punctate epithelial keratitis (PEK) is a nonspecific term that encompasses a spectrum of biomicroscopic changes, from punctate epithelial granularity to erosive and inflammatory changes (Fig 3-6). Punctate epithelial erosions (PEE) are lesions of abnormal or degenerated corneal epithelial cells that stain with fluorescein.

Inflammatory cells can enter the stroma from the tear film, through an epithelial defect; less often, they enter by direct interlamellar infiltration of leukocytes at the limbus (eg, after laser in situ keratomileusis [LASIK]). In the presence of endothelial injury, inflammatory cells enter from aqueous humor. Stromal inflammation may be manifested by the presence of new blood vessels. In a vascularized cornea, inflammatory cells can enter the stroma directly from infiltrating blood and lymphatic vessels.

Stromal inflammation is characterized as *suppurative* or *nonsuppurative* (Fig 3-7). It is further described by distribution (*focal* or *multifocal* infiltrates) and by location (*central,*

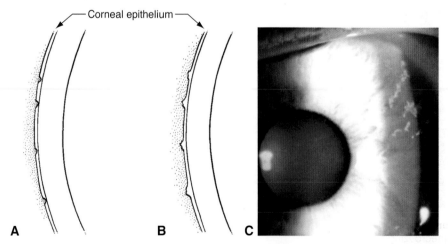

Corneal epithelium

A   **B**   **C**

Figure 3-6 Punctate lesions of the corneal epithelium. **A,** Punctate epithelial erosions. **B,** Punctate epithelial keratitis. **C,** Slit-lamp photograph from a patient with epithelial keratitis due to herpes zoster. *(Part C courtesy of Robert S. Feder, MD.)*

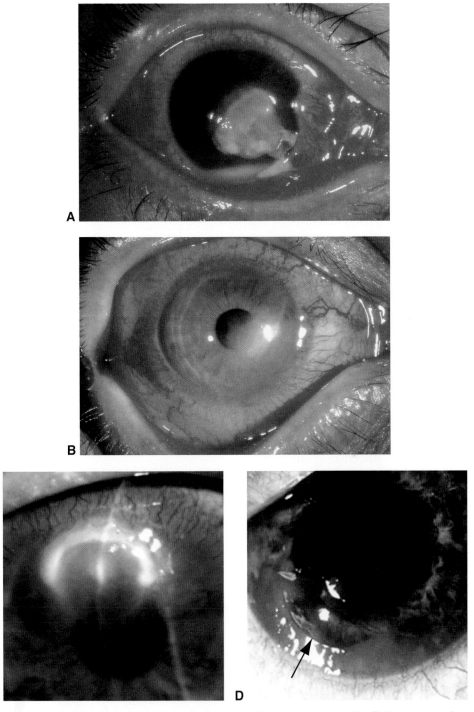

Figure 3-7 Inflammation of the corneal stroma. **A,** Suppurative keratitis. **B,** Nonsuppurative, nonnecrotizing (disciform) stromal keratitis. **C,** Immune ring. **D,** Peripheral ulcerative keratitis. An ovoid area of thinning *(arrow)* can be seen in the inferonasal quadrant. *(Parts C and D courtesy of Robert S. Feder, MD.)*

paracentral, or *peripheral*). The differential diagnosis for suppurative corneal inflammation or necrotizing stromal keratitis includes microbial keratitis due to bacteria, fungi,
or acanthamoeba; retained foreign body; and topical anesthetic abuse. Nonsuppurative
stromal keratitis can be caused by reactive arthritis, Cogan syndrome, viral keratitis, congenital or acquired syphilis, Lyme disease, tuberculosis, leprosy (Hansen disease), and
onchocerciasis.

Endothelial dysfunction often leads to epithelial and stromal edema. Swollen endothelial cells called *inflammatory pseudoguttae* are visible by specular reflection as dark
areas of the normal endothelial mosaic pattern. *Keratic precipitates (KPs)* are clumps of
inflammatory cells that adhere to the back of the cornea and come from the anterior uvea
during the course of keratitis or uveitis. The clinical appearance of KPs depends on their
composition:

- Fibrin and other proteins coagulate into small dots and strands.
- Neutrophils and lymphocytes aggregate into punctate opacities.
- Macrophages form larger "mutton-fat" clumps.

Corneal inflammation can lead to opacification. Altered stromal keratocytes fail to
produce some water-soluble factors and, consequently, make new collagen fibers that are
disorganized, scatter light, and form a nontransparent scar. Scarring can incorporate calcium complexes, lipids, and proteinaceous material. Dark pigmentation of a residual corneal opacity is often a result of incorporated melanin or iron salts.

Corneal inflammation can also lead to neovascularization. Superficial stromal blood
vessels originate as capillary buds of limbal vascular arcades in the palisades of Vogt. New
lymphatic vessels may also form but cannot be seen clinically. Subepithelial fibrous ingrowth into the peripheral cornea is called a *pannus* or *vascularized pannus* (Fig 3-8).
Neovascularization may invade the cornea at deeper levels depending on the nature and
location of the inflammatory stimulus.

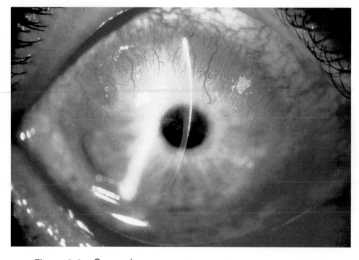

Figure 3-8 Corneal pannus. *(Courtesy of Kirk R. Wilhelmus, MD.)*

Ciralsky J, Lai E, Waring GO III, Bouchard CS. A matrix of pathologic responses in the cornea. In: Mannis MJ, Holland EJ, eds. *Cornea*. Vol 1. 4th ed. Philadelphia: Elsevier; 2017:46–71.

Leibowitz HM, Waring GO III, eds. *Corneal Disorders: Clinical Diagnosis and Management.* 2nd ed. Philadelphia: Saunders; 1998:432–479.

Clinical Approach to Dry Eye

In 2007, the International Dry Eye Workshop defined *dry eye* as "a multifactorial disease of the tears and ocular surface that results in symptoms of discomfort, visual disturbance, and tear film instability with potential damage to the ocular surface." Dry eye represents a disturbance of the lacrimal functional unit, an integrated system comprising the lacrimal glands, ocular surface (cornea, conjunctiva, and limbus), and eyelids, as well as the sensory and motor nerves connecting these components. See Chapter 1 for a discussion and illustration of the lacrimal functional unit.

Dry eye is one of the most common reasons for ophthalmic consultation. It becomes increasingly prevalent with age, affecting approximately 10% of individuals 30–60 years of age and 15% of adults older than 65 years. Most epidemiologic studies have demonstrated a higher prevalence among women; dry eye seems to affect all racial and ethnic groups equally.

The psychological problems associated with a highly symptomatic, incurable, chronic disease can require considerable support. Results of quality-of-life studies have shown that the impact of moderate to severe dry eye on affected patients is similar to that of moderate to severe angina. Organizations such as the Sjögren's Syndrome Foundation (www.sjogrens.org) can provide valuable resources for these patients. For certain patients, consultation with physicians who specialize in pain management can be very helpful.

The definition and classification of dry eye disease: report of the Definition and Classification Subcommittee of the International Dry Eye WorkShop (2007). *Ocul Surf.* 2007;5(2):75–92.

Mechanisms of Dry Eye

Dry eye results from a combination of factors. Tear hyperosmolarity stresses the surface epithelium and leads to the release of inflammatory mediators, which disrupt the junctions between the superficial epithelial cells. T cells can then infiltrate the epithelium and in turn produce cytokines such as tumor necrosis factor-α and interleukin-1. These cytokines promote accelerated detachment of the epithelial cells and apoptosis (programmed cell death). This results in further disruption of junctions and influx of inflammatory cells, creating a vicious cycle. The cycle of events is shown in Figure 3-9.

One diagnostic classification scheme divides dry eye patients into those with aqueous tear deficiency and those with evaporative dry eye (Fig 3-10). An individual patient may have elements of both conditions, however. In aqueous tear deficiency, T-cell–mediated inflammation of the lacrimal gland occurs, leading to diminished tear production and the propagation of inflammatory mediators on the ocular surface. In evaporative dry eye, the primary abnormality is meibomian gland dysfunction, in which altered lipid metabolism of the meibum causes a transition from unsaturated to saturated fats, resulting in

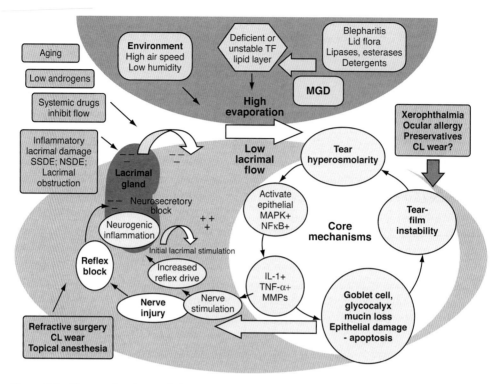

Figure 3-9 The mechanisms of dry eye. *(Modified with permission from The definition and classification of dry eye disease: report of the Definition and Classification Subcommittee of the International Dry Eye WorkShop (2007). Ocul Surf. 2007;5(2):75–92.)*

obstruction of the glands. This leads to tear film instability as well as tear evaporation and hyperosmolarity, initiating the inflammatory cycle.

Tear film instability can also be initiated by other conditions, including xerophthalmia, ocular allergy, contact lens wear, a high ratio of dietary n-6 to n-3 essential fatty acids, diabetes mellitus, cigarette smoking, prolonged use of video displays, and long-term use of medications with topical preservatives such as benzalkonium chloride.

Epithelial injury stimulates corneal nerve endings, leading to symptoms such as ocular discomfort, increased blinking, and, potentially, compensatory reflex lacrimal tear secretion. Loss of normal mucins at the ocular surface contributes to symptoms by increasing frictional resistance between the eyelids and globe. During this period of corneal nerve stimulation, the high reflex input may cause neurogenic inflammation within the lacrimal gland.

Tear delivery may be obstructed by cicatricial conjunctival scarring or reduced by a loss of sensory reflex drive to the lacrimal gland from the ocular surface. The etiology of dry eye may include refractive surgery (eg, LASIK), contact lens wear, and chronic topical anesthetic abuse. The pathogenesis of dry eye may involve several interacting mechanisms.

American Academy of Ophthalmology Cornea/External Disease Panel. Preferred Practice Pattern Guidelines. *Dry Eye Syndrome.* San Francisco: American Academy of Ophthalmology; 2013. Available at www.aao.org/ppp.

The definition and classification of dry eye disease: report of the Definition and Classification Subcommittee of the International Dry Eye WorkShop (2007). *Ocul Surf.* 2007;5(2):75–92.

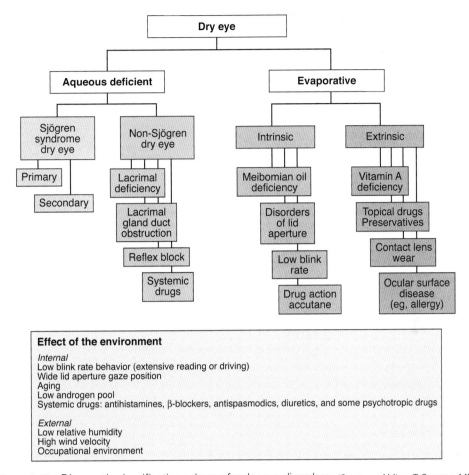

Figure 3-10 Diagnostic classification scheme for dry eye disorders. *(Courtesy of Minas T. Coroneo, MD.)*

Bohm KJ, Djalilian AR, Pflugfelder SC, Starr CE. Dry eye. In: Mannis MJ, Holland EJ, eds. *Cornea.* Vol 1. 4th ed. Philadelphia: Elsevier; 2017:377–396.

Nichols KK, Foulks GN, Bron AJ, et al. The International Workshop on Meibomian Gland Dysfunction: Executive Summary. *Invest Ophthalmol Vis Sci.* 2011;52(4):1922–1929.

Pflugfelder SC. Tear dysfunction and the cornea: LXVIII Edward Jackson Memorial Lecture. *Am J Ophthalmol.* 2011;152(6):900–909.

Stevenson W, Chauhan SK, Dana R. Dry eye disease: an immune-mediated ocular surface disorder. *Arch Ophthalmol.* 2012;130(1):90–100.

Aqueous Tear Deficiency

The clinical presentation of aqueous tear deficiency (ATD) ranges from mild ocular irritation with minimal ocular surface disease to severe and disabling disease. Patients commonly report burning, a dry sensation, photophobia, and blurred vision. Symptoms tend to be worse toward the end of the day, with prolonged use of the eyes (exacerbated by the reduced blink rate associated with computer use), or with exposure to environmental extremes (eg, lower levels of humidity associated with indoor heating or air conditioning). The clinician can quickly assess dry eye by conducting the "stare test": after a few blinks, the patient is asked to look at a visual acuity chart; the time until the image blurs should be more than 8 seconds.

Signs of ATD include bulbar conjunctival hyperemia, a decreased tear meniscus, an irregular corneal surface, and debris in the tear film. Slit-lamp examination of the inferior tear meniscus (which is normally 1.0 mm in height and convex) is an additional, important evaluation. A significantly reduced tear meniscus is considered abnormal. Epithelial keratopathy, which can be fine and granular, coarse, or confluent, is best demonstrated following the instillation of lissamine green, rose bengal, or fluorescein dye. Rose bengal and lissamine green staining can be more sensitive than fluorescein staining in revealing early or mild cases of keratoconjunctivitis sicca (KCS) because they stain devitalized epithelium. The staining may be seen at the nasal and temporal limbus and/or inferior paracentral cornea *(exposure staining)*. Mucous discharge is common in patients with moderate to severe ATD and in those with infectious conjunctivitis; consequently, ATD is frequently misdiagnosed as infectious conjunctivitis.

In severe ATD, filaments (strands of degenerating epithelial cells attached to the corneal surface over a core of mucus) and mucous plaques may be seen. Filamentary keratopathy can be quite painful, as these strands are firmly attached to the richly innervated surface epithelium (Fig 3-11). Marginal or paracentral corneal thinning and even perforation can occur in severe dry eye. Incomplete blinking is frequently noted. Advanced disease may also involve corneal calcification (band keratopathy), particularly in association with certain topical medications (especially glaucoma medications), and keratinization of the cornea and conjunctiva. A grading scheme for dry eye severity is presented in Table 3-4. See Chapter 2 for a discussion on tear production evaluation and tear film quantitative tests.

Sjögren syndrome

Patients with ATD are considered to have Sjögren syndrome if they have associated hypergammaglobulinemia, collagen vascular disease, or circulating autoantibodies (eg, SS-A, SS-B). The revised international classification criteria for Sjögren syndrome appear

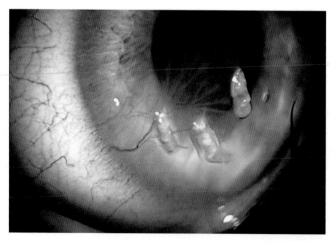

Figure 3-11 Filamentary keratopathy in a vascularized cornea. *(Courtesy of Minas T. Coroneo, MD.)*

Table 3-4 Dry Eye Severity Grading Scheme

Signs and Symptoms	Dry Eye Severity Level			
	1	2	3	4*
Discomfort, severity and frequency	Mild and/or episodic; occurs under environmental stress	Moderate episodic or chronic, stress or no stress	Severe frequent or constant without stress	Severe and/or disabling and constant
Visual symptoms	None or episodic mild fatigue	Annoying and/ or activity-limiting episodic	Annoying, chronic and/ or constant, limiting activity	Constant and/ or possibly disabling
Conjunctival injection	None to mild	None to mild	+/–	+/++
Conjunctival staining	None to mild	Variable	Moderate to marked	Marked
Corneal staining (severity/location)	None to mild	Variable	Marked central	Severe punctate erosions
Corneal/tear signs	None to mild	Mild debris, ↓ tear meniscus	Filamentary keratitis, mucus clumping, ↑ tear debris	Filamentary keratitis, mucus clumping, ↑ tear debris, ulceration
Eyelid/ meibomian glands	MGD variably present	MGD variably present	MGD frequently present	Trichiasis, keratinization, symblepharon
TBUT (seconds)	Variable	≤10	≤5	Immediate
Schirmer score (mm wetting after 5 min)	Variable	≤10	≤5	≤2

MGD = meibomian gland dysfunction; TBUT = fluorescein tear break-up time; ↓ = reduced; ↑ = increased.
*Must have signs AND symptoms.

Modified with permission from The definition and classification of dry eye disease: report of the Definition and Classification Subcommittee of the International Dry Eye Workshop (2007). *Ocul Surf.* 2007;5(2):75–92. Permission conveyed through Copyright Clearance Center, Inc.

in Table 3-5. Although the precise causes of ATD in Sjögren syndrome are unknown, ATD is generally considered to be a T-cell–mediated inflammatory disease leading to destruction of the lacrimal glands, in part by increasing the rate of programmed cell death.

Involvement of the salivary glands is common in Sjögren syndrome, resulting in dry mouth and predisposing the patient to periodontal disease. Mucous membranes throughout the body (ie, vaginal, gastric, and respiratory mucosae) may also be affected, which would have a great impact on the patient's quality of life.

Sjögren syndrome can be divided into 2 clinical subsets. In primary Sjögren syndrome, patients either have ill-defined systemic immune dysfunction or lack any evidence of immune dysfunction or connective tissue disease. In secondary Sjögren syndrome, patients have a well-defined, generalized connective tissue disease, most commonly rheumatoid

Table 3-5 Criteria for the Classification of Sjögren Syndrome

1. Ocular symptoms
   Definition: A positive response to at least 1 of the following 3 questions:
   a. Have you had daily, persistent, troublesome dry eyes for more than 3 months?
   b. Do you have a recurrent sensation of sand or gravel in the eyes?
   c. Do you use tear substitutes more than 3 times a day?
2. Oral symptoms
   Definition: A positive response to at least 1 of the following 3 questions:
   a. Have you had a daily feeling of dry mouth for more than 3 months?
   b. Have you had recurrent or persistently swollen salivary glands as an adult?
   c. Do you frequently drink liquids to aid in swallowing dry foods?
3. Ocular signs
   Definition: Objective evidence of ocular involvement, determined on the basis of a positive
   result on at least 1 of the following 2 tests:
   a. Schirmer I test (<5.5 mm after 5 minutes)
   b. Rose bengal score (>4 van Bijsterveld score)
4. Histopathologic features
   Definition: Focus score >1 on minor salivary gland biopsy (*focus* defined as a conglomeration of at
   least 50 mononuclear cells; *focus score* defined as the number of foci in 4 mm² of glandular tissue)
5. Salivary gland involvement
   Definition: Objective evidence of salivary gland involvement, determined on the basis of a
   positive result on at least 1 of the following 3 tests:
   a. Salivary scintigraphy: delayed uptake and/or secretion
   b. Parotid sialography: diffuse sialectasis without obstruction
   c. Unstimulated salivary flow (<1.5 mL in 15 minutes)
6. Autoantibodies
   Definition: Presence of at least 1 of the following serum autoantibodies:
   a. Antibodies to Ro/SS-A
   b. Antibodies to La/SS-B antigens
Exclusion criteria: Preexisting lymphoma, acquired immunodeficiency syndrome, sarcoidosis,
or chronic graft-vs-host disease, prior head and neck irradiation, hepatitis C, use of
anticholinergic medications
Primary Sjögren syndrome: Presence of 4 out of 6 items or presence of 3 of 4 objective criteria
(items 3–6)
Secondary Sjögren syndrome: A combination of a positive response to item 1 or 2 plus a positive
response to at least 2 items from among 3, 4, and 5

Modified with permission from Vitali C, Bombardieri S, Jonnson R, et al; European Study Group on
Classification Criteria for Sjögren's Syndrome. Classification criteria for Sjögren's syndrome: a revised
version of the European criteria proposed by the American-European Consensus Group. *Ann Rheum Dis.*
2002;61(6):557.

arthritis; however, many other autoimmune and systemic diseases are associated with secondary Sjögren syndrome (Table 3-6).

Evaporative Dry Eye

The symptoms in evaporative dry eye consist of burning, foreign-body sensation, redness of the eyelids and conjunctiva, and filmy vision that is worse in the morning. The clinical signs associated with evaporative disease are usually confined to the posterior eyelid margins, although patients may occasionally have associated seborrheic changes on the anterior eyelid margin. The posterior eyelid margins are often irregular and have prominent, telangiectatic blood vessels coursing from the posterior to anterior eyelid margins. The meibomian gland

---

Table 3-6 Systemic Diseases and Other Conditions Associated With Dry Eye

Autoimmune disorders
  Primary Sjögren syndrome
  Secondary Sjögren syndrome associated with
    Rheumatoid arthritis
    Systemic lupus erythematosus
    Progressive systemic sclerosis (scleroderma)
    Polymyositis and dermatomyositis
    Primary biliary cirrhosis
  Graft-vs-host disease
  Immune reactions after radiation to head and neck
Infiltrative processes
  Lymphoma
  Amyloidosis
  Hemochromatosis
  Sarcoidosis
Infectious processes
  HIV-diffuse infiltrative lymphadenopathy syndrome
  Trachoma
Neuropathic dysfunction
  Multiple sclerosis
  Cranial neuropathies (Bell palsy, vasculitis)
  Parkinson disease
  Alzheimer disease
Endocrine dysfunction
  Androgen deficiency
Miscellaneous
  Familial dysautonomia (Riley-Day syndrome)
  Congenital alacrima
  Anhidrotic ectodermal dysplasia
  Adie syndrome
  Shy-Drager syndrome (idiopathic autonomic dysfunction with orthostatic hypotension and
    multiple system atrophy)

---

orifices may pout or show metaplasia, with white material extending through the glandular orifice (Fig 3-12). They also may become posteriorly displaced on the eyelid margin. In active disease, meibomian secretions may be turbid, more viscous, or even cheesy.

As discussed, the primary abnormality in evaporative dry eye is meibomian gland dysfunction (MGD), which the International Workshop on Meibomian Gland Dysfunction has classified as high delivery (ie, hypersecretory) or low delivery. Low delivery is further divided into hyposecretory or obstructive. Obstructive MGD can be cicatricial (eg, trachoma, mucous membrane pemphigoid, or atopy), or noncicatricial (eg, seborrheic dermatitis, rosacea, or atopy). MGD is more common in people of Asian ethnicity than it is in whites.

Occasionally, a patient is symptomatic but lacks obvious clinical signs of meibomian gland disease. The meibomian glands appear normal; however, with mild compression, obstruction of the glands is detected. More forceful expression produces a thin filamentous secretion, which is due to narrowing of the distal portion of the ducts, near the orifice. This condition is believed to be a precursor to clinically apparent disease. Gland expression can be performed using a cotton swab or a commercially available handheld device.

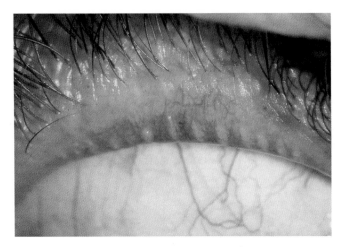

Figure 3-12   Meibomian gland dysfunction.

Extensive atrophy of the meibomian gland acini may develop after years of inflamma-tion from MGD, so that eyelid compression does not result in expression of meibomian gland secretions. Atrophy of meibomian gland acini and derangement of glandular ar-chitecture can be demonstrated by shortening or absence of the vertical lines of the mei-bomian glands, which may be revealed by transillumination of the everted eyelid using a muscle light or infrared photography (see Chapter 2).

Tear breakup is a functional measure of tear film stability. In MGD, the stability is disrupted, causing a rapid tear breakup time (TBUT). After a fluorescein strip moistened with sterile saline has been applied to the tarsal conjunctiva, the tear film is evaluated using a broad beam of the slit lamp with cobalt blue illumination. This should be done before any manipulation of the eyelids or instillation of other drops. Fluorescein-anesthetic com-bination drops are not recommended for this purpose, because excessive fluorescein is typically instilled and the anesthetic may affect the ocular surface. The time lapse between the last blink and the appearance of the first randomly distributed dry spot on the cornea is the TBUT. The appearance of dry spots in less than 10 seconds is considered abnormal.

Additional clinical findings in MGD include foam in the tear meniscus along the lower eyelid, bulbar and tarsal conjunctival injection, papillary reaction on the inferior tarsus, linear staining along the inferior cornea and inferior conjunctiva, episcleritis, marginal epithelial and subepithelial infiltrates, corneal neovascularization or pannus, and corneal scarring or thinning. Corneal vascularization is more typical of MGD, while punctate staining is more typical of staphylococcal blepharitis.

Patients with MGD frequently have acne rosacea. Rosacea is discussed later in this chapter.

American Academy of Ophthalmology Cornea/External Disease Panel. Preferred Practice Pattern Guidelines. *Blepharitis.* San Francisco: American Academy of Ophthalmology; 2013. Available at www.aao.org/ppp.

Foulks GN. Meibomian gland dysfunction. *Focal Points: Clinical Modules for Ophthalmologists.* San Francisco: American Academy of Ophthalmology; 2014, module 12.

Treatment of Dry Eye

Before treatment of dry eye is initiated, the eye should be carefully examined for conjunctivochalasis, floppy eyelid syndrome, superior limbic keratoconjunctivitis, nighttime lagophthalmos, and other structural and exogenous disorders that can cause symptoms similar to those of dry eye. In addition, the clinician must determine whether the patient has any associated systemic conditions (eg, Parkinson disease or mucous membrane pemphigoid) or uses medications that can contribute to dry eye, such as drugs with antihistaminic or anticholinergic properties (see "Medical management of aqueous tear deficiency").

ATD and evaporative dry eye frequently coexist. Certain therapeutic interventions, such as artificial tear supplements, topical cyclosporine, short pulses of topical corticosteroids, and omega-3 fatty acid supplements, are helpful for both conditions. However, certain treatments for ATD can exacerbate evaporative dry eye. For example, punctal occlusion in the presence of active MGD increases the retention of the toxic meibum secretions.

Medical management of aqueous tear deficiency

Selection of the treatment modalities for patients with ATD depends largely on the severity of their disease (Table 3-7). Since smoking is a risk factor for dry eye, advice should be given regarding cessation. It may also be appropriate to modify the patient's environment in an effort to reduce evaporation of the tear film; a humidifier and/or moisture shields on glasses can be helpful in severe cases.

Changing or discontinuing any topical or systemic medications that may contribute to the condition should be considered, although this is not always practical. Topical β-blockers have been associated with an increased incidence of dry eye, and many systemic

Table 3-7 Therapeutic Options for Aqueous Tear Deficiency

Severity of ATD	Therapeutic Options
Mild	Tear substitutes with preservatives up to 4× daily
	Lubricating ointment at bedtime
	Hot compresses and eyelid massage
Moderate	Tear substitutes without preservatives 4× daily to hourly
	Lubricating ointment at bedtime
	Topical anti-inflammatory treatment (cyclosporine A 0.05% 2× daily)
	Omega-3 supplement
	Reversible occlusion (plugs), lower puncta
	Systemic immunosuppression if ATD is associated with inflammatory connective tissue disease
Severe	All of the above, plus one or more of the following:
	Punctal occlusion (upper and lower puncta); consider permanent occlusion
	Autologous serum drops (20%) 4–6× daily
	Topical corticosteroids (nonpreserved if available) on a short-term basis
	Humidifier
	Moisture-retaining eyewear
	Tarsorrhaphy (lateral and/or medial)
	Bandage lenses (rarely)
	Scleral contact lens
	Systemic cholinergic agonist (eg, pilocarpine)

ATD = aqueous tear deficiency.

medications (diuretics, antihistamines, and anticholinergic and psychotropic drugs) decrease aqueous tear production and increase dry eye symptoms. These drugs should be avoided as much as possible in patients with symptoms of ATD (Table 3-8).

The mainstay of treatment for ATD is the use of tear substitutes (drops, gels, and ointments). Preservative-free tear substitutes are recommended to avoid the toxic effects that can arise with dosing more than 4 times daily. Demulcents are polymers added to artificial tear solutions to improve their lubricant properties. Demulcent solutions are

Table 3-8 Medications With Anticholinergic Side Effects That Decrease Tear Production

Antihypertensives
Clonidine
Diuretics, sometimes in combination with other antihypertensive drugs
Guanethidine, methyldopa
Prazosin
Propranolol
Reserpine

Antidepressants and psychotropic drugs
Amitriptyline, nortriptyline
Amoxapine, trimipramine
Clomipramine, desipramine, imipramine
Diazepam, nitrazepam
Doxepin
Phenelzine, tranylcypromine
Phenothiazines

Cardiac antiarrhythmia drugs
Amiodarone
Disopyramide
Mexiletine

Parkinson disease medications
Benztropine
Biperiden
Procyclidine
Trihexyphenidyl

Antiulcer agents
Atropine-like agents
Metoclopramide, other drugs that decrease gastric motility

Muscle spasm medications
Cyclobenzaprine
Methocarbamol

Decongestants (nonprescription cold remedies)
Ephedrine
Pseudoephedrine

Antihistamines

Anesthetics
Bisphosphonates
Enflurane
Halothane
Nitrous oxide

Hormonal: estrogen replacement, androgen antagonists

mucomimetic agents that can briefly substitute for glycoproteins lost late in the disease process. Demulcents alone, however, cannot restore lost glycoproteins or conjunctival goblet cells, reduce corneal cell desquamation, or decrease tear film osmolarity. Until relatively recently, all demulcent solutions contained preservatives. Preservative-free demulcent solutions were introduced after it was recognized that preservatives increase corneal desquamation. The elimination of preservatives from traditional demulcent solutions has led to improved corneal barrier function in patients using these agents, and subsequent attempts have been made to improve function even further by adding various ions to the solutions. Liposomal sprays, applied to the closed eyelids by a sterile spray mechanism, may help support the tear film. Hydroxypropyl cellulose inserts are occasionally helpful for patients unable to frequently instill artificial tears.

Topical cyclosporine A 0.05% addresses the inflammatory component of moderate to severe ATD and is thus being used earlier in the disease course. Therapy is often initiated in combination with a short course of topical corticosteroids to provide an initial reduction in surface inflammation. Patients should be advised that it may take many months of consistent twice-daily use before they obtain symptomatic relief, which results from the anti-inflammatory benefits of cyclosporine.

Lifitegrast 5% eyedrops, used twice daily from unit-dose vials, was approved by the US Food and Drug Administration (FDA) in 2016 to treat the symptoms and signs of dry eye disease. Lifitegrast may inhibit the migration and activation of T-cells and the subsequent release of inflammatory cytokines by blocking the interaction of intercellular adhesion molecule-1 and lymphocyte function-associated antigen-1. Patients generally know within a few weeks whether this treatment will be beneficial. Lifitegrast can cause mild irritation, transient blurred vision, and altered taste perception. Contact lenses should not be inserted for at least 15 minutes after eyedrop instillation.

Other treatments that have been successful in patients with severe ATD are dilute solutions of hyaluronic acid and autologous serum drops. Autologous serum drops require blood draws of 3 or 4 red-top tubes. The tubes are spun to separate the serum; they are then placed on dry ice and sent to a compounding pharmacy, which prepares the solution for the patient. Besides its use in the treatment of ATD, autologous serum may be helpful for patients with persistent epithelial defects and neurotrophic keratopathy.

Treatment of filamentary keratopathy associated with severe ATD can be challenging. Filaments should be debrided with a jeweler's forceps or a cotton swab soaked with topical anesthetic. Treatment directed at enhancing the tear film reduces the severity of recurrence. In addition to tear supplementation and punctal occlusion, acetylcysteine 10%, dispensed with an eyedrop container, can serve as a mucolytic agent and may further reduce filament formation. Topical low-dose corticosteroids, cyclosporine, and therapeutic soft contact lenses may be helpful. While therapeutic soft contact lenses may be beneficial for treatment of filamentary keratitis due to other causes, bandage soft contact lenses are rarely used to reduce symptoms in patients with ATD, because they may be associated with an increased risk of infection. Patients who use them should therefore be observed carefully. Scleral contact lenses have been found to be extremely helpful in patients with advanced dry eye symptoms.

In severe cases of ATD, use of moisture-retaining eyewear, also called moisture chamber glasses (glasses, goggles, or sunglasses incorporating a moisture shield or seal), can decrease tear evaporation; however, all but the most severely affected patients may find this therapy cosmetically objectionable.

Pharmacologic stimulation of tear secretion has been attempted using many compounds, with varying degrees of success. The cholinergic agonists pilocarpine and cevimeline hydrochloride stimulate muscarinic receptors present in salivary and lacrimal glands, thereby increasing secretion. Although studies have shown the 2 agents to be effective in treating both xerostomia and dry eye in patients with Sjögren syndrome, they are approved by the FDA only for the treatment of xerostomia. It is uncertain whether these agents provide long-term benefits, and they are associated with significant adverse effects, which may affect patient adherence.

Dietary supplementation with omega-3 fatty acids has been shown to increase average tear production and tear volume. Certain fish (eg, salmon, tuna, cod, flounder) and crustaceans (shrimp and crab), flaxseed oil, dark leafy greens, and walnuts are rich in omega-3 fatty acids, which block proinflammatory eicosanoids and cytokines. Commercial preparations of omega-3 fatty acids are also available and include TheraTears Eye Nutrition (Akorn Consumer Health, Lake Forest, IL), Dry Eye Omega Benefits (PRN Physician Recommended Nutriceuticals, Plymouth Meeting, PA), HydroEye (ScienceBased Health, Houston, TX), and Systane Vitamin (Alcon, Fort Worth, TX).

Epitropoulos AT, Donnenfeld ED, Shah ZA, et al. Effect of oral re-esterified omega-3 nutritional supplementation on dry eyes. *Cornea.* 2016;35(9):1185–1191.

Kojima T, Higuchi A, Goto E, Matsumoto Y, Dogru M, Tsubota K. Autologous serum eye drops for the treatment of dry eye diseases. *Cornea.* 2008;27(Suppl 1):S25–S30.

Wojtowicz JC, Butovich I, Uchiyama E, Aronowicz J, Agee S, McCulley JP. Pilot, prospective, randomized, double-masked, placebo-controlled clinical trial of an omega-3 supplement for dry eye. *Cornea.* 2011;30(3):308–314.

Surgical management of aqueous tear deficiency

Surgical treatment is generally reserved for patients with severe disease for whom medical treatment is either inadequate or impractical. Patients with moderate to severe ATD may benefit from punctal occlusion, which can be temporary, semipermanent, or permanent. Reversible punctal occlusion can be performed using collagen implants or silicone punctal plugs and has varying degrees of effectiveness (Fig 3-13). Collagen plugs usually dissolve within days and do not provide complete canalicular occlusion. Intracanalicular plugs made of polydioxanone (eg, VisiPlug; Lacrimedics Inc, Eastsound, WA) provide occlusion for up to 6 months. These plugs can be seen by transilluminating the eyelid, enabling the clinician to determine whether they have become displaced or eroded. The Extend plug, another absorbable implant (Beaver-Visitec International, Waltham, MA), dissolves over a 3-month period. Permanent intracanalicular plugs have been associated with infectious canaliculitis and sterile inflammation, which in some cases have required canaliculotomy and dacryocystorhinostomy. The absorbable intracanalicular plugs may be less likely to cause such problems; however, clinicians should be aware of the risk of intracanalicular inflammation.

Silicone plugs may remain in place for months or years unless they are inadequately sized or are manually displaced. For example, Parasol plugs (Beaver-Visitec International) have a high retention rate. Some plugs have a small hole bored through the center to

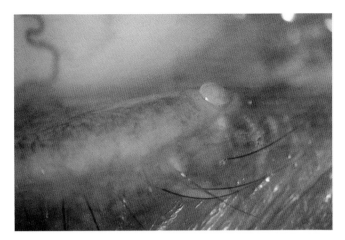

Figure 3-13 Silicone punctal plug. *(Courtesy of Robert W. Weisenthal, MD.)*

reduce the likelihood of epiphora. Most silicone plugs are continuously visible at the slit lamp, making it obvious if they become displaced or eroded.

If inserted too forcefully, punctal plugs can be inadvertently inserted into the canaliculus and may require surgical removal. If a plug protrudes from the punctum, conjunctival irritation or abrasion may occur. Granuloma formation at the punctal opening has been seen and may require removal of the plug and possible excision.

The most cost-effective manner of performing irreversible punctal occlusion is with a disposable cautery, a hyfrecator, or a radiofrequency probe. Although the procedure is usually permanent, the canaliculi and puncta may subsequently recanalize.

The value of punctal occlusion for ocular surface disease other than tear deficiency is unproven. The procedure is recommended primarily for patients who have minimal basal tear secretion and punctate keratopathy but no significant ocular surface inflammation or infection. Correction of eyelid malpositions such as entropion and ectropion may also be beneficial in managing patients with dry eye symptoms. Reduction of the palpebral aperture by means of lateral and/or medial tarsorrhaphy can be performed in severe KCS when more conservative measures have failed. However, lateral tarsorrhaphy may limit the temporal visual field and produce an undesirable cosmetic deformity.

American Academy of Ophthalmology Cornea/External Disease Panel. Preferred Practice Pattern Guidelines. *Dry Eye Syndrome.* San Francisco: American Academy of Ophthalmology; 2013. Available at www.aao.org/ppp.

The definition and classification of dry eye disease: report of the Definition and Classification Subcommittee of the International Dry Eye WorkShop. *Ocul Surf.* 2007;5(2):75–92.

Marcet MM, Shtein RM, Bradley EA. Safety and efficacy of lacrimal drainage system plugs for dry eye syndrome: a report by the American Academy of Ophthalmology. *Ophthalmology.* 2015;122(8):1681–1687.

Mazow ML, McCall T, Prager TC. Lodged intracanalicular plugs as a cause of lacrimal obstruction. *Ophthal Plast Reconstr Surg.* 2007;23(2):138–142.

Stevenson W, Chauhan SK, Dana R. Dry eye disease: an immune-mediated ocular surface disorder. *Arch Ophthalmol.* 2012;130(1):90–100.

Medical management of evaporative dry eye

Management is based on the stage of MGD; see Tables 3-9 and 3-10. Eyelid hygiene is the mainstay of treatment. Application of warm compresses to the eyelids twice daily for 3–5 minutes liquefies thickened meibomian gland secretions and softens adherent crusts on the eyelid margins. The patient should be warned to avoid excessive or uneven heat

Table 3-9 Clinical Summary of the MGD Staging Used to Guide Treatment

Stage	MGD Grade	Symptoms	Corneal Staining
1	+ (minimally altered expressibility and secretion quality)	None	None
2	++ (mildly altered expressibility and secretion quality)	Minimal to mild	None to limited
3	+++ (moderately altered expressibility and secretion quality)	Moderate	Mild to moderate; mainly peripheral
4	++++ (severely altered expressibility and secretion quality)	Marked	Marked; central in addition
"Plus" disease	Coexisting or accompanying disorders of the ocular surface and/or eyelids		

Reproduced with permission from Nichols KK, Foulks GN, Bron AJ, et al. The International Workshop on Meibomian Gland Dysfunction: Executive Summary. *Invest Ophthalmol Vis Sci.* 2011;52(4):1922–1929.

Table 3-10 Treatment Algorithm for Meibomian Gland Dysfunction

Stage	Clinical Description	Treatment
1	No *symptoms* of ocular discomfort, itching, or photophobia *Clinical signs* of MGD based on gland expression • Minimally altered secretions: grade ≥2 to 4 • Expressibility: 1 • No ocular surface *staining*	*Inform* patient about MGD, the potential impact of diet, the effect of work/home environments on tear evaporation, and the possible drying effect of certain systemic medications *Consider* eyelid hygiene, including warming/expression as described below (±)
2	Minimal to mild *symptoms* of ocular discomfort, itching, or photophobia Minimal to mild MGD *clinical signs* • Scattered eyelid margin features • Mildly altered secretions: grade ≥4 to <8 • Expressibility: 1 • None to limited ocular surface *staining*: DEWS grade 0–7; Oxford grade 0–3*	*Advise* patient on improving ambient humidity, optimizing workstations, and increasing dietary omega-3 fatty acid intake (±) *Institute* eyelid hygiene with eyelid warming (a minimum of 4 minutes, once or twice daily) followed by moderate to firm massage and expression of MG secretions (+) *All the above, plus* (±) • Artificial lubricants (for frequent use, nonpreserved preferred) • Topical azithromycin • Topical emollient lubricant or liposomal spray • Consider oral tetracycline derivatives

Table 3-10 *(continued)*

Stage	Clinical Description	Treatment
3	Moderate *symptoms* of ocular discomfort, itching, or photophobia with limitation of activities Moderate MGD *clinical signs* • ↑ Eyelid margin features: plugging, vascularity • Moderately altered secretions: grade ≥8 to <13 • Expressibility: 2 • Mild to moderate conjunctival and peripheral corneal *staining,* often inferior: DEWS grade 8–23; Oxford grade 4–10	*All the above, plus* • Oral tetracycline derivatives (+) • Lubricant ointment at bedtime (±) • Anti-inflammatory therapy for dry eye as indicated (±)
4	Marked *symptoms* of ocular discomfort, itching, or photophobia with definite limitation of activities Severe MGD *clinical signs* • ↑ Eyelid margin features: dropout, displacement • Severely altered secretions: grade ≥13 • Expressibility: 3 • Increased conjunctival and corneal *staining,* including central staining: DEWS grade 24–33; Oxford grade 11–15 • ↑ Signs of inflammation: ≥moderate conjunctival hyperemia, phlyctenules	*All the above, plus* • Anti-inflammatory therapy for dry eye (+)
"Plus" disease	Specific conditions occurring at any stage and requiring treatment. May be causal of, or secondary to, MGD or may occur incidentally 1. Exacerbated inflammatory ocular surface disease 2. Mucosal keratinization 3. Phlyctenular keratitis 4. Trichiasis (eg, in cicatricial conjunctivitis, mucous membrane pemphigoid) 5. Chalazion 6. Anterior blepharitis 7. *Demodex*-related anterior blepharitis, with cylindrical dandruff	1. Pulsed soft steroid as indicated 2. Bandage contact lens/scleral contact lens 3. Steroid therapy 4. Epilation, electrolysis using radiofrequency 5. Intralesional steroid or excision 6. Topical antibiotic or antibiotic/steroid 7. Tea tree oil scrubs

DEWS = Dry Eye Workshop; MG = meibomian gland; MGD = meibomian gland dysfunction.
Meibum quality is assessed in each of eight glands of the central third of the lower eyelid on a scale of 0 to 3 for each gland: 0, clear; 1, cloudy; 2, cloudy with debris (granular); and 3, thick, like toothpaste (total score range, 0–24). *Expressibility* is assessed on a scale of 0 to 3 in five glands in the lower or upper eyelid, according to the number of glands expressible: 0, all glands; 1, three to four glands; 2, one to two glands; and 3, no glands. *Staining scores* are obtained by summing the scores of the exposed cornea and conjunctiva. Oxford staining score range, 1–15; DEWS staining score range, 0–33.
*Oxford grade: see Anthony.bron@eye.ex.ac.uk.

Modified with permission from Nichols KK, Foulks GN, Bron AJ, et al. The International Workshop on Meibomian Gland Dysfunction: Executive Summary. *Invest Ophthalmol Vis Sci.* 2011;52(4):1922–1929.

if a microwave is used for the compress. The application of heat should be followed by moderate to firm massage of the eyelids to express retained meibomian secretions. Eyelid massage can be followed by cleansing of the closed eyelid margin with a clean wash-cloth or a commercially available pad. A solution prepared with a nonirritating shampoo and water or a commercially available solution designed for this purpose may facilitate cleansing.

Short-term or periodic use of topical antibiotics reduces the bacterial load on the eyelid margin. Topical azithromycin ophthalmic solution may be particularly efficacious, as it is a lipophilic antibiotic that reduces the production of bacterial lipases and improves the composition of meibomian lipids. The high viscosity of the drop prolongs the contact time and aids its penetration into the glands. Long-term use of topical antibiotics or sub-therapeutic dosing can result in the development of resistant organisms.

Topical corticosteroids may be required for short periods in cases with moderate to severe inflammation, particularly if corneal infiltrates and vascularization are present. Patients treated with topical corticosteroids should be warned about the potential complications associated with long-term use.

Patients with blepharitis and obstructive MGD benefit from dietary changes and omega-3 supplementation. In one study, the use of 1000-mg omega-3 nutritional supplements 3 times a day for 1 year was found to improve symptoms, tear film stability, and meibomian secretions. In another study, supplementation with fish oil showed no significant effect on meibum lipid composition or aqueous tear evaporation rate, but average tear production and tear volume increased. Therefore, the mechanism of action of omega-3 supplementation for MGD is not yet established.

Treatment with oral tetracyclines can be very effective; however, patients with MGD should be informed that therapy may only control their condition, not eliminate it. Because tetracycline must be taken on an empty stomach and requires more frequent dosing, doxycycline and minocycline are increasingly used. The dosages for doxycycline and minocycline are 100 mg and 50 mg, respectively, every 12 hours for 1–2 weeks; the dose for each drug is tapered to 50 mg daily. Even lower doses may be equally effective. Therapy must often be repeated to achieve long-term control. If long-term therapy is required, a 1-week structured treatment interruption each month may reduce the risk of yeast infection. Erythromycin can be used as alternative therapy in children or in patients with known hypersensitivity to tetracycline.

Adverse effects of oral tetracyclines include photosensitization, gastrointestinal upset, and, in rare instances, azotemia. Long-term use may lead to oral or vaginal candidiasis in susceptible patients. The use of tetracyclines is contraindicated during pregnancy, in women who are breastfeeding, and in patients with a known hypersensitivity to these agents. These agents should be used with caution in women of childbearing age, women with a family history of breast cancer, and patients with a history of liver disease. Oral tetracyclines can also potentiate the effect of certain anticoagulants (eg, warfarin). In addition, these antibiotics should be avoided in children younger than 8 years because they cause permanent discoloration of teeth and bones in this population. Tetracyclines may reduce the efficacy of oral contraceptives. Oral azithromycin is an alternative treatment, but it may be hazardous when used in patients with cardiovascular problems. In March 2013, the FDA issued a warning that oral azithromycin may lead to abnormalities in the electrical activity of the heart, with the potential to create serious irregularities in heart rhythm.

Recently, several new modalities have been introduced for the treatment of MGD. Mechanical meibomian gland probing using special instruments (Maskin Meibomian Gland Intraductal Probe; Rhein Medical Inc, St Petersburg, FL) lyses a fibrovascular membrane growing into the duct and may facilitate gland function, permitting normal secretion of meibum. The LipiFlow thermal pulsation system (TearScience, Morrisville, NC), which combines gentle pulsatile pressure and thermal energy to increase blood flow to the eyelid and open obstructed meibomian gland ductules, may be an appropriate alternative when conventional treatment has failed to improve symptoms. Variable improvement in dry eye symptoms has been achieved with this treatment modality; however, it is expensive and may need to be repeated. Adverse effects of LipiFlow, which are self-limited, include conjunctival hyperemia, edema, hemorrhage, and surface staining. The safety and efficacy of LipiFlow have not been established in moderate to severe allergic or vernal conjunctivitis, in the presence of severe eyelid inflammation, or for dry eye related to systemic disease. LipiFlow should not be used in the presence of active infection, postoperatively, or in the presence of functional abnormalities of the eyelid. The MiBoFlo Thermoflo (Mibo Medical Group, Dallas, TX) utilizes a thermoelectric heat pump to promote liquefaction of meibum; the device is applied to the eyelid skin manually, supplying continuous heat. Intense pulsed-light (IPL) therapy (Lumenis, San Jose, CA), a concentrated heat treatment, may also be used to treat MGD. The efficacy of these treatments has not been proven in well-designed, prospective, randomized, controlled studies.

American Academy of Ophthalmology Cornea/External Disease Panel. Preferred Practice Pattern Guidelines. *Blepharitis.* San Francisco: American Academy of Ophthalmology; 2013. Available at www.aao.org/ppp.

Foulks GN, Lemp MA. Meibomian gland dysfunction and seborrhea. In: Mannis MJ, Holland EJ, eds. *Cornea.* Vol 1. 4th ed. Philadelphia: Elsevier; 2017:357–365.

Macsai MS. The role of omega-3 dietary supplementation in blepharitis and meibomian gland dysfunction. *Trans Am Ophthalmol Soc.* 2008;106:336–356.

Eyelid Diseases Associated With Ocular Surface Disease

Rosacea

PATHOGENESIS Rosacea (sometimes called *acne rosacea*) is a chronic dermatological disease that can affect both the skin and the eyes. It has no proven cause, but bacteria associated with *Demodex* mites have been implicated. The condition may be related to the overexpression of cathelicidin. Cathelicidins, cationic peptides with antimicrobial activity, contribute to neutrophil recruitment, angiogenesis, and cytokine release, which may play a role in the inflammatory skin changes seen in patients with rosacea. Rosacea is associated with cutaneous sebaceous gland dysfunction of the face, neck, and shoulders. Although rosacea has generally been thought to be more common in fair-skinned individuals, it may simply be more difficult to diagnose in patients with dark skin. It is important to look for the sometimes subtle clinical findings by external examination in a brightly lit room.

Although alcohol consumption can contribute to a worsening of this disorder because of its effect on vasomotor stability, most patients with rosacea do not have a history of excessive alcohol intake. In some patients, exacerbation can be triggered by emotional stress, ingestion of hot or spicy foods, or a hot or cold environment.

CLINICAL PRESENTATION Rosacea frequently involves the eyes. It affects individuals aged 30–60 years most commonly and women slightly more often than men, although ocular rosacea can occur in young patients and is often underdiagnosed. Rosacea is characterized by excessive sebum secretion with frequently recalcitrant chronic blepharitis. Eyelid margin telangiectasia is very common, and the often-associated meibomian gland distortion, disruption, and dysfunction can lead to recurrent chalazia. The ocular condition can progress, leading to chronic conjunctivitis, severe stromal keratitis (Fig 3-14), marginal keratitis (Fig 3-15A), sterile ulceration, episcleritis, or iridocyclitis. If properly treated, these lesions can resolve with few sequelae. Repeated bouts of ocular surface inflammation can cause corneal neovascularization and scarring (Fig 3-15B).

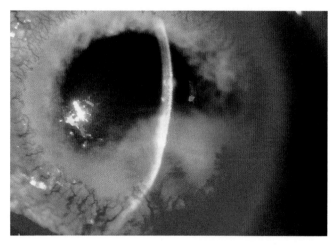

Figure 3-14 Stromal keratitis associated with rosacea.

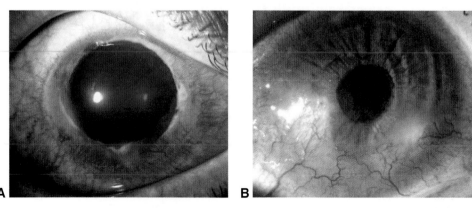

Figure 3-15 A, Rosacea-associated marginal keratitis with possible episcleritis. B, Corneal neovascularization and scarring associated with rosacea. *(Courtesy of Mark Mannis, MD.)*

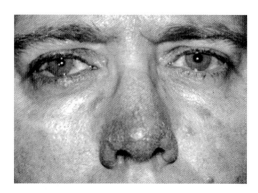

Figure 3-16 Facial characteristics of moderate acne rosacea, including facial erythema, papules, and rhinophyma. *(Courtesy of Robert S. Feder, MD.)*

Facial lesions consist of telangiectasias, recurrent papules and pustules, and midfacial erythema (Fig 3-16). Rosacea is characterized by a malar rash with unpredictable flushing episodes. Rhinophyma, thickening of the skin and connective tissue of the nose, is a characteristic and obvious sign associated with this disorder, but such hypertrophic cutaneous changes occur relatively late in the disease process.

MANAGEMENT The ocular and systemic diseases are managed simultaneously, and oral tetracyclines are the mainstay of therapy. Tetracyclines have anti-inflammatory properties that include suppression of leukocyte migration, reduced production of nitric oxide and reactive oxygen species, inhibition of matrix metalloproteinases, and inhibition of phospholipase A2. In addition, tetracyclines may reduce irritative free fatty acids and diglycerides by suppressing bacterial lipases. Erythromycin or azithromycin may be used when tetracyclines are not appropriate. Oral azithromycin should not be used in patients prone to cardiac arrhythmia.

With time, oral therapy with doxycycline or minocycline can be tapered. In addition to oral therapy, topical therapy with metronidazole gel 0.75%, metronidazole cream 1%, or azelaic acid gel 15% applied to the affected facial areas can significantly reduce facial erythema. Azelaic acid 15%, the only gel approved by the FDA for the treatment of papulopustular rosacea, is thought to suppress rosacea through anti-inflammatory and antimicrobial mechanisms.

Ulcerative keratitis in rosacea can be associated with infection or due to a sterile inflammatory response. Once it is ascertained that ulceration is noninfectious, topical corticosteroids, used judiciously, can play a significant role in reducing sterile inflammation and enhancing epithelialization of the cornea. In advanced cases with scarring and neovascularization, conservative therapy is generally recommended. Penetrating keratoplasty is a high-risk procedure in the rosacea patient, and the prognosis may be poor, particularly if the ocular surface is severely compromised.

Intense pulsed-light therapy may help reduce eyelid erythema as well as symptoms related to meibomian gland dysfunction. See "Medical management of evaporative dry eye," earlier in the chapter.

National Rosacea Society website. Available at www.rosacea.org. Accessed February 3, 2017.

Schittek B, Paulmann M, Senyürek I, Steffen H. The role of antimicrobial peptides in human skin and in skin infectious diseases. *Infect Disord Drug Targets.* 2008;8(3):135–143.

Seborrheic Blepharitis

CLINICAL PRESENTATION Seborrheic blepharitis may occur alone or in combination with staphylococcal blepharitis, MGD, or seborrheic dermatitis. Inflammation occurs primarily at the anterior eyelid margin; a variable amount of scaling or scurf (Fig 3-17), typically of an oily or greasy consistency, may be found on the eyelids, eyelashes, eyebrows, and scalp. Patients with seborrheic blepharitis often have increased meibomian gland secretions that appear turbid when expressed. Additional signs and symptoms include chronic eyelid redness, burning, and, occasionally, foreign-body sensation. In a small percentage of patients (approximately 15%), an associated keratitis or conjunctivitis develops. The keratitis is characterized by punctate epithelial erosions distributed over the inferior one-third of the cornea. Approximately one-third of patients with seborrheic blepharitis have evaporative dry eye. See Table 3-11 for additional information on seborrheic and other types of blepharitis.

MANAGEMENT Eyelid hygiene (discussed elsewhere in this chapter) is the primary treatment for seborrheic blepharitis as well as the associated MGD or staphylococcal blepharitis. Concurrent treatment of the scalp disease with selenium sulfide shampoos is recommended.

Demodicosis should be considered in patients who do not improve with traditional blepharitis treatments. Eyelash sleeves are typically seen (Fig 3-18A; also see Fig 3-17). In a recent small case series, improvement in symptoms and signs was seen when weekly 50% tea tree oil eyelid scrubs and daily tea tree oil shampoo scrubs were used for a minimum of 6 weeks in a group of patients who had not improved with eyelid hygiene and concurrent scalp treatment. Oral ivermectin has also been reported to be of benefit in some cases of recalcitrant *Demodex* blepharitis.

Staphylococcal Blepharitis

PATHOGENESIS In general, the term *staphylococcal blepharitis* (caused usually by *Staphylococcus aureus* but occasionally by other species) refers to cases in which bacterial infection of the eyelids (and frequently the conjunctiva) is predominant. MGD and seborrheic

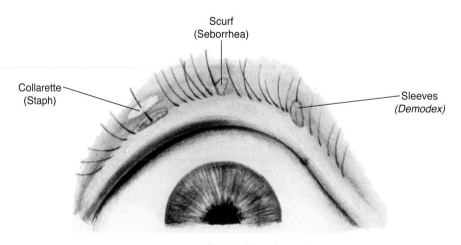

Figure 3-17 Blepharitis schematic.

Table 3-11 Types of Blepharitis

	Staphylococcal	Meibomian Gland Dysfunction	Seborrheic
Location	Anterior eyelid margin	Posterior eyelid margin	Anterior eyelid margin
Loss and whitening of eyelashes	Varying degrees	(−)	Rare
Eyelid crusting	Hard, fibrinous scales; hard, matted crusts (often accompany ulcerative form)	+/−	Oily or greasy
Eyelid ulceration	Occasional	(−)	(−)
Conjunctivitis	Papillary (occasionally with mucopurulent discharge)	Mild to moderate injection, papillary tarsal reaction	Mild injection, follicular or papillary tarsal reaction
Keratitis	Inferior PEE, marginal infiltrates, vascularization, phlyctenulosis	Inferior PEE, marginal infiltrates, vascular pannus	Inferior PEE
Rosacea	(−)	Common	Less common

PEE = punctate epithelial erosions.

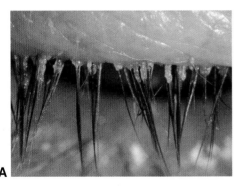 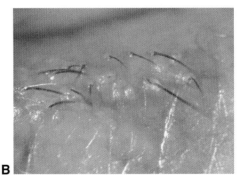

Figure 3-18 **A,** Eyelash sleeves typical of demodicosis. **B,** Staphylococcal blepharitis. *(Part A courtesy of Robert S. Feder, MD; part B courtesy of Robert W. Weisenthal, MD.)*

blepharitis, in contrast, are primarily inflammatory. Clinical features that may help in the differential diagnosis of these conditions are summarized in Table 3-11.

CLINICAL PRESENTATION Staphylococcal blepharitis is seen more commonly in younger individuals. Symptoms include burning, itching, foreign-body sensation, and crusting, particularly upon awakening. Symptoms of irritation and burning tend to peak in the morning and improve as the day progresses, presumably as the crusted material that accumulates on the eyelid margin overnight is liberated.

Typical clinical manifestations include hard, brittle fibrinous scales and hard, matted crusts surrounding individual cilia (collarettes) on the anterior eyelid margin (Fig 3-18B). Small ulcers of the anterior eyelid margin may be seen when the hard crusts are removed (see Fig 3-17). Injection and telangiectasis of the anterior and posterior eyelid margins, white lashes (poliosis), lash loss (madarosis), and trichiasis may be seen in varying degrees, depending on the severity and duration of the blepharitis.

Staphylococcal blepharoconjunctivitis may present as a chronic (>4-week duration) unilateral or bilateral conjunctivitis. Clinical findings include a papillary reaction of the tarsal conjunctiva, particularly the inferior tarsal conjunctiva near the eyelid margin, as well as injection of the bulbar and tarsal conjunctivae. Conjunctival injection is mild and mucopurulent discharge scant. Concomitant ATD and/or lipid-induced tear film instability may also occur. If unilateral signs or symptoms persist, the clinician should consider obstruction of the nasolacrimal system and perform a dye disappearance test or perhaps irrigation of the nasolacrimal system.

Specific clinical signs in patients with chronic conjunctivitis may implicate certain bacterial species. *Staphylococcus aureus* is often associated with matted, honey-colored crusts and ulcers on the anterior eyelid margin, inferior punctate keratopathy, marginal corneal infiltrates, and, in rare cases, conjunctival or corneal phlyctenules. *Moraxella lacunata* may cause a chronic angular blepharoconjunctivitis, with crusting and ulceration of the skin in the lateral canthal angle and a papillary or follicular reaction on the tarsal conjunctiva, sometimes with adjacent keratitis. *Moraxella* angular blepharoconjunctivitis is frequently associated with concomitant *S aureus* blepharoconjunctivitis.

Several forms of keratitis may develop in association with staphylococcal blepharoconjunctivitis. Punctate epithelial keratopathy manifests as erosions that stain with fluorescein; these erosions are often distributed across the inferior cornea, coinciding with the contour of the eyelids across the corneal surface. A diffuse pattern may also be observed, and asymmetric or unilateral keratopathy is not uncommon. The degree of corneal involvement can be markedly disproportionate to the severity of the eyelid disease, a circumstance that can lead to diagnostic confusion. Marginal corneal infiltrates may be the most distinctive clinical finding, with creamy white elliptical opacities typically separated from the limbus by a relatively lucent zone. They most often occur near the point of intersection of the eyelid margin and the limbus, that is, at 10, 2, 4 and 8 o'clock (Fig 3-19; also see Fig 3-15A).

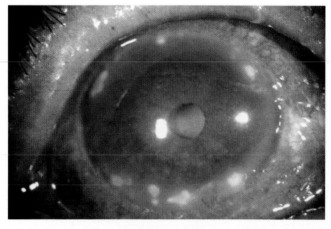

Figure 3-19 Staphyloccocal marginal corneal infiltrates are typically oval, white opacities; usually, there is a clear zone between the lesions and the limbus. *(Courtesy of David Rootman, MD.)*

Phlyctenulosis is a local corneal and/or conjunctival inflammation that is believed to represent a cell-mediated, or delayed, hypersensitivity response induced by microbial antigens such as the cell wall components of staphylococcus. Phlyctenulosis is frequently associated with *S aureus* in developed countries and is classically associated with *Mycobacterium tuberculosis* infection affecting malnourished children in tuberculosis-endemic areas of the world.

Phlyctenules are hyperemic, focal nodules consisting of chronic inflammatory cells. They often present unilaterally at or near the limbus, on the bulbar conjunctiva or cornea, as small, round, elevated, gray or yellow nodules accompanied by a zone of engorged hyperemic vessels (Fig 3-20A). Phlyctenules typically become necrotic and ulcerate centrally; they then spontaneously involute over a period of 2–3 weeks. Conjunctival phlyctenules do not lead to scarring, but residual wedge-shaped fibrovascular corneal scars form along the limbus; when such scars are bilateral and inferior, they may suggest previous phlyctenulosis. Corneal involvement is recurrent, and centripetal migration of successive inflammatory lesions may eventually occur, affecting vision if untreated (Fig 3-20B). Occasionally, such inflammation leads to corneal thinning and, in rare cases, perforation.

LABORATORY EVALUATION Eyelid and conjunctival cultures can be performed in suspected cases of staphylococcal blepharoconjunctivitis when the initial diagnosis is in doubt, the treatment response is poor, or the infection is worsening. An antibiotic washout period of at least a week should be employed prior to culture. In chronic unilateral conjunctivitis refractory to therapy, conjunctival malignancy (eg, sebaceous cell carcinoma) and factitious illness should be ruled out.

The characteristic laboratory finding in staphylococcal blepharoconjunctivitis is a heavy, confluent growth of *S aureus*. Nevertheless, the finding of a light to moderate growth of bacteria and/or the isolation of staphylococcal species other than *S aureus* does not exclude the diagnosis, particularly if a predominant manifestation of the disease is punctate epithelial keratopathy, marginal infiltrates, or phlyctenulosis. Susceptibility testing may be useful in guiding treatment in cases that have been refractory to empiric antibiotic therapy.

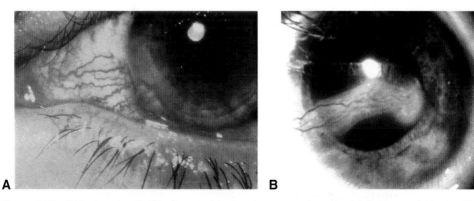

Figure 3-20 Phlyctenule. **A,** Confluent phlyctenules secondary to staphylococcal blepharitis. **B,** Recurrent phlyctenular involvement may result in fibrovascular scarring that progresses across the cornea and into the visual axis. *(Part B courtesy of Robert S. Feder, MD.)*

MANAGEMENT Effective treatment addresses both the infection and the associated inflammation. Eyelid hygiene, with either commercially available eyelid scrub kits or warm water mixed with baby shampoo, may help reduce bacterial colonization and the accumulation of sebaceous secretions. With these treatments, patients should focus their attention on the base of the lashes, where colonization and seborrhea are the greatest. Aggressive scrubbing should be discouraged. Topical bacitracin, erythromycin, azithromycin, or tobramycin may be applied to the eyelid margin to reduce both the bacterial load and associated inflammation. As stated earlier, ATD and/or lipid-induced tear film instability may occur concomitantly; these should be treated to improve patient comfort. Because many strains of bacteria have developed resistance to sulfa drugs, these antibiotics are less efficacious in the treatment of staphylococcal blepharitis.

In selected cases, anti-inflammatory therapy consists of limited use of mild doses of topical corticosteroids. Phlyctenulosis and staphylococcal marginal keratitis readily respond to judicious use of topical steroids used in concert with antibiotic therapy and eyelid hygiene. If epithelial defects are noted over the infiltrates, diagnostic cultures should be considered before corticosteroid treatment is begun. Long-term or indiscriminate use of corticosteroids should always be avoided.

Patients with routine staphylococcal blepharitis or blepharoconjunctivitis obtain more rapid symptomatic relief with adjunct topical corticosteroids; however, punctate epithelial keratopathy related to drug toxicity is unlikely to respond. The long-term use of topical corticosteroids should be weighed against the risk of adverse effects and, less likely, further proliferation of the pathogen.

Hordeola and Chalazia

CLINICAL PRESENTATION Hordeola present as painful, tender, red nodular masses near the eyelid margin (Fig 3-21). Those occurring on the anterior eyelid in the glands of Zeis or lash follicles are called *external hordeola,* or *styes.* Hordeola occurring on the posterior eyelid from meibomian gland inspissation are termed *internal hordeola.* Both types are associated with a localized purulent abscess, usually caused by *S aureus,* and may rupture, producing a purulent drainage. Hordeola are generally self-limited, improving spontaneously over the course of 1–2 weeks.

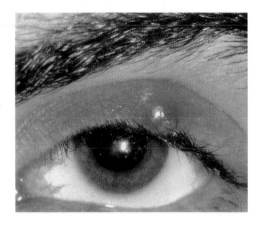

Figure 3-21 Hordeolum. *(Courtesy of Vincent P. deLuise, MD.)*

Internal hordeola occasionally evolve into chalazia, which are chronic lipogranulomatous nodules involving either the meibomian glands or the glands of Zeis. The lesion disappears in weeks to months, when the sebaceous contents drain either externally through the eyelid skin or internally through the tarsus or when the extruded lipid is phagocytosed and the granuloma dissipates. A small amount of scar tissue may remain. Occasionally, patients with a chalazion experience blurred vision secondary to astigmatism induced by its pressure on the globe. Basal cell, squamous cell, and sebaceous cell carcinoma can masquerade as chalazia or chronic blepharitis. The histologic examination of persistent, recurrent, or atypical chalazia is therefore important. Lash loss occurring over a chronic lesion is suggestive of malignancy.

MANAGEMENT Cultures are not indicated for isolated, uncomplicated cases of hordeolum or chalazion. Warm compresses can facilitate drainage. Topically applied antibiotics are generally not effective and, therefore, are not indicated unless an accompanying infectious blepharoconjunctivitis is present. Systemic antibiotics are generally indicated only in cases of secondary eyelid cellulitis. If the patient has a prominent and chronic accompanying meibomitis, oral doxycycline may be necessary.

If an internal hordeolum evolves into a chalazion that fails to respond to warm compresses and eyelid hygiene, intralesional injection of a corticosteroid (eg, 0.1–0.2 mL of triamcinolone 40 mg/mL), incision and curettage, or both may be necessary. In general, intralesional corticosteroid injection works best with small chalazia, chalazia on the eyelid margin, and multiple chalazia. Intralesional corticosteroid injection in patients with dark skin may lead to depigmentation of the overlying eyelid skin and thus should be used with caution. Oral doxycycline can be helpful for a patient with recurrent chalazia.

Large chalazia are best treated with surgical drainage and curettage. Internal chalazia require vertical incisions through the tarsal conjunctiva along the meibomian gland to facilitate drainage and avoid horizontal scarring of the tarsal plates. Surgical drainage usually requires perilesional anesthesia. A biopsy should be performed for recurrent chalazia to rule out meibomian gland carcinoma.

See also BCSC Section 7, *Orbit, Eyelids, and Lacrimal System,* for further discussion of chalazion.

CHAPTER 4

Structural and Exogenous Conditions Associated With Ocular Surface Disorders

Highlights

- Exposure keratopathy is common in patients with Parkinson syndrome, who exhibit poor blinking, and in patients after blepharoplasty, who show incomplete blinking.
- Patients with floppy eyelids should be examined for obstructive sleep apnea and keratoconus.
- Recurrent corneal erosion can usually be successfully treated with anterior stromal puncture or epithelial debridement.
- Patching followed by topical lubrication may be considered to reverse stromal thinning associated with dellen.

Exposure Keratopathy

PATHOGENESIS Exposure keratopathy can develop as a result of any disease associated with poor blinking or any process that limits eyelid closure. Lagophthalmos can be caused by the following:

- neurogenic disease such as seventh nerve palsy
- degenerative neurologic conditions such as Parkinson disease
- cicatricial or restrictive eyelid diseases such as ectropion
- drug abuse
- blepharoplasty
- skin disorders (eg, Stevens-Johnson syndrome, dermatomyositis, and xeroderma pigmentosum)
- proptosis (eg, due to thyroid eye disease or other inflammatory or infiltrative orbital disease)

CLINICAL PRESENTATION When corneal sensation is normal, the symptoms of exposure keratopathy are similar to those associated with dry eye, including foreign-body sensation and photophobia. Exposure keratopathy is characterized by punctate epithelial erosions that usually involve the inferior one-third of the cornea; however, the entire corneal surface can be involved in severe cases. Large, coalescent epithelial defects may result, which may in turn lead to infectious or sterile ulceration and perforation. The risk of a stromal melt is greater when exposure is associated with a neurotrophic or anesthetic cornea (see the section Neurotrophic Keratopathy and Persistent Corneal Epithelial Defects).

MANAGEMENT Therapy is similar to that for severe evaporative dry eye. In the earliest stages, nonpreserved artificial tears instilled during the day and ointment applied at bedtime may suffice. Taping the eyelid shut at bedtime can help if the exposure occurs mainly during sleep. Bandage contact lenses should be used with caution in patients with exposure keratopathy because of the risk of desiccation and infection. For cases in which the problem is likely to be temporary or self-limited, temporary tarsorrhaphy using tissue adhesive or sutures may be helpful. However, if the problem is likely to be long-standing, definitive surgical therapy to correct the exposure is recommended.

Most commonly, surgical management consists of permanent lateral and/or medial tarsorrhaphy (see Chapter 13). Insertion of gold or platinum weights into the upper eyelid is also an effective, more cosmetic approach to promote eyelid closure. Reported complications of gold weight implants include infection, implant malposition, extrusion, induced astigmatism, unacceptable ptosis, and noninfectious inflammatory response to the gold. The weights remain stable during magnetic resonance imaging. In addition, correction of any associated eyelid abnormalities, such as ectropion, entropion, and/or trichiasis, is indicated. For example, in cases of paralytic ectropion of the lower eyelid, a horizontal tightening procedure may also be beneficial.

See BCSC Section 7, *Orbit, Eyelids, and Lacrimal System,* for further discussion of thyroid eye disease, lagophthalmos, and proptosis.

Neurotrophic Keratopathy and Persistent Corneal Epithelial Defects

PATHOGENESIS There are a number of causes of neurotrophic keratopathy, one being damage to cranial nerve V, which results in corneal hypoesthesia or anesthesia (Table 4-1). Probably the most common cause of neurotrophic keratopathy is herpetic keratitis, which can be associated with persistent or recurrent corneal epithelial defects in the absence of replicating virus or active inflammation. A neurotrophic cornea can also occur after penetrating keratoplasty or deep anterior lamellar keratoplasty, in the early postoperative period.

Some medications used to treat ocular surface disease and glaucoma may impair epithelial wound healing, resulting in the formation of persistent corneal epithelial defects. The drugs most frequently implicated include topical anesthetics, topical nonsteroidal anti-inflammatory drugs (NSAIDs), trifluridine, β-blockers, carbonic anhydrase inhibitors, and, in sensitive individuals, all eyedrops containing the preservative benzalkonium chloride (BAK). Some authors refer to the condition as *toxic ulcerative keratopathy.* This clinical problem usually presents as a diffuse punctate keratopathy, and the cause

Table 4-1 Causes of Neurotrophic Keratopathy and Persistent Corneal Epithelial Defects

Aneurysms
Cerebrovascular accident
Damage to cranial nerve V (due to surgical trauma, large limbal incisions, corneal nerve damage after penetrating keratoplasty and LASIK)
Diabetes mellitus (types 1 and 2)
Familial dysautonomia (Riley-Day syndrome)
Herpes simplex keratitis
Herpes zoster keratitis
Leprosy (Hansen disease)
Multiple sclerosis
Topical medication toxicity (eg, anesthetics, β-blockers, carbonic anhydrase inhibitors, NSAIDs)
Tumors (acoustic neuroma, angioma, neurofibroma)

LASIK = laser in situ keratomileusis; NSAIDs = nonsteroidal anti-inflammatory drugs.

may be unrecognized by the ophthalmologist. In some instances, pericentral pseudodendritiform lesions and pseudogeographic defects may occur. These clinical findings are often misinterpreted as a worsening of the underlying disease and thus may lead to more frequent dosing of the offending medication.

In patients with diabetic retinopathy, persistent epithelial defects often occur following epithelial debridement in the course of vitreoretinal procedures. Diabetic neuropathy is thought to be a potential cause of neurotrophic keratopathy and nonhealing epithelial defects.

CLINICAL PRESENTATION Persistent corneal epithelial defects typically occur in the central or paracentral cornea and tend to be located inferiorly or inferonasally because of the protective effect of the Bell phenomenon on the superior cornea. The round or oval lesions frequently have elevated gray-white edges of "heaped-up" epithelium, which are associated with underlying stromal inflammation (Fig 4-1). Left untreated, persistent corneal epithelial defects can progress to vascularization and corneal opacification or corneal thinning and possible perforation. Secondary bacterial keratitis may also occur in this setting.

MANAGEMENT Management of neurotrophic keratopathy with or without persistent epithelial defect starts with eliminating or limiting the use of potentially aggravating topical medications to the degree possible. Frequent lubrication with nonpreserved drops, gels, or ointments is suggested. Autologous serum drops (20%), which contain growth factors and fibronectin, can be useful. In cases involving significant dry eye, temporary or permanent punctal occlusion can be effective in improving the volume and stability of the tear film and restoring the ocular surface.

Patching, low-water-content bandage lenses (soft, thin, highly oxygen-permeable lenses), or scleral contact lenses with a fluid-filled reservoir may facilitate reepithelialization or improve the keratopathy.

In cases associated with stromal melting, medications with specific activity against matrix metalloproteinases (MMPs), such as a tetracycline administered orally, may help

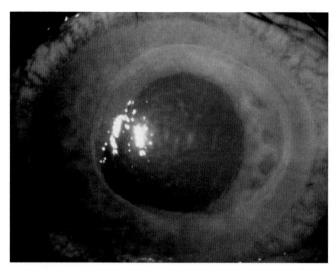

Figure 4-1 Neurotrophic ulcer. Ovoid corneal ulceration with typical "heaped-up" gray-white epithelial edges. *(Courtesy of Stephen Orlin, MD.)*

prevent or halt keratolysis. Corneal crosslinking performed early in the course of stromal ulceration has been reported to be useful in a small number of patients. Amniotic membrane transplantation has been reported to encourage healing of persistent epithelial erosions. Lateral and/or medial tarsorrhaphy may be required to prevent ocular surface desiccation. Tarsorrhaphy, which can be performed in a temporary or permanent manner, decreases the ocular surface area and tear film evaporation. Partial or total conjunctival flaps prevent corneal melting, but they should be used as a last resort. See Chapter 13 for further discussion of surgical management of ocular surface disorders.

Goins KM. New insights into the diagnosis and treatment of neurotrophic keratopathy. *Ocul Surf.* 2005;3(2):96–110.

Jeng BH. Use of autologous serum in the treatment of ocular surface disorders. *Arch Ophthalmol.* 2011;129(12):1610–1612.

Jeng BH. Persistent epithelial defects. *Focal Points: Clinical Practice Perspectives.* San Francisco: American Academy of Ophthalmology; 2016, module 9.

Floppy Eyelid Syndrome

Floppy eyelid syndrome is an ophthalmic disorder consisting of chronic ocular irritation and inflammation and characterized by a lax upper tarsus that everts with minimal upward force applied to the upper eyelid. The syndrome is most frequently seen in obese individuals, who often have obstructive sleep apnea. Clinical findings include small to large papillae on the upper palpebral conjunctiva, mucous discharge, and corneal involvement ranging from mild punctate epitheliopathy to superficial vascularization (Fig 4-2). Keratoconus has also been reported in patients with floppy eyelid syndrome. The problem may result from spontaneous eversion of the upper eyelid when it comes into contact

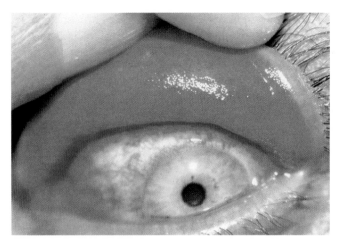

Figure 4-2 Floppy eyelid syndrome with a papillary response on the superior tarsus. *(Courtesy of Vincent P. deLuise, MD.)*

with the pillow or other bed linens during sleep. This may result in trauma to the upper tarsal conjunctiva, inducing inflammation and chronic irritation. The condition is most often bilateral but can be asymmetric or unilateral if the patient always sleeps on the same side. The differential diagnosis includes vernal conjunctivitis, giant papillary conjunctivitis, atopic keratoconjunctivitis, bacterial conjunctivitis, and toxic keratopathy. Treatment consists of covering the affected eye with a metal shield, taping the eyelids closed at night, or performing a surgical procedure to tighten the upper eyelid. See also BCSC Section 7, *Orbit, Eyelids, and Lacrimal System.*

Pham TT, Perry JD. Floppy eyelid syndrome. *Curr Opin Ophthalmol.* 2007;18(5):430–433.
Stern GA. Chronic conjunctivitis, Parts 1–2. *Focal Points: Clinical Modules for Ophthalmologists.* San Francisco: American Academy of Ophthalmology; 2012, modules 11–12.

Superior Limbic Keratoconjunctivitis

Superior limbic keratoconjunctivitis (SLK) is a chronic, recurrent inflammatory condition involving the superior tarsal and bulbar conjunctiva, as well as the superior limbus and superior cornea.

PATHOGENESIS The pathogenesis of SLK has not been established, but the condition is thought to result from mechanical trauma transmitted from the upper eyelid to the superior bulbar and tarsal conjunctiva. An association with autoimmune thyroid disease has been observed. In addition, SLK has been associated with graft-vs-host disease and has been seen following blepharoplasty.

CLINICAL PRESENTATION SLK is a chronic, recurrent condition characterized by ocular irritation and injection superiorly. It is most frequently seen in women between 20 and 70 years of age and may recur over a period of 1–10 years. Vision is not usually affected. SLK is often bilateral but can be asymmetric. The condition can be associated with aqueous tear deficiency (ATD) or blepharospasm. Ocular findings may include the following:

- a fine papillary reaction on the superior tarsal conjunctiva
- injection and thickening of the superior bulbar conjunctiva (Fig 4-3A)
- hypertrophy of the superior limbus
- fine punctate fluorescein, lissamine green, or rose bengal staining of the superior bulbar conjunctiva above the limbus with involvement of the superior cornea just below the limbus (Fig 4-3B)
- superior filamentary keratitis

This condition must be differentiated from contact lens–induced keratoconjunctivitis (CLK), which is in effect a focal limbal stem cell deficiency. Unlike in SLK, vision in CLK may be impaired by punctate keratopathy, which extends through the visual axis. Also, in CLK, filamentary keratitis does not typically occur, and contact lens wear is a cause, not a treatment.

LABORATORY EVALUATION Hyperproliferation, acanthosis, loss of goblet cells, and keratinization are seen in histologic sections of the superior bulbar conjunctiva. SLK can often be diagnosed clinically. However, scrapings or impression cytology of the superior bulbar conjunctiva showing characteristic features of nuclear pyknosis with "snake nuclei," increased epithelial cytoplasm–nucleus ratio, goblet cell loss, or keratinization may be helpful in the diagnosis of mild or confusing cases. Patients with SLK should undergo thyroid function tests, including free thyroxine (T_4), thyroid-stimulating hormone (TSH), and thyroid antibodies.

MANAGEMENT A variety of therapies have been reported to provide temporary or permanent relief of symptoms, but in general, medical treatment of SLK is less effective than surgical treatment. Medical treatment options include topical anti-inflammatory agents, topical cyclosporine, autologous serum eyedrops, and large-diameter bandage contact lenses. Surgical options include thermocauterization of the superior bulbar conjunctiva, resection of the superior limbal bulbar conjunctiva, amniotic membrane transplantation, and conjunctival fixation sutures.

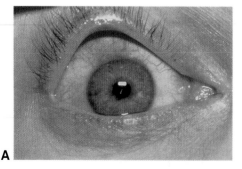
A

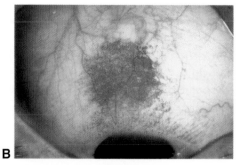
B

Figure 4-3 Superior limbic keratoconjunctivitis. **A,** Note the conjunctival injection, primarily superiorly. **B,** Rose bengal staining pattern in superior limbic keratoconjunctivitis. *(Courtesy of Vincent P. deLuise, MD.)*

Kim SK, Couriel DR, Ghosh S, Pflugfelder SC. Superior limbic keratoconjunctivitis in ocular graft vs. host disease. *Invest Ophthalmol Vis Sci.* 2005;46:2661.

Sahin A, Bozkurt B, Irkec M. Topical cyclosporine A in the treatment of superior limbic keratoconjunctivitis: a long-term follow-up. *Cornea.* 2008;27(2):193–195.

Sheu MC, Schoenfield L, Jeng BH. Development of superior limbic keratoconjunctivitis after upper eyelid blepharoplasty surgery: support for the mechanical theory of its pathogenesis. *Cornea.* 2007;26(4):490–492.

Stern GA. Chronic conjunctivitis, Parts 1–2. *Focal Points: Clinical Modules for Ophthalmologists.* San Francisco: American Academy of Ophthalmology; 2012, modules 11–12.

Theodore FH, Ferry AP. Superior limbic keratoconjunctivitis. Clinical and pathological correlations. *Arch Ophthalmol.* 1970;84(4):481–484.

Udell IJ, Kenyon KR, Sawa M, Dohlman CH. Treatment of superior limbic keratoconjunctivitis by thermocauterization of the superior bulbar conjunctiva. *Ophthalmology.* 1986; 93(2):162–166.

Yamada M, Hatou S, Mochizuki H. Conjunctival fixation sutures for refractory superior limbic keratoconjunctivitis. *Br J Ophthalmol.* 2009;93(12):1570–1571.

Conjunctivochalasis

Conjunctivochalasis is a term used to describe laxity or redundancy of the otherwise normal conjunctiva. The condition is typically seen in the inferior bulbar conjunctiva (Fig 4-4). The tissue may roll up on the eyelid margin or over the lacrimal punctum, in which case it may obstruct tear outflow.

PATHOGENESIS The pathogenesis has not been established but may be similar to that of SLK (see the section Superior Limbic Keratoconjunctivitis). Histologic studies have revealed elastosis and chronic nongranulomatous inflammation. In addition, collagenolysis may explain the conjunctival laxity.

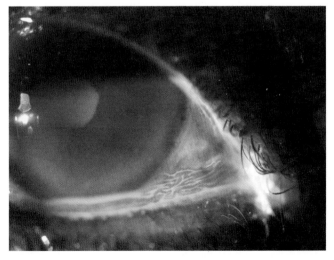

Figure 4-4 "Redundant" conjunctiva of conjunctivochalasis. *(Courtesy of Cornea Service, Paulista School of Medicine, Federal University of São Paulo.)*

CLINICAL PRESENTATION Patients typically present with chronic ocular irritation that does not respond to treatment with topical lubricants or topical corticosteroid. They may also present with epiphora. In addition to the conjunctival folds on the eyelid margin, punctate staining may be observed. This surface disruption is presumably caused by conjunctival tissue chafing against itself with movement of the eye. These patients may be predisposed to recurrent subconjunctival hemorrhages. A grading system has been proposed (see Meller and Tseng reference) that may help characterize the findings in this underrecognized condition.

MANAGEMENT It is reasonable to try topical lubricants, antihistamines, a short course of topical corticosteroid, or nocturnal patching. Cauterization of the redundant folds is sometimes effective. Alternatively, the clinician may consider excision of excess conjunctival tissue with primary closure to relieve the chronic ocular irritation and, in some cases, the epiphora. Tissue adhesive may facilitate wound closure without the need for sutures. Amniotic tissue grafting and conjunctival fixation are alternative surgical procedures. See Chapter 13 for further discussion of surgical management.

Meller D, Tseng SCG. Conjunctivochalasis: literature review and possible pathophysiology. *Surv Ophthalmol.* 1998;43(3):225–232.

Yamamoto Y, Yokoi N, Ogata M, et al. Correlation between recurrent subconjunctival hemorrhages and conjunctivochalasis by clinical profile and successful surgical outcome. *Eye Contact Lens.* 2015;41(6):367–372.

Recurrent Corneal Erosion

Recurrent erosions typically occur either in eyes that have suffered a sudden, sharp, abrading corneal injury (eg, from a fingernail, paper cut, tree branch), in patients with a history of herpetic keratitis, or in those with preexisting epithelial basement membrane dystrophy or other dystrophy involving the epithelial basement membrane complex. The superficial injury produces an epithelial abrasion that heals rapidly, frequently leaving no clinical evidence of damage. After an interval ranging from days to years, symptoms suddenly recur without any obvious precipitating event. Symptoms subside spontaneously in most cases, only to recur periodically. In contrast to shearing injuries, small, superficial lacerating injuries involving the cornea rarely result in recurrent erosions.

PATHOGENESIS Poor adhesion of the corneal epithelium is thought to be caused by underlying abnormalities in the epithelial basement membrane complex. The precise nature of these abnormalities has yet to be fully determined.

CLINICAL PRESENTATION Recurrent corneal erosions are characterized by the sudden onset of eye pain, usually during the night or upon first awakening, accompanied by redness, photophobia, and tearing. Individual episodes may vary in severity and duration. Minor episodes usually last from 30 minutes to several hours; typically, the cornea has an intact epithelial surface at the time of examination. More severe episodes may last for several days and are often associated with greater pain, eyelid edema, decreased vision, and extreme photophobia. Many patients seem to experience ocular discomfort that is out of proportion to the degree of observable pathology. However, slit-lamp examination using retroillumination frequently reveals subtle corneal abnormalities (eg, epithelial cysts). The corneal epithelium is loosely attached to the underlying basement membrane and Bowman layer, both at the time of a recurrent attack and between attacks, when the cornea appears to be entirely healed. During an acute attack, the epithelium in the involved area often appears heaped up and edematous. Although no frank epithelial defect may be present, significant pooling of fluorescein around the affected area is often visible.

A key to distinguishing between posttraumatic erosion and dystrophic erosion in a patient who has no clear-cut history of superficial trauma is careful examination of the contralateral eye following maximal pupillary dilation. Occasionally, subtle areas of loosely adherent corneal epithelium can be identified by applying gentle pressure with a surgical sponge following instillation of topical anesthetic. The presence of basement membrane changes in the *unaffected* eye implicates a primary basement membrane defect in the pathogenesis, whereas the absence of such findings suggests a posttraumatic etiology. Other clinical conditions with associated abnormalities of the epithelial basement membrane include diabetes mellitus and dystrophies of the stroma and Bowman layer (see also the discussion on corneal dystrophies in Chapter 7).

MANAGEMENT Traditional therapy for the acute phase of this condition consists of frequent lubrication or patching with antibiotic ointments and cycloplegia, followed by use of non-preserved lubricants or hypertonic saline solution (5% sodium chloride) during the day and ointment at bedtime for at least 6 weeks to facilitate epithelial attachment. Hypertonic agents provide lubrication and may transiently produce an osmotic gradient, drawing fluid from the epithelium and theoretically promoting the adherence of epithelial cells to the underlying tissue. Some patients find hypertonic medications unacceptably irritating, but many others do quite well with this therapy indefinitely. Low-dose oral doxycycline and short-term use of topical corticosteroids have been shown to be very efficacious. The mode of action is thought to be localized inhibition of MMPs.

Although use of a bandage contact lens may be helpful, proper patient education and judicious monitoring are crucial to a successful outcome. The ideal bandage lens fits without excessive movement and has high oxygen transmissibility (Dk). New-generation soft contact lenses with lens-surface treatments that decrease bacterial adherence may offer a better safety profile than older lens designs. Concomitant use of a topical broad-spectrum antibiotic 2–4 times daily may reduce the possibility of secondary infection but increase the risk of toxicity and bacterial resistance over the long term. Some cornea specialists prefer not to prescribe topical antibiotics for a patient using a bandage contact lens.

When consistent conservative management fails to control the symptoms, surgical therapy may be indicated. Surgical management of recurrent corneal erosion includes epithelial debridement and anterior stromal puncture. Some clinicians prefer to use debridement for central erosions or erosions related to corneal dystrophy, and stromal puncture in patients with posttraumatic recurrent erosions. An alternative to these procedures is excimer laser ablation either with phototherapeutic keratectomy (PTK) or photorefractive keratectomy (PRK). See Chapter 13 in this volume and BCSC Section 13, *Refractive Surgery*, for further discussion.

Ewald M, Hammersmith KM. Review of diagnosis and management of recurrent erosion syndrome. *Curr Opin Ophthalmol.* 2009;20(4):287–291.

Reidy JJ, Paulus MP, Gona S. Recurrent erosions of the cornea: epidemiology and treatment. *Cornea.* 2000;19(6):767–771.

Wang L, Tsang H, Coroneo M. Treatment of recurrent corneal erosion syndrome using the combination of oral doxycycline and topical corticosteroid. *Clin Experiment Ophthalmol.* 2008;36(1):8–12.

Wong VW, Chi SC, Lam DS. Diamond burr polishing for recurrent corneal erosions: results from a prospective randomized controlled trial. *Cornea.* 2009;28(2):152–156.

Trichiasis and Distichiasis

Trichiasis is an acquired condition in which eyelashes emerging from their normal anterior origin curve inward toward the cornea. It can be idiopathic or secondary to chronic inflammatory conditions such as mucous membrane pemphigoid, Stevens-Johnson syndrome, blepharitis, or chemical burns. Most cases are probably the result of subtle cicatricial entropion of the eyelid margin.

Distichiasis is a congenital (often autosomal dominant) or acquired condition in which an extra row of eyelashes emerges from the ducts of meibomian glands. These eyelashes can be fine and well tolerated or coarser and a threat to corneal integrity.

Aberrant eyelashes and poor eyelid position and movement should be corrected. Aberrant eyelashes may be removed by mechanical epilation, electrolysis with a radiofrequency probe, or cryotherapy. Mechanical epilation is temporary because the eyelashes normally grow back in as few as 3 weeks. Electrolysis works well for removing only a few eyelashes; however, it may be preferable in younger patients for cosmetic reasons. Cryotherapy is still a common treatment for aberrant eyelashes, but freezing can result in eyelid margin thinning, loss of skin pigmentation, loss of adjacent normal eyelashes, and persistent lanugo (hairs), which may continue to abrade the cornea. Treatment at –20°C should be limited to less than 30 seconds to minimize complications. The preferred surgical technique for aberrant eyelashes due to marginal cicatricial entropion is tarsotomy with eyelid margin rotation. See BCSC Section 7, *Orbit, Eyelids, and Lacrimal System*, for additional discussion of trichiasis and cicatricial entropion.

Woreta F, Muñoz B, Alemayehu W, West SK. Three-year outcomes of the Surgery for Trichiasis, Antibiotics to Prevent Recurrence trial. *Arch Ophthalmol.* 2012;130(4):427–431.

Factitious Ocular Surface Disorders

Factitious disorders include a spectrum of self-induced injuries with symptoms or physical findings. Factitious conjunctivitis usually shows evidence of mechanical injury to the inferior and nasal quadrants of the cornea and conjunctiva. The areas of involvement show sharply delineated borders. The conjunctival tissues usually show no evidence of inflammation on pathologic examination.

Mucus-Fishing Syndrome

Mucus-fishing syndrome is characterized by a well-circumscribed pattern of rose bengal or lissamine green staining on the nasal and inferior bulbar conjunctiva. All patients have a history of increased mucus production as a nonspecific response to ocular surface damage. The inciting event is typically keratoconjunctivitis sicca. Patients usually demonstrate vigorous eye rubbing and compulsive removal of strands of mucus from the fornix (mucus fishing). The resultant epithelial injury heightens the ocular surface irritation, which in turn stimulates additional mucus production, resulting in a vicious cycle.

Topical Anesthetic Abuse

Clinical application of topical anesthetics has become an integral part of the modern practice of ophthalmology. However, indiscriminate use of topical anesthetics can cause serious ocular surface toxicity and complications. Local anesthetics are known to inhibit epithelial cell migration and division. Loss of microvilli, reduction of desmosomes and other intercellular contacts, and swelling of mitochondria and lysosomes have been reported in ultrastructural studies. The characteristic clinical feature of anesthetic abuse is failure of the presenting condition, for example, corneal abrasion or keratitis, to respond to appropriate therapy.

Initially, a punctate keratopathy is seen. As the abuse continues, the eye becomes more injected and epithelial defects appear or take on a neurotrophic appearance. As the process continues, keratic precipitates and hypopyon develop, thus mimicking an infectious course. Diffuse stromal edema, dense stromal infiltrates, and a large ring opacity are common presenting signs (Fig 4-5). Stromal vascularization may occur in chronic abuse, and secondary infection may ensue. Because of the presence of corneal infiltrates and anterior segment inflammation, infectious keratitis and corneal scraping, culture, or biopsy should be considered.

The differential diagnosis includes bacterial, fungal, herpetic, and amebic keratitis. Suspicion of anesthetic abuse should be raised in any patient with negative culture results

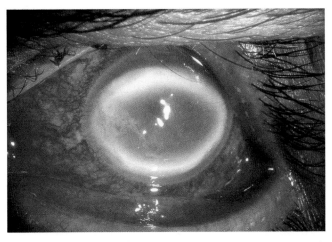

Figure 4-5 Topical anesthetic overuse with persistent corneal epithelial defect and necrotic ring opacity. *(Courtesy of Kirk R. Wilhelmus, MD.)*

who does not respond to appropriate therapy. A trial of patching in suspected cases, with the patch appropriately labeled to detect removal, may be therapeutic as well as diagnostic. Often, the condition is diagnosed only when the patient is discovered concealing the anesthetic drops. Once the diagnosis is made and the offending anesthetics are removed, corneal healing usually ensues. In advanced cases, permanent corneal scarring or perforation may occur. Psychiatric counseling is sometimes helpful. Health care workers and others with access to topical anesthetics may be more likely to abuse these agents.

Toxic Reactions to Topical Ophthalmic Medications

PATHOGENESIS Toxic ocular surface disease can occur as a complication of exposure to various substances (Table 4-2). Epithelial keratopathy secondary to use of topical ophthalmic medications can result in a dose-dependent cytotoxic effect on the ocular surface. One of the most toxic ingredients in these preparations is the preservative, usually BAK. The corneal and conjunctival epithelial cells absorb and retain preservatives, with residual amounts of preservative being detectable in the corneal epithelium days after a single application of a topical preserved medication.

CLINICAL PRESENTATION Punctate staining of the corneal or conjunctival epithelium, erosive changes, and subepithelial corneal infiltrates are all indicative of direct toxicity. Conjunctival injection, a follicular response, mild to severe papillary reaction, and mucopurulent discharge may be seen. Occasionally, the discharge may be copious and mimic bacterial conjunctivitis. Infrequently, a monocular reaction occurs despite the medication being applied to both eyes.

More severe cases of toxic keratitis can present with a diffuse punctate epitheliopathy, occasionally in a whorl pattern called *vortex* or *hurricane keratopathy*. The most severe cases may present with a corneal epithelial defect of the inferior or central cornea, stromal

Table 4-2 Toxic Reactions to Topical Ophthalmic Medications

Toxic Keratoconjunctivitis	Toxic Follicular Conjunctivitis
Aminoglycosides	Glaucoma medications
Gentamicin sulfate	*Miotics*
Neomycin	Carbachol
Tobramycin sulfate	Pilocarpine
Antiviral agents	*Adrenergic agonists*
Trifluridine (trifluorothymidine)	Apraclonidine HCl
Antineoplastic agent	Brimonidine tartrate
Mitomycin C	Dipivefrin
Topical anesthetics	Epinephrine
Proparacaine	Cycloplegics
Tetracaine	Atropine sulfate
Preservatives	Homatropine hydrobromide
Benzalkonium chloride	
Thimerosal	

HCl = hydrochloride.

opacification, and neovascularization and may be associated with extensive damage to the limbal stem cells. A sign of limbal stem cell deficiency is effacement of the palisades of Vogt, which can be seen with prolonged use of preserved topical medications or agents that block fibrin formation (eg, mitomycin C). Mitomycin C, even when used with care, has been associated with prolonged, irreversible stem cell damage with a resultant chronic keratopathy. Localized application of mitomycin (applied only to the surgical site) using a cellulose surgical sponge, as in trabeculectomy or pterygium excision, followed by copious irrigation is believed to reduce the risk of limbal stem cell damage and is, therefore, the preferred approach.

Toxic keratitis manifesting as peripheral corneal infiltrates in the epithelium and anterior stroma, with a clear zone between the lesions and the limbus, is typically associated with aminoglycoside antibiotics, antiviral agents, or medications preserved with BAK or thimerosal.

Chronic follicular conjunctivitis generally involves both the upper and the lower palpebral conjunctivae but is usually most prominent inferiorly. Bulbar follicles are uncommon but, when present, are highly suggestive of a toxic etiology (Fig 4-6). The medications most commonly associated with toxic follicular conjunctivitis include atropine, antiviral agents, miotics, sulfonamides, epinephrine (including dipivefrin), α-adrenergic agonists (eg, apraclonidine, brimonidine tartrate), and vasoconstrictors. Inferior punctate epithelial erosions may occasionally accompany toxic follicular conjunctivitis.

Contact lens solutions can also cause severe epithelial damage and pain when contact lenses soaked in cleaning or preservative-laden solutions are inadvertently placed in the eye without rinsing. The alkaline cleaning material or preservative (often thimerosal) can cause chemical injury of the cornea.

Asymptomatic subconjunctival fibrosis is sometimes associated with the long-term use of topical ophthalmic drugs (eg, miotics); however, in a small minority of affected patients, a more severe type of progressive subconjunctival scarring develops, which can lead to contraction of the conjunctival fornix, symblepharon formation, punctal stenosis, and corneal pannus formation. This entity is called *drug-induced cicatricial pemphigoid.*

MANAGEMENT Treatment of ocular toxicity requires that the offending topical medications be discontinued. Severe cases may take months to resolve completely; thus, failure of symptoms and signs to resolve within a period of days to a few weeks is not inconsistent

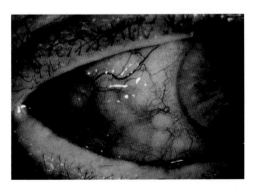

Figure 4-6 Bulbar follicles seen in drug-induced chronic follicular conjunctivitis. *(Courtesy of James J. Reidy, MD.)*

with a toxic etiology. Patients who are experiencing significant ocular irritation may find relief with nonpreserved topical lubricant drops or ointment. It is important to stress that toxic reactions to ocular medications can lead to irreversible changes, for example, conjunctival scarring and/or shrinkage.

Drug-induced pemphigoid should be confirmed with a conjunctival biopsy, which often (but not always) demonstrates the characteristic diffuse, nonlinear immunofluorescent staining indicative of antibody deposition. Withdrawal of the medication is generally followed by a lag of weeks before progressive scarring can be stabilized (see Chapter 11).

Dellen

Dellen are saucerlike depressions in the corneal surface due to focal stromal dehydration. Desiccation of the corneal epithelium and subepithelial tissues occurs at or near the limbus, adjacent to conjunctival surface elevations such as those produced after recession–resection surgery or in the presence of large filtration blebs. Normal blinking does not wet the involved area properly because the tear film is interrupted by these surface elevations. Patching followed by frequent topical lubrication is most effective in rapidly restoring stromal hydration, although resolution of conjunctival chemosis or bleb revision may be necessary for permanent resolution of dellen.

Limbal Stem Cell Deficiency

The ocular surface comprises populations of epithelial cells, which are replaced throughout life via proliferation of a distinct subpopulation of cells known as *stem cells*. Corneal stem cells are located in the basal cell layer of the limbus, whereas conjunctival stem cells may be uniformly distributed throughout the bulbar surface or located in the fornices. Stem cells have an unlimited capacity for self-renewal and are slow cycling (ie, they have low mitotic activity). Once stem cell differentiation begins, it is irreversible. The process of differentiation occurs by means of transit amplification. Transit-amplifying cells, which have a limited capacity for self-renewal, can be found at the limbus as well as at the basal layer of the corneal epithelium. Each of these cells is able to undergo a finite number of cell divisions. Corneal and conjunctival stem cells can be identified only by indirect means, such as clonal expansion and identification of slow cycling.

Approximately 25%–33% of the limbus must be intact to ensure normal ocular resurfacing. The normal limbus acts as a barrier against corneal vascularization from the conjunctiva and invasion of conjunctival cells from the bulbar surface.

PATHOGENESIS When the limbal stem cells are congenitally absent, injured, or destroyed, conjunctival cells migrate onto the ocular surface, often accompanied by surface irregularity and superficial neovascularization. The absence of limbal stem cells reduces the effectiveness of epithelial wound healing, as evidenced by compromised ocular surface integrity with an irregular ocular surface and recurrent epithelial breakdown.

Stem cell deficiency states result from both primary and secondary causes. Primary causes include *PAX6* gene mutations (aniridia), ectodactyly–ectodermal dysplasia–clefting syndrome, sclerocornea, keratitis-ichthyosis-deafness (KID) syndrome, and congenital erythrokeratodermia. Secondary causes include chemical burns, thermal burns, radiation, contact lens wear, ocular surgery, immune-based mucous membrane conjunctivitis (eg, mucous membrane pemphigoid, Stevens-Johnson syndrome), mucous membrane conjunctivitis related to infection (eg, trachoma), pterygia, long-term use of topical medications (pilocarpine, β-blockers, antibiotics, antimetabolites), and dysplastic or neoplastic lesions of the limbus.

See Table 4-3 for an etiologic classification of limbal stem cell deficiency.

CLINICAL PRESENTATION Clinically, stem cell deficiency of the cornea can be found in several ocular surface disorders. Affected patients usually have recurrent ulceration and decreased vision as a result of the irregular corneal surface. Corneal neovascularization is invariably present in the involved cornea. A whorl-like irregularity of the ocular surface emanating from the limbus can be more easily observed following the instillation of topical fluorescein (Fig 4-7).

Table 4-3 Etiologic Classification of Limbal Stem Cell Deficiency

Idiopathic

Trauma
Chemical or thermal burns

Iatrogenic
Local
  Contact lens use
  Ocular surgery (cryotherapy, excessive conjunctival resection, multiple ocular surface operations)
  Radiation and radiotherapy
  Topical medications (eg, mitomycin C)
Systemic
  Graft-vs-host disease
  Medications: hydroxyurea

Autoimmune disease
Mucous membrane pemphigoid
Stevens-Johnson syndrome

Ocular disease
Anterior segment ischemic syndrome
Atopic keratoconjunctivitis
Infections (eg, herpetic, trachoma)
Neoplasia and degeneration (eg, pterygium)
Neurotrophic keratitis
Peripheral corneal ulcers (eg, Fuchs marginal keratitis)

Congenital and hereditary conditions
Aniridia
Ectrodactyly–ectodermal dysplasia–clefting syndrome
Erythrokeratodermia
KID (keratitis-ichthyosis-deafness) syndrome (due to mutations in the *GJB2* gene coding for connexin-26)
LADD (lacrimo-auriculo-dento-digital) syndrome/Levy-Hollister syndrome
Multiple endocrine neoplasia
Sclerocornea
Xeroderma pigmentosa

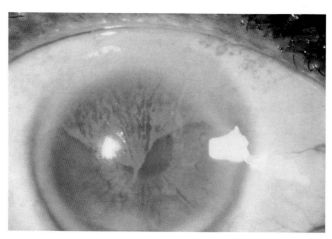

Figure 4-7 Mild stem cell deficiency secondary to contact lens wear. A whorl-like irregularity of the ocular surface is seen following instillation of topical fluorescein. *(Courtesy of James J. Reidy, MD.)*

MANAGEMENT In mild or focal cases associated with local factors such as contact lens use or topical medications, any possible inciting cause should be discontinued. In these cases, treatment with topical corticosteroids is advocated by some clinicians. If the stem cell deficiency is sectoral and mild, the abnormal epithelium can be debrided, allowing for resurfacing of the denuded area with cells derived from the remaining intact limbal epithelium.

In more extensive or severe cases of limbal stem cell deficiency, initial therapy with a scleral contact lens may be helpful. If this is not effective, replacement of stem cells by limbal transplantation is an alternative. When the limbus is focally affected in 1 eye (eg, pterygium), a limbal or conjunctival autograft can be harvested from the same eye. For unilateral, moderate or severe chemical injuries, a limbal autograft can be obtained from the healthy fellow eye. For bilateral limbal deficiency, as with Stevens-Johnson syndrome or bilateral chemical burns, a limbal allograft from a human leukocyte antigen–matched living related donor (or, if unavailable, an eye bank donor eye) can be considered; however, systemic immunosuppression is required following limbal allograft transplantation (see the discussion of ocular surface surgery in Chapter 13). Another alternative in cases of severe limbal cell deficiency is a keratoprosthesis (see Chapter 15).

Zhao Y, Ma L. Systematic review and meta-analysis of transplantation of ex vivo cultivated limbal epithelial stem cell on amniotic membrane in limbal stem cell deficiency. *Cornea.* 2015;34(5):592–600.

CHAPTER 5

Congenital Anomalies of the Cornea and Sclera

▶ *This chapter includes a related video, which can be accessed by scanning the QR code provided in the text or going to www.aao.org/bcscvideo_section08.*

Highlights

- Megalocornea can be associated with poor zonular integrity and predispose the eye to complications in cataract surgery.
- Anterior segment dysgenesis disorders are undergoing reclassification based on underlying genetic factors and the recognition that widely variable phenotypes may share common genotypes.
- Patients with congenital glaucoma can present with enlarged corneas, which may be misdiagnosed as megalocornea.

Developmental Anomalies of the Anterior Segment

See Table 5-1 for a summary of developmental anomalies of the anterior segment. Congenital anomalies are discussed in depth in BCSC Section 6, *Pediatric Ophthalmology and Strabismus*. See also BCSC Section 2, *Fundamentals and Principles of Ophthalmology*.

Anomalies of Size and Shape of the Cornea

Microcornea

Microcornea refers to a clear cornea of normal thickness with a diameter of less than 10 mm (or <9 mm in a newborn). The cause is unknown and may be related to fetal arrest of corneal growth in the fifth month of gestation. Alternatively, it may be related to overgrowth of the anterior tips of the optic cup, which leaves less space for the cornea to develop. Microcornea is inherited as an autosomal dominant (most commonly) or recessive trait and has been associated with mutations in paired box gene 6 *(PAX6)*. There is no sex predilection. Because the cornea is relatively flat in microcornea, these eyes are usually hyperopic, and there is an increased incidence of angle-closure glaucoma. Open-angle glaucoma develops later in life in 20% of patients in whom angle-closure glaucoma does

Table 5-1 Developmental Anomalies of the Anterior Segment

Anomaly	Unilateral/ Bilateral	Clinical Findings	Associated Ocular Anomalies	Associated Systemic Anomalies	Inheritance	Gene Loci
Microcornea	Unilateral or bilateral	Corneal diam. <10 mm or <9 mm in newborn; flat corneas with narrow anterior chamber; hyperopia	Persistent fetal vasculature, congenital cataracts, anterior segment dysgenesis, optic nerve hypoplasia, cornea plana	Myotonic dystrophy, fetal alcohol syndrome, achondroplasia, Ehlers-Danlos syndrome	Autosomal dominant (more common) or recessive	—
Megalocornea	Bilateral	Corneal diam. ≥13 mm; typically seen in males	Iris hypoplasia, miosis, goniodysgenesis, glaucoma, cataract, ectopia lentis, iridodonesis, arcus juvenilis, central cloudy dystrophy	Craniosynostosis, frontal bossing, hypertelorism, facial anomalies, facial hemiatrophy, hypotonia, dwarfism, intellectual disability, Down syndrome, Marfan syndrome, Alport syndrome, osteogenesis imperfecta, mucolipidosis II	X-linked recessive Autosomal dominant and recessive (rare)	Xq23: *CHRDL1*
Cornea plana	Bilateral	Corneal curvature <43 D, typically 30–35 D; peripheral corneal haze; high hyperopia is typical	Cataracts, anterior and posterior colobomas, narrow angle, angle closure, microcornea or sclerocornea	Ehlers-Danlos syndrome	Autosomal dominant and recessive; Finnish ancestry	12q22: *KERA*

Anomaly	Unilateral/ Bilateral	Clinical Findings	Associated Ocular Anomalies	Associated Systemic Anomalies	Inheritance	Gene Loci
Posterior embryotoxon	Usually bilateral	Thickened, anteriorly displaced Schwalbe line; seen in 8%–30% of normal eyes	Usually none	Alagille syndrome, X-linked ichthyosis, familial aniridia	Usually autosomal dominant	—
Axenfeld-Rieger syndrome	Unilateral or bilateral	Anteriorly displaced Schwalbe line with attached iris strands	Iris hypoplasia and atrophy, corectopia, pseudopolycoria, glaucoma	Skeletal, cranial, facial, dental, and umbilical anomalies	Usually autosomal dominant, may be sporadic	6p25: *FOXC1* 4q25: *PITX2* 13q14: *FOX01A* 11p13: *PAX6*
Peters anomaly	80% bilateral	Central corneal opacity present at birth; variable degrees of iridocorneal adhesion (type I); cataractous lens or corneolenticular adhesions (type II)	Congenital glaucoma, microcornea, aniridia, persistent fetal vasculature, retinal detachment	Intellectual disability, heart defects, external ear anomalies, hearing loss, CNS deficits, GI and GU anomalies, facial clefts, skeletal anomalies, spinal defects, short stature	Most cases sporadic; autosomal dominant and recessive inheritance patterns reported	11p13: *PAX6* 4q25-26: *PITX2* 2p22-21: *CYP1B1* 6p25: *FOXC1* 1p32: *FOXE3*
Posterior keratoconus	Typically unilateral	Localized central or paracentral indentation of posterior cornea with normal anterior topography; overlying stromal haze; focal pigment deposits and guttae often present at margins of the opacity	Astigmatism and amblyopia may occur	Usually none	Sporadic	—

(Continued)

Table 5-1 *(continued)*

Anomaly	Unilateral/ Bilateral	Clinical Findings	Associated Ocular Anomalies	Associated Systemic Anomalies	Inheritance	Gene Loci
Sclerocornea	90% bilateral; often asymmetric	Nonprogressive, noninflammatory scleralization of cornea; may be partial or complete; ill-defined limbus; vascularization	Cornea plana, angle anomalies	Multiple systemic anomalies reported	Usually sporadic; autosomal dominant and recessive inheritance patterns reported	22q11 2p25
Congenital anterior staphyloma	Typically unilateral	Large, ectatic cornea protruding between the eyelids at birth; lined by uveal tissue	Anterior segment anomalies, glaucoma, cataract	None	Sporadic	—
Keratectasia	Typically unilateral	Large, ectatic cornea protruding between the eyelids at birth	Anterior segment anomalies, glaucoma, cataract	None	Sporadic	—

CNS = central nervous system; GI = gastrointestinal; GU = genitourinary.

not occur. Important ocular anomalies often associated with microcornea include persistent fetal vasculature (PFV), congenital cataracts, anterior segment dysgenesis, and optic nerve hypoplasia. Significant systemic associations include myotonic dystrophy, fetal alcohol syndrome, achondroplasia, and Ehlers-Danlos syndrome.

When microcornea occurs as an isolated finding, the visual prognosis is excellent if spectacles are used to treat the hyperopia resulting from the flat cornea. Concurrent ocular pathologic conditions such as refractive amblyopia, cataract, PFV, and glaucoma may require treatment consisting of the usual procedures for those conditions.

Wang P, Sun W, Li S, Xiao X, Guo X, Zhan Q. *PAX6* mutations identified in 4 of 35 families with microcornea. *Invest Ophthalmol Vis Sci.* 2012;53(10):6338–6342.

Megalocornea

Megalocornea is a bilateral, nonprogressive enlargement of the cornea. It may be inherited as an X-linked recessive trait and is associated with mutations in the chordlin-like 1 gene *(CHRDL1)* (see Table 5-1). Rare cases of autosomal recessive and autosomal dominant inheritance have been reported. The cornea is histologically normal but measures 13.0–16.5 mm in diameter (Fig 5-1). Males are affected more often than females, but in heterozygous females, corneal diameter may be slightly increased.

The etiology may be related to failure of the optic cup to grow and of its anterior tips to close, leaving a larger space for the cornea to fill. Alternatively, megalocornea may represent arrested buphthalmos and exaggerated growth of the cornea in relation to the rest of the eye. An abnormality in collagen production is suggested by the association of megalocornea with systemic disorders of collagen synthesis (eg, Marfan syndrome).

Associated ocular anomalies may include iris translucency (diaphany), miosis, goniodysgenesis, cataract, ectopia lentis, arcus juvenilis, and glaucoma (but not congenital glaucoma). Nonocular and systemic associations may include craniosynostosis, frontal bossing, hypertelorism, facial anomalies, facial hemiatrophy, dwarfism, intellectual disability, hypotonia, Down syndrome, Marfan syndrome, Alport syndrome, osteogenesis imperfecta, mucolipidosis II, or occasionally other genetic syndromes.

The differential diagnosis is primarily congenital glaucoma (discussed later in the chapter), which can be ruled out by intraocular pressure measurement and careful biomicroscopy. The presence of pigmentary dispersion, iris transillumination defects, and/or

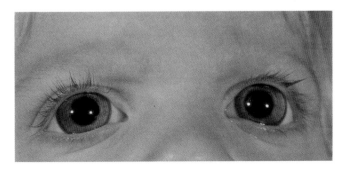

Figure 5-1 Megalocornea.

a Krukenberg spindle and the absence of Haab striae and previous breaks in Descemet membrane can also help distinguish megalocornea from congenital glaucoma. Ultrasonography may be of value in demonstrating the short vitreous length, deep lens and iris position, and normal axial length that distinguish megalocornea from buphthalmos caused by congenital glaucoma. Myopia and with-the-rule astigmatism, which are common in megalocornea, are managed as in patients without this anomaly.

Lens instability and subluxation, iridodonesis, and poor zonular integrity are also associated with megalocornea and present additional risks and challenges in the management of cataracts, particularly in terms of the selection and placement of an intraocular lens (IOL) after cataract surgery. If the lens is of normal size, an IOL can be inserted in the capsular bag. A capsular tension ring may be placed to reduce stress on the zonular fibers (Video 5-1). Standard-sized posterior chamber lenses are typically too short to be fixated in the ciliary sulcus, and anterior chamber lenses are similarly problematic in the enlarged anterior chamber. If zonular support is insufficient or capsular volume too great to allow stable IOL centration, an iris clip or iris-sutured lens may be the best option.

 VIDEO 5-1 Phacoemulsification with intraocular lens implantation for megalocornea.
Courtesy of Robert W. Weisenthal, MD.
Access all Section 8 videos at www.aao.org/bcscvideo_section08.

Smith JEH, Traboulsi EI. Malformations of the anterior segment of the eye. In: Traboulsi EI, ed. *Genetic Diseases of the Eye.* 2nd ed. Cary, NC: Oxford University Press; 2011:92–93.

Webb TR, Matarin M, Gardner JC, et al. X-linked megalocornea caused by mutations in *CHRDL1* identifies an essential role for ventroptin in anterior segment development. *Am J Hum Genet.* 2012;90(2):247–259.

Welder J, Oetting TA. Megalocornea. EyeRounds.org. September 17, 2010. Available at www.EyeRounds.org/cases/121-megalocornea.htm. Accessed February 3, 2017.

Cornea plana

Cornea plana, literally "flat cornea," is a rare condition in which the radius of curvature is less than 43 D and keratometry readings of 30–35 D are common (see Table 5-1). Additional hallmarks of cornea plana include high hyperopia (usually >10 D) and peripheral corneal haze or arcus. Corneal curvature that is the same as the curvature of the adjacent sclera is pathognomonic of this condition. Sclerocornea also features flat corneas, but it is distinguished by the loss of corneal transparency (see Fig 5-6).

Both autosomal recessive and dominant forms of cornea plana have been associated with mutations of the *KERA* gene (12q22), which codes for keratan sulfate proteoglycans (keratocan, lumican, and mimecan). These proteins are thought to play an important role in the regular spacing of corneal collagen fibrils. Investigators have speculated that mutations in the *KERA* gene cause an alteration of the tertiary structure of the keratan sulfate proteoglycans that leads to the cornea plana phenotype.

Cornea plana is often seen in association with sclerocornea (discussed later in the chapter) or microcornea. Other associated ocular or systemic abnormalities may include central corneal clouding, cataracts, anterior and posterior colobomas, and Ehlers-Danlos syndrome. Because of the morphologically shallow anterior chamber, angle-closure glaucoma occurs; open-angle glaucoma may develop because of angle abnormalities. Most isolated cases of cornea plana appear in patients of Finnish ancestry.

Treatment of cornea plana consists of correction of refractive errors and control of glaucoma, either medically or surgically. Loss of central corneal clarity may require deep anterior lamellar keratoplasty (DALK) or penetrating keratoplasty (PK), which has the added risk of endothelial rejection.

Khan AO. Cornea plana. In: Traboulsi EI, ed. *Genetic Diseases of the Eye*. 2nd ed. Cary, NC: Oxford University Press; 2011:85–91.

Lehmann OJ, El-Ashry MF, Ebenezer ND, et al. A novel keratocan mutation causing autosomal recessive cornea plana. *Invest Ophthalmol Vis Sci*. 2001;42(13):3118–3122.

Tahvanainen E, Villanueva AS, Forsius H, Salo P, de la Chapelle A. Dominantly and recessively inherited cornea plana congenita map to the same small region of chromosome 12. *Genome Res*. 1996;6(4):249–254.

Anomalies of Corneal and Associated Anterior Segment Structures

Beginning around the sixth week of gestation, anterior ocular structures are formed by 3 waves of neural crest migration that differentiate into corneal endothelium, corneal stroma, and iris stroma. Disruption at any point in this process can hinder subsequent development and differentiation of anterior segment structures. *Anterior segment dysgenesis* is the term used to describe a spectrum of congenital anomalies that arise from miscues during anterior segment embryogenesis and affect any or all of the anterior segment structures, including the cornea, anterior chamber angle, iris, and lens. Historically, this mixed group of anomalies was categorized by phenotypic, clinical, and anatomical presentation. Updated reclassification of anterior segment dysgenesis disorders is based on underlying genetic factors and the recognition that widely variable phenotypes may share common genotypes. For further discussion, see the chapter on ocular development in BCSC Section 2, *Fundamentals and Principles of Ophthalmology*.

Mihelec M, St Heaps L, Flaherty M, et al. Chromosomal rearrangements and novel genes in disorders of eye development, cataract and glaucoma. *Twin Res Hum Genet*. 2008;11(4): 412–421.

Nischal KK. Genetics of congenital corneal opacification–impact on diagnosis and treatment. *Cornea*. 2015;34(10 Suppl):S24–S34.

Reis LM, Semina EV. Genetics of anterior segment dysgenesis disorders. *Curr Opin Ophthalmol*. 2011;22(5):314–324.

Smith JEH, Traboulsi EI. Malformations of the anterior segment of the eye. In: Traboulsi EI, ed. *Genetic Diseases of the Eye*. 2nd ed. Cary, NC: Oxford University Press; 2011:92–108.

Posterior embryotoxon

Posterior embryotoxon involves a thickened and anteriorly displaced Schwalbe line (Fig 5-2). The Schwalbe line, which represents the junction of the trabecular meshwork and the termination of Descemet membrane, is visible in 8%–30% of normal eyes as an irregular, opaque ridge 0.5–2.0 mm central to the limbus. The term *posterior embryotoxon* is used when the Schwalbe line is visible on external examination. Posterior embryotoxon is usually bilateral and inherited as a dominant trait. Posterior embryotoxon may occur as

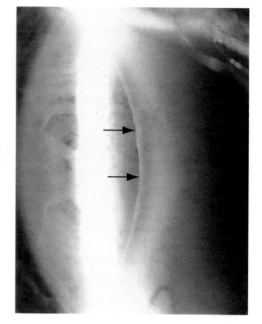

Figure 5-2 Posterior embryotoxon displaying a prominent and anteriorly displaced Schwalbe line *(arrows).*

an isolated finding or with other anterior segment anomalies that are part of ocular or systemic syndromes, such as Axenfeld-Rieger syndrome, arteriohepatic dysplasia (Alagille syndrome), X-linked ichthyosis, and familial aniridia.

Axenfeld-Rieger syndrome

The conditions previously referred to as *Axenfeld anomaly* or *syndrome* and *Rieger anomaly* or *syndrome* overlap genotypically and phenotypically and are now considered a single entity, *Axenfeld-Rieger syndrome.* This syndrome represents a spectrum of disorders characterized by an anteriorly displaced Schwalbe line (posterior embryotoxon) with attached iris strands, iris hypoplasia, corectopia, and glaucoma (in 50% of the cases occurring in late childhood or in adulthood) (Fig 5-3). Associated craniofacial, dental, skeletal, and umbilical abnormalities are often present.

Autosomal dominant inheritance is most common (75% of cases) for the Axenfeld-Rieger group, but transmission can be sporadic. The syndrome can be caused by mutations in the forkhead box C1 gene *(FOXC1),* the pituitary homeobox 2 gene *(PITX2),* or *PAX6.*

Nishimura DY, Searby CC, Alward WL, et al. A spectrum of *FOXC1* mutations suggests gene dosage as a mechanism for developmental defects of the anterior chamber of the eye. *Am J Hum Genet.* 2001;68(2):364–372.

Peters anomaly

Peters anomaly is characterized by the presence, at birth, of a central or paracentral corneal opacity, which is due to the localized absence of the corneal endothelium and Descemet membrane beneath the area of opacity. Eighty percent of cases are bilateral. Most cases occur sporadically, but autosomal recessive and dominant modes of inheritance have been reported.

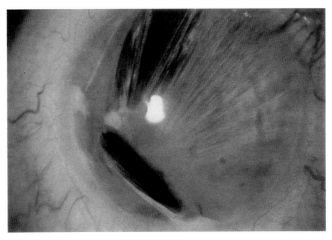

Figure 5-3   Axenfeld-Rieger syndrome exhibiting iris atrophy, corectopia, and pseudopolycoria. *(Courtesy of Vincent P. deLuise, MD.)*

Peters anomaly type I is characterized by iridocorneal adhesions and a corneal opacity that is usually avascular and may be central, eccentric, or less commonly total. The syndrome is associated with mutations in *PITX2, FOXC1, CYP1B1, PAX6,* and other genes. Peters anomaly type II is characterized by corneolenticular adhesions and/or cataract, along with a central or total corneal opacity that is usually vascularized (Fig 5-4). Peters anomaly type II is presumed to be due to a developmental failure in separation of the invaginating lens vesicle from the overlying surface ectoderm. Mutations in the gene *FOXE3* have been implicated in lens malformation in Peters anomaly type II. The same genetic mutation can cause Peters type I to occur in one eye and type II in the contralateral eye. High-frequency ultrasonography can be very useful in differentiating Peters types I and II, and sclerocornea.

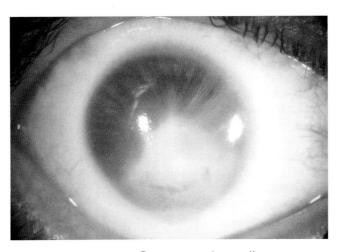

Figure 5-4   Peters anomaly type II.

Glaucoma is present in 50% of Peters anomaly cases. Additional associated ocular abnormalities include microcornea, aniridia, retinal detachment, and PFV. The prognosis for vision rehabilitation with corneal transplantation is better for patients with Peters anomaly type I than for those with type II (see Chapter 15).

Peters plus syndrome refers to Peters anomaly associated with systemic abnormalities. Systemic involvement is variable and may include cleft lip/palate, short stature, external ear abnormalities, hearing loss, intellectual disability, heart defects, central nervous system deficits, spinal defects, gastrointestinal and genitourinary defects, and skeletal anomalies. Although the systemic malformations in this syndrome may be associated with genetically transmitted syndromes (trisomy 13–15, Kivlin syndrome, Pfeiffer syndrome), these associations are the exception rather than the rule.

See also BCSC Section 4, *Ophthalmic Pathology and Intraocular Tumors,* Section 6, *Pediatric Ophthalmology and Strabismus,* and Section 10, *Glaucoma.*

Bhandari R, Ferri S, Whittaker B, Liu M, Lazzaro DR. Peters anomaly: review of the literature. *Cornea.* 2011;30(8):939–944.

Nischal KK. Genetics of congenital corneal opacification—impact on diagnosis and treatment. *Cornea.* 2015;34(10 Suppl):S24–S34.

Traboulsi EI, Maumenee IH. Peters anomaly and associated congenital malformations. *Arch Ophthalmol.* 1992;110(12):1739–1742.

Posterior keratoconus

Posterior keratoconus is characterized by a usually localized central or paracentral indentation of the posterior cornea without protrusion of the anterior corneal surface, as is seen in typical keratoconus. Posterior excavation can occur in multiple areas; there is also a generalized form of this disease that can involve much of the cornea. Classification of posterior keratoconus as a congenital anomaly is supported by its association with abnormal anterior banding of Descemet membrane and its presence at birth. Loss of stromal substance can lead to corneal thinning that approaches one-third of normal (Fig 5-5). The ectasia is usually stable but can gradually progress. Focal deposits of pigment and guttae are often present at the involved margins. Subtle anterior corneal irregularities overlying the area of posterior involvement can contribute to irregular astigmatism and amblyopia, which should be sought and treated appropriately. Corneal tomography can confirm the corneal thinning and posterior elevation.

Most cases of posterior keratoconus are unilateral and sporadic. An autosomal recessive form of disease is associated with bilateral corneal changes, short stature, intellectual disability, cleft lip and palate, and vertebral anomalies. Acquired posterior keratoconus can also occur, usually following trauma.

Charles N, Charles M, Croxatto JO, Charles DE, Wertheimer D. Surface and Orbscan II slit-scanning elevation topography in circumscribed posterior keratoconus. *J Cataract Refract Surg.* 2005;31(3):636–639.

Krachmer JH, Rodrigues MM. Posterior keratoconus. *Arch Ophthalmol.* 1976;96:1867–1873.

Zare MA, Mehrjardi HZ, Zare F, Oskoie J. Visante in atypical posterior keratoconus. *Iran J Ophthalmol.* 2011;23(4):61–64.

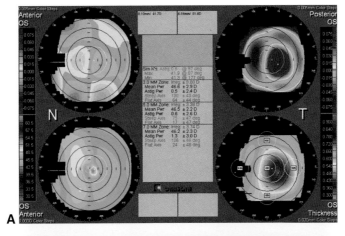

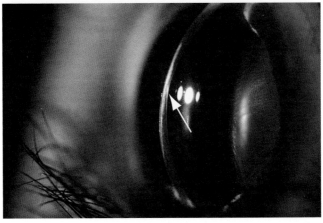

Figure 5-5 Posterior keratoconus. **A,** Scanning-slit corneal topography shows a nasally displaced anterior corneal apex *(top left),* temporal paracentral posterior corneal vaulting *(top right),* normal anterior keratometry reading *(bottom left),* and significant loss of stromal thickness *(bottom right).* **B,** This slit-lamp photograph shows loss of stromal thickness, stromal haze, and a craterlike depression in the posterior cornea *(arrow). (Courtesy of Kenneth M. Goins, MD.)*

Sclerocornea

Sclerocornea is a nonprogressive, noninflammatory scleralization of the cornea. The scleralization may be limited to the corneal periphery, or the entire cornea may be involved. The limbus is usually ill defined, and superficial vessels that are extensions of normal scleral, episcleral, and conjunctival vessels cross the cornea (Fig 5-6). Sclerocornea is usually sporadic, but both autosomal dominant and recessive patterns of inheritance have been reported. No sex predilection is evident, and 90% of cases are bilateral.

The most common associated ocular finding is cornea plana, which occurs in 80% of cases. Angle structures are also commonly malformed. Multiple systemic anomalies have been reported in association with sclerocornea.

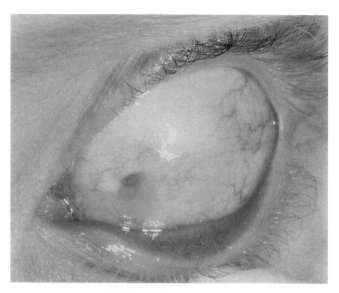

Figure 5-6 Sclerocornea.

Ali M, Buentello-Volante B, McKibbin M, et al. Homozygous *FOXE3* mutations cause non-syndromic, bilateral, total sclerocornea, aphakia, microphthalmia and optic disc coloboma. *Mol Vis.* 2010;16:1162–1168.

Congenital anterior staphyloma and keratectasia

Congenital anterior staphyloma is a rare developmental anomaly characterized by an opaque cornea protruding between the eyelids and partial or complete absence of Descemet membrane and endothelium (Fig 5-7). A thin layer of uveal tissue lines the posterior cornea. The anterior segment is usually markedly abnormal, often with iridocorneal adhesions, iris hypoplasia, and lens opacity. Exposure may promote corneal scarring and keratinization. Inflammation is markedly absent. Unlike Peters anomaly, congenital anterior staphyloma is usually unilateral, but the contralateral eye frequently has some form of anterior segment abnormality. Typically, cases are sporadic, with no familial or systemic association.

Keratectasia differs from congenital anterior staphyloma histologically only by the absence of a thin layer of uveal tissue lining the posterior cornea. Keratectasia is possibly

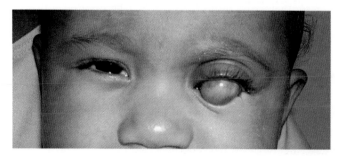

Figure 5-7 Congenital anterior staphyloma. *(Courtesy of Denise de Freitas, MD.)*

the result not of abnormal development but rather of intrauterine keratitis or vitamin deficiency and subsequent corneal perforation.

Except in very mild cases, the visual prognosis for both congenital anterior staphyloma and keratectasia is poor because of associated severe damage to the anterior segment. Penetrating keratoplasty and sclerokeratoplasty may be useful to preserve the globe and improve cosmesis; however, enucleation may be required for a painful, blind glaucomatous eye.

Congenital Corneal Opacities in Hereditary Syndromes and Corneal Dystrophies

The *mucopolysaccharidoses (MPS)* and the *mucolipidoses* are disorders caused by abnormal carbohydrate metabolism. Affected patients present with corneal clouding and haziness. These conditions are discussed further in Chapter 8 of this volume and in BCSC Section 6, *Pediatric Ophthalmology and Strabismus*.

See Chapter 7 in this volume for discussion of congenital hereditary stromal dystrophy and congenital hereditary endothelial dystrophy.

Secondary Abnormalities Affecting the Fetal Cornea

Intrauterine Keratitis: Bacterial and Syphilitic

Infections acquired in utero or during delivery can cause ocular damage in several ways:

- through direct action of the infecting agent, which damages tissue
- through a teratogenic effect resulting in malformation
- through a delayed reactivation of the infectious agent after birth, with inflammation that damages developed tissue

Congenital syphilis is acquired in utero and caused by infection with the spirochete *Treponema pallidum*. It can lead to fetal death or premature delivery. A variety of systemic manifestations have been widely described. In children with untreated congenital syphilis, onset of interstitial keratitis is typically between 6 and 12 years of age. The keratitis presents as rapidly progressive corneal edema, followed by abnormal vascularization in the deep stroma adjacent to Descemet membrane. The cornea may assume a salmon-pink color because of intense vascularization, giving rise to the term *salmon patch*. Over several weeks to months, blood flow through these vessels gradually ceases, leaving empty "ghost" vessels in the corneal stroma. See Chapter 11 in this volume for a more complete discussion of interstitial keratitis, as well as BCSC Section 6, *Pediatric Ophthalmology and Strabismus*, for additional discussion of congenital syphilis.

Congenital Corneal Keloid

Corneal keloids are relatively rare lesions, most commonly occurring following corneal perforation, trauma, or surgery. Congenital corneal keloids, which are often bilateral, have been described in Lowe (oculocerebrorenal) syndrome (an X-linked recessive disorder characterized by cataracts, renal failure, intellectual disability, and seizures),

Rubinstein-Taybi syndrome, and the ACL syndrome (*a*cromegaly, *c*utis verticis gyrata, corneal *l*eukoma syndrome). Autosomal dominant inheritance has been observed in the ACL syndrome. Corneal keloids can occur in association with cataracts, aniridia, and glaucoma and may represent a developmental anomaly with failure of normal differentiation of corneal tissue. Histologic examination reveals thick collagen bundles haphazardly arranged, with focal areas of myofibroblastic proliferation.

Congenital Corneal Anesthesia

Congenital corneal anesthesia is a rare, usually bilateral, condition that is often misdiagnosed as herpes simplex virus keratitis, recurrent corneal erosion, or dry eye. Most patients present with painless corneal opacities and sterile epithelial ulcerations during infancy or childhood. Rosenberg classified the disorder into 3 distinct groups: Group I is associated with isolated trigeminal anesthesia, which is probably due to primary hypoplasia of the hindbrain. Group II is associated with mesenchymal anomalies, which include Goldenhar syndrome, Möbius syndrome, and familial dysautonomia (FD; also known as *Riley-Day syndrome*). Group III is associated with focal brainstem signs without evidence of mesenchymal dysplasia.

A thorough systemic examination, including neuroradiologic studies, is performed to rule out associated systemic conditions. In family linkage studies, FD (also called *hereditary sensory and autonomic neuropathy type III*) is an autosomal recessive disorder that maps to 9q31-q33. CIPA (congenital insensitivity to pain with anhidrosis), another rare autosomal recessive condition associated with congenital corneal anesthesia, is linked to mutations in the *NTRK1* gene, located at 1q23.

Treatment options for congenital corneal anesthesia include frequent topical lubrication, punctal occlusion, nighttime eyelid splinting, permanent lateral tarsorrhaphy, amniotic membrane transplantation, scleral contact lenses, and, in recalcitrant cases, conjunctival flap to stabilize the ocular surface.

Ramappa M, Chaurasia S, Chakrabarti S, Kaur I. Congenital cornea anesthesia. *J AAPOS.* 2014;18(5):427–432.

Verpoorten N, De Jonghe P, Timmerman V. Disease mechanisms in hereditary sensory and autonomic neuropathies. *Neurobiol Dis.* 2006;21(2):247–255.

Congenital Glaucoma

Primary congenital glaucoma (PCG) is evident either at birth or within the first few years of life. It is believed to be caused by dysplasia of the anterior chamber angle without other ocular or systemic abnormalities. In more than 10% of cases, PCG is inherited as an autosomal recessive trait associated with mutations in *CYP1B1,* located at 2p22; *MYOC,* at 1q25; and numerous other genes. Characteristic findings in newborns with PCG include the triad of epiphora, photophobia, and blepharospasm. External eye examination may reveal buphthalmos, with the cornea enlarging to more than 12 mm in diameter during the first year of life. (In full-term infants, the normal horizontal corneal diameter is 9.5–10.5 mm.) Corneal edema, present in 25% of affected infants at birth and in more than 60% by the sixth month of life, may range from mild haze to dense opacification in the corneal stroma because of elevated intraocular pressure. Tears in Descemet membrane *(Haab striae)* may occur acutely as a result of corneal stretching and are typically oriented horizontally or concentric to the limbus. For additional discussion, see BCSC Section 6, *Pediatric Ophthalmology and Strabismus,* and Section 10, *Glaucoma.*

Wiggs JL, Langgurth AM, Allen KF. Carrier frequency of CYP1B1 mutations in the United States (an American Ophthalmological Society thesis). *Trans Am Ophthalmol Soc.* 2014; 112(July):94–102.

Birth Trauma

Progressive corneal edema developing during the first few postnatal days, accompanied by vertical or oblique posterior striae, may be caused by birth trauma (Fig 5-8). Ruptures occur in the Descemet membrane and the corneal endothelium. These ruptures usually heal but leave a hypertrophic ridge of Descemet membrane. The edema may or may not clear; if it does clear, the cornea can again become edematous at any time later in life. High astigmatism and amblyopia may be associated findings. Congenital glaucoma can present with similar findings and should be considered in the differential diagnosis.

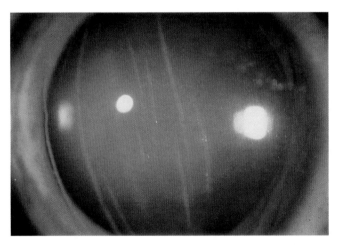

Figure 5-8   Vertical ruptures of Descemet membrane secondary to traumatic delivery. *(Courtesy of Vincent P. deLuise, MD.)*

CHAPTER 6

Clinical Approach to Depositions and Degenerations of the Conjunctiva, Cornea, and Sclera

Highlights

- Pterygium, a fibrovascular degeneration of the conjunctiva with a characteristic appearance, should be evaluated for neoplastic disease if there is atypical pigmentation, elevation, or vascularization.
- The presence of band keratopathy can have systemic implications as well as an effect on the patient's vision and comfort. Proper evaluation can therefore be particularly important for patients with band keratopathy, as it may help uncover associated systemic disease.
- The 3 clinical variants of iridocorneal endothelial (ICE) syndrome can be easily remembered as follows: the first letter of each variant, when combined, also produces the acronym ICE—*i*ris nevus syndrome, *C*handler syndrome, and *e*ssential (progressive) iris atrophy.

Degenerations of the Conjunctiva

Degeneration of a tissue refers to decomposition and deterioration of tissue elements and functions. For a proper diagnosis, it is important to distinguish corneal degenerations, which infrequently exhibit an inheritance pattern, from corneal dystrophies (Table 6-1).

Table 6-1 Differences Between Corneal Degenerations and Corneal Dystrophies

Degeneration	Dystrophy
Opacity often peripherally located	Opacity often centrally located
May be bilateral but asymmetric	Is bilateral and symmetric
Presents later in life, usually associated with aging but may be related to a specific disease	Presents early in life, hereditary
Progression can be very slow or rapid	Progression is usually slow

Age-Related Changes

As a result of aging, the conjunctiva loses transparency and becomes thinner. The *substantia propria* (stroma) becomes less elastic, causing conjunctival laxity. In older individuals, the conjunctival vessels may become more prominent. Saccular telangiectasias, fusiform dilatory changes, or tortuosities may appear in the vessels. These changes are not necessarily uniform; they tend to be more pronounced in the region of the interpalpebral fissure, corresponding to the area most commonly exposed to the environment.

Pinguecula

A pinguecula is a common conjunctival condition that occurs typically on the nasal side of the bulbar conjunctiva, adjacent to the limbus in the interpalpebral zone. It is usually bilateral, appears as a yellow-white elevated mass (Fig 6-1), and occurs as a result of the effects of aging, UV light exposure, and environmental insults such as dust and wind. Pingueculae represent an elastotic degeneration (the material stains for elastin but is not broken down by elastase) of subepithelial collagen with hyalinized connective tissue. The mass may enlarge gradually over long periods of time. There may be recurrent inflammation and ocular irritation. Lubricant therapy to alleviate ocular irritation is the mainstay of treatment. Excision is indicated only when pingueculae are cosmetically unacceptable, when they become chronically inflamed, or when they interfere with contact lens wear. Judicious use of topical corticosteroids may be considered for patients with inflammation, but their use as long-term therapy for pingueculae is strongly discouraged because of their adverse effects.

Pterygium

A pterygium is a wing-shaped growth of conjunctiva and fibrovascular tissue on the superficial cornea (Fig 6-2). As with pingueculae, the pathogenesis of pterygia is strongly correlated with UV light exposure, although environmental insults such as exposure to

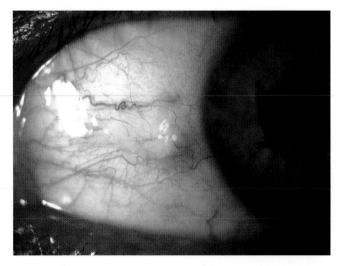

Figure 6-1 A pinguecula, shown in its typical location, on the nasal side of the bulbar conjunctiva. *(Courtesy of Cornea Service, Paulista School of Medicine, Federal University of São Paulo.)*

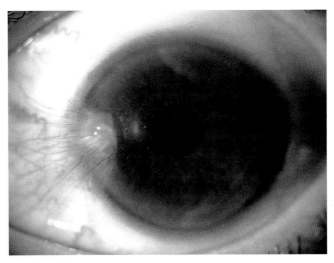

Figure 6-2 A pterygium, a wing-shaped growth of conjunctiva and fibrovascular tissue on the superficial cornea. *(Courtesy of Cornea Service, Paulista School of Medicine, Federal University of São Paulo.)*

dust, wind, or other irritants causing chronic ocular inflammation may also be factors. The predominance of pterygia on the nasal side in the interpalpebral zone is theorized to result from light passing medially through the cornea, focusing on the nasal limbus area, while the shadow of the nose reduces the intensity of light transmitted to the temporal limbus. The prevalence of pterygia increases steadily with proximity to the equator, and the condition is more common in men than women, in persons 20–30 years of age (the most common age range for onset of pterygia), and in people who work outdoors. The histopathology of pterygia is similar to that of pingueculae (basophilic degeneration of elastotic fibers), except that a pterygium invades the superficial cornea, which is preceded by dissolution of the Bowman layer. For further discussion of the histopathology of both pingueculae and pterygia, see BCSC Section 4, *Ophthalmic Pathology and Intraocular Tumors.*

Astigmatism (regular and irregular), as well as corneal scarring, occurs in proportion to pterygium size. A pigmented iron line *(Stocker line)* may be seen in the cornea, anterior to the edge of the pterygium. A pterygium must be distinguished from a pseudopterygium, which may occur after trauma or chemical burns or secondary to inflammatory corneal disease. It is important to maintain an index of suspicion for carcinoma in situ or squamous cell carcinoma, primarily in patients with atypical presentations.

Treatment with artificial tears can alleviate associated ocular irritation, but as with pingueculae, long-term use of topical corticosteroids is contraindicated. Excision is indicated if the pterygium causes persistent discomfort or chronic irritation; exhibits progressive growth toward the central cornea or visual axis (>3–4 mm), causing blurred vision or irregular astigmatism; is cosmetically unacceptable; or restricts ocular motility. See Chapter 13 for discussion of the surgical treatment of pterygium.

Conjunctival Concretions

Concretions appear to be epithelial inclusion cysts filled with epithelial and keratin debris, as well as mucopolysaccharide and mucin. They are seen as small, yellow-white dots in the palpebral conjunctiva of older patients or patients who have had chronic conjunctivitis. Concretions are almost always asymptomatic, but they may erode the overlying epithelium, causing foreign-body sensation. If symptomatic, concretions can be easily removed under topical anesthesia.

Conjunctival Epithelial Inclusion Cysts

Conjunctival epithelial inclusion cysts are clear lesions that appear in either the bulbar conjunctiva or the conjunctival fornix and are typically incidental findings on examination (Fig 6-3). As these cysts are usually asymptomatic, they do not require treatment. If the cyst is symptomatic, simple drainage is not sufficient, because the inner epithelial cell wall remains, allowing the cyst to re-form. Complete excision is necessary to prevent recurrence.

Conjunctival inclusion cysts can be congenital or acquired. Most acquired cysts of the conjunctiva are derived from an inclusion of conjunctival epithelium in the substantia propria. The implanted cells proliferate to form a central fluid-filled cavity that is lined by nonkeratinized conjunctival epithelium. Conjunctival cysts may also form from ductal epithelium of the accessory lacrimal glands; these cysts are lined by a double layer of epithelium. Stimuli for cyst formation include chronic inflammation, trauma, and surgery. Dilated lymphatic channels may mimic an inclusion cyst of the bulbar conjunctiva.

Conjunctivochalasis

Poor adherence of the bulbar conjunctiva leading to redundancy of conjunctiva is referred to as conjunctivochalasis. This condition is described in Chapter 4, and its treatment is discussed in Chapter 13.

Conjunctival Vascular Tortuosity and Hyperemia

There are many causes of conjunctival vascular tortuosity and hyperemia. A differential diagnosis is outlined in Table 6-2.

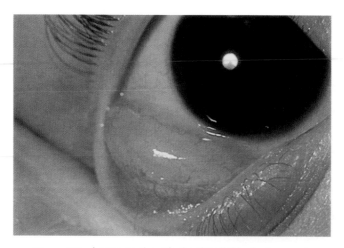

Figure 6-3 Large conjunctival epithelial inclusion cyst.

Table 6-2 Causes of Conjunctival Vascular Tortuosity, Hyperemia, and Telangiectasia and Subconjunctival Hemorrhage

Diffuse vascular tortuosity and hyperemia: blood hyperviscosity disorders, carcinoid tumor, carotid-cavernous sinus fistula (trauma) and dural shunts, diabetes mellitus, Fabry disease, hypertension, mucolipidosis I, polycythemia vera, sickle cell anemia, Sturge-Weber syndrome, venous obstruction, and use of systemic vasodilators such as alcohol, cannabis, oxygen

Segmented vascular tortuosity and hyperemia: choristoma, epithelial cysts, ocular tumor, pinguecula, pterygium

Telangiectasia: ataxia-telangiectasia (Louis-Barr syndrome), concomitant telangiectasia of conjunctiva and skin, galactosialidosis (Goldenberg syndrome), hereditary hemorrhagic telangiectasia, local conditions that dilate the conjunctival vessels, Rendu-Osler-Weber syndrome

Subconjunctival hemorrhage: *(ocular causes)* allergy, conjunctival amyloidosis, conjunctivitis, conjunctivochalasis, contact lens wear, idiopathic, orbital injury, trauma, tumor; *(systemic causes)* acute febrile systemic diseases, anticoagulant use, arteriosclerosis, blood dyscrasia, carotid-cavernous fistula, diabetes mellitus, hypertension, Valsalva maneuver

---

Degenerations of the Cornea

Age-Related Changes

As a result of aging, the cornea gradually becomes flatter in the vertical meridian, thinner, and slightly less transparent. Its refractive index increases, and the Descemet membrane becomes thicker, increasing from 3 μm at birth to 13 μm in adults. With age, occasional peripheral endothelial guttae, sometimes known as *Hassall-Henle bodies,* may form (discussed later in the chapter). Age-related attrition of corneal endothelial cells results in a loss of approximately 100,000 cells during the first 50 years of life, from a cell density of about 4000 cells/mm² at birth to a density of 2500–3000 cells/mm² in older adults.

Epithelial and Subepithelial Degenerations

Coats white ring

Coats white ring (Fig 6-4) refers to a small (1 mm or less in diameter) circular or oval area of discrete gray-white dots seen in the superficial corneal stroma and representing iron-containing fibrotic remnants of a metallic foreign body. Once these lesions mature and are free of any associated inflammation, they do not change; hence, therapy with corticosteroids or other anti-inflammatory agents is not indicated.

Spheroidal degeneration

Spheroidal degeneration is characterized by the appearance in the cornea, and sometimes in the conjunctiva, of translucent, golden-brown, spheroidal deposits in the subepithelium, Bowman layer, or superficial stroma (Fig 6-5). The condition has been reported under different names, including *actinic keratopathy, climatic droplet keratopathy, Bietti nodular dystrophy,* and *Labrador keratopathy.* In *primary spheroidal degeneration,* the deposits are bilateral and initially located in the nasal and temporal cornea. With age, they can extend onto the conjunctiva in the interpalpebral zone. The primary degeneration is unrelated to the coexistence of other ocular disease. In rare cases, generally in childhood,

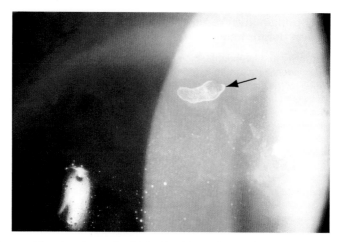

Figure 6-4   Coats white ring *(arrow)*, which should not be confused with map-dot-fingerprint dystrophy. *(Courtesy of W. Craig Fowler, MD.)*

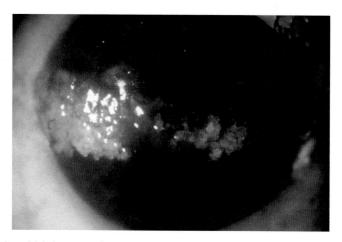

Figure 6-5   Spheroidal degeneration. *(Courtesy of Cornea Service, Paulista School of Medicine, Federal University of São Paulo.)*

the spheroidal deposits extend across the interpalpebral zone of the cornea, producing a noncalcific band-shaped keratopathy. The etiology is controversial, but the deposits may develop from UV radiation–induced alteration of preexisting structural connective tissue components or from the synthesis of abnormal extracellular material in limbal conjunctiva. *Secondary spheroidal degeneration* is associated with ocular injury or inflammation. The deposits aggregate near the area of corneal scarring or vascularization. All cases show extracellular, proteinaceous, hyaline deposits with characteristics of elastotic degeneration; these deposits are thought to be secondary to the combined effects of genetic predisposition, actinic exposure associated with temperature extremes, age, and perhaps various kinds of environmental trauma other than sunlight, such as dust and wind. The deposit composition is not lipid, despite its "oil droplet" appearance. Medical therapy is not of much value, but ocular lubrication is recommended to address uneven layering of the tear film over affected areas. In cases of central corneal involvement, superficial keratectomy or phototherapeutic keratectomy (PTK) using an excimer laser may be indicated.

Iron deposition

Most iron lines are related to abnormalities of tear pooling due to ocular surface irregularities (Fig 6-6). Often, the clinician can see these lines only by using red-free or diffuse illumination with a cobalt-blue filter before instilling fluorescein. A *Fleischer ring*, representing iron deposition in keratoconus, is one of many corneal iron lines associated with epithelial irregularities (see Chapter 7, Fig 7-27). This ring is extremely useful as a diagnostic sign in mild or early cases of keratoconus. The *Hudson-Stähli line*, generally located at the junction of the upper two-thirds and lower one-third of the cornea, is ubiquitous. Iron lines are also associated with keratorefractive surgery. Following radial keratotomy, visually insignificant iron lines are noted in the inferior paracentral cornea in approximately 80% of patients and are commonly characterized as a "tear star." Corneal iron lines are summarized in Table 6-3.

Calcific band keratopathy

Calcific band keratopathy is a degeneration of the superficial cornea that involves mainly the Bowman layer. The degeneration begins as fine, dustlike, basophilic deposits in the Bowman layer. These changes are usually first seen peripherally, in the 3- and 9-o'clock positions. Eventually, the deposits may coalesce to form a horizontal band of dense calcific plaques across the interpalpebral zone of the cornea (Fig 6-7). Small cracks can occur in the band as a result of fractures in the calcium deposits. In addition, small, lucent holes, representing corneal nerves that penetrate the Bowman layer, can be seen throughout the opacity.

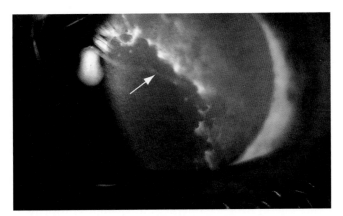

Figure 6-6 Iron deposition (iron line) *(arrow)* due to irregularity of the tear film, which results from subepithelial fibrosis. *(Courtesy of Robert W. Weisenthal, MD.)*

Table 6-3 Corneal Deposits

Location in Cornea	Pigment	Clinical Findings	Characteristics
Epithelium	Iron	Ferry line	Anterior to filtering bleb
		Fleischer ring	Surrounding base of cone in keratoconus
			Can also be seen in iatrogenic keratectasia after refractive surgery
		Hudson-Stähli line	Horizontal line at junction of upper two-thirds and lower one-third of the aging cornea
		Stocker line	Anterior to head of pterygium
		LASIK line	Line, ring, or patch at the margin of the ablation zone or centrally in the flatter area of the cornea. In hyperopia, has been considered pseudo-Fleischer ring
Epithelium and superficial stroma	Melanin-like pigment (alkapton)	Ochronosis	Peripherally; occurs in the metabolic disease alkaptonuria
Between basement membrane and Bowman layer	Melanin-like pigment (oxidized epinephrine)	Adrenochrome deposition	Occurs in patients using topical epinephrine compounds for glaucoma or in those given tetracycline or minocycline therapy
Stroma	Iron	Blood staining	Chiefly stroma; epithelium in some cases; occurs in some cases of hyphema
	Iron (foreign body)	Siderosis	Chiefly stroma; epithelium in some cases
	Carbon	Corneal tattoo	In the keratocytes or between collagen fibrils
	Gold	Chrysiasis	More often in the periphery
Deep stroma and Descemet membrane	Silver	Argyriasis	Slate-gray or silver discoloration
Descemet membrane	Copper	Kayser-Fleischer ring	Peripherally; in patients with hepatolenticular degeneration (Wilson disease)
		Chalcosis	Usually occurs with copper-containing foreign body
Endothelium	Melanin	Krukenberg spindle	In a vertical ellipse; sometimes associated with pigmentary glaucoma; most often bilateral

The condition can be idiopathic, but the chief known causes are

- chronic ocular (usually inflammatory) disease such as uveitis in children, interstitial keratitis, severe superficial keratitis, and phthisis bulbi
- hypercalcemia due to hyperparathyroidism, vitamin D toxicity, milk-alkali syndrome, sarcoidosis, or other systemic disorders
- hereditary transmission (primary hereditary band keratopathy, with or without other anomalies)

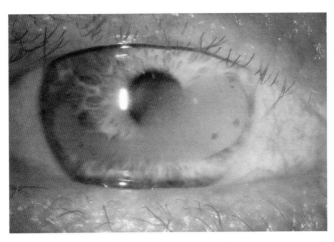

Figure 6-7 Band keratopathy, displaying a horizontal calcific plaque with a lucid interval between the limbus and small lucent holes representing corneal nerves that penetrate the Bowman layer.

- elevated serum phosphorus level with normal serum calcium level (may occur in patients with renal failure, particularly if they are not receiving appropriate treatment to lower serum phosphate concentrations)
- chronic exposure to mercurial vapors or to mercurial preservatives (phenylmercuric nitrate or acetate) in ophthalmic medications (the mercury causes changes in corneal collagen that result in the deposition of calcium)
- silicone oil, instilled in an aphakic eye

Band keratopathy may also result from the deposition of urates in the cornea. The urates appear brown, unlike the gray-white calcific deposits, and may be associated with gout or hyperuricemia.

A workup (eg, serum electrolytes and urinalysis) to rule out associated metabolic or renal disease should be considered. Underlying conditions, such as keratoconjunctivitis sicca or renal failure, should be treated or controlled as much as possible, which may reduce or control the deposition of calcium or at least help reduce the recurrence of band keratopathy. The calcium can usually be removed from the Bowman layer by chelation with a neutral solution of disodium EDTA, which can be warmed to speed up the chemical chelation. The usual concentration of EDTA (0.05 mol/L), 0.5%–1.5%, can be obtained through a compounding pharmacy. The epithelium overlying the calcium needs to be removed before the chelating solution is applied. Any cylindrical tube that approximates the corneal diameter (eg, corneal trephine) can facilitate the process by acting as a reservoir to confine the chelating solution to the desired treatment area; however, this is not always necessary. With the reservoir in place, very gentle surface agitation with a truncated cellulose sponge (mechanical debridement) may further enhance the release of the impregnated calcium. Certain types of calcium deposits can be removed with forceps alone. In any case, the deposit should be excised carefully to avoid further damage to the Bowman layer. A fibrous pannus may be present along with extensive calcific band keratopathy, especially if silicone oil is responsible; neither EDTA nor scraping will remove such fibrous tissue. A bandage contact lens can be helpful postoperatively until the epithelium has healed. Band keratopathy can recur but may not do so for years, at which time the treatment may be repeated. PTK using an excimer laser is not advised as primary treatment, because calcium ablates at a different rate than stroma and thus could produce a severely irregular surface. If there is residual opacification after the initial EDTA chelation, PTK may be used.

Jhanji V, Rapuano CJ, Vajpayee RB. Corneal calcific band keratopathy. *Curr Opin Ophthalmol.* 2011;22(4):283–289.

Stromal Degenerations

White limbal girdle of Vogt

Two forms of the white limbal girdle of Vogt have been described. Type I is a narrow, concentric, whitish superficial band running along the limbus in the palpebral fissure and is generally thought to represent early calcific band keratopathy. A lucid interval appears between the limbus and the girdle. This girdle is a degenerative change of the anterior limiting membrane, with chalklike opacities and small clear areas resembling the holes in Swiss cheese. Type II consists of small, white, flecklike, and needlelike deposits that are often seen at the nasal and temporal limbus in older patients. No clear interval separates this girdle from the limbus (Fig 6-8). Histologically, there is epithelial elastotic degeneration of collagen, sometimes with particles of calcium.

Corneal arcus

Corneal arcus, or *arcus senilis,* is most often an involutional change that is modified by genetic factors and caused by the deposition of lipid in the peripheral corneal stroma.

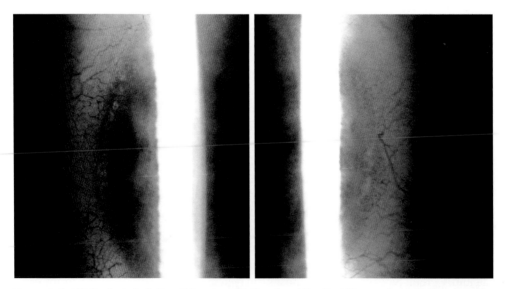

Figure 6-8 White limbal girdle of Vogt type II. Small, white, flecklike, and needlelike deposits at the nasal and temporal limbus, seen by retroillumination. *(Courtesy of Cornea Service, Paulista School of Medicine, Federal University of São Paulo.)*

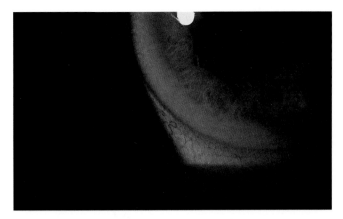

Figure 6-9   Corneal arcus. *(Courtesy of Robert W. Weisenthal, MD.)*

Arcus starts at the inferior and superior poles of the cornea and, in the late stages, involves the entire circumference. The prevalence of corneal arcus is higher in African Americans and males. The arcus has a hazy white appearance, a sharp outer border, and an indistinct central border; it is denser superiorly and inferiorly (Fig 6-9). A lucid interval is usually present between the peripheral edge of the arcus and the limbus. The lipid is found to be concentrated mainly in 2 areas of the peripheral corneal stroma: one adjacent to the Bowman layer and another near the Descemet membrane.

In patients younger than 40 years, the presence of arcus may be indicative of a hyperlipoproteinemia (involving low-density lipoproteins) with elevated serum cholesterol level (see Chapter 8). Corneal arcus may also occur as a congenital anomaly *(arcus juvenilis)*.

Unilateral corneal arcus is a rare condition associated with contralateral carotid artery disease or ocular hypotony. Arcus is also seen in Schnyder corneal dystrophy and osteogenesis imperfecta.

Crocodile shagreen

Anterior crocodile shagreen, or *mosaic degeneration,* is a bilateral, usually visually insignificant condition with a characteristic mosaic pattern. It consists of centrally located polygonal, gray opacities at the level of the Bowman layer that are separated by clear zones. Histologically, the Bowman layer is indented, forming ridges, and may be calcified. In posterior crocodile shagreen, there are similar changes in the deep stroma, near the Descemet membrane.

Cornea farinata

Cornea farinata is an involutional change, most likely dominantly transmitted, in which the deep corneal stroma shows many subtle dotlike and comma-shaped opacities (Fig 6-10). These opacities are often best seen in retroillumination. The opacities in pre-Descemet corneal dystrophy are similar but larger and more polymorphous. Confocal microscopy reveals highly reflective particles in the cytoplasm of keratocytes in the deep stroma, adjacent to the corneal endothelial layer. No abnormalities are detected in the epithelial layer, in the mid-stromal layer, at the level of the Descemet membrane, or in the endothelial

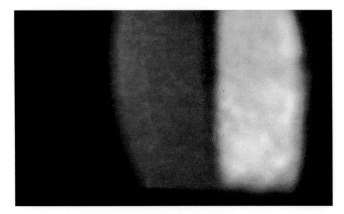

Figure 6-10 Cornea farinata, as seen in direct illumination. *(Courtesy of Robert W. Weisenthal, MD.)*

layer. The deposits may consist of lipofuscin, a degenerative pigment that appears in some aging cells. The condition does not affect vision and has no clinical significance, except that it is sometimes mistaken for a progressive dystrophy.

Polymorphic amyloid degeneration

Polymorphic amyloid degeneration is a bilaterally symmetric, primarily axial, and slowly progressive corneal degeneration that appears late in life and is characterized by amyloid deposition. The deposits, which can resemble some of those seen in early lattice corneal dystrophy type 3, form corneal opacities, appearing as stellate flecks in mid- to deep stroma and as irregular filaments. The opacities are gray to white and somewhat refractile, but they appear translucent in retroillumination (Fig 6-11). The intervening stroma appears clear, and vision is usually normal. There is also an *acquired* (secondary localized) corneal amyloidosis; see Chapter 8 for a discussion of the amyloidoses.

Senile furrow degeneration

Senile furrow degeneration is seen in older patients with corneal arcus and refers to an appearance of peripheral thinning in the lucid interval of the arcus (see the section "Corneal arcus," earlier in this chapter). Although slight thinning is occasionally present, it is usually more apparent than real. True thinning can eventually occur in the affected area and should be considered by the cataract surgeon, particularly with placement of the clear corneal incision, because of the risk of wound leak. The corneal epithelium is intact. There is no inflammation, vascularization, or potential for perforation. Vision is rarely affected, and no treatment is required.

Terrien marginal degeneration

Terrien marginal degeneration is a noninflammatory, slowly progressive thinning of the peripheral cornea. It is usually bilateral but can be very asymmetric. Although individuals of any age can be affected, this degeneration appears primarily in those older than 40 years. Males and females are affected equally, with men affected slightly more frequently. The cause of this condition is unknown. Initially presenting in the superonasal area, the thinning spreads circumferentially; in rare cases, it involves the central cornea or

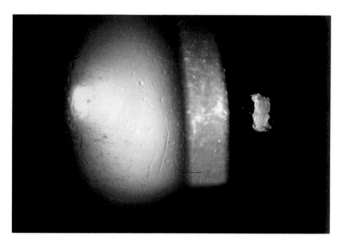

Figure 6-11 Polymorphic amyloid degeneration. *(Courtesy of Robert W. Weisenthal, MD.)*

inferior limbus. Affected patients are usually asymptomatic until the thinning results in increased astigmatism and subsequent reduction in vision.

The corneal epithelium remains intact, and a fine pannus traverses the area of stromal thinning. A line of lipid deposits appears at the leading edge of the pannus (central edge of the furrow) (Fig 6-12). Spontaneous perforation is rare, although it can easily occur with minor trauma. Ruptures in the Descemet membrane can result in acute corneal hydrops or even a corneal cyst. Corneal topography reveals flattening of the peripheral thinned cornea, with steepening of the corneal surface approximately 90° away from the midpoint of the thinned area. This pattern usually results in high against-the-rule or oblique astigmatism.

An inflammatory condition of the peripheral cornea that may resemble Terrien marginal degeneration occurs in rare instances in children and young adults and is also known as *Fuchs superficial marginal keratitis.* This condition may represent different clinical features of the same disease process.

Surgical correction is indicated when perforation is imminent because of progressive thinning, or when marked astigmatism significantly limits vision. Crescent-shaped

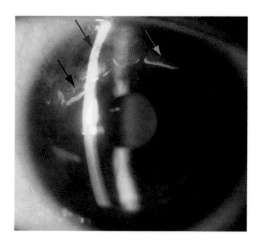

Figure 6-12 Terrien marginal degeneration with a fine vascular pannus *(black arrow),* superior thinning *(red arrow),* and lipid deposits *(green arrow)* at the leading edge of the pannus. *(Courtesy of Cornea Service, Paulista School of Medicine, Federal University of São Paulo.)*

lamellar or full-thickness corneoscleral patch grafts may be used; they have been reported to arrest the progression of severe against-the-rule astigmatism for up to 20 years. Annular lamellar keratoplasty grafts may be required in severe cases of 360° marginal degeneration.

Chan AT, Ulate R, Goldich Y, Rootman DS, Chan CC. Terrien marginal degeneration: clinical characteristics and outcomes. *Am J Ophthalmol.* 2015;160(5):867–872.e1.

Keenan JD, Mandel MR, Margolis TP. Peripheral ulcerative keratitis associated with vasculitis manifesting asymmetrically as Fuchs superficial marginal keratitis and Terrien marginal degeneration. *Cornea.* 2011;30(7):825–827.

Salzmann nodular degeneration

Salzmann nodular degeneration is a noninflammatory corneal degeneration that some-times occurs as a late sequela to long-standing keratitis such as phlyctenulosis, trachoma, and interstitial keratitis; it may also be idiopathic. The degeneration may not appear until years after the active keratitis has subsided. It can be bilateral and is more common in middle-aged and older women. The nodules are gray-white or blue-white and elevated (Fig 6-13). They often develop in a roughly circular configuration in the central or para-central cornea and at the ends of vessels of a pannus.

Histologic examination reveals localized replacement of the Bowman layer with hya-line and fibrillar material, probably representing basement membrane and material similar to that found in spheroidal degeneration (discussed earlier). Confocal microscopy reveals elongated basal epithelial cells and activated keratocytes in the anterior stroma, near the nodules; occasionally, subbasal nerves and tortuous stromal nerve bundles are also seen.

Treatment for mild cases is ocular lubrication; manual superficial keratectomy may be indicated in more severe cases (those causing decreased vision secondary to irregular astigmatism). This degeneration may recur after removal of the nodules.

A variant of Salzmann nodular degeneration, called *peripheral hypertrophic subepi-thelial corneal degeneration,* has been described. It is most common in women. Bilateral, fairly symmetric, peripheral, and hypertrophic subepithelial corneal opacification is pres-ent. Adjacent superficial limbal vascularization with occasional pseudopterygium has

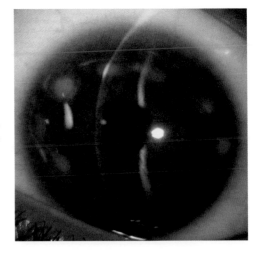

Figure 6-13 Slit-lamp biomicroscopy image shows elevated gray-white Salzmann nodules in a roughly circular configuration in the para-central cornea. *(Courtesy of Cornea Service, Paulista School of Medicine, Federal University of São Paulo.)*

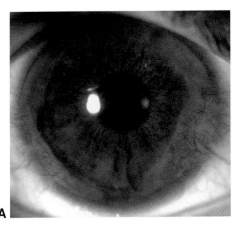 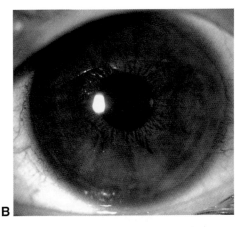

A   **B**

Figure 6-14 Peripheral hypertrophic subepithelial corneal degeneration, with elevated circumferential corneal opacities. **A,** Pseudopterygia are present in the right eye. **B,** The left eye shows fairly symmetric opacification. *(Courtesy of Cornea Service, Paulista School of Medicine, Federal University of São Paulo.)*

been noted (Fig 6-14). Underlying chronic ocular surface inflammation is absent, and minimal relief of ocular irritation is achieved with topical corticosteroids.

> Gore DM, Iovieno A, Connell BJ, Alexander R, Meligonis G, Dart JK. Peripheral hypertrophic subepithelial corneal degeneration: nomenclature, phenotypes, and long-term outcomes. *Ophthalmology.* 2013;120(5):892–898.
>
> Roszkowska AM, Aragona P, Spinella R, Pisani A, Puzzolo D, Micali A. Morphologic and confocal investigation on Salzmann nodular degeneration of the cornea. *Invest Ophthalmol Vis Sci.* 2011;52(8):5910–5919.

Corneal keloid

Corneal keloids are superficial, sometimes protuberant, glistening, white corneal masses that can eventually involve the entire corneal surface. They are thought to be secondary to a vigorous fibrotic response to corneal injury or chronic ocular surface inflammation. Keloids can be congenital or primary, and they have been reported in association with many congenital conditions, such as Lowe disease (oculocerebrorenal syndrome). They have sometimes been confused with hypertrophic scars, Salzmann degeneration, or dermoids. Treatment of symptomatic patients may include superficial keratectomy or penetrating or lamellar keratoplasty.

> Bakhtiari P, Agarwal DR, Fernandez AA, et al. Corneal keloid: report of natural history and outcome of surgical management in two cases. *Cornea.* 2013;32(12):1621–1624.

Lipid keratopathy

In lipid keratopathy, yellow or cream-colored lipids containing cholesterol, neutral fats, and glycoproteins are deposited in the superficial or deeper cornea, usually after prolonged corneal inflammation with scarring and corneal vascularization (eg, herpes simplex or herpes zoster keratitis, interstitial keratitis, including syphilitic). This form is best described as *secondary lipid keratopathy* (Fig 6-15). In rare instances, lipid keratopathy

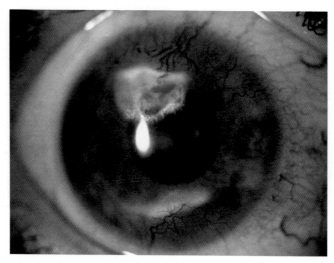

Figure 6-15 Lipid keratopathy secondary to corneal vascularization. *(Courtesy of Cornea Service, Paulista School of Medicine, Federal University of São Paulo.)*

has been reported with no evidence of an antecedent infection, inflammatory process, or corneal damage. These cases are best described as *primary lipid keratopathy*. Treatment is indicated in cases of decreased vision or compromised cosmetic appearance. Lipid keratopathy should be distinguished from Schnyder corneal dystrophy, a rare autosomal dominant stromal dystrophy characterized by bilateral corneal opacification resulting from an abnormal accumulation of cholesterol and lipid. Controlling the neovascularization with topical corticosteroids may reduce or even stop progression of the keratopathy. Argon laser treatment with and without fluorescein, photodynamic therapy with verteporfin, and subconjunctival and topical bevacizumab have been reported to reduce corneal neovascularization and lipid deposition.

Chang JH, Garg NK, Lunde E, Han KY, Jain S, Azar DT. Corneal neovascularization: an anti-VEGF therapy review. *Surv Ophthalmol.* 2012;57(5):415–429.

Goh YW, McGhee CN, Patel DV, Barnes R, Misra S. Treatment of herpes zoster–related corneal neovascularization and lipid keratopathy by photodynamic therapy. *Clin Exp Optom.* 2014;97(3):274–277.

Endothelial Degenerations

Iridocorneal endothelial syndrome

Iridocorneal endothelial (ICE) syndrome is a spectrum of disorders characterized by varying degrees of iris changes, pupillary anomalies, structural and proliferative abnormalities of the corneal endothelium, and peripheral anterior synechiae. Three clinical variants of ICE syndrome have been described in the literature. When the disease is confined to the inner corneal surface, corneal edema may occur as a result of subnormal endothelial pump function *(Chandler syndrome)*. When the abnormal endothelium spreads onto the surface of the iris, the resulting contractile membrane may produce iris atrophy, corectopia, and polycoria—hallmarks of *essential (progressive) iris atrophy* (Fig 6-16). The third

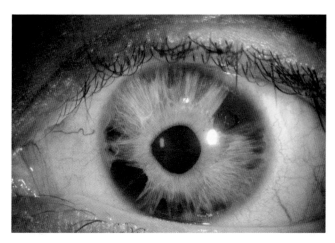

Figure 6-16 Iridocorneal endothelial syndrome, essential iris atrophy variant, with corectopia. *(Courtesy of Stephen Orlin, MD.)*

variant, *Cogan-Reese syndrome (iris nevus syndrome)* is characterized by the presence of multiple pigmented iris nodules, which are also produced by the contracting endothelial membrane. The syndrome occurs most commonly in middle-aged women and is almost always unilateral.

The pathogenesis of ICE syndrome is unknown but appears to involve abnormal cloning of endothelial cells, which take on the ultrastructural characteristics of epithelial cells ("ICE cells"). It is not clear when the abnormal cloning occurs, however. Herpesvirus may be causative, as viral DNA has been identified in some corneal biopsy specimens following keratoplasty and in the aqueous humor of some ICE patients. ICE cells seen with specular microscopy are typically abnormal, large, rounded, and pleomorphic. They show a characteristic reversal of the normal "light-dark" pattern; thus, the surface appears dark with an occasional central light spot, and the intercellular borders appear light. In vivo confocal microscopy shows ICE cells to be pleomorphic epithelial-like endothelial cells with hyperreflective nuclei and cell borders that appear brighter than cell surfaces.

Varying degrees of progressive endothelialization take place in the cornea, in the anterior chamber angle, and on the iris surface. Gonioscopy demonstrates broad-based iridotrabecular synechiae, which are due to the proliferation and migration of abnormal endothelium over the anterior chamber angle and which result in outflow obstruction and secondary glaucoma. Ultrasound biomicroscopy (UBM) is useful for detecting changes in angle structures in ICE syndrome, especially in the presence of corneal edema that does not allow visualization with gonioscopy.

The differential diagnosis of ICE syndrome should include asymmetric posterior polymorphous dystrophy and other causes of unilateral corneal edema.

Treatment options for the corneal component of this syndrome are penetrating keratoplasty and endothelial keratoplasty. Treatment of the glaucoma can be challenging, as filtering surgery may fail because of the progressive growth of the abnormal endothelial membrane extending over the trabecular meshwork and filtration site. Implanted tube shunts may overcome regrowth of the membrane in the filtration site. Long-term graft clarity depends on the successful control of intraocular pressure, which can be difficult (see BCSC Section 10, *Glaucoma*). Definitive keratoprosthesis may be an alternative to repeated traditional keratoplasty.

Carpel EF. Iridocorneal endothelial syndrome. In: Mannis MJ, Holland EJ, eds. *Cornea.* Vol 1. 4th ed. Philadelphia: Elsevier; 2017:844–855.

Phillips DL, Goins KM, Greiner MA, Alward WL, Kwon YH, Wagoner MD. Boston type 1 keratoprosthesis for iridocorneal endothelial syndromes. *Cornea.* 2015;34(11): 1383–1386.

Quek DT, Wong CW, Wong TT, et al. Graft failure and intraocular pressure control after keratoplasty in iridocorneal endothelial syndrome. *Am J Ophthalmol.* 2015;160(3): 422–429.e1.

Sacchetti M, Mantelli F, Marenco M, Macchi I, Ambrosio O, Rama P. Diagnosis and management of iridocorneal endothelial syndrome. *Biomed Res Int.* 2015;2015:763093.

Peripheral cornea guttae

Peripheral cornea guttae (Hassall-Henle bodies) are small wartlike excrescences that appear in the peripheral portion of the Descemet membrane. A normal change with aging, they result from thickening of the Descemet membrane, which takes place throughout life, and occur on the posterior part of the membrane, protruding toward the anterior chamber. With the slit lamp, Hassall-Henle bodies have the appearance of small, dark dimples within the endothelial mosaic; these are best seen by specular reflection. Rarely seen before age 20 years, Hassall-Henle bodies then increase steadily in number with age. When they appear in the central cornea, they are pathologic and are called *cornea guttae.* Central cornea guttae associated with progressive stromal and eventually epithelial edema represent Fuchs endothelial corneal dystrophy (see Chapter 7).

Melanin pigmentation

Deposits of melanin on the corneal endothelium can be seen in patients with glaucoma associated with pigment dispersion syndrome. The cluster of vertically oriented spindle-shaped pigment deposits is usually referred to as *Krukenberg spindle* (see Table 6-3). Transillumination defects in the midperipheral iris can also be seen.

Degenerations of the Sclera

The sclera becomes less elastic with age, and there is a relative decrease in scleral hydration and the amount of mucopolysaccharide. These changes are accompanied by subconjunctival deposition of fat, which gives the sclera a yellowish appearance. Calcium may also be deposited either diffusely among the scleral collagen fibers in granular or crystalline form or focally in a plaque anterior to the horizontal rectus muscle insertions. This senile plaque *(Cogan plaque)* is visible as an ovoid or rectangular zone of grayish translucency (Fig 6-17) and is sometimes mistaken for a pigmented tumor. Histologically, the midportion of the involved sclera contains a focal calcified plaque surrounded by relatively acellular collagen. These plaques do not elicit inflammation and rarely extrude. If sufficiently dense, they may be visualized on a computed tomography scan.

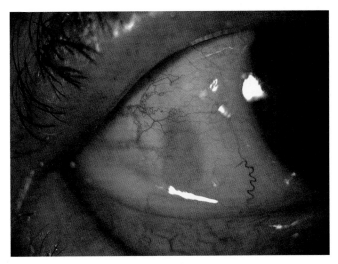

Figure 6-17 Senile scleral plaque (Cogan plaque) anterior to the horizontal rectus muscle insertions. *(Courtesy of Cornea Service, Paulista School of Medicine, Federal University of São Paulo.)*

Drug-Induced Deposition and Pigmentation

Ocular medications deposit within the cornea as a result of their concentration within the tear film, limbal vasculature, or aqueous humor or because of their chemical properties' specific affinity to corneal tissue. Certain drugs deposit in a characteristic fashion and particular corneal layer. The deposition of the drug may reduce vision, induce photosensitivity, or cause ocular irritation. Cessation of the drug often eliminates the symptoms and resolves the drug deposits. Most drug-induced deposition is not symptomatic, however, and does not require cessation of the medication (Table 6-4).

Table 6-4 Systemic Drugs Associated With Cornea Verticillata

Aminoquinolines (amodiaquine, chloroquine, hydroxychloroquine)	Monobenzone (topical skin ointment)
	Naproxen
Amiodarone	Perhexiline maleate
Antacids	Phenothiazines (eg, chlorpromazine)
Atovaquone	Phenylbutazone
Clarithromycin	Practolol
Clofazimine	Retinoids (isotretinoin)
Gentamicin (subconjunctival)	Silver
Gold	Suramin
Ibuprofen	Tamoxifen
Immunoglobulins	Thioxanthenes (chlorprothixene, thiothixene)
Indomethacin	
Mepacrine	

Information from Hollander DA, Aldave AJ. Drug-induced corneal complications. *Curr Opin Ophthalmol.* 2004;15(6):541–548; and Tyagi AK, Kayarkar VV, McDonnell PJ. An unreported side effect of topical clarithromycin when used successfully to treat *Mycobacterium avium*-intracellulare keratitis. *Cornea.* 1999;18(5):606–607.

Corneal Epithelial Deposits

Cornea verticillata

Cornea verticillata, or *vortex keratopathy*, manifests as a clockwise whorl-like pattern of golden-brown or gray deposits in the inferior interpalpebral portion of the cornea (Fig 6-18). A variety of medications bind with the cellular lipids of the basal epithelial layer of the cornea because of their cationic, amphiphilic properties. Amiodarone, an antiarrhythmic drug, is the most common cause of cornea verticillata, followed by chloroquine, hydroxychloroquine, indomethacin, and the phenothiazines (eg, chlorpromazine). See Table 6-4 for a comprehensive list of systemic drugs associated with cornea verticillata.

It is unusual for these deposits to result in reduced vision or ocular symptoms, although this has occurred in some patients. The deposits typically resolve with discontinuation of the responsible drugs. If there is reduced vision with the use of amiodarone or tamoxifen, the possibility of optic neuropathy should be considered. Retinal toxicity associated with the use of drugs belonging to the aminoquinoline family can also reduce vision (see BCSC Section 12, *Retina and Vitreous,* for further discussion of retinal toxicity). The differential diagnosis of cornea verticillata should also include Fabry disease, a disorder of sphingolipid metabolism.

Epithelial cysts

Due to the rapid turnover of epithelial cells, drugs that inhibit DNA synthesis may be toxic to the epithelium when used in high doses systemically. Cytarabine, for example, may cause punctate keratopathy and refractile epithelial microcysts, which are associated with pain, photophobia, foreign-body sensation, and reduced vision.

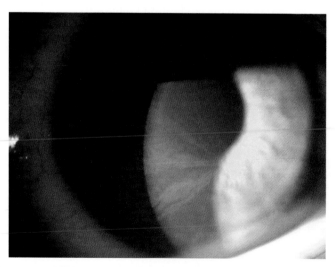

Figure 6-18 Cornea verticillata. A clockwise whorl-like pattern of golden-brown deposits can be seen in the inferior interpalpebral portion of the cornea. *(Courtesy of Cornea Service, Paulista School of Medicine, Federal University of São Paulo.)*

Ciprofloxacin deposits

Therapy with topical ciprofloxacin (and, less often, other fluoroquinolones) can result in the deposition of a chalky white precipitate composed of ciprofloxacin crystals within an epithelial defect (Fig 6-19). Although white plaques predominate, a crystalline pattern may also be seen. The deposits resolve after discontinuation of the medication.

Adrenochrome deposits

Long-term administration of epinephrine compounds, tetracycline, or minocycline may lead to adrenochrome deposition in the conjunctiva and cornea. Adrenochrome is an oxidation product of the basic epinephrine compound. The black or very dark-brown melanin-like deposits can accumulate in conjunctival cysts and concretions (Fig 6-20) and

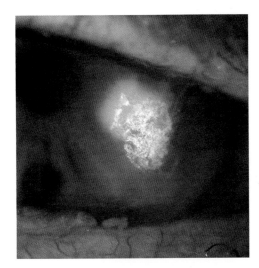

Figure 6-19 Ciprofloxacin deposits in the cornea. *(Courtesy of Robert W. Weisenthal, MD.)*

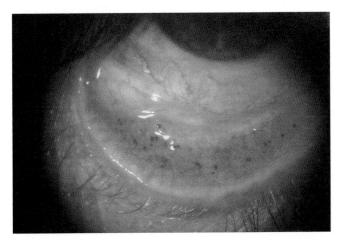

Figure 6-20 Adrenochrome deposits in the inferior cul-de-sac.

may also discolor the cornea or contact lenses. The deposits are harmless but are occasionally misdiagnosed as conjunctival melanoma or other conditions.

Kaiser PK, Pineda R, Albert DM, Shore JW. "Black cornea" after long-term epinephrine use. *Arch Ophthalmol.* 1992;110(9):1273–1275.

Stromal and Descemet Membrane Pigmentation

Chlorpromazine, a member of the phenothiazine family, may cause corneal pigmentation in up to a third of patients on long-term chlorpromazine therapy. It probably enters the cornea through the aqueous; therefore, the brown opacities are first found in the posterior stroma, Descemet membrane, and endothelium. The drug later spreads to the anterior stroma and epithelium. Chlorpromazine can also deposit on the anterior lens capsule. Clofazimine may produce anterior stromal opacities or crystalline deposits. Isotretinoin is typically associated with fine, diffuse, gray deposits in the central and peripheral cornea.

Certain classes of metallic compounds can produce characteristic deep stromal or Descemet opacities. Long-term use of silver compounds, which were commonly used in the preantibiotic era to treat external infections, can result in a condition known as *argyriasis,* a potentially permanent slate-gray or silver discoloration of the bulbar and palpebral conjunctiva. Silver nitrate, which is applied to the bulbar conjunctiva in the treatment of superior limbic keratoconjunctivitis, can also cause argyriasis if this compound is applied excessively. Gold salts are one of the drugs that can be used in the treatment of rheumatoid arthritis. With long-term usage and cumulative doses exceeding 1 g, posterior stromal deposits that spare the Descemet membrane and corneal endothelium develop in a high percentage of patients. See Table 6-3 for a list of corneal deposits that may be of diagnostic importance.

Palay DA. Corneal deposits. In: Mannis MJ, Holland EJ, eds. *Cornea.* Vol 1. 4th ed. Philadelphia: Elsevier; 2017:251–264.

Endothelial Manifestations

In rare instances, rifabutin has been described as causing stellate, refractile corneal endothelial deposits. These appear initially in the periphery but may extend to the central cornea.

Hollander DA, Aldave AJ. Drug-induced corneal complications. *Curr Opin Ophthalmol.* 2004; 15(6):541–548.

CHAPTER 7

Corneal Dystrophies and Ectasias

Highlights

- Recurrent erosions are typical of the keratoepithelin dystrophies affecting the epithelial basement membrane complex.
- Genetic analysis has dramatically reshaped our understanding of the corneal dystrophies.
- The location of stromal thinning relative to the area of corneal protrusion is important for identifying the specific ectatic disorder.

Corneal Dystrophies

General Considerations

Corneal dystrophies are commonly defined as bilateral, symmetric, inherited conditions that appear to have little or no relationship to environmental or systemic factors. Dystrophies begin early in life, are slowly progressive, increase with age, and may not become clinically apparent until years later. They are often characterized by the progressive accumulation of deposits. These deposits result from genetic mutations that lead to transcription of aberrant proteins. Mutations in the transforming growth factor beta–induced gene *(TGFBI),* which leads to production of the keratoepithelin protein, are an important example.

Many patients with corneal dystrophies associated with deposits present with symptoms of recurrent corneal erosion or blurred vision due to either irregular astigmatism or stromal opacification. This is particularly true when the pathology is more superficial, encroaching on the epithelial basement membrane complex. However, there are patients who experience blurred vision because of corneal edema (eg, as in Fuchs endothelial corneal dystrophy) or because of dystrophies not associated with deposits (eg, epithelial basement membrane dystrophy); the latter example may in fact be a degeneration rather than a dystrophy. In general, these conditions are in the process of redefinition and recharacterization.

To more accurately reflect the evolving genetic, clinical, and histologic characteristics of the dystrophies, the International Committee for the Classification of Corneal Dystrophies (IC3D) revised the dystrophy nomenclature. In this reclassification, recently updated, each dystrophy is classified into 1 of 4 groups: epithelial and subepithelial dystrophies, epithelial–stromal *TGFBI* dystrophies, stromal dystrophies, and endothelial

133

dystrophies. The dystrophies are described according to a template consisting of clinical, pathologic, and genetic information. The system is upgradable and can be retrieved at www.corneasociety.org.

In addition, the strength of evidence for each dystrophy is described using 1 of 4 assigned categories (Table 7-1). The category assignment may change as more information about an individual dystrophy is obtained. It is hoped that, over time, all valid corneal dystrophies will attain category 1 status. The IC3D classification of major corneal dystrophies is summarized in Table 7-2. A fairly comprehensive treatment of all corneal dystrophies is available in the IC3D publication and is beyond the scope of the BCSC. This chapter provides a basic discussion of the more common dystrophies for which there is the best evidence.

The genetics of major corneal dystrophies is summarized in Table 7-3. Although learning the genetics of each dystrophy is not critical to developing a basic understanding of these diseases, it is important to appreciate the significance of particular genetic mutations. For example, mutations in the *TGFBI* gene lead to most of the stromal corneal dystrophies associated with recurrent corneal erosions. In addition, there are dystrophies that appear the same phenotypically but differ genetically; conversely, dystrophies due to mutations in the same gene may have different phenotypes.

During the clinical examination, the ophthalmologist is encouraged to consider the following questions to determine whether a dystrophy is present and to differentiate between the corneal dystrophies:

- Are other family members affected?
- Are there signs of inflammation (eg, stromal cells or neovascularization)? If so, the condition may not be a dystrophy.
- Are the corneal opacities in both eyes and, if so, are they symmetric or asymmetric?
- In which corneal layer(s) do the opacities appear?
- Are there clear zones between the lesions?
- Do the lesions extend to the limbus?
- Is the cornea abnormally thick, thin, or of normal thickness?
- Is the morphology of the lesions suggestive of a corneal dystrophy?

Table 7-1 The IC3D Categories of Evidence for the Corneal Dystrophies

Category 1: A well-defined corneal dystrophy in which the gene has been mapped and identified and the specific mutations are known.

Category 2: A well-defined corneal dystrophy that has been mapped to one or more specific chromosomal loci, but the gene(s) remains to be identified.

Category 3: A well-defined corneal dystrophy in which the disorder has not yet been mapped to a chromosomal locus.

Category 4: Reserved for a suspected, new, or previously documented corneal dystrophy, although the evidence for its being a distinct entity is not yet convincing.

IC3D = International Committee for the Classification of Corneal Dystrophies.

Information taken from Weiss JS, Møller HU, Aldave A, et al. IC3D classification of corneal dystrophies—edition 2. *Cornea.* 2015;34(2):119.

Table 7-2 Major Corneal Dystrophies in the IC3D Classification

Epithelial and subepithelial dystrophies
1. Epithelial basement membrane dystrophy (EBMD): thought to be degenerative, C1 in rare cases
2. Meesmann epithelial corneal dystrophy (MECD): C1
3. Lisch epithelial corneal dystrophy (LECD): C2
4. Gelatinous droplike corneal dystrophy (GDLD): C1
5. Subepithelial mucinous corneal dystrophy (SMCD): C4
6. Epithelial recurrent erosion dystrophies (EREDs): C3

Epithelial–stromal *TGFBI* dystrophies
1. Reis-Bücklers corneal dystrophy (RBCD), atypical granular corneal dystrophy: C1
2. Thiel-Behnke corneal dystrophy (TBCD): C1
3. Lattice corneal dystrophy
   a. Lattice corneal dystrophy type 1 (LCD1): C1
   b. Lattice corneal dystrophy variants (III, IIIA, I/IIIA, and IV): C1
4. Granular corneal dystrophy
   a. Granular corneal dystrophy type 1 (GCD1): C1
   b. Granular corneal dystrophy type 2 (GCD2): C1

Stromal dystrophies
1. Macular corneal dystrophy (MCD): C1
2. Schnyder corneal dystrophy (SCD): C1
3. Congenital stromal corneal dystrophy (CSCD): C1
4. Fleck corneal dystrophy (FCD): C1
5. Posterior amorphous corneal dystrophy (PACD): C1
6. Pre-Descemet corneal dystrophy (PDCD): C1 associated with X-linked ichthyosis; C4

Endothelial dystrophies
1. Fuchs endothelial corneal dystrophy (FECD): C1, C2, or C3
2. Posterior polymorphous corneal dystrophy (PPCD): C1 or C2
3. Congenital hereditary endothelial dystrophy (CHED): C1

C = category; TGFBI = transforming growth factor beta–induced.

Adapted with permission from Weiss JS, Møller HU, Aldave A, et al. IC3D classification of corneal dystrophies—edition 2. *Cornea*. 2015;34(2):120.

Obtaining a family history is essential. Examination of biological relatives who have accompanied the patient to the office may be revealing, and genetic testing of the patient or affected family members may also be helpful.

For further discussion of genetics, see the genetics section in BCSC Section 2, *Fundamentals and Principles of Ophthalmology.* See also Section 4, *Ophthalmic Pathology and Intraocular Tumors,* Chapter 6.

Weiss JS, Møller HU, Aldave AJ, et al. IC3D classification of corneal dystrophies—edition 2. *Cornea*. 2015;34(2):117–159.

Epithelial and Subepithelial Dystrophies

Epithelial basement membrane dystrophy (EBMD)

Alternative names Map-dot-fingerprint dystrophy, Cogan microcystic epithelial dystrophy, anterior basement membrane dystrophy

Table 7-3 Genetics of the Major Corneal Dystrophies

Dystrophy	Gene Locus	Gene	Category
Epithelial basement membrane	5q31	Transforming growth factor beta–induced (TGFBI) in 2 families	Sporadic in most cases, C1 in rare cases
Meesmann	12q13	Keratin K3 (KRT3)	C1
Stocker-Holt variant	17q12	Keratin K12 (KRT12)	C1
Lisch	Xp22.3	Unknown	C2
Gelatinous droplike	1p32	Tumor-associated calcium signal transducer 2 (TACSTD2)	C1
Reis-Bücklers	5q31	TGFBI	C1
Thiel-Behnke	5q31	TGFBI	C1
Lattice type 1	5q31	TGFBI	C1
Granular type 1	5q31	TGFBI	C1
Granular type 2	5q31	TGFBI	C1
Macular	16q22	Carbohydrate sulfotransferase 6 (CHST6)	C1
Schnyder	1p36	UbiA prenyltransferase domain-containing protein 1 (UBIAD1)	C1
Congenital stromal	12q21.33	Decorin (DCN)	C1
Fleck	2q34	Phosphoinositide kinase, FYVE finger containing–PIKFYVE (PIKFYVE)	C1
Posterior amorphous	12q21.33	Deletion of keratocan (KERA), lumican (LUM), decorin (DCN), and epiphycan (EPYC)	C1
Pre-Descemet	Unknown	Unknown	C1 or C4
Fuchs	None (most commonly)	None (most commonly)	C3 (Fuchs in patients with no known inheritance)
	13pter-q12.13 (FECD2), 18q21.2-q21.3 (FECD3), 20p13-p12 (FECD4), 5q33.1-q35.2 (FECD5), 10p11.2 (FECD6), 9p24.1-p22.1 (FECD7), 15q25 (FECD8)	Unknown, transcription factor 4 (TCF4) on chromosome 18	C2 (Fuchs with known genetic loci but gene not yet localized)
Early-onset variant	1p34.3-p32	Collagen, type VIII, alpha-2 (COL8A2)	C1
Posterior polymorphous: PPCD1	20p11.2-q11.2	Unknown	C2
PPCD2	1p34.3-p32.3	Collagen, type VIII, alpha-2 (COL8A2)	C1
PPCD3	10p11.22	Zinc finger E box–binding homeobox 1 (ZEB1)	C1
Congenital hereditary endothelial*	20p13 (telomeric portion)	Solute carrier family 4, sodium borate transporter, member 11 (SLC4A11)	C1

C = category.

*Formerly divided into CHED1 and CHED2; no convincing evidence of autosomal dominant form.

Modified with permission from Weiss JS, Møller HU, Lisch W, et al. The IC3D classification of the corneal dystrophies. *Cornea.* 2008;27(Suppl 2):S1–S83.

Inheritance No well-documented inheritance; may be degenerative

Category Most cases are sporadic; however, category 1 in rare cases

PATHOLOGY EBMD is an abnormality of epithelial turnover, maturation, and production of basement membrane. Histologic findings include the following:

- sheets of intraepithelial, multilamellar basal lamina material (maps)
- intraepithelial extension of basal laminar material (fingerprint lines)
- intraepithelial pseudocysts containing cytoplasmic debris (dots)
- irregular, subepithelial accumulation of fibrogranular material (bleb)

CLINICAL PRESENTATION Epithelial basement membrane dystrophy occurs in 6%–18% of the population, more commonly in women, with increasing frequency in patients older than 50 years. Gray patches, pseudocysts, and/or fine lines in the corneal epithelium are noted on examination and are best seen by using a broad oblique slit-lamp beam or with retroillumination. (See Chapter 2 for a discussion of slit-lamp biomicroscopy.) The clinician can also identify EBMD by using the sclerotic scatter illumination technique or by using the slit lamp with a cobalt-blue filter after instilling fluorescein. Four kinds of patterns are seen:

- fingerprint lines
- maps
- dots
- bleb pattern (Bron)

These abnormalities occur in varying combinations and can change in number and distribution over time. *Fingerprint lines* are thin, relucent, parallel, hairlike lines; several of them can be arranged in a concentric pattern so that they resemble fingerprints or a horse's tail. *Maps* are geographic, irregular coastlines or islands of thickened, gray, hazy epithelium with scalloped, circumscribed borders (Fig 7-1). *Dots* are irregular round, oval,

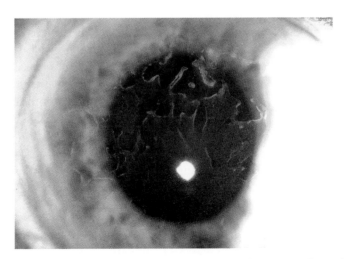

Figure 7-1 Epithelial basement membrane dystrophy (EBMD), seen using sclerotic scatter, demonstrates characteristic geographic maps. *(Courtesy of Robert S. Feder, MD.)*

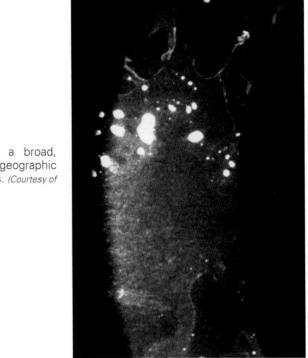

Figure 7-2 EBMD (seen using a broad, oblique slit beam) demonstrates geographic map areas and putty-gray opacities. *(Courtesy of Robert S. Feder, MD.)*

or comma-shaped intraepithelial opacities containing the debris of epithelial cells that collapsed and degenerated before reaching the epithelial surface (Fig 7-2). The *bleb pattern (Bron)* resembles pebbled glass and is best seen with retroillumination. The gray-white dots have discrete edges.

Symptoms are typically related to recurrent epithelial erosions and/or blurred vision, ghosting, or monocular diplopia, and while more common in patients older than 30 years, they can occur at any age. The impact of EBMD on vision correlates with the degree of surface disruption and induced irregular astigmatism, which can be detected on keratometry or corneal topography. Symptoms of recurrent erosions typically occur in the morning; however, discomfort in the morning may also occur in patients with nighttime lagophthalmos. Punctate erosions are usually noted in the inferior cornea in this setting. It is estimated that only 10% of patients with EBMD will have corneal erosions but that 50% of patients with recurrent epithelial erosions have evidence of this anterior dystrophy. Both eyes must be examined because evidence of the dystrophy may be found in the uninvolved eye. Unilateral dystrophic changes may be related to focal trauma rather than a dystrophy. In some cases, clinical findings may mimic corneal intraepithelial dysplasia; therefore, consideration should be given to submitting removed material for histologic study.

MANAGEMENT Asymptomatic patients may not require treatment. For patients with irregular astigmatism, epithelial debridement may be necessary. See Chapter 4 for a discussion of recurrent erosions.

Meesmann epithelial corneal dystrophy (MECD)

Variant Stocker-Holt

Inheritance Autosomal dominant (AD)

Category 1 (including the Stocker-Holt variant)

PATHOLOGY Intraepithelial cysts consisting of degenerated epithelial cell products (cellular debris that is periodic acid–Schiff [PAS] positive and fluoresces) are present. The epithelial cells contain an electron-dense accumulation of fibrogranular material surrounded by tangles of cytoplasmic filaments ("peculiar substance"). There are frequent mitoses and a thickened basement membrane with projections into the basal epithelium; the basal epithelial cells have increased levels of glycogen. On confocal microscopy, hyporeflective areas ranging from 40 to 150 µm in diameter are seen in the basal epithelium and contain potential reflective spots.

CLINICAL PRESENTATION Meesmann corneal dystrophy appears very early in life. Tiny intraepithelial vesicles are seen—most easily with retroillumination—extending to the limbus. These appear as minute bubblelike blebs (Fig 7-3). In 85% of eyes, the entire epithelium is affected. The epithelium surrounding the cyst is clear. Whorled and wedge-shaped epithelial patterns may be seen. The cornea may be slightly thinned, and corneal sensation may be reduced. Symptoms are usually limited to mild ocular irritation and a slight decrease in vision. Some patients report glare and light sensitivity. Painful recurrent erosions may occur.

The Stocker-Holt variant, which maps to a different gene, may have an earlier onset and demonstrate more severe signs and symptoms.

MANAGEMENT Most patients require no treatment, but soft contact lens wear may be helpful if symptoms are frequent.

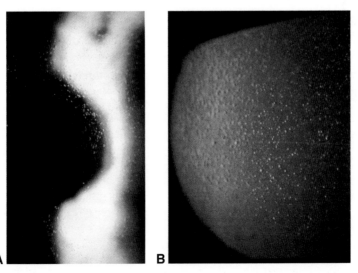

Figure 7-3   A, Meesmann corneal dystrophy, appearing as tiny bubblelike blebs with indirect slit-lamp illumination. **B,** Blebs are also well seen against the red reflex. *(Part A courtesy of Robert S. Feder, MD; part B courtesy of Richard Abbott, MD.)*

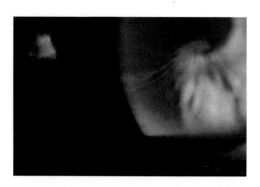

Figure 7-4 Lisch epithelial corneal dystrophy, characterized by bands of feathery, gray opacities. Retroillumination shows sectorial, densely crowded, clear microcysts in a feathery shape. *(Courtesy of Robert W. Weisenthal, MD.)*

Lisch epithelial corneal dystrophy (LECD)

Inheritance X-chromosomal dominant

Category 2

PATHOLOGY Diffuse cytoplasmic vacuolization of affected cells, which are PAS positive, is seen in light and transmission electron microscopy. On immunohistochemistry, there is scattered staining on Ki67 without evidence of increased mitotic activity. Confocal microscopy shows highly reflective cytoplasm and hyporeflective nuclei.

CLINICAL PRESENTATION On direct slit-lamp examination, discrete sectorial, band-shaped and feathery gray lesions are seen in whorled, flame-shaped, or feathery patterns. Retroillumination reveals intraepithelial, densely crowded, clear microcysts (Fig 7-4). The surrounding epithelium is clear. In Meesmann dystrophy, such band-shaped, feathery lesions do not exist, and the corneal involvement is more diffuse. Also, the intraepithelial cysts of Meesmann dystrophy are not as densely crowded as in Lisch dystrophy but are isolated, with clear spaces between the cysts.

MANAGEMENT Patients with Lisch dystrophy are pain free. There may be an associated decrease in vision. Corneal debridement may be attempted but often results in recurrence. Contact lenses may be helpful for more severe cases. There is one case report on the successful treatment of Lisch dystrophy (one eye) using photorefractive keratectomy (PRK) with mitomycin.

Alvarez-Fischer M, de Toledo JA, Barraquer RI. Lisch corneal dystrophy. *Cornea.* 2005;24(4): 494–495.

Lisch W, Büttner A, Oeffner F, et al. Lisch corneal dystrophy is genetically distinct from Meesmann corneal dystrophy and maps to xp22.3. *Am J Ophthalmol.* 2000;130(4): 461–468.

Wessel MM, Sarkar JS, Jakobiec FA, et al. Treatment of Lisch corneal dystrophy with photorefractive keratectomy and mitomycin C. *Cornea.* 2011;30(4):481–485.

Gelatinous droplike corneal dystrophy (GDLD)

Alternative names Subepithelial amyloidosis, primary familial amyloidosis

Inheritance Autosomal recessive (AR)

Category 1

PATHOLOGY Light microscopy shows subepithelial and stromal amyloid deposits. Disruption of epithelial tight junctions leads to abnormally high epithelial permeability. Confocal microscopy shows irregular, elongated epithelial cells with large accumulations of brightly reflective material noted within or beneath the epithelium and within the anterior stroma. Amyloid deposition is noted in the basal epithelial layer on transmission electron microscopy. See also Chapter 8 for discussion of amyloidosis.

CLINICAL PRESENTATION Onset occurs in the first to second decade of life with groups of multiple small nodules (mulberry configuration) or with subepithelial lesions that may appear similar to those of band keratopathy (Fig 7-5A, B). The lesions are visible on fluorescein staining. There is a significant decrease in vision, with photophobia, irritation, and tearing, as well as progression of protruding subepithelial lesions. Superficial vascularization is often seen. Stromal opacification or larger nodular lesions (kumquat-like lesions) may develop (Fig 7-5C).

MANAGEMENT The lesions recur within a few years in all patients following superficial keratectomy, lamellar keratoplasty (LK), or penetrating keratoplasty (PK). Soft contact lenses are effective in reducing the abnormal epithelial permeability to decrease recurrences.

Ide T, Nishida K, Maeda N, et al. A spectrum of clinical manifestations of gelatinous drop-like corneal dystrophy in Japan. *Am J Ophthalmol.* 2004;137(6):1081–1084.

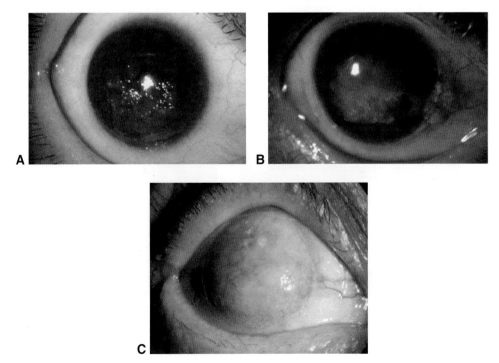

Figure 7-5 Gelatinous droplike corneal dystrophy. **A,** Mulberry type. **B,** Band keratopathy type. **C,** Kumquat-like type. *(Reproduced with permission from Weiss JS, Møller HU, Aldave AJ, et al. IC3D classification of corneal dystrophies—edition 2. Cornea. 2015;34(2):130).*

Epithelial–Stromal *TGFBI* Dystrophies

Reis-Bücklers corneal dystrophy (RBCD)

Alternative names Corneal dystrophy of Bowman layer type 1 (CDB1), atypical granular corneal dystrophy

Inheritance AD

Category 1

PATHOLOGY On light microscopy, the Bowman layer is disrupted or absent and replaced by a sheetlike connective tissue layer with granular deposits that stain red with Masson trichrome stain. Transmission electron microscopy shows subepithelial electron-dense, rod-shaped bodies. The rod-shaped bodies are immunopositive for the *TGFBI* protein, keratoepithelin. Electron microscopy is needed to histologically distinguish RBCD from Thiel-Behnke corneal dystrophy (TBCD), which has curly fibers (see the next section). On confocal microscopy, distinct deposits are found in the epithelium and Bowman layer. The basal epithelial cell layer shows high reflectivity associated with small granular deposits without any shadows (Fig 7-6A), as is seen in TBCD. The Bowman layer is replaced with highly reflective irregular material. Greater hyperreflectivity is seen at the Bowman layer in RBCD than in TBCD.

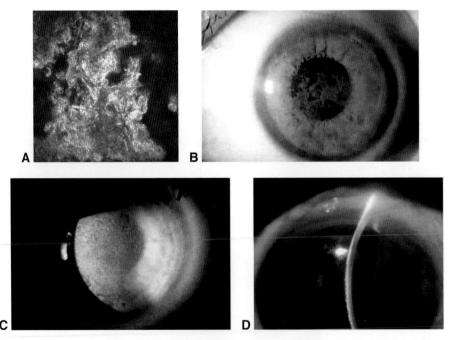

Figure 7-6 Reis-Bücklers corneal dystrophy. **A,** Confocal microscopy reveals highly reflective material without shadows in the basal epithelium. **B,** Coarse geographic opacity of the superficial cornea. **C,** Broad, oblique illumination shows a dense, reticular, superficial opacity. **D,** Slit-lamp photograph showing irregularities at the level of the Bowman layer. *(Part A reproduced with permission from Weiss JS, Møller HU, Aldave AJ, et al. IC3D classification of corneal dystrophies—edition 2. Cornea. 2015;34(2):132. Parts B–D reproduced with permission from Weiss JS, Møller HU, Lisch W, et al. The IC3D classification of the corneal dystrophies. Cornea. 2008;27(suppl 2):S1–S42.)*

CLINICAL PRESENTATION Reis-Bücklers corneal dystrophy appears in the first few years of life and mainly affects the Bowman layer. Confluent, irregular, and coarse geographic opacities with varying densities develop at the level of the Bowman layer and superficial stroma, mostly centrally (Fig 7-6B). With time, the opacities may extend to the limbus and deeper stroma (Fig 7-6C, D).

The posterior cornea appears normal. In advanced cases, stromal scarring can lead to surface irregularity. Symptoms often begin in the first or second decade of life with painful recurrent epithelial erosions. The erosions in RBCD are usually more severe and more frequent than those in TBCD, but they recur less often over time. Anterior scarring and associated surface irregularity both contribute to reduced vision.

MANAGEMENT Initial treatment is aimed at the recurrent erosions. Superficial keratectomy, LK, phototherapeutic keratectomy (PTK), or, in rare instances, PK may be performed. Recurrence in the graft is common.

Laibson PR. Anterior corneal dystrophies. In: Mannis MJ, Holland EJ, eds. *Cornea*. Vol 1. 4th ed. Philadelphia: Elsevier; 2017:770–780.

Thiel-Behnke corneal dystrophy (TBCD)

Alternative names Corneal dystrophy of Bowman layer type 2 (CDB2), honeycomb-shaped corneal dystrophy, Waardenburg-Jonkers corneal dystrophy

Inheritance AD

Category 1 (*TGFBI* variant), 2 (10q24 variant)

PATHOLOGY Light microscopy shows irregular thickening and thinning of the epithelial layer, which offset the ridges and furrows in the underlying stroma and the focal absences of the epithelial basement membrane. The Bowman layer is replaced with fibrocellular material in a pathognomonic wavy, "sawtoothed" pattern. On electron microscopy, curly fibers (9–15 nm) are apparent, distinguishing this dystrophy from RBCD. These curly fibers are immunopositive for the *TGFBI* protein, keratoepithelin, which is associated with the 5q31 locus. On confocal microscopy, distinct deposits are found in the epithelium and Bowman layer. The deposits in the basal epithelial cell layer show reflectivity, with round edges and dark shadows not seen in RBCD (Fig 7-7A). The Bowman layer is replaced with irregular reflective material that is less reflective than in RBCD. Optical coherence tomography (OCT) shows hyperreflective material at the level of the Bowman layer in the characteristic sawtoothed configuration that also distinguishes TBCD from RBCD (Fig 7-7B).

CLINICAL PRESENTATION Onset is in the first or second decade of life as solitary flecks at the level of the Bowman layer. Over time, symmetric subepithelial reticular opacities develop in a honeycomb pattern, sparing the peripheral cornea (Fig 7-7C). The opacities may progress to the deep stromal layers and the corneal periphery. Clinically distinguishing TBCD from RBCD is difficult, but noninvasive OCT and confocal microscopy may help differentiate these entities. Recurrent erosions in TBCD, which are less frequent and less

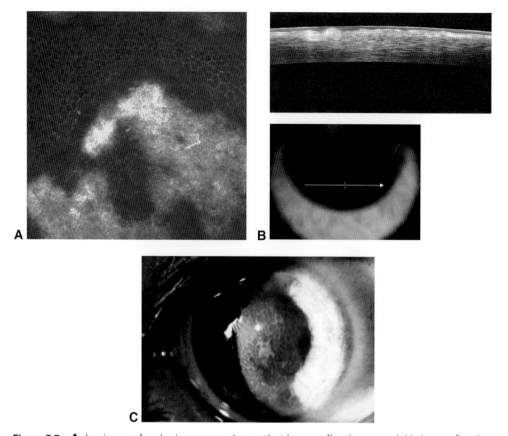

Figure 7-7 **A,** In vivo confocal microscopy shows that hyperreflective material is less reflective in Thiel-Behnke corneal dystrophy than in Reis-Bücklers dystrophy and reveals dark shadows in the basal epithelium not seen in Reis-Bücklers dystrophy. **B,** Anterior segment optical coherence tomography shows typical hyperreflective deposits in the characteristic sawtoothed configuration at the level of the Bowman layer. **C,** Subepithelial reticular (honeycomb) opacities of Thiel-Behnke corneal dystrophy. *(Parts A and B reproduced with permission from Weiss JS, Møller HU, Aldave AJ, et al. IC3D classification of corneal dystrophies—edition 2. Cornea. 2015;34(2):134. Part C reproduced with permission from Weiss JS, Møller HU, Lisch W, et al. The IC3D classification of the corneal dystrophies. Cornea. 2008;27(suppl 2):S1–S42.)*

severe than those in RBCD, cause ocular discomfort and pain. Vision decreases secondary to increased corneal opacification.

MANAGEMENT Management is similar to the approach used in RBCD.

Kobayashi A, Sugiyama K. In vivo laser confocal microscopy findings for Bowman's layer dystrophies (Thiel-Behnke and Reis-Bücklers corneal dystrophies). *Ophthalmology.* 2007; 114(1):69–75.

Küchle M, Green WR, Völcker HE, Barraquer J. Reevaluation of corneal dystrophies of Bowman's layer and the anterior stroma (Reis-Bücklers and Thiel-Behnke types): a light and electron microscopic study of eight corneas and a review of the literature. *Cornea.* 1995;14(4):333–354.

Weiss JS, Møller HU, Aldave AJ, et al. IC3D classification of corneal dystrophies—edition 2. *Cornea.* 2015;34(2):117–159.

Lattice corneal dystrophy type 1 (classic) (LCD1) and variants

Alternative names Biber-Haab-Dimmer

Inheritance AD

Category 1

PATHOLOGY Light microscopy of classic lattice dystrophy shows arborizing amyloid deposits concentrated most heavily in the anterior stroma. Amyloid may also accumulate in the subepithelial area, giving rise to poor epithelial–stromal adhesion. Epithelial atrophy and disruption, with degeneration of basal epithelial cells, and focal thinning or absence of the Bowman layer increase progressively with age. An eosinophilic layer develops between the epithelial basement membrane and Bowman layer, with stromal deposition of the amyloid substance distorting the corneal lamellar architecture. Amyloid stains rose to orange-red with Congo red dye and metachromatically with crystal violet dye (Table 7-4). It exhibits dichroism (shift from red-orange to apple green in response to a single rotating polarizing filter) and birefringence. (See BCSC Section 4, *Ophthalmic Pathology and Intraocular Tumors*, Chapter 6, for a discussion on birefringence [property of amyloid to change the axis of light polarization]). Electron microscopy reveals extracellular masses of fine 8–10-μm fibrils that are electron dense and randomly aligned. In vivo confocal microscopy reveals characteristic linear images that should be differentiated from those seen in infection with fungal hyphae (Fig 7-8). Corneal deposits caused by monoclonal gammopathy may resemble lattice lines.

CLINICAL PRESENTATION Lattice dystrophy is relatively common and is characterized by refractile branching lines in the corneal stroma. The spectrum of corneal changes is broad, and the classic branching lattice lines may not be present in all cases. Subtle refractile lines, central and subepithelial ovoid white dots, and diffuse anterior stromal haze appear early in life and, in a corneal graft, these may be the first signs of recurrence. The typical branching

---

Table 7-4 Histologic Differentiation of Granular, Lattice, Schnyder, and Macular Dystrophies

Dystrophy	Deposited Material	Masson Trichrome	Alcian Blue and Colloidal Iron	PAS	Oil red O and Sudan Black B	Congo Red
Granular type 1	Hyaline	+	–	–	–	–
Granular type 2 (granular-lattice)	Hyaline, amyloid*	+	–	–	–	+
Lattice type 1	Amyloid*	+	–	+	–	+
Schnyder	Phospholipid, cholesterol	–	–	–	+	–
Macular	Glycosaminoglycans (acid mucopolysaccharide)	–	+	–	–	–

PAS = periodic acid–Schiff.

*Amyloid also stains with thioflavine T and metachromatically with crystal violet. It demonstrates dichroism and birefringence with polarizing filters.

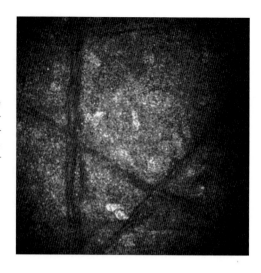

Figure 7-8 In vivo confocal microscopy image demonstrates filamentous lines that correspond to corneal stromal lattice lines. *(Reproduced with permission from Weiss JS, Møller HU, Aldave AJ, et al. IC3D classification of corneal dystrophies—edition 2. Cornea. 2015;34(2):136.)*

refractile lines, so-called lattice lines, develop as the condition progresses and are best seen against a red reflex or with indirect illumination (Fig 7-9). These lines start centrally and superficially and spread centrifugally, becoming deeper. The stroma can take on a "ground-glass" appearance, but the peripheral cornea typically remains clear. Epithelial erosions recur often and may occur as early as the first decade of life. Stromal haze and epithelial surface irregularity may decrease vision, typically in the fourth decade. Familial amyloidosis with lattice corneal changes (formerly lattice corneal dystrophy type 2) is no longer considered a dystrophy (see Chapter 8). Variant lattice dystrophy type IIIA is associated with severe erosions occurring later in life. Thick, ropy lattice lines and heavy amyloid deposits are seen (Fig 7-10). The findings in lattice dystrophy type IV occur more posteriorly than those in type IIIA and therefore type IV is less likely to be associated with erosions.

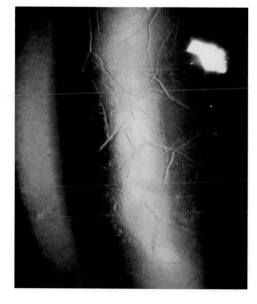

Figure 7-9 Classic lattice corneal dystrophy (LCD1).

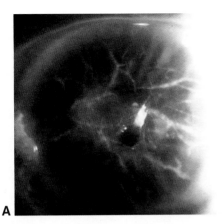 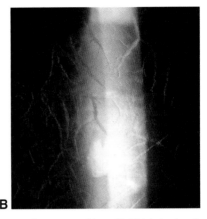

Figure 7-10 Variant lattice dystrophy type IIIA. **A,** Coarse linear opacities. **B,** Thick lattice lines are well seen on retroillumination. *(Courtesy of Robert S. Feder, MD.)*

MANAGEMENT Recurrent erosions are managed with therapeutic contact lenses, superficial keratectomy, or PTK. Severe cases of lattice dystrophy with vision loss are treated with deep anterior lamellar keratoplasty (DALK) or PK. Recurrence of this dystrophy in the corneal graft is common.

> Aldave AJ, Vo RC, de Sousa LB, Mannis MJ. The stromal dystrophies. In: Mannis MJ, Holland EJ, eds. *Cornea.* Vol 1. 4th ed. Philadelphia: Elsevier; 2017:781–799.
>
> Pradhan MA, Henderson RA, Patel D, McGhee CN, Vincent AL. Heavy chain amyloidosis in TGFBI-negative and Gelsolin-negative atypical lattice corneal dystrophy. *Cornea.* 2011; 30(10):1163–1166.
>
> Stock EL, Feder RS, O'Grady RB, Sugar J, Roth SI. Lattice corneal dystrophy type IIIA: clinical and histopathologic correlations. *Arch Ophthalmol.* 1991;109(3):354–358.

Granular corneal dystrophy type 1 (classic) (GCD1)

See Table 7-4 for information on the histologic identification of granular corneal dystrophy.

Alternative names Groenouw corneal dystrophy type I

Inheritance AD

Category 1

PATHOLOGY Microscopically, the granular material is hyaline, and it stains bright red with Masson trichrome stain. An electron-dense material made up of rod-shaped bodies immersed in an amorphous matrix is seen on electron microscopy. Histochemically, the deposits are noncollagenous protein that may derive from the corneal epithelium and/or keratocytes. Hyperreflective opacities are seen on confocal microscopy. Although the exact cause is unknown, a mutation different from that in RBCD, LCD1, and granular corneal dystrophy type 2 (GCD2; granular-lattice) has been identified in the *TGFBI* gene on 5q31, which is responsible for the formation of keratoepithelin.

CLINICAL PRESENTATION Onset occurs early in life with crumblike opacities in the superficial cornea. With direct illumination, the opacities appear white; however, indirect

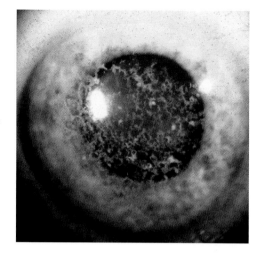

Figure 7-11 Granular corneal dystrophy type 1. *(Courtesy of Robert S. Feder, MD.)*

illumination reveals small translucent dots with vacuoles and a glassy splinter or "crushed bread crumb" appearance. The lesions are separated by clear spaces early in the disease process but later become more confluent. The lesions do not extend to the limbus but can extend anteriorly through focal breaks in the Bowman layer (Fig 7-11). The dystrophy is slowly progressive, with most patients maintaining good vision and visual acuity, and only rarely dropping to 20/200 after age 50 years. Patients report glare and photophobia. Recurrent erosions occur and vision decreases as the opacities become more confluent.

MANAGEMENT Early in the disease process, no treatment is needed. Recurrent erosions may be treated with therapeutic contact lenses and superficial keratectomy. PTK may be effective temporarily. When vision is affected, DALK or PK has a good prognosis. The disease may recur in the graft after several years, presenting as fine subepithelial opacities anteriorly and peripherally in contrast to the original presentation. Laser refractive surgery should be avoided in patients with granular dystrophy because of the risk of haze.

Granular corneal dystrophy type 2 (GCD2)

Alternative names Avellino corneal dystrophy

Inheritance AD

Category 1

PATHOLOGY Pathologically, both the hyaline deposits typical of granular dystrophy and the amyloid deposits typical of lattice dystrophy are seen. These lesions extend from the basal epithelium to the deep corneal stroma. Individual opacities stain with the Masson trichrome or Congo red stain. The deposits appear as rod-shaped bodies on electron microscopy; randomly aligned fibrils of amyloid are also seen. Findings on confocal microscopy are a combination of those seen in GCD1 and LCD.

CLINICAL PRESENTATION Affected patients have a granular dystrophy both histologically and clinically, with shorter, whiter lattice lesions in addition to the granular lesions. Clinical findings in GCD2 differ from those in GCD1. Stellate-shaped, snowflake-like, and

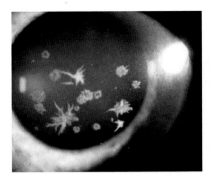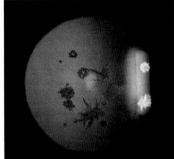

Figure 7-12 Granular corneal dystrophy type 2. Stellate-shaped opacities with intervening clear spaces can be seen in direct illumination *(left)* and in retroillumination *(right)*. *(Reproduced with permission from Weiss JS, Møller HU, Aldave AJ, et al. IC3D classification of corneal dystrophies—edition 2. Cornea. 2015;34(2):141.)*

icicle-like opacities appear between the superficial stroma and midstroma (Fig 7-12). Lattice lines are also seen deeper than the snowflake opacities. Older patients have anterior stromal haze between deposits, which reduces vision. Pain may occur with mild corneal erosions.

MANAGEMENT Lamellar or penetrating keratoplasty may be useful, depending on the depth of the deposits. PTK may be considered as an alternative to reduce surface irregularity and increase corneal clarity. Laser in situ keratomileusis (LASIK) and PRK are contraindicated.

Aldave AJ, Vo RC, de Sousa LB, Mannis MJ. The stromal dystrophies. In: Mannis MJ, Holland EJ, eds. *Cornea.* Vol 1. 4th ed. Philadelphia: Elsevier; 2017:781–799.

Holland EJ, Daya SM, Stone EM, et al. Avellino corneal dystrophy. Clinical manifestations and natural history. *Ophthalmology.* 1992;99(10):1564–1568.

Kim TI, Hong JP, Ha BJ, Stulting RD, Kim EK. Determination of treatment strategies for granular corneal dystrophy type 2 using Fourier-domain optical coherence tomography. *Br J Ophthalmol.* 2010;94(3):341–345.

Weiss JS, Møller HU, Aldave AJ, et al. IC3D classification of corneal dystrophies—edition 2. *Cornea.* 2015;34(2):117–159.

Stromal Dystrophies

Macular corneal dystrophy (MCD)

Alternative names Groenouw corneal dystrophy type II

Inheritance AR

Category 1

PATHOLOGY The deposits in macular dystrophy are glycosaminoglycans (GAGs), or acid mucopolysaccharides, and they stain with colloidal iron and alcian blue (see Table 7-4). They accumulate in the endoplasmic reticulum and not in lysosomal vacuoles, as seen in systemic mucopolysaccharidoses. Electron microscopy reveals keratocytes and endothelial cells that stain positive for GAGs, as well as extracellular clumps of fibrogranular material that also stains for GAGs. On confocal microscopy, blurred accumulations of light-reflective material are seen in the anterior corneal stroma.

CLINICAL PRESENTATION Macular dystrophy occurs less frequently than the stromal dystrophies associated with mutations in the *TGFBI* gene. Unlike most corneal dystrophies, it has an autosomal recessive inheritance, involves the entire corneal stroma and periphery, and may involve the corneal endothelium. The corneas are clear at birth and begin to cloud between 3 and 9 years of age.

Patients with macular dystrophy initially show superficial, irregular, whitish, flecklike opacities that evolve into focal, gray-white, superficial stromal opacities with intervening haze. Unlike in GCD, the lesions progress to involve all layers of the cornea and extend to the corneal periphery. The opacities tend to be more superficial centrally and more posterior peripherally. Macular spots have indefinite edges (Fig 7-13). Involvement of the Descemet membrane and endothelium is indicated by the presence of guttate excrescences, but corneal edema does not occur. Dystrophic opacities in the periphery may also appear similar to keratic precipitates. Epithelial erosions rarely develop, but a severe decrease in vision typically occurs between 10 and 30 years of age. Hypoesthesia has been noted. Central corneal thinning is common and may appear similar to long-standing interstitial keratitis (IK), but the ghost vessels and thickened Descemet membrane seen in IK help differentiate the conditions.

There are 3 variants of macular dystrophy, and they are distinguished based on biochemical differences. In type I, the most prevalent form of macular dystrophy, antigenic keratan sulfate (AgKS) is lacking in the cornea, serum, and cartilage. In affected patients, there is normal synthesis of dermatan sulfate proteoglycan. Errors occur in the synthesis of keratan sulfate and in the activity of specific sulfotransferases involved in the sulfation of the keratan sulfate lactose aminoglycan side chain. In type IA, keratocytes show AgKS reactivity, but the extracellular material does not. There is no AgKS in the serum.

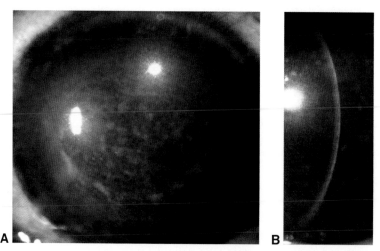

Figure 7-13 Macular dystrophy. **A,** Diffuse illumination shows involvement to the limbus with diffuse haze. **B,** Slit view. Typically, the cornea is thin with dense opacities that occur more posteriorly in the periphery. *(Courtesy of Robert S. Feder, MD.)*

In macular dystrophy type II, all of the abnormal deposits react positively with AgKS, and the serum has normal or lower levels of AgKS.

An enzyme-linked immunosorbent assay (ELISA) measures sulfated keratan sulfate. This test can help in the diagnosis of macular dystrophy, even in preclinical forms and carriers.

MANAGEMENT Recurrent erosions should be treated, and photophobia may be reduced with tinted contact lenses. PTK may be used for symptomatic anterior macular dystrophy. Definitive treatment requires PK or DALK, and recurrences are uncommon.

Aldave AJ, Vo RC, de Sousa LB, Mannis MJ. The stromal dystrophies. In: Mannis MJ, Holland EJ, eds. *Cornea*. Vol 1. 4th ed. Philadelphia: Elsevier; 2017:781–799.

Weiss JS, Møller HU, Aldave AJ, et al. IC3D classification of corneal dystrophies— edition 2. *Cornea*. 2015;34(2):117–159.

Schnyder corneal dystrophy (SCD)

Inheritance AD

Category 1

PATHOLOGY This condition is thought to be a local disorder of corneal lipid metabolism. Pathologically, the opacities are accumulations of unesterified and esterified cholesterol and phospholipids. Lipids stain with oil red O and Sudan black B (see Table 7-4). In the normal process of embedding tissue in paraffin, cholesterol and other fatty substances are dissolved; therefore, fresh tissue should be submitted to the pathologist for special lipid stains. Electron microscopy shows abnormal accumulation of lipid and dissolved cholesterol in the corneal epithelium, in the Bowman layer, and throughout the stroma. Confocal microscopy reveals disruption of the basal epithelial/subepithelial nerve plexus, with highly reflective intracellular and extracellular deposits.

CLINICAL PRESENTATION Schnyder corneal dystrophy is a rare, slowly progressive stromal dystrophy that may become apparent as early as in the first year of life. The diagnosis is usually made by the second or third decade of life, although it may be further delayed in patients who have the crystalline form of the disease. Central subepithelial crystals are seen in only 50% of patients and do not involve the epithelium. For this reason, the name Schnyder crystalline dystrophy has been replaced. Vision and corneal sensation decrease with age. Glare increases because of progressive corneal haze.

Changes are progressive and predictable by age, beginning with central corneal opacification:

1. ring or disclike central corneal opacification (can affect the entire corneal stromal thickness) ± subepithelial crystals (Fig 7-14A); individuals younger than 23 years
2. dense corneal arcus lipoides (Fig 7-14B); third decade of life
3. midperipheral corneal opacification (affects entire corneal stromal thickness); fourth decade
4. corneal sensation that decreases with age
5. abnormal lipid profile

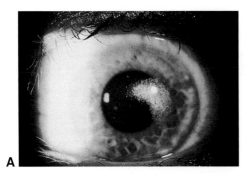 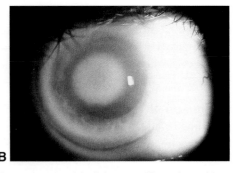

A **B**

Figure 7-14 Schnyder corneal dystrophy. **A,** Central subepithelial crystalline deposition. **B,** Central panstromal corneal opacity and arcus lipoides. No crystals are present. *(Courtesy of Jayne S. Weiss, MD.)*

MANAGEMENT Schnyder corneal dystrophy disproportionately reduces photopic vision (despite maintenance of excellent scotopic vision); thus, most SCD patients older than 50 years require corneal transplant surgery. The dystrophy can recur after PK or DALK. PTK has been used to treat decreased vision from subepithelial crystals, but it does not reduce panstromal haze. A fasting lipid profile should be done to detect possible hyperlipoproteinemia or hyperlipidemia. Patients with abnormal serum lipid levels are managed with dietary changes and/or medication, but the progression of the corneal dystrophy is unaltered. Unaffected family members may also have an abnormal lipid profile.

> Weiss JS. Visual morbidity in thirty-four families with Schnyder crystalline corneal dystrophy (an American Ophthalmological Society thesis). *Trans Am Ophthalmol Soc.* 2007;105:616–648.

Congenital stromal corneal dystrophy (CSCD)

Inheritance AD

Category 1

PATHOLOGY The stromal lamellae are separated from each other in a regular manner, sometimes with areas of amorphous deposition. On electron microscopy, the collagen fibril diameter is approximately half the normal size in all lamellae. Abnormal lamellar layers consisting of thin filaments arranged in an electron-lucent ground substance separate the lamellae of normal appearance. The keratocytes and endothelium are normal. The absence of the anterior banded zone of Descemet membrane has been reported. The epithelial cells are normal on confocal microscopy. Stromal evaluation is not possible because of increased reflectivity.

CLINICAL PRESENTATION Congenital diffuse, bilateral corneal clouding with flakelike, whitish opacities is found throughout the stroma (Fig 7-15). The corneas are thickened. The course is nonprogressive or slowly progressive, with moderate to severe vision loss.

MANAGEMENT Penetrating keratoplasty is recommended in advanced cases.

> Bredrup C, Knappskog PM, Majewski J, Rødahl E, Boman H. Congenital stromal dystrophy of the cornea caused by a mutation in the decorin gene. *Invest Ophthalmol Vis Sci.* 2005; 46(2):420–426.

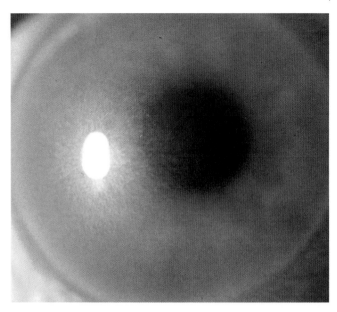

Figure 7-15 Congenital stromal corneal dystrophy: diffuse bilateral clouding with flakelike opacities throughout the stroma. *(Reproduced with permission from Weiss JS, Møller HU, Lisch W, et al. The IC3D classification of the corneal dystrophies. Cornea. 2008;27(10:Suppl 2):S22.)*

Fleck corneal dystrophy (FCD)

Alternative names François-Neetens speckled corneal dystrophy

Inheritance AD

Category 1

PATHOLOGY Affected keratocytes are vacuolated and contain 2 abnormal substances: excess glycosaminoglycan, which stains with alcian blue and colloidal iron; and lipids, which stain with Sudan black B and oil red O. Transmission electron microscopy shows membrane-based inclusions with delicate granular material. Confocal microscopy shows an accumulation of pathologic material in stromal cells and inclusions in the basal nerves.

CLINICAL PRESENTATION Fleck corneal dystrophy is a nonprogressive condition that may be congenital or may present early in the first decade of life. Discrete, flat, gray-white, dandrufflike (sometimes ring-shaped) opacities appear throughout the corneal stroma to its periphery (Fig 7-16). The epithelium, Bowman layer, Descemet membrane, and endothelium are not involved. Fleck dystrophy may be unilateral or bilateral but asymmetric. Symptoms are minimal, and vision is usually not reduced. Fleck dystrophy may be associated with decreased corneal sensation, limbal dermoid, keratoconus, central cloudy dystrophy, punctate cortical lens changes, pseudoxanthoma elasticum, or atopy.

MANAGEMENT None is required.

Purcell JJ Jr, Krachmer JH, Weingeist TA. Fleck corneal dystrophy. *Arch Ophthalmol.* 1977; 95(3):440–444.

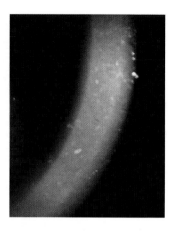

Figure 7-16 Dandrufflike opacities seen in Fleck corneal dystrophy. *(Reproduced with permission from Weiss JS, Møller HU, Lisch W, et al. The IC3D classification of the corneal dystrophies. Cornea. 2008;27(10:Suppl 2):S23.)*

Posterior amorphous corneal dystrophy (PACD)

Inheritance AD

Category 3; may be a mesodermal dysgenesis rather than a corneal dystrophy

PATHOLOGY Focal attenuation of corneal endothelial cells and irregular stromal architecture anterior to the Descemet membrane are seen on light microscopy. On electron microscopy, there is disorganization of the posterior stromal lamellae. A fibrillar layer interrupts the Descemet membrane. On confocal microscopy, there are microfolds and a hyperreflective layer in the posterior stroma.

CLINICAL PRESENTATION Posterior amorphous dystrophy presents in the first decade of life with a diffuse, sheetlike, gray-white opacity, usually in the posterior cornea (Fig 7-17). The condition is usually nonprogressive. The cornea is flat (<41 D) and thin (as thin as 380 μm),

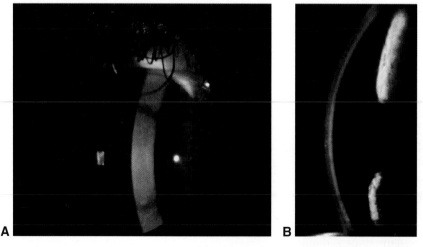

A   B

Figure 7-17 Posterior amorphous corneal dystrophy. **A,** Central, deep stromal pre-Descemet opacity. **B,** Slit-lamp photograph shows a diffusely thin, flat cornea with a posterior stromal opacity. *(Part A reproduced with permission from Weiss JS, Møller HU, Lisch W, et al. The IC3D classification of the corneal dystrophies. Cornea. 2008;27(Suppl 2):S24.)*

and there is associated hyperopia. Cornea plana, a bilateral familial disease caused by a mutation in the *KERA* gene, also has marked flattening of the cornea and is also stationary. In PACD, the Descemet membrane and the corneal endothelium may be indented by opacities. Focal endothelial abnormalities, a prominent Schwalbe line, fine iris processes, pupillary remnant, iridocorneal adhesions, corectopia, pseudopolycoria, and anterior stromal tags have been noted. There is no associated glaucoma. Visual acuity is usually 20/40 or better.

MANAGEMENT Although usually no treatment is required, PK is sometimes performed.

Dunn SP, Krachmer JH, Ching SS. New findings in posterior amorphous corneal dystrophy. *Arch Ophthalmol.* 1984;102(2):236–239.

Johnson AT, Folberg R, Vrabec MP, Florakis GJ, Stone EM, Krachmer JH. The pathology of posterior amorphous corneal dystrophy. *Ophthalmology.* 1990;97(1):104–109.

Pre-Descemet corneal dystrophy (PDCD)

Inheritance No definite pattern of inheritance, although PDCD has been described in families through 2–4 generations

Category 1 (PDCD associated with X-linked ichthyosis), 4 (isolated PDCD)

PATHOLOGY Large keratocytes are seen in the posterior stroma, with vacuoles and intracytoplasmic inclusions containing lipidlike material. On electron microscopy, there are membrane-bound intracellular vacuoles containing electron-dense material suggestive of secondary lysosomes, and there are inclusions consistent with lipofuscin-like lipoprotein, suggesting a degenerative process.

CLINICAL PRESENTATION Onset is usually after 30 years of age, but it has been reported in children as young as 3 years old. Focal fine, polymorphic, gray opacities that may be central, annular, or diffuse are seen in the deep stroma just anterior to the Descemet membrane (Fig 7-18). The rest of the cornea is unaffected. Vision is normal. Similar opacities

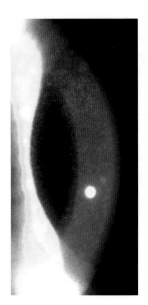

Figure 7-18 Pre-Descemet corneal dystrophy: punctate opacities just anterior to the Descemet membrane. *(Courtesy of Robert S. Feder, MD.)*

have been described in pseudoxanthoma elasticum, X-linked and recessive ichthyosis, keratoconus, posterior polymorphous corneal dystrophy, and EBMD.

MANAGEMENT None is indicated.

Endothelial Dystrophies

Fuchs endothelial corneal dystrophy (FECD)

Alternative names Endothelial corneal dystrophy

Inheritance Cases without known inheritance are most common; some cases with AD inheritance have been reported

Category 1 (early-onset FECD); 2 (FECD with known genetic loci but gene not yet localized, although transcription factor 4 [TCF4] may be implicated in these patients); 3 (FECD in patients with no known inheritance)

PATHOLOGY Microscopically, the endothelial cells are noted to be more varied in size (polymegethism) and more irregular in shape (pleomorphism) than normal and are disrupted by excrescences of collagen. Primary dysfunction of the endothelial cells manifests as increased corneal swelling and deposition of collagen and extracellular matrix in the Descemet membrane, which is thickened. There is a reduction in the number of Na^+,K^+-ATPase pump sites or in pump function. It is not clear whether the reduction in the posterior nonbanded zone and the increase in thickness of the abnormal posterior collagenous layer are primary effects of endothelial dysfunction or are secondary to chronic corneal edema.

CLINICAL PRESENTATION Findings vary with the severity of the disease. Cornea guttata is first evident centrally and then spreads toward the periphery (stage 1). In some patients, cornea guttata develops, and the disease never progresses beyond this stage (Fig 7-19). Cornea guttae may become confluent and take on a "beaten metal" appearance. Cornea guttae in late-onset FECD are larger than those seen in early-onset FECD. Stage 2 is characterized by endothelial decompensation and stromal edema (Fig 7-20). As the disease progresses, the Descemet membrane may become thickened, and stromal edema may worsen, causing epithelial bullae and bullous keratopathy (stage 3). The central corneal thickness may approach 1 mm (0.50–0.60 mm is typically considered normal). Subepithelial fibrosis, scarring, and peripheral superficial vascularization secondary to chronic edema occur in end-stage disease (stage 4).

Fuchs dystrophy usually presents in the fourth decade of life or later (except in the case of the early-onset variant, which may present as early as the first decade of life). Symptoms are rare before 50 years of age and are related to the edema, which causes a decrease in vision, contrast sensitivity, and/or glare. Pain may result from ruptured bullae or microcystic edema. Symptoms are often worse upon awakening because of decreased surface evaporation during sleep. Painful episodes may subside once subepithelial fibrosis occurs.

MANAGEMENT Initial treatment is aimed at reducing corneal edema, which typically begins in the morning, and relieving pain. Use of sodium chloride drops and ointment (5%),

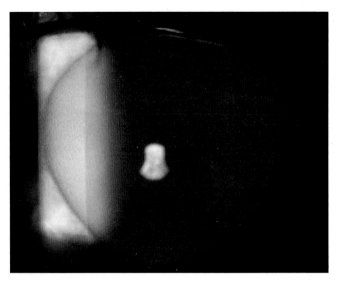

Figure 7-19 Fuchs endothelial corneal dystrophy. Cornea guttae are seen with indirect illumination over the iris and with the red reflex. *(Courtesy of Robert S. Feder, MD.)*

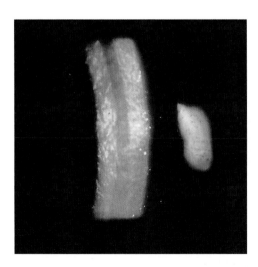

Figure 7-20 Fuchs endothelial corneal dystrophy showing the "beaten metal" appearance of the endothelium with mild stromal edema. *(Courtesy of Vincent P. deLuise, MD.)*

as well as measures taken to lower intraocular pressure (IOP), may temporarily help the edema. A bandage contact lens may be useful in treating ruptured bullae. In advanced cases, anterior stromal puncture, placement of amniotic membrane, or a conjunctival flap may be considered to relieve pain, but restoration of vision requires a corneal transplant. In the past, full-thickness (penetrating) keratoplasty was the standard procedure, but this has been largely replaced by endothelial keratoplasty (EK), as the latter targets the pathologic endothelial cells. In one recent case series, removal of a relatively small area of abnormal Descemet membrane and endothelium (descemetorhexis) resulted in mitosis of normal endothelial cells from the periphery, leading to resolution of the edema and improvement in vision. In the future, more traditional keratoplasty may be replaced with descemetorhexis combined with topical and/or intracameral Rho kinase (ROCK) inhibitor to stimulate endothelial proliferation. Another future treatment may be injection of the patient's own cultured endothelial cells. In advanced cases where there has been anterior corneal scarring, a full-thickness procedure may still be indicated. The prognosis for graft survival is good, especially if the procedure is done before vascularization occurs. See Chapter 15 for detailed discussion of corneal transplantation as well as new therapeutic modalities.

COMMENT Specular microscopy may be helpful in the initial evaluation of Fuchs dystrophy and in following the clinical course for loss of corneal endothelial cells; however, it is not necessary in the presence of diffuse confluent guttae. Corneal pachymetry may indicate relative corneal endothelial function, and the readings may change with progression of the disease; pachymetry can also be helpful in determining the relative safety of cataract or other intraocular surgery in a patient with FECD. Endothelial cell counts less than $1000/mm^2$, morning increase in corneal thickness, or the presence of epithelial edema suggests that the cornea may decompensate following intraocular surgery (see Chapter 2); thus, appropriate precautionary measures should be taken. See BCSC Section 11, *Lens and Cataract*.

Baratz KH, Tosakulwong N, Ryu E, et al. E2-2 protein and Fuchs's corneal dystrophy. *N Engl J Med.* 2010;363(11):1016–1024.

Borkar DS, Veldman P, Colby KA. Treatment of Fuchs endothelial dystrophy by Descemet stripping without endothelial keratoplasty. *Cornea.* 2016;35(10):1267–1273.

Gottsch JD, Sundin OH, Liu SH, et al. Inheritance of a novel *COL8A2* mutation defines a distinct early-onset subtype of Fuchs corneal dystrophy. *Invest Ophthalmol Vis Sci.* 2005; 46(6):1934–1939.

Li YJ, Minear MA, Rimmler J, et al. Replication of *TCF4* through association and linkage studies in late-onset Fuchs endothelial corneal dystrophy. *PLoS One* [serial online]. 2011; 6(4):e18044. Available at http://journals.plos.org/plosone/article?id=10.1371/journal.pone.0018044. Accessed November 20, 2017.

Posterior polymorphous corneal dystrophy (PPCD)

Alternative names Posterior polymorphous dystrophy (PPMD), Schlichting dystrophy

Inheritance AD (isolated unilateral cases with similar phenotype but no heredity reported)

Category 2 (PPCD1); 1 (PPCD2, PPCD3)

PATHOLOGY The most distinctive microscopic finding is the appearance of abnormal, multilayered corneal endothelial cells that look and behave like epithelial cells or fibroblasts. These endothelial cells have the following features or characteristics:

- microvilli
- positive immunohistochemical staining for keratin
- rapid and easy growth in cell culture
- intercellular desmosomes
- proliferative tendencies

A diffuse abnormality of Descemet membrane is common, including thickening of the posterior nonbanded layer, a multilaminated appearance, and polymorphous alterations.

Similar changes that are not limited to the cornea are seen in iridocorneal endothelial (ICE) syndrome (see Chapter 6). ICE, however, is sporadic and almost always unilateral. Specular microscopy may show typical vesicles and bands, in contrast to the involved cells in ICE syndrome, which appear as dark areas with central highlights and light peripheral borders. Opinion is divided on the value of relying on specular microscopy alone in making the diagnosis. Confocal microscopy reveals vesicular lesions and railroad track, band-like dark areas with irregular edges.

CLINICAL PRESENTATION Careful examination of the posterior corneal surface will show any or all of the following:

- isolated grouped endothelial vesicles (Fig 7-21A)
- geographic-shaped, discrete, gray lesions
- broad endothelial bands with scalloped edges (Fig 7-21B)

Various degrees of stromal edema, corectopia, and broad iridocorneal adhesions may also be seen (Fig 7-22). Fine, glasslike iridocorneal adhesions may be seen on gonioscopy. Both angle-closure and open-angle glaucoma can occur, and 14% of patients with PPCD have elevated IOP.

MANAGEMENT Most patients are asymptomatic. Mild corneal edema may be managed in the same manner as early Fuchs dystrophy. Anterior stromal puncture can be used to induce focal subepithelial fibrosis in cases of localized swelling. With more severe disease, keratoplasty may be required and, if present, glaucoma must be managed. If peripheral anterior synechiae, glaucoma, or both are present preoperatively, the prognosis for successful corneal transplant is reduced. PPCD may recur in the graft. In cases with limited stromal opacification, EK is the preferred approach for targeting the abnormal endothelial cells.

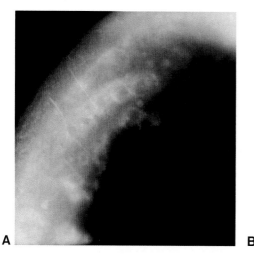 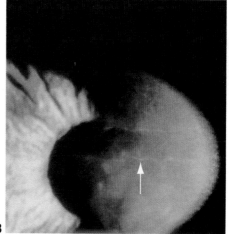

A   B

Figure 7-21 Findings in posterior polymorphous corneal dystrophy. **A,** Broad, oblique view shows clusters of endothelial vesicles, which are commonly seen. **B,** Scallop-edged endothelial band *(arrow)*. *(Part A courtesy of Robert S. Feder, MD.)*

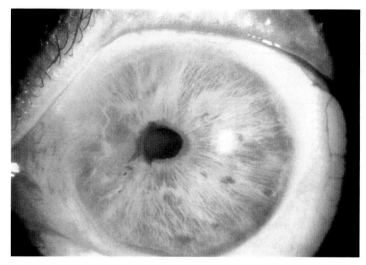

Figure 7-22 Posterior polymorphous corneal dystrophy showing iridocorneal adhesion and corectopia.

Weinstein JE, Weiss JS. Descemet membrane and endothelial dystrophies. In: Mannis MJ, Holland EJ, eds. *Cornea*. Vol 1. 4th ed. Philadelphia: Elsevier; 2017:800–817.

Congenital hereditary endothelial dystrophy (CHED)

Alternative names Formerly divided into 2 forms, CHED1 (AD) and CHED2 (AR); however, a careful review of the findings from reported families suggests that CHED1 is actually indistinct from CHED2.

Inheritance AR

Category 1

PATHOLOGY There is diffuse thickening and lamination of the Descemet membrane, with sparse atrophic corneal endothelial cells. On electron microscopy, multiple layers of basement membrane–like material are seen on the posterior part of the Descemet membrane, along with degeneration of the endothelial cells, which show many vacuoles. Stromal thickening with severe disorganization and disruption of the lamellar pattern is evident.

CLINICAL PRESENTATION This dystrophy is a congenital, usually nonprogressive condition with asymmetric corneal clouding and edema that ranges from a diffuse haze to a ground-glass appearance; focal gray spots are occasionally seen. Thickening of the cornea (2–3 times normal) occurs (Fig 7-23), with rare subepithelial band keratopathy and IOP elevation. Blurred vision and nystagmus occur with minimal to no tearing or photophobia.

MANAGEMENT Due to marked corneal edema present in more severe cases, corneal transplant (PK or EK) is required.

Weinstein JE, Weiss JS. Descemet membrane and endothelial dystrophies In: Mannis MJ, Holland EJ, eds. *Cornea*. Vol 1. 4th ed. Philadelphia: Elsevier; 2017:800–817.

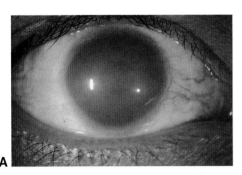
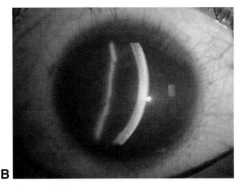

A **B**

Figure 7-23 Congenital hereditary endothelial dystrophy. **A,** Milky appearance of the cornea with diffuse illumination. **B,** Slit view shows diffuse stromal thickening. *(Reproduced with permission from Weiss JS, Møller H, Aldave A, et al. IC3D classification of corneal dystrophies—edition 2. Cornea. 2015;34(2):156.)*

Ectatic Disorders

Keratoconus

Keratoconus is a common disorder (incidence of about 1 per 2000) in which the central or paracentral cornea undergoes progressive thinning and protrusion, resulting in a cone-shaped cornea (Fig 7-24; see also Fig 7-35). A hereditary pattern is not prominent or predictable, but positive family histories have been reported in 6%–8% of cases. Multiple chromosomal loci for keratoconus have been reported, but the identification of specific genes remains elusive. Clinically unaffected first-degree relatives have a higher chance of showing subclinical topographic abnormalities associated with keratoconus than does the general population. The prevalence of keratoconus in first-degree relatives has been shown to be 3.34%. There is a slight female preponderance, and the incidence is higher in South Asia and the Middle East. Genetic predisposition and environmental risk factors such as eye rubbing, inflammation, atopy, hard contact lens wear, and oxidative stress all play a role in the onset and progression of keratoconus.

Onset occurs during puberty, and the progression rate is greatest in young people. Progression typically slows in the fourth decade of life and is unusual after age 40 years but

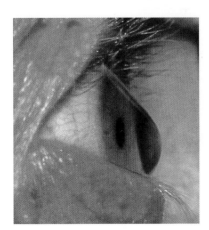

Figure 7-24 Keratoconus. Note the marked corneal protrusion, a hallmark of keratoconus.

can occur. The presence of hyperelastic joints may be as high as 50% in these patients. Keratoconus can be associated with ocular diseases such as vernal keratoconjunctivitis, Leber tapetoretinal degeneration, retinitis pigmentosa, and floppy eyelids. It can also be associated with systemic diseases, including atopic disease, Down syndrome, Ehlers-Danlos syndrome, osteogenesis imperfecta, sleep apnea, and mitral valve prolapse.

Feder RS, Neems LC. Noninflammatory ectatic disorders. In: Mannis MJ, Holland EJ, eds. *Cornea.* Vol 1. 4th ed. Philadelphia: Elsevier; 2017:820–843.

Kiliç A, Colin J. Advances in the surgical treatment of keratoconus. *Focal Points: Clinical Modules for Ophthalmologists.* San Francisco: American Academy of Ophthalmology; 2012, module 2.

McMonnies CW. Abnormal rubbing and keratectasia. *Eye Contact Lens.* 2007;33(6 Pt 1): 265–271.

Saidel MA, Paik JY, Garcia C, Russo P, Cao D, Bouchard C. Prevalence of sleep apnea syndrome and high-risk characteristics among keratoconus patients. *Cornea.* 2012;31(6): 600–603.

Wang Y, Rabinowitz YS, Rotter JI, Yang H. Genetic epidemiological study of keratoconus: evidence for major gene determination. *Am J Med Genet.* 2000;93(5):403–409.

PATHOLOGY Histologically, keratoconus shows the following:

- iron deposition in the basal epithelium at the base of the cone
- fragmentation or breaks of the Bowman layer
- thinning of the corneal stroma and overlying epithelium
- folds or breaks in the Descemet membrane
- variable amounts of apical scarring

CLINICAL PRESENTATION Nearly all cases are bilateral, but asymmetry is common. Early biomicroscopic and histologic findings include breaks in the Bowman layer followed by fibrous growth through the break, leading to reticular scarring (Fig 7-25). As progression

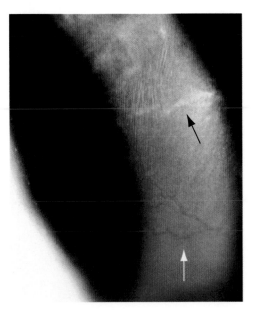

Figure 7-25 Broad, oblique slit-lamp image (high magnification). Breaks at the level of the Bowman layer *(white arrow)* are apparent. The *black arrow* indicates where collagen has presumably filled in a previous break. Vogt striae are also seen. This is the mechanism of the superficial reticular scarring seen in keratoconus. *(Reprinted from Shapiro MB, Rodrigues MM, Mandel MR, Krachmer JH. Anterior clear spaces in keratoconus. Ophthalmology. 1986;93(10):1316–1319.)*

occurs, the apical thinning of the central cornea worsens, as does the degree of irregular astigmatism. There is generally no associated keratitis or corneal neovascularization.

Scissoring of the red reflex on retinoscopy is commonly associated with irregular astigmatism and is an early sign of keratoconus. *Rizzutti sign,* a focusing of the light within the nasal limbus when a penlight is shone from the temporal side, is another early but nonspecific finding. *Munson sign,* an inferior deviation of the lower eyelid contour on downgaze (Fig 7-26), is also nonspecific and is a late sign. Iron deposition within the basal epithelium at the base of the cone forms a *Fleischer ring* (Fig 7-27), best seen with the slit lamp using a broad, oblique beam and the cobalt-blue filter. The line becomes narrower and increasingly well defined as the disease progresses. Fine, parallel stress lines, *Vogt striae,* can be observed in the posterior stroma at the apex of the cone and may clear with application of external pressure (Fig 7-28).

Spontaneous perforation in keratoconus is extremely rare. However, a tear can occur in the Descemet membrane, usually late in the disease course, resulting in the sudden development of corneal edema, or *acute hydrops* (Fig 7-29). Allergy and eye rubbing are

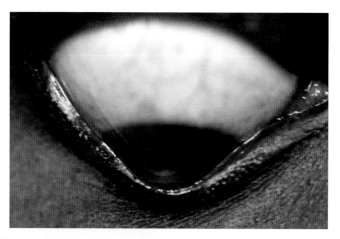

Figure 7-26 Munson sign. Note the angulation of the lower eyelid with the eye in downgaze. *(Courtesy of Woodford S. Van Meter, MD.)*

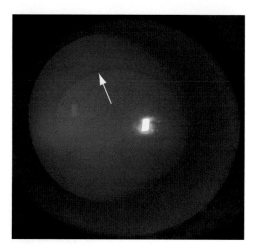

Figure 7-27 Fleischer ring *(arrow),* demonstrated using diffuse illumination with a cobalt-blue filter. *(Courtesy of James J. Reidy, MD.)*

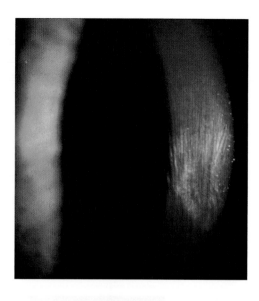

Figure 7-28 Vogt striae are fine folds in the posterior stroma at the cone apex. Striae become less apparent when external pressure is applied. *(Courtesy of Robert S. Feder, MD.)*

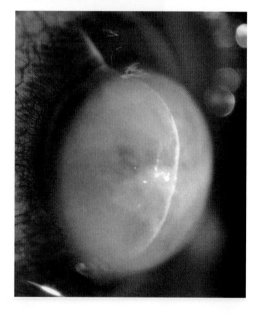

Figure 7-29 Corneal edema in keratoconus due to a sudden rupture of the Descemet membrane (acute hydrops). *(Courtesy of Robert S. Feder, MD.)*

risk factors for the development of hydrops, which is more common in patients with Down syndrome. The break in the posterior cornea usually heals spontaneously within 3 months; the corneal edema then disappears, but posterior stromal scarring occurs. Some patients experience improved vision following the resolution of hydrops because of apical flattening. The improved vision will depend on the extent and location of the scar. Occasionally, stromal clefts can be seen in association with hydrops. Even large clefts usually close, but corneal neovascularization can develop.

EVALUATION Keratometry can be used to detect keratoconus even at an early stage. Irregular astigmatism, indicated by the inability to superimpose the mires, is commonly seen. Inferior steepening, an early finding in keratoconus, can be detected by comparing measurements obtained with the patient in primary gaze to those in upgaze. Corneal topography and corneal tomography (Fig 7-30) have become indispensable in the management of keratoconus and are used by clinicians in several ways, such as detecting early keratoconus, following its progression, fitting contact lenses, and managing the postoperative patient. Important power map findings include superior flattening, inferior steepening, increase in I–S ratio (inferior to superior power), and significant skewing of the radial axes of the bow tie, in contrast to the normal symmetric bow-tie pattern of regular astigmatism. Findings obtained via slit-scanning devices, Scheimpflug imaging, or anterior segment OCT include decentered islands of elevation anteriorly and/or posteriorly. The elevation map is developed in reference to a computer-generated best-fit sphere.

These devices can also identify abnormal corneal thinning and/or decentration of the thinnest cornea, which is particularly significant when it is coincident with an island of

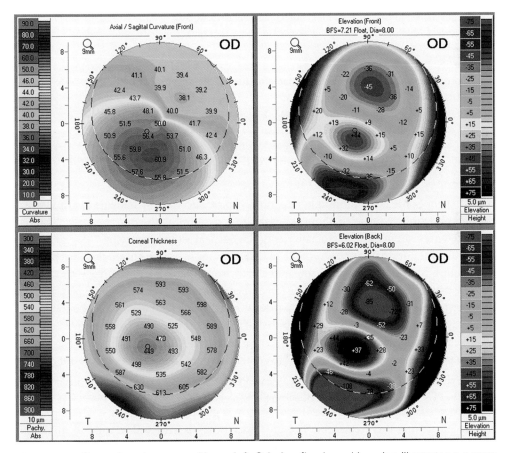

Figure 7-30 Corneal contour map. *Upper left:* Scheimpflug-based imaging illustrates a power map with inferior steepening and superior flattening. *Upper right:* An isolated island of anterior elevation above a best-fit sphere coincident with the maximum steepness. *Lower right:* An isolated island of posterior elevation. *Lower left:* Marked thinning in an area coincident with steepening and elevation. *(Courtesy of Robert S. Feder, MD.)*

elevation. Scheimpflug imaging and OCT have largely supplanted ultrasonic pachymetry. Accurate measurement of corneal thickness and elevation has been the cornerstone of recent advances in keratoconus detection programs. Examples of other advances are the various indices and graphic representations of both the change in thickness from thinnest cornea to limbus (more dramatic in keratoconus) and the impact of calculations of the best-fit sphere when the thinnest cornea is included or eliminated from the calculation. Serial evaluations over time are necessary to determine whether the changes noted are unlikely to progress (forme fruste keratoconus) or whether subclinical or suspected keratoconus is progressing and likely to become symptomatic. Corneal ectasia can also occur in association with ablative keratorefractive surgery (eg, LASIK or PRK). Risk factors for ectasia after LASIK or PRK are young age, high myopia, thin residual stromal bed, thin preoperative cornea, and abnormal preoperative contour. A young patient with a suspicious corneal contour who is considering refractive surgery should be observed over time to determine whether keratoconus will develop.

Feder RS. Corneal topography. In: Feder RS, ed. *The LASIK Handbook: A Case-based Approach.* 2nd ed. Philadelphia: Wolters Kluwer; 2013:32–39.

Gomes JA, Tan D, Rapuano CJ, et al. Global consensus on keratoconus and ectatic diseases. *Cornea.* 2015;34(4):359–369.

Rao SN, Raviv T, Majmudar PA, Epstein RJ. Role of Orbscan II in screening keratoconus suspects before refractive corneal surgery. *Ophthalmology.* 2002;109(9): 1642–1646.

Weisenthal R. Optical coherence tomography. In: Feder RS, ed. *The LASIK Handbook: A Case-based Approach.* 2nd ed. Philadelphia: Wolters Kluwer; 2013:40–46.

Yeu E, Belin MW, Khachikian SS. Topographic analysis in keratorefractive surgery. In: Mannis MJ, Holland EJ, eds. *Cornea.* Vol 1. 4th ed. Philadelphia: Elsevier; 2017: 1728–1735.

MANAGEMENT Some cases of mild keratoconus can be successfully managed with glasses. Patients should be counseled about the risk of progression with continued eye rubbing. Contact lenses can mask the associated irregular corneal astigmatism (Fig 7-31), and their use results in a dramatic improvement in vision in most cases. Although most patients will require hard or rigid gas-permeable lenses, some patients, particularly those with mild disease, may achieve improved vision and comfortable wear with soft lenses. Hybrid (gas-permeable contact lenses with a soft lens "skirt") or scleral lenses may be helpful in more advanced disease. A central subepithelial scar can, on occasion, be removed (superficial keratectomy), allowing continued comfortable wear of contact lenses. Intrastromal corneal ring segments can be implanted to center the cone and facilitate successful contact lens wear. The procedure does not prevent progression, however, and is not intended to reduce dependence on glasses or contact lenses. Corneal crosslinking is used in patients with progressive disease. The risk of progression is greater in adolescents, who may benefit the most from this treatment. The greatest efficacy is achieved in mild to moderate cases. Corneal crosslinking may not work as well in cases of post-LASIK ectasia or in patients with more severe disease. Crosslinking may be performed in concert with intrastromal ring insertion. See also BCSC Section 13, *Refractive Surgery.*

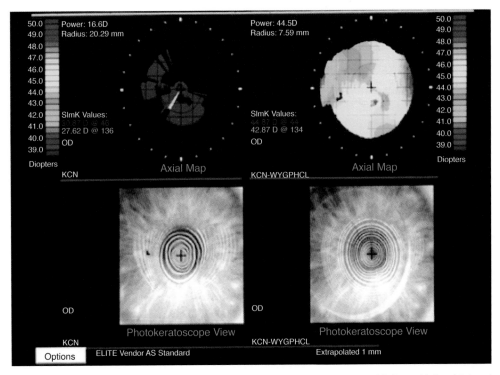

Figure 7-31 Hard contact lens effect on the keratoconus power map; with lens *(right side)* and without lens *(left side)*. *Upper left:* Apical scarring has resulted in flattening, as noted in the power map. *Lower left:* The corresponding videokeratoscopic image is irregular, and the rings are widely spaced. *Upper right:* The power map appears much more normal when acquired with the patient wearing a contact lens. *Lower right:* The videokeratoscopic image is also much more regular, with narrower spacing. *(Courtesy of Robert S. Feder, MD.)*

Keratoplasty becomes an important option under the following circumstances:

- poor vision even with a comfortable contact lens fit (usually due to scarring)
- contact lens intolerance even with good vision
- unstable contact lens fit (even with good vision and tolerance)
- progressive thinning to the corneal periphery approaching the limbus, requiring a very large graft (with increased risk)
- corneal hydrops that fails to clear after several months

PK is still the most widely performed surgical procedure for the treatment of keratoconus, and the prognosis is excellent. Some surgeons prefer DALK for keratoconus. Endothelial cell counts are significantly higher at 6 months following DALK compared with PK. Endothelial rejection does not occur after DALK, but stromal rejection is still possible. Postostoperative wound integrity in the case of postoperative trauma is better with DALK than with PK. (See Chapter 15 for further discussion of PK and DALK.)

Hydrops is treated conservatively with topical hypertonic agents and/or a soft contact lens for several months. A cycloplegic agent may help with pain relief. Aqueous suppressants may decrease the flow of fluid into the cornea. Intracameral injection of air or gas (SF_6 or C_3F_8) may help in speeding the resolution of hydrops. Pupil dilation and/or inferior peripheral iridectomy may reduce the risk of pupillary block. Hydrops is not an indication for emergency keratoplasty.

Feder RS, Neems LC. Noninflammatory ectatic disorders. In: Mannis MJ, Holland EJ, eds. *Cornea.* Vol 1. 4th ed. Philadelphia: Elsevier; 2017:820–843.

Kiliç A, Colin J. Advances in the surgical treatment of keratoconus. *Focal Points: Clinical Modules for Ophthalmologists.* San Francisco: American Academy of Ophthalmology; 2012, module 2.

Panda A, Aggarwal A, Madhavi P, et al. Management of acute corneal hydrops secondary to keratoconus with intracameral injection of sulfur hexafluoride (SF6). *Cornea.* 2007;26(9): 1067–1069.

Raiskup-Wolf F, Hoyer A, Spoerl E, Pillunat L. Collagen crosslinking with riboflavin and ultraviolet-A light in keratoconus: long-term results. *J Cataract Refract Surg.* 2008;34: 796–801.

Terry M, Ousley P. Deep lamellar endothelial keratoplasty visual acuity, astigmatism, and endothelial survival in a large prospective series. *Ophthalmology.* 2005;112(9):1541–1548.

Pellucid Marginal Degeneration

Pellucid marginal degeneration (PMD) is an uncommon, nonhereditary, and bilateral condition. It is associated with inferior, peripheral corneal thinning in the absence of inflammation. The etiology is unknown. PMD and keratoconus can occur in the same family or even in the same eye.

CLINICAL PRESENTATION Protrusion of the cornea occurs above the band of thinning (Fig 7-32), which occurs 1–2 mm from the limbus and extends up to 4 clock-hours. In keratoconus, the cornea protrudes at the point of maximal thinning, which is typically just below the center. In contrast, PMD is associated with peripheral thinning (Fig 7-33) and exhibits protrusion central to the area of maximum thinning. At times, a clear distinction between PMD and keratoconus is not possible. In PMD, no vascularization or lipid deposition occurs, but posterior stromal scarring has been noted within the thinned area. PMD

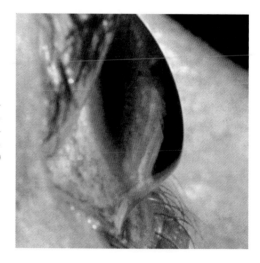

Figure 7-32 Typically in pellucid marginal degeneration there is inferior protrusion of the cornea above the band of thinning, which occurs 1–2 mm from the limbus and extends up to 4 clock-hours. *(Courtesy of Vincent P. deLuise, MD.)*

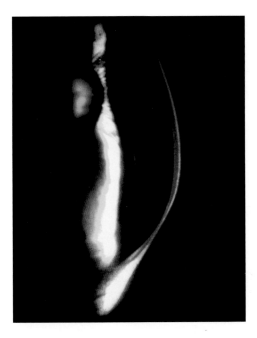

Figure 7-33 Slit view demonstrates protrusion of the cornea above a band of stromal thinning in pellucid marginal degeneration. *(Reproduced with permission from Feder RS, Neems LC. Noninflammatory ectatic disorders. In: Mannis MJ, Holland EJ, eds.* Cornea. *Vol 1. 4th ed. Philadelphia: Elsevier; 2017:836.)*

is diagnosed in most patients between 20 and 40 years of age, and men and women are affected equally. Decreased vision results from high irregular astigmatism. Acute hydrops has been reported, and, though rare, spontaneous corneal perforation has also occurred. While the "crab claw" pattern is the typical map appearance in PMD (Fig 7-34), inferior keratoconus has a similar appearance. Clinical correlation and review of elevation and pachymetric maps are important for more accurate differentiation.

MANAGEMENT Treatment consists of contact lens fitting early in the disease, although the fit is more difficult to achieve in PMD than in keratoconus. Hybrid or scleral lenses may be options. Eventually, PK may be required to restore vision. Because of the location of the thinning, the grafts tend to be large and close to the limbus, making surgery technically more difficult and the graft more prone to rejection. Wedge resection and lamellar tectonic grafts have been advocated as alternative or adjunctive procedures. Corneal crosslinking may also be considered for some of these patients.

Belin MW, Asota IM, Ambrosio R Jr, Khachikian SS. What's in a name: keratoconus, pellucid marginal degeneration, and related thinning disorders. *Am J Ophthalmol.* 2011;152(2): 157–162.

Rasheed K, Rabinowitz YS. Surgical treatment of advanced pellucid marginal degeneration. *Ophthalmology.* 2000;107(10):1836–1840.

Keratoglobus

Keratoglobus is a rare, bilateral, noninflammatory condition that is typically present at birth, unlike keratoconus and PMD. It is usually not hereditary. Keratoglobus manifests as a globular rather than a conical deformation of the cornea (Fig 7-35).

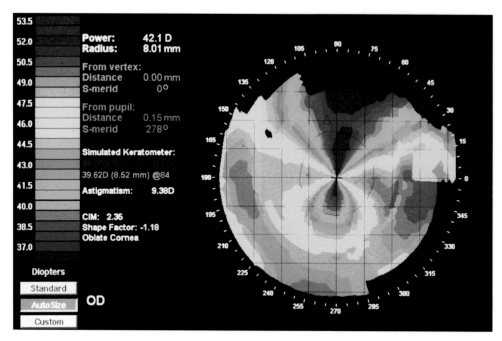

53.5	
52.0	**Power:** 42.1 D
	Radius: 8.01 mm
50.5	
	From vertex:
49.0	**Distance** 0.00 mm
	S-merid 0°
47.5	
	From pupil:
46.0	**Distance** 0.15 mm
	S-merid 278°
44.5	
	Simulated Keratometer:
43.0	49.00D (6.89 mm) @174
41.5	39.62D (8.52 mm) @84
	Astigmatism: 9.38D
40.0	
38.5	**CIM:** 2.35
	Shape Factor: -1.18
37.0	**Oblate Cornea**

Diopters

Standard
AutoSize OD
Custom

Figure 7-34 Power map shows the typical "crab claw" pattern seen in pellucid marginal degeneration, which can also be seen in keratoconus with inferior apical decentration. *(Courtesy of Robert S. Feder, MD.)*

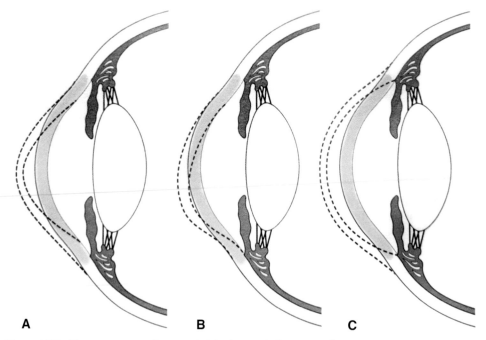

A   B   C

Figure 7-35 The presence of corneal thinning and the type of contour abnormality can be helpful to the clinician in recognizing the type of ectatic disorder. **A,** Keratoconus. **B,** Pellucid marginal degeneration. **C,** Keratoglobus. *(Reproduced with permission from Feder RS, Neems LC. Noninflammatory ectatic disorders. In: Mannis MJ, Holland EJ, eds. Cornea. Vol 1. 4th ed. Philadelphia: Elsevier; 2017:822.)*

PATHOLOGY Keratoglobus is strongly associated with blue sclerae and Ehlers-Danlos syndrome type VI (see Chapter 8), and it may represent a defect in collagen synthesis. Histologically, it is characterized by an absent or fragmented Bowman layer, thinned stroma with normal lamellar organization, and a thin Descemet membrane. Unlike keratoconus, keratoglobus is not associated with atopy or hard contact lens wear.

CLINICAL PRESENTATION The corneas have a globular shape with a deep anterior chamber. The corneal curvature may be as steep as 50–60 D, and generalized thinning appears, especially in the periphery. This is in contrast to keratoconus, which typically has inferior paracentral thinning and protrusion with thinning at the apex. Spontaneous rupture of the Descemet membrane and corneal hydrops can occur, but iron lines, stress lines, and anterior scarring are not typically seen. The corneal diameter may be slightly increased. Fleischer rings are usually not present, but prominent folds and areas of thickening in Descemet membrane are common.

MANAGEMENT Contact lenses, especially scleral lenses, may be of benefit. The prognosis for PK is much poorer in keratoglobus than in the other corneal ectasias. Tectonic lamellar keratoplasty followed by PK could be considered in cases requiring intervention to maintain functional vision. Spontaneous corneal rupture has been reported; thus, patients must be counseled regarding the importance of protective eyewear. High myopia is treated with spectacles to prevent amblyopia in children.

Feder RS, Neems LC. Noninflammatory ectatic disorders. In: Mannis MJ, Holland EJ, eds. *Cornea.* Vol 1. 4th ed. Philadelphia: Elsevier; 2017:820–843.

CHAPTER 8

Systemic Disorders With Corneal and Other Anterior Segment Manifestations

Highlights

- A Kayser-Fleischer ring is found not only in Wilson disease but also in primary biliary cirrhosis, chronic active hepatitis, and exogenous chalcosis. It should not be confused with a Fleischer ring, an iron ring seen in keratoconus.
- Crystals in the cornea are often related to amyloid deposition but may also be related to cystinosis and dysproteinemia.
- Patients with diabetes mellitus may have problems with epithelial healing after debridement and are at risk for recurrent corneal erosion.
- The differential diagnosis for prominent corneal nerves includes multiple endocrine neoplasia.

Introduction

Corneal clarity can be affected by the accumulation of a variety of substances, such as carbohydrates, lipids, and amino or nucleic acids. The anterior segment can be affected by autoimmune, dermatologic, musculoskeletal, and other disease processes. Recognition of the manifestations of these disorders requires prompt medical intervention. This chapter reviews common systemic conditions affecting the anterior segment, particularly the cornea. See also BCSC Section 2, *Fundamentals and Principles of Ophthalmology,* and Section 6, *Pediatric Ophthalmology and Strabismus.*

Mannis MJ, Holland EJ, eds. *Cornea.* Vol 1. 4th ed. Philadelphia: Elsevier; 2017.

Poll-The BT, Maillette de Buy Wenniger-Prick CJ. The eye in metabolic disease: clues to diagnosis. *Eur J Paediatr Neurol.* 2011;15(3):197–204.

Inherited Metabolic Diseases

Lysosomal Storage Diseases

Lysosomes are cellular organelles containing acid hydrolase enzymes that break down waste materials and cellular debris, including proteins, carbohydrates, lipids, and nucleic acids. Mutations in the genes that synthesize the lysosomal enzymes are responsible for more than 30 different human genetic diseases, collectively known as lysosomal storage diseases. Each of these disorders is due to deficiency of a single lysosomal enzyme that prevents breakdown of target molecules.

Systemic mucopolysaccharidoses

Systemic mucopolysaccharidoses (MPSs) are rare, inherited lysosomal storage diseases that can cause corneal clouding as a result of the accumulation of incompletely degraded glycosaminoglycans (GAGs; previously called mucopolysaccharides) within the keratocytes, corneal epithelium, and endothelium, as well as within the extracellular matrix of the cornea. These disorders result from defects in various lysosomal enzymes and are associated with other ophthalmic and systemic manifestations (Table 8-1). The incidence of the MPSs is approximately 1 in 10,000 births.

PATHOGENESIS At least 8 MPS syndromes have been described, most of which are autosomal recessive. The exception is Hunter syndrome, which is X-linked recessive. Specific enzyme defects and genetic mutations have been identified for each of these syndromes. There is variation in phenotypic expression. For example, the three MPS I disorders (Hurler, Scheie, and Hurler-Scheie syndromes) arise from different amino acid substitutions that result in a deficiency of α-L-iduronidase. Hurler-Scheie is thought to result from the transmission of 1 Hurler gene and 1 Scheie gene.

CLINICAL PRESENTATION Hurler syndrome (also termed MPS IH, MPS 1-H) is the most serious of the three MPS I disorders, with severe cognitive impairment and with corneal clouding appearing by 1 year of age (Fig 8-1). The life span of patients with Hurler syndrome is very limited unless a bone marrow transplant is performed. In contrast, symptoms of Scheie syndrome (also called MPS IS, MPS 1-S) do not appear until age 5–15 years. As in Hurler syndrome, corneal clouding occurs in Scheie syndrome, but children with Scheie syndrome generally have normal intelligence and a normal life span. Hurler-Scheie syndrome (MPS IH/S) is an intermediate form. Ophthalmic manifestations of most MPSs include not only corneal clouding, but also retinopathy and optic atrophy. The clouding generally involves the entire cornea and may or may not be present at birth. It is often slowly progressive from the periphery toward the center and can cause serious reduction in vision.

LABORATORY EVALUATION Urine can be screened for the presence of GAGs, but the most precise method of diagnosing the various MPSs is through a leukocyte or plasma enzyme assay. Confirmation of the disease can also be demonstrated using a conjunctival biopsy, although this is rarely necessary.

MANAGEMENT Penetrating keratoplasty (PK) or deep anterior lamellar keratoplasty (DALK) may be considered in the management of corneal clouding in the MPSs, although the

Table 8-1 Summary of Mucopolysaccharidosis Syndromes

MPS Syndrome	Inheritance	Enzyme Defect	Accumulated Material	Corneal Changes	Other Ophthalmic Changes
MPS IH (Hurler syndrome)	Autosomal recessive	α-L-Iduronidase	Dermatan and heparan sulfate	Severe clouding within first few years of life; diffuse punctate stromal opacities; epithelium and endothelium not affected	Pigmentary retinopathy, glaucoma, optic nerve swelling and atrophy, hypertelorism
MPS IS (Scheie syndrome)	Autosomal recessive	α-L-Iduronidase	Dermatan and heparan sulfate	Slowly progressive corneal opacification causing decreased vision by second decade of life; corneal edema; corneal changes may be more prominent in periphery	Glaucoma may occur
MPS IH/S (Hurler-Scheie syndrome)	Autosomal recessive	α-L-Iduronidase	Dermatan and heparan sulfate	Diffuse corneal opacification	Retinopathy
MPS II (Hunter syndrome)	X-linked recessive	Iduronate-2-sulfatase	Dermatan and heparan sulfate	Does not present as a congenital corneal opacity; corneal opacity may occur later in life in milder phenotypes	Exophthalmos, hypertelorism, optic nerve swelling and atrophy, retinopathy
MPS III A–D (Sanfilippo syndrome)	Autosomal recessive	Multiple enzyme defects	Heparan sulfate	Uncommon	Moderate to severe pigmentary retinopathy with abnormal ERG response
MPS IV A–B (Morquio syndrome)	Autosomal recessive	Galactose-6-sulfatase (MPS IV A) β-Galactosidase (MPS IV B)	Keratan sulfate (MPS IV A and IV B) Chondroitin sulfate (MPS IV A)	Opacities after age 10 years in 10% of patients; usually mild	Retinopathy, shallow orbits
MPS VI (Maroteaux-Lamy syndrome)	Autosomal recessive	N-Acetylgalactosamine-4-sulfatase	Dermatan sulfate	Severe corneal clouding within first years of life; corneal edema	Narrow-angle glaucoma, optic neuropathy
MPS VII (Sly syndrome)	Autosomal recessive	β-Glucuronidase	Dermatan sulfate, keratan sulfate, chondroitin sulfate	Corneal clouding	—
MPS IX (Natowicz syndrome)	Autosomal recessive	Hyaluronidase 1	Chondroitin sulfate	None reported	—

ERG = electroretinogram; MPS = mucopolysaccharidosis.

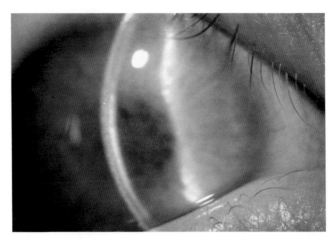

Figure 8-1 Slit-lamp photograph from a patient with Hurler syndrome, showing diffuse, patchy corneal clouding. *(Courtesy of Stephen E. Orlin, MD.)*

patient's mental status or retinal or optic nerve abnormalities may limit visual improvement. The visual prognosis for patients with MPS who have undergone PK is considered guarded, as the abnormal storage material may accumulate in the graft. Some regression of corneal clouding occurs in approximately one-third of patients following successful allogeneic bone marrow transplant. Enzyme replacement therapy is being used for several MPSs, and gene transfer therapy is under investigation.

> Ashworth JL, Biswas S, Wraith E, Lloyd IC. Mucopolysaccharidoses and the eye. *Surv Ophthalmol.* 2006;51(1):1–17.

Sphingolipidoses

Sphingolipidoses are rare inherited disorders of complex lipids (gangliosides and sphingomyelin) that involve the cornea. They comprise 4 conditions:

- Fabry disease (angiokeratoma corporis diffusum), X-linked recessive
- multiple sulfatase deficiency, autosomal recessive
- generalized gangliosidosis (GM$_1$ gangliosidosis type I), autosomal recessive
- Tay-Sachs disease (GM$_2$ gangliosidosis), autosomal recessive

PATHOGENESIS Fabry disease is caused by a deficiency of α-galactosidase A, which leads to the accumulation of ceramide trihexoside in the renal and cardiovascular systems. Generalized gangliosidosis is characterized by deficiencies of β-galactosidases and the resultant accumulation of ganglioside GM$_1$ in the central nervous system and of keratan sulfate in somatic tissues. It has been linked to 3p12–p13. Tay-Sachs disease is related to the generalized gangliosidoses but results from β-hexosaminidase A deficiency, which causes accumulation of ganglioside GM$_2$.

CLINICAL PRESENTATION In the sphingolipidoses, the cornea exhibits distinctive changes consisting of whorl-like lines *(cornea verticillata)* in the basal layers of the epithelium that appear to converge at the inferior central corneal epithelium (Fig 8-2).

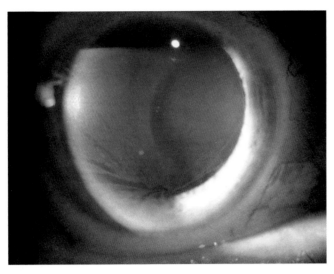

Figure 8-2 Slit-lamp photograph from a patient with Fabry disease, showing cornea verticillata in the basal layers of the epithelium. *(Courtesy of Stephen E. Orlin, MD.)*

Periorbital edema occurs in 25% of cases, posterior spokelike cataracts in 50%, and conjunctival aneurysms in 60%. Other ocular signs include papilledema, retinal or macular edema, optic atrophy, and retinal vascular dilation. The corneal changes resemble those noted in patients after long-term oral chloroquine or amiodarone therapy.

Hemizygous males with Fabry disease are more seriously affected than heterozygous females and show the typical corneal changes. A heterozygous female patient with Fabry disease will show the same corneal changes. Fabry disease is also characterized by renal failure, peripheral neuropathy with painful dysesthesias in the lower extremities, and skin lesions (angiokeratomas). The skin lesions are small, round, vascular eruptions that later become hyperkeratotic. They consist of an accumulation of sphingolipid within the vascular endothelium.

The clinical phenotype of multiple sulfatase deficiency combines features of metachromatic leukodystrophy and MPS. Affected children have subtle diffuse corneal opacities, macular changes, optic atrophy, and progressive psychomotor retardation. They die in the first decade of life.

The ocular findings in Tay-Sachs disease primarily involve the retina; however, the corneal endothelial cells can appear distended and filled with single membrane–bound vacuoles.

LABORATORY EVALUATION In patients with Fabry disease, levels of α-galactosidase A are markedly decreased in urine and plasma. The conjunctival biopsy result may be positive before cornea verticillata are apparent. Prenatal diagnosis can be performed with chorionic villus sampling. Gene sequencing may help in diagnosing Fabry disease in suspected female carriers, as enzyme levels may be close to normal in heterozygotes.

MANAGEMENT If a female patient is found to be an asymptomatic heterozygous carrier of Fabry disease, genetic counseling should be considered. Enzyme replacement with infusion of α-galactosidase A is a therapeutic option, but long-term benefit has not been proven. Corneal deposits have been cleared with enzyme replacement therapy. The addition of agents that help stabilize native enzymes may improve the efficacy of enzyme replacement therapy.

Fledelius HC, Sandfeld L, Rasmussen ÅK, Madsen CV, Feldt-Rasmussen U. Ophthalmic experience over 10 years in an observational nationwide Danish cohort of Fabry patients with access to enzyme replacement. *Acta Ophthalmol.* 2015;93(3):258–264.

Samiy N. Ocular features of Fabry disease: diagnosis of a treatable life-threatening disorder. *Surv Ophthalmol.* 2008;53(4):416–423.

Mucolipidoses

Mucolipidoses (MLs) are autosomal recessive conditions that have features common to both MPSs and lipidoses. Currently recognized diseases in this class are the following:

- ML I (dysmorphic sialidosis)
- ML II (inclusion cell disease)
- ML III (pseudo-Hurler polydystrophy)
- ML IV

See Table 28-2 in BCSC Section 6, *Pediatric Ophthalmology and Strabismus,* which lists ocular findings in the mucolipidoses.

PATHOGENESIS The MLs are inherited disorders of carbohydrate and lipid metabolism combined. Incompletely degraded GAGs (mucopolysaccharides) accumulate in the cornea and viscera, and sphingolipids are deposited in the retina and central nervous system.

The ML IV gene has been mapped to the short arm of chromosome 19. Histologic examination of corneal scrapings has revealed the accumulation of intracytoplasmic storage material in the corneal epithelium. All are caused by a defect in lysosomal acid hydrolase enzymes.

CLINICAL PRESENTATION All of the MLs are characterized by varying degrees of corneal clouding, which is often progressive. A retinal cherry-red spot and retinal degeneration are also associated with many of these disorders.

LABORATORY EVALUATION Plasma cells are vacuolated, and levels of plasma lysosomal hydrolases are elevated. In ML IV, in which corneal clouding is present from birth, conjunctival biopsy shows fibroblast inclusion bodies that are

- single membrane–limited cytoplasmic vacuoles containing both fibrillogranular material and membranous lamellae
- lamellar and concentric bodies resembling those of Tay-Sachs disease

There is no evidence of mucopolysacchariduria or cellular metachromasia. Chorionic villus sampling has been used for prenatal diagnosis of ML II.

MANAGEMENT Both PK and lamellar keratoplasty (LK) have been associated with generally poor results, probably because resurfacing is impaired by the abnormal epithelial cells. Allograft limbal stem cell transplantation may be an option. Bone marrow transplantation has been reported.

Miscellaneous lysosomal storage diseases

A number of the lysosomal storage diseases do not fit into a specific category. These include

- galactosialidosis (Goldberg syndrome)
- mannosidosis
- fucosidosis

Goldberg syndrome is a cathepsin-related disorder and has features of β-galactosidase and sialidase deficiencies. Mannosidosis is caused by deficient activity of the enzyme mannosidase. There are 2 subsets, α- and β-mannosidosis. Both galactosialidosis and mannosidosis are associated with corneal clouding.

Fucosidosis is due to mutations in the *FUCA1* gene, which result in reduction in activity of the α-L-fucosidase enzyme. Histologic studies have revealed that even when the cornea appears clinically normal in fucosidosis, corneal endothelial cells show the presence of cytoplasmic, membrane-bound, confluent areas of fibrillar, granular, and multilaminated deposits.

Disorders of Lipoprotein Metabolism

Hyperlipoproteinemias

Hyperlipoproteinemias are common conditions associated with premature coronary artery and peripheral vascular disease. Recognition of the ocular hallmarks of these diseases, such as xanthelasma and corneal arcus, can result in early intervention and reduced morbidity.

Schnyder corneal dystrophy, a dominantly inherited category 1 corneal dystrophy, can be associated with hyperlipoproteinemia. Corneal dystrophies are discussed in Chapter 7.

See BCSC Section 1, *Update on General Medicine,* for additional information about hyperlipoproteinemias.

PATHOGENESIS Extracellular deposits consist of cholesterol, cholesterol esters, phospholipids, and triglycerides.

CLINICAL PRESENTATION Corneal arcus is a very common degenerative change in older patients and does not require systemic evaluation (see Chapter 6 for further discussion of corneal arcus). However, corneal arcus in individuals younger than 40 years or asymmetric corneal arcus may be associated with a hyperlipoproteinemia with elevated serum cholesterol level. These patients should have a systemic workup. Unilateral or asymmetric corneal arcus may be secondary to carotid atherosclerotic disease on the less affected side.

LABORATORY EVALUATION A fasting and alcohol-restricted lipid profile that includes cholesterol, triglycerides, and high-density and low-density lipoproteins (HDL and LDL, respectively) is typically considered. The clinician can then classify these patients phenotypically to assess their risk for atherosclerotic disease.

MANAGEMENT Early detection of a hyperlipoproteinemia by the ophthalmologist allows time for the patient to be referred for dietary or drug treatment.

Hypolipoproteinemias

Abnormal reductions in serum lipoprotein levels occur in 5 disorders:

- lecithin–cholesterol acyltransferase (LCAT) deficiency
- fish eye disease
- Tangier disease
- familial hypobetalipoproteinemia
- Bassen-Kornzweig syndrome

The last 2 disorders do not result in corneal disease; the discussion in this section focuses on the other 3 disorders.

PATHOGENESIS LCAT promotes transfer of excess cholesterol from peripheral tissues to the liver, and a deficiency of this enzyme results in accumulation of unesterified cholesterol in the plasma and tissues. This, in turn, leads to atherosclerosis, renal insufficiency, early corneal arcus, and nebular corneal clouding composed of minute focal lipid deposits.

LCAT deficiency and fish eye disease are allelic variants of the same genetic locus on band 16q22.1. In fish eye disease, LCAT levels are normal, but the enzyme does not function properly. Tangier disease is characterized by a complete absence of serum high-density α-lipoproteins. The gene responsible for this disease maps to 9q22–q31.

CLINICAL PRESENTATION LCAT deficiency, fish eye disease, and Tangier disease are rare autosomal recessive conditions. Familial LCAT deficiency is characterized by peripheral arcus and nebular stromal haze made up of myriad minute focal deposits of lipid that appear early in childhood but do not interfere with vision (Fig 8-3). Fish eye disease features obvious corneal clouding from minute gray-white-yellow dots that progress from the periphery to the central cornea to decrease vision. Tangier disease features very large orange

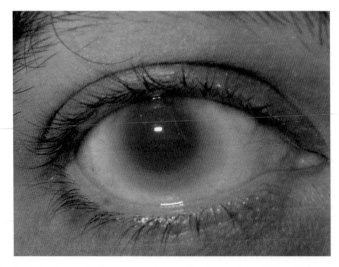

Figure 8-3 Clinical photograph from a patient with familial lecithin-cholesterol acyltransferase (LCAT) deficiency, showing peripheral arcus and nebular stromal haze. *(Courtesy of Gerald Zaidman, MD.)*

tonsils; enlarged liver, spleen, and lymph nodes; hypocholesterolemia; and abnormal chylomicron remnants. Affected corneas show diffuse clouding and posterior focal stromal opacities but no arcus. Neuropathy leads to lagophthalmos and corneal sequelae.

LABORATORY EVALUATION AND MANAGEMENT The serum lipid profile shows characteristic low levels of HDL (markedly low in Tangier disease). Recognition of hypolipoproteinemia can allow the clinician to make appropriate referrals and encourage the patient to seek genetic counseling.

Disorders of Amino Acid, Nucleic Acid, Protein, and Mineral Metabolism

Cystinosis

Cystinosis is a rare autosomal recessive metabolic disorder, affecting 3.5 infants per 1 million births. The disease is characterized by the accumulation of the amino acid cystine within lysosomes. The defective gene in cystinosis, *CTNS,* has been mapped to 17p13. See also BCSC Section 6, *Pediatric Ophthalmology and Strabismus.*

PATHOGENESIS A defect in transport across the lysosomal membrane leads to intracellular accumulation of cystine.

CLINICAL PRESENTATION Cystinosis is categorized on the basis of the patient's age at diagnosis and the severity of symptoms. *Nephropathic cystinosis* is divided into infantile (classic) and intermediate (juvenile or adolescent) forms. Dwarfism and progressive renal dysfunction are prominent in infantile cystinosis and less severe in the juvenile disease. Life expectancy is normal in *nonnephropathic cystinosis* (formerly called *adult cystinosis*). All 3 types are characterized by the deposition of fine iridescent and polychromatic cystine crystals in the conjunctiva, cornea, iris, and other parts of the eye. The crystals are densest in the peripheral cornea but are present throughout the anterior stroma, even within the central cornea (Fig 8-4), and can be seen in the trabecular meshwork with gonioscopy. Patients

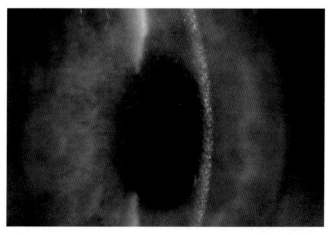

Figure 8-4 Nonnephropathic cystinosis. Slit-lamp photograph showing diffuse stromal refractile crystals. *(Courtesy of Stephen E. Orlin, MD.)*

with cystinosis often have photophobia, and the crystals can recur following PK. Table 8-2 lists other causes of corneal crystals; Table 8-3 summarizes the ocular and systemic findings in disorders of amino acid metabolism.

Liang H, Baudouin C, Tahiri JHR, Brignole-Baudouin F, Labbe A. Photophobia and corneal crystal density in nephropathic cystinosis: an in vivo confocal microscopy and anterior segment optical coherence tomography study. *Invest Ophthalmol Vis Sci.* 2015;56(5): 3218–3225.

LABORATORY EVALUATION Cystine crystals may be seen in conjunctiva, blood leukocytes, or bone marrow.

MANAGEMENT Topical cysteamine 0.44% is a commercially available agent used to reduce the density of the crystals and diminish corneal pain, possibly by reducing the frequency of corneal erosions. Cysteamine is thought to react with intracellular cystine, forming a cysteine–cysteamine disulfide that resembles lysine and is transported through the lysosome by the normal lysine transport system. Posterior segment manifestations such as pigmentary retinopathy and optic nerve involvement may be treated with oral cysteamine, which may also prevent or delay other manifestations of the disease, including death.

Table 8-2 Differential Diagnosis of Corneal Crystals

Medical Disorders	Specific Conditions and Medications
Lipid keratopathies	Familial lipoprotein disorders LCAT deficiency Schnyder corneal dystrophy Tangier disease
Disorders of protein metabolism	Cystinosis Gout Hyperuricemia Tyrosinemia
Immunoglobulin disorders	Benign monoclonal gammopathy Cryoglobulinemia Multiple myeloma Rheumatoid arthritis Waldenström macroglobulinemia
Infectious crystalline keratopathy	Bacterial infection *(Streptococcus viridans)* Fungal infection Viral infection
Medication toxicity	Chloroquine Chlorpromazine Topical ciprofloxacin
Miscellaneous causes	Bietti corneal dystrophy Calcium deposits *Dieffenbachia* plant sap Oxalosis Porphyria

LCAT = lecithin–cholesterol acyltransferase.

Table 8-3 Disorders of Amino Acid Metabolism

Type	Heredity	Ocular Findings	Associated Nonocular Conditions
Cystinosis	Rare autosomal recessive	Polychromatic cystine crystals in conjunctiva, trabecular meshwork, corneal stroma, and iris Photophobia (usually)	Dwarfism Renal dysfunction
Tyrosinemia	Autosomal recessive	Photophobia, tearing, conjunctival injection, tarsal papillary hypertrophy, pseudodendrites Epithelial breakdown with secondary corneal neovascularization and scarring	Hyperkeratotic lesions of palms, soles, and elbows Cognitive impairment
Alkaptonuria	Rare autosomal recessive	Ochronotic (brownish) deposits of alkapton in corneal epithelium or in Bowman layer near limbus Rectus muscle tendons and adjacent sclera develop smudgelike pigmentation	Arthropathy Renal calculi Pigmentation of cartilaginous structures, including earlobes, trachea, nose, and tendons

Tyrosinemia

Tyrosinemia encompasses a group of inborn errors in the metabolism of the amino acid tyrosine. Tyrosinemia type I, caused by fumarylacetoacetate deficiency, is not associated with corneal pathology. Tyrosinemia type II (Richner-Hanhart syndrome) is characterized by hyperkeratotic lesions of the palms, soles, and elbows, as well as eventual cognitive impairment; corneal manifestations of this syndrome are discussed under Clinical Presentation.

PATHOGENESIS Tyrosinemia type II is an autosomal recessive disorder resulting from defective tyrosine aminotransferase, which leads to excess tyrosine in the blood and urine. The elevated tyrosine level likely has a direct effect on lysosomal membranes, leading to enzyme release. The gene defect is located at 16q22.1–22.3.

CLINICAL PRESENTATION Ocular changes include marked photophobia, tearing, conjunctival injection, and tarsal papillary hypertrophy. Affected patients experience recurrent episodes of corneal erosions and pseudodendrites (Fig 8-5), which usually do not stain well with fluorescein or rose bengal. Continued episodes of epithelial breakdown can result in corneal vascularization and scarring. It is important to consider this disorder in young children who may carry a diagnosis of recurrent herpes simplex virus keratitis.

LABORATORY EVALUATION Hypertyrosinemia and tyrosinuria with normal phenylalanine levels and conjunctival biopsy showing soluble tyrosine aminotransferase deficiency are diagnostic.

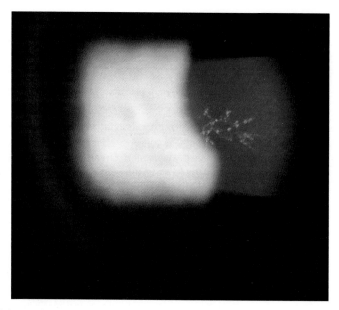

Figure 8-5 Slit-lamp photograph showing a pseudodendrite in a patient with tyrosinemia. *(Courtesy of Robert W. Weisenthal, MD.)*

MANAGEMENT Restriction of dietary intake of tyrosine and phenylalanine can reduce the severity of both the corneal and systemic changes, including cognitive impairment. The institution of appropriate dietary restrictions, even later in life, can improve mental status.

Alkaptonuria

Alkaptonuria is a rare autosomal recessive disorder caused by deficiency of the enzyme homogentisic acid oxidase, which leads to an accumulation of homogentisic acid. The defect is caused by mutations in the *HGD* gene, which maps to 3q13.33. The frequency of alkaptonuria is unusually high in the Dominican Republic and Slovakia.

PATHOGENESIS Homogentisate 1,2-dioxygenase, the enzyme necessary to degrade tyrosine and phenylalanine, is deficient in patients with this disorder. Phenylalanine and tyrosine cannot be metabolized beyond homogentisic acid, which is oxidized and polymerized into alkapton, a brown-black material similar to melanin. Alkapton binds to collagen and is then deposited in connective tissues as a dark pigment; this process is known as *ochronosis*.

CLINICAL PRESENTATION Systemic findings include arthropathy; renal calculi; and pigmentation of cartilaginous structures, including earlobes, trachea, nose, tendons, dura mater, heart valves, and prostate. Eventually, medial and lateral rectus muscle tendons and the sclera adjacent to the tendon insertions develop a smudgelike bluish-black pigmentation (Fig 8-6). Darkly pigmented, dotlike opacities, similar to those seen in spheroidal degeneration, may appear in the corneal epithelium or in the Bowman layer, near the limbus.

LABORATORY EVALUATION The urine of affected patients turns dark on standing. Alkaptonuria is diagnosed by finding elevated levels of homogentisic acid in the urine.

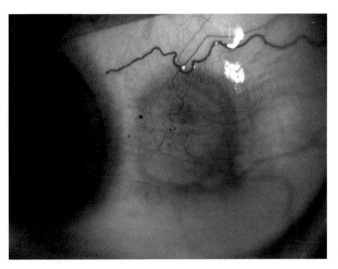

Figure 8-6 Slit-lamp photograph from a female patient with alkaptonuria, showing ochronosis (scleral pigmentation) at the insertion of the lateral rectus muscle. *(Courtesy of Irving M. Raber, MD.)*

MANAGEMENT No specific therapy is available, but high-dose ascorbic acid may reduce arthropathy in young patients. Gene therapy may be a future treatment.

Srinivasan S, Shehadeh-Mashor R, Slomovic AR. Corneal manifestations of metabolic diseases. In: Mannis MJ, Holland EJ, eds. *Cornea.* Vol 1. 4th ed. Philadelphia: Elsevier; 2017:620–644.

Amyloidosis

The amyloidoses are a heterogeneous group of diseases characterized by the extracellular accumulation of amyloid in various tissues and organs, including the cornea and conjunctiva. Amyloid deposits may be composed of many different types of proteins, including immunoglobulin fragments. The deposits are insoluble and inert, but they interfere with the normal structure and function of tissues and organs.

Amyloid has the following staining characteristics:

- positive staining with Congo red dye
- dichroism and birefringence
- metachromasia with crystal violet dye
- fluorescence in ultraviolet light with thioflavin T stain
- typical filamentous appearance on electron microscopy

CLASSIFICATION AND CLINICAL PRESENTATION Ocular amyloidosis is classified as either primary (idiopathic) or secondary (to a chronic disease) and as either localized or systemic. A useful classification of amyloidosis considers these 4 types. Each type is summarized in Table 8-4.

Primary localized amyloidosis is the most common form of ocular amyloidosis. Conjunctival amyloid plaques occur in the absence of systemic involvement (Fig 8-7). Gelatinous droplike corneal dystrophy (formerly primary familial amyloidosis), classic lattice corneal dystrophy (LCD1), and lattice variants are special forms of primary localized

Table 8-4 Amyloid in the Eye

Type	Heredity	Ocular Distribution/Findings	Other Associated Ocular and Systemic Conditions
Primary localized amyloidosis	Nonfamilial	Conjunctival plaque Polymorphic amyloid degeneration	None
	Familial	Lattice corneal dystrophy and lattice variants Granular corneal dystrophy type 2 (Avellino) Gelatinous droplike dystrophy	
Primary systemic amyloidosis	Nonfamilial	Eyelid skin and conjunctiva (very rare)	Occult plasma cell dyscrasias
	Familial	Ophthalmoplegia (orbital and muscle infiltrates), ptosis, vitreous veils, dry eye, pupillary abnormalities Meretoja syndrome, cranial neuropathies	Cardiomyopathy, peripheral neuropathy, gastrointestinal disease Skin involvement Meretoja syndrome (facial palsies, skin nodules, rarely renal involvement)
Secondary localized amyloidosis	Nonfamilial Familial	Conjunctiva, eyelid skin, cornea None	Trachoma, psoriasis, trauma, phlyctenulosis, retinopathy of prematurity, keratoconus, bullous keratopathy, interstitial keratitis, Hansen disease (leprosy), trichiasis, tertiary syphilis, uveitis, climatic droplet keratopathy
Secondary systemic amyloidosis	Nonfamilial	Vitreous body (rare) (Corneal deposits are not amyloid) Conjunctiva, eyelid skin (rare)	Multiple myeloma Infectious diseases (tuberculosis, Hansen disease [leprosy], syphilis) Inflammatory diseases (rheumatoid arthritis, other connective tissue disorders) Hodgkin disease
	Familial	(Corneal nerve enlargement is not due to amyloid)	Multiple endocrine neoplasia type 2A

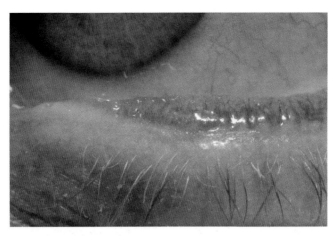

Figure 8-7 Clinical photograph of the inferior palpebral conjunctiva, showing moderate thickening with yellowish amyloid deposition. *(Courtesy of Stephen E. Orlin, MD.)*

amyloidosis and are discussed in Chapter 7. Polymorphic amyloid degeneration is discussed in Chapter 6.

Primary systemic amyloidosis is a heterogeneous group of diseases in which waxy, ecchymotic eyelid papules occur in association with vitreous veils and opacities as well as with pupillary anomalies such as light–near dissociation. Orbital involvement, extraocular muscle involvement with ophthalmoplegia, and scleral infiltration with uveal effusion have been reported. The most common form of primary systemic amyloidosis is an autosomal dominant group of diseases linked to mutations in the transthyretin gene (*TTR*, prealbumin) on chromosome 18 (18q11.2–q12.1); more than 40 mutations in this gene have been described.

Familial amyloidosis, Finnish type, or *gelsolin type (Meretoja syndrome)* is an example of primary systemic amyloidosis. This condition was initially described in persons of Finnish descent but was later reported in individuals of other ethnicities. Previously called lattice corneal dystrophy type 2, it has been excluded as a corneal dystrophy by the International Committee for the Classification of Corneal Dystrophies (IC3D) because of its systemic associations.

Familial amyloidosis presents in the third to fourth decade of life. Because the ocular symptoms are the first to arise, the ophthalmologist is often the first physician to see patients with this condition, who typically present with corneal findings. Affected patients have a characteristic facial mask; dermatochalasis; lagophthalmos; pendulous ears; cranial and peripheral nerve palsies; and dry, lax skin with amyloid deposition (Fig 8-8). The classic corneal lattice lines are less numerous and more peripheral, and they spread centripetally from the limbus. The central cornea is relatively spared; corneal sensation is reduced. The risk of open-angle glaucoma may be increased, and dry eye and recurrent erosions may occur late in life.

PATHOLOGY OF FAMILIAL AMYLOIDOSIS Light microscopy shows amyloid in the lattice lines as a discontinuous band under the Bowman layer and within the sclera. The amyloid in this condition is related to gelsolin and does not stain for type AA or AP. The mutated gelsolin

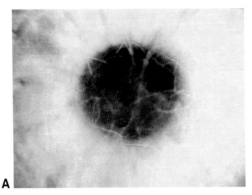 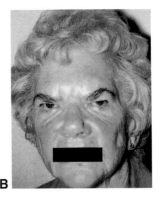

Figure 8-8 **A,** Diffuse lattice lines in Meretoja syndrome. **B,** Typical facies. *(Reproduced with permission from Weiss JS, Møller H, Lisch W, et al. The ICD3 classification of the corneal dystrophies. Cornea. 2008; 27(10 Suppl 2):S16.)*

is observed to be deposited in the conjunctiva, sclera, and ciliary body; along the choriocapillaris; in the ciliary nerves and vessels; and in the optic nerve. Extraocularly, amyloid is detected in arterial walls, peripheral nerves, and glomeruli. On confocal microscopy, deposits are observed along the basal epithelial cells and stromal nerves.

Reidy JJ. Corneal and conjunctival degenerations. In: Mannis MJ, Holland EJ, eds. *Cornea.* Vol 1. 4th ed. Philadelphia: Elsevier; 2017:856–874.

Srinivasan S, Shehadeh-Mashor R, Slomovic AR. Corneal manifestations of metabolic diseases. In: Mannis MJ, Holland EJ, eds. *Cornea.* Vol 1. 4th ed. Philadelphia: Elsevier; 2017: 620–644.

Gout

Disorders of purine metabolism cause *hyperuricemia* (increased uric acid). *Gout* results from deposition of urate crystals in the joints or kidney.

PATHOGENESIS Hyperuricemia may be familial, arising from an enzyme deficiency (eg, hypoxanthine phosphoribosyltransferase in Lesch-Nyhan syndrome). More commonly, gout is polygenic or secondary to obesity, cytotoxic chemotherapy, myeloproliferative disease, diuretic therapy, or excessive alcohol consumption.

CLINICAL PRESENTATION Acute inflammation of the sclera, episclera, or conjunctiva can occur. Fine corneal epithelial and stromal deposits may appear in the absence of inflammation. Either an orange-brown band keratopathy or a typical whitish band keratopathy is seen in rare cases.

LABORATORY EVALUATION Serum uric acid level is typically elevated. However, in urate keratopathy, the uric acid level may be normal in the presence of keratopathy if there is no concurrent inflammation.

MANAGEMENT Indomethacin, colchicine, or phenylbutazone is used for acute treatment; long-term reduction in uric acid levels should be pursued with medications such as allopurinol. Superficial corneal deposits can be removed mechanically with scraping or keratectomy.

Wilson disease

PATHOGENESIS Wilson disease *(hepatolenticular degeneration)* is an autosomal recessive disorder caused by multiple allelic substitutions or deletions in a Cu^{2+}-ATPase-transporting β-polypeptide, linked to mutations in the *ATP7B* gene on chromosome 13 (13q14.3–q21). Copper is deposited first in the liver, then in the kidneys, and eventually in the brain and the cornea at the Descemet membrane (Fig 8-9).

CLINICAL PRESENTATION Muscular rigidity increases, and tremor and involuntary movement gradually occur in a fluctuating course resembling parkinsonism. Unintelligible speech and mild dementia usually occur concomitantly. Equal numbers of patients (40%) present with hepatic or nervous system symptoms. In the cornea, a golden-brown, ruby-red, or green pigment ring (Kayser-Fleischer ring) consisting of copper deposits appears in peripheral Descemet membrane (see Fig 8-9), although not all patients with Wilson disease manifest this ring. Copper deposition occurs in the posterior Descemet membrane, first superiorly, then gradually spreading to meet inferior deposits. Gonioscopy may assist in visualizing the ring. A "sunflower" cataract may be present.

The differential diagnosis includes primary biliary cirrhosis, chronic active hepatitis, exogenous chalcosis, and progressive intrahepatic cholestasis of childhood. These and other non-Wilsonian hepatic disorders can also be associated with Kayser-Fleischer rings, but only Wilson disease is characterized by decreased serum ceruloplasmin levels and neurologic symptoms.

LABORATORY EVALUATION Patients with Wilson disease can be differentiated from patients with other diseases that show Kayser-Fleischer rings by their inability to incorporate radioactive copper into ceruloplasmin. Low serum ceruloplasmin, high non-ceruloplasmin-bound serum copper, and high urinary copper suggest the diagnosis, which can be confirmed with liver biopsy. Nonspecific findings of proteinuria, aminoaciduria, glycosuria, uricaciduria, hyperphosphaturia, and hypercalciuria are seen.

MANAGEMENT Wilson disease can be treated with penicillamine. Liver transplantation is reserved for patients with fulminant liver failure. The Kayser-Fleischer ring disappears gradually with therapy, including liver transplant, and the disappearance of the rings can

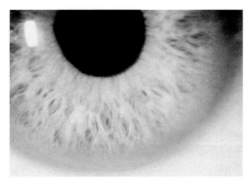

Figure 8-9 Wilson hepatolenticular degeneration. Deposits of copper in the Descemet membrane (Kayser-Fleischer ring). *(Reproduced with permission from Krachmer JH, Mannis MJ, Holland EJ, eds. Cornea. 3rd ed. Vol 1. Philadelphia: Elsevier/Mosby; 2011:299.)*

be used to help monitor therapy. Electrophysiologic abnormalities from retinal dysfunction have been shown to reverse after treatment of the disease.

Porphyria

The porphyrias are a group of disorders characterized by excess production and excretion of porphyrins, which are pigments involved in the synthesis of heme.

PATHOGENESIS *Porphyria cutanea tarda,* the form most commonly associated with ocular surface disease, is either sporadic or inherited in an autosomal dominant pattern (band 1p34). The enzyme uroporphyrinogen decarboxylase is deficient, resulting in an accumulation of porphyrins in the liver and in the circulation. Typically, a second insult to the liver, such as alcoholism or drug metabolism, triggers the condition in late middle age.

A severe form of porphyria, called *hepatoerythropoietic porphyria (HEP),* is a homozygous presentation of the same enzymatic defect, but onset of the disease is in infancy.

CLINICAL PRESENTATION Hyperpigmentation, erythema, scleroderma-like changes, increased fragility, and vesicular and ulcerative lesions occur on sun-exposed surfaces of the body. There is interpalpebral injection, and the conjunctiva may develop vesicles, scarring, and symblepharon mimicking bullous pemphigoid; conjunctival necrosis may also occur. Necrotizing scleritis has been reported. The cornea may be affected by exposure or by thinning and perforation at the limbus. Skin and ocular lesions may fluoresce.

LABORATORY EVALUATION Urine turns dark on standing. Reduced liver and red cell uroporphyrinogen decarboxylase activity confirms the diagnosis. Hepatic biopsy shows liver parenchymal cells filled with porphyrins that fluoresce bright red in ultraviolet light.

MANAGEMENT Protection from ultraviolet light and reduction of iron by phlebotomy or subcutaneous deferoxamine are the principal treatments. No specific ocular treatment is available, although artificial tears may help wash away porphyrins. Corneal thinning and perforation are treated in standard ways.

Srinivasan S, Shehadeh-Mashor R, Slomovic AR. Corneal manifestations of metabolic diseases. In: Mannis MJ, Holland EJ, eds. *Cornea.* Vol 1. 4th ed. Philadelphia: Elsevier; 2017:620–644.

Skeletal and Connective Tissue Disorders

Many musculoskeletal and connective tissue diseases affect the cornea. The corneal manifestations of these diseases are outlined in Table 8-5.

Ehlers-Danlos Syndrome

Ehlers-Danlos syndrome (EDS), a heterogeneous group of diseases, is characterized by hyperextensibility of joints and skin, tendency to bruise easily, and formation of "cigarette paper" scars.

PATHOGENESIS There are more than 20 known types of EDS, which are classified as autosomal dominant, autosomal recessive, or X-linked recessive. Multiple genetic loci have been

Table 8-5 Skeletal and Connective Tissue Disorders of Interest to the Ophthalmologist

Name (OMIM #)	Corneal Findings	Other Ocular Findings
Albright hereditary osteodystrophy (300800)	None	Zonular cataracts with multicolored flecks in 25% of affected patients
Apert syndrome (101200)	Exposure keratitis with severe proptosis Keratoconus (very rare) Megalocornea (very rare)	Strabismus (exotropia with V pattern) Absence of extraocular muscles; proptosis, ocular hypopigmentation, optic atrophy Rare: nystagmus, ptosis, cataract, ectopia lentis, coloboma of iris
Carpenter syndrome; acrocephalopolysyndactyly type II (201000)	Exposure keratitis secondary to severe proptosis Microcornea (rare) Corneal leukoma (rare)	Epicanthal folds, downward slant, hypertelorism or hypotelorism, optic atrophy, strabismus Rare: coloboma of the iris and choroid, congenital cataract, lens subluxation, nystagmus, retinal detachment
Cockayne syndrome Type A (216400) Type B (133540)	Raised inferior corneal lesion, band keratopathy, recurrent erosions	Cataracts, retinal dystrophy, nystagmus, iris atrophy, hyperopia, enophthalmos, strabismus
Crouzon syndrome (123500)	Exposure keratitis with severe proptosis Keratoconus (very rare) Microcornea (very rare)	Strabismus (exotropia with V pattern) Exophthalmos, hypertelorism, optic atrophy in 30% of affected patients Rare: nystagmus, glaucoma, cataract, ectopia lentis, aniridia, anisocoria, myelinated nerve fibers
Ehlers-Danlos syndrome (EDS) EDS I (130000) EDS II (130010) EDS III (130020) EDS IV (130050) EDS V (305200) EDS VI (225400) EDS VII–AD (130060) EDS VII–AR (225410) EDS VIII (130080)	Brittle cornea in type VI Keratoconus in types I and VI Keratoglobus in type VI	Epicanthal folds, blue sclera, retinal detachment, glaucoma, ectopia lentis, angioid streaks (rare)
Goldenhar-Gorlin syndrome; oculoauriculovertebral sequence; hemifacial microsomia (164210)	Limbal dermoid	Upper > lower eyelid coloboma, strabismus (25% of affected patients), Duane retraction syndrome, microphthalmos, anophthalmos, lacrimal system dysfunction, optic nerve hypoplasia, tortuous retinal vessels, macular hypoplasia and heterotropia, choroidal hyperpigmentation, iris and retinal colobomas
Hallermann-Streiff-François syndrome; oculomandibulodyscephaly (234100)	One case of sclerocornea	Congenital cataracts, spontaneous resorption of lens cortex with secondary membranous cataract formation, glaucoma, uveitis, retinal folds, optic nerve dysplasia, microphthalmos

(Continued)

Table 8-5 (continued)

Name (OMIM #)	Corneal Findings	Other Ocular Findings
Hypophosphatasia Infantile (241500) Childhood (241510) Adult (146300)	Band keratopathy with conjunctival calcifications in infantile form	Blue sclera, cataracts, optic atrophy secondary to craniostenosis, atypical retinitis pigmentosa; ocular complications present only in infantile and childhood forms, not in adult form
Marfan syndrome (154700)	Megalocornea (uncommon) Flat cornea Keratoconus (uncommon)	Ectopia lentis, strabismus, cataracts, myopia, retinal detachment, glaucoma, blue sclera
Nail–patella syndrome; onycho-osteodysplasia (161200)	Microcornea	Cataracts, microphthalmos
Oculodento-osseous dysplasia AD (164200) AR (257850)	Microcornea	Hypotelorism, convergent strabismus, anterior segment dysgenesis, glaucoma, cataracts, remnants of the hyaloid system
Osteogenesis imperfecta Type I (259400) Type II (166200) Type III (259420) Type IV (166220)	Decreased central corneal thickness Keratoconus (rare) Megalocornea (rare) Posterior embryotoxon (rare)	Blue sclera Rare: congenital glaucoma, cataract, choroidal sclerosis, subhyaloid hemorrhage, hyperopia, ectopia lentis
Parry-Romberg syndrome; progressive facial hemiatrophy (141300)	Neuroparalytic keratitis	Enophthalmos, oculomotor palsies, pupillary abnormalities, Horner syndrome, heterochromia, intraocular inflammation, optic nerve hypoplasia, choroidal atrophy
Pierre Robin malformation (261800)	Megalocornea (rare)	Congenital glaucoma, high myopia, vitreoretinal degeneration, retinal detachment, esotropia, congenital cataracts, microphthalmos
Rothmund-Thomson syndrome (268400)	Degenerative lesions of cornea	Cataracts
Treacher Collins syndrome; mandibulofacial dysostosis (154500)	Microcornea	Lower eyelid coloboma, bony orbit dysplasia, absent lower eyelid cilia, absent lower eyelid lacrimal puncta, iris coloboma, microphthalmos, strabismus, downward slant
Werner syndrome (277700)	Corneal edema secondary to endothelial decompensation following cataract surgery Poor wound healing	Presenile posterior subcapsular cataracts (age 20–30 years), proptosis, blue sclera Rare: nystagmus, astigmatism, telangiectasia of iris, macular degeneration, pigmentary retinopathy

AD = autosomal dominant; AR = autosomal recessive; OMIM = Online Mendelian Inheritance in Man.

identified. Specific defects occur in collagen type I and III synthesis; lysyl hydroxylase deficiency may occur as well.

CLINICAL PRESENTATION Ehlers-Danlos syndrome type VI (EDS VI), or the ocular–scoliotic type, is autosomal recessive and associated with only moderate joint and skin extensibility, brittle cornea easily ruptured upon minor trauma, blue sclera, keratoconus and keratoglobus, and severe scoliosis. Type VIA shows lysyl hydroxylase deficiency, but type VIB shows normal production of lysyl hydroxylase.

LABORATORY EVALUATION Traditionally, clinical diagnosis of EDS VI is confirmed by an insufficiency of hydroxylysine on analysis of hydrolyzed dermis and/or reduced enzyme activity in cultured skin fibroblasts. However, the diagnosis can also be confirmed by an altered urinary ratio of lysyl pyridinoline to hydroxylysyl pyridinoline, which is characteristic of EDS VI.

MANAGEMENT Recognition of EDS VI is essential. In addition, the clinician must be aware of the syndrome's association with mitral valve prolapse, spontaneous bowel rupture, and strabismus surgery complications, as well as the potential to confuse the brittle cornea with injury due to child abuse. Use of patch grafts for repair of corneoscleral ruptures has been successful. Genetic counseling should be considered.

Marfan Syndrome

Marfan syndrome is a common autosomal dominant disorder associated with disorders of the eye (ectopia lentis) (Fig 8-10), heart (dilation of the aortic root and aneurysms of the aorta), and skeletal system (arachnodactyly, pectus excavatum, and kyphoscoliosis).

PATHOGENESIS Fibrillin and glycoprotein make up the microfibrillar system of the extracellular matrix. Fibrillin is found in corneal basement membrane, zonular fibers of the lens

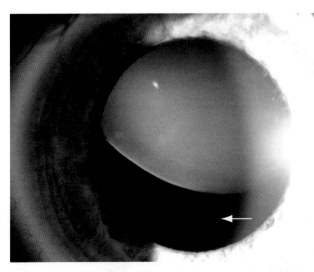

Figure 8-10 Slit-lamp photograph from a patient with Marfan syndrome, showing superior displacement of the lens. Note the stretched zonular fibers *(arrow)*. *(Courtesy of Stephen E. Orlin, MD.)*

and capsule, and sclera. The syndrome is caused by mutations in the *FBN1* gene, which encodes fibrillin-1 and maps to 15q21.1.

CLINICAL PRESENTATION Defects in fibrillin synthesis lead to thinning of the sclera (blue sclera), subluxation of the lens, and flattening of the cornea. Open-angle glaucoma and cataract occur at a higher rate and at an earlier age than in the population without Marfan syndrome. Megalocornea and keratoconus are uncommon, but excessive flattening, in the range of 35 diopters (D), occurs in up to 20% of patients.

MANAGEMENT Cardiac evaluation is typically considered, given that premature mortality is associated with aortic complications. Treatment of lens subluxation may require the use of advanced cataract surgery techniques such as capsular tension rings or scleral fixation; in severe cases of subluxation, a pars plana approach may be a better way to safely remove the lens. BCSC Section 11, *Lens and Cataract,* discusses the lens subluxation caused by Marfan syndrome and its treatment.

Osteogenesis Imperfecta

Osteogenesis imperfecta is a rare, dominantly inherited condition occurring in 1 in 20,000 live births. There are 4 types resulting from mutations in the *COL1A1* and *COL1A2* genes. The disease results in defects in the skeleton and teeth, hearing deficits, and ocular anomalies.

PATHOGENESIS The genetic mutation causes abnormalities of the α1 or α2 chain of type I collagen. As a result, the collagen fibrils fail to mature to their normal diameters.

CLINICAL PRESENTATION Patients with osteogenesis imperfecta are susceptible to brittle bones and multiple skeletal fractures. Hearing loss is common; the prevalence ranges from 50% to 92% in some studies. Hearing loss may be conductive, mixed, or sensorineural and is more common after adolescence. Patients are also predisposed to brittle teeth. Ocular manifestations include blue sclera (Fig 8-11) and reduced central corneal thickness (average of 450 μm). The blue sclera is present throughout life in type I osteogenesis imperfecta, but fades within the first few years of life in the other 3 types. Other rare ocular findings include optic nerve damage due to fractures in the calvarial bones, keratoconus, and megalocornea. Table 8-6 summarizes other conditions associated with blue sclera.

MANAGEMENT Treatment with oral bisphosphonates reduces bone resorption, and aggressive orthopedic management of fractures is indicated. Low-impact exercise might help preserve bone and muscle integrity.

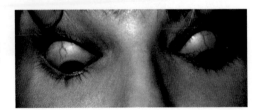

Figure 8-11 Clinical photograph showing blue sclera in a patient with osteogenesis imperfecta. *(Courtesy of Stephen E. Orlin, MD.)*

Table 8-6 Conditions and Medications Associated With Blue Sclera

Local
High myopia
Inactive scleritis
Oculodermal melanocytosis (nevus of Ota)
Previous eye surgeries
Thin sclerae in neonates

Systemic
Alkaptonuria
Brittle cornea syndrome
Ehlers-Danlos syndrome type VI
Hypophosphatasia
Marfan syndrome
Osteogenesis imperfecta
Primary adrenal insufficiency (Addison disease)

Medications
Amiodarone
Antimalarials
Minocycline
Phenothiazines

Goldenhar-Gorlin Syndrome

Goldenhar-Gorlin syndrome, also known as *oculoauriculovertebral (OAV) syndrome,* is a rare congenital condition characterized by incomplete development of the ear, nose, soft palate, lip, and mandible. It is associated with anomalous development of the first branchial arch and second branchial arch.

PATHOGENESIS The cause of Goldenhar-Gorlin syndrome is uncertain, but it may have a genetic component.

CLINICAL PRESENTATION Common clinical manifestations include limbal dermoids (Fig 8-12A), preauricular skin tags (Fig 8-12B), and strabismus. Affected patients also have hemifacial

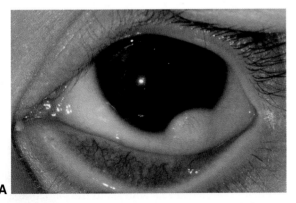
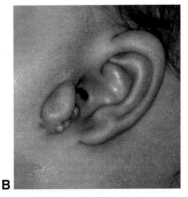

A

B

Figure 8-12 **A,** Clinical photograph showing an inferotemporal limbal dermoid in a patient with Goldenhar-Gorlin syndrome. Note the multiple hair follicles. **B,** External photograph showing preauricular skin tags in a patient with Goldenhar-Gorlin syndrome. *(Courtesy of Stephen E. Orlin, MD.)*

microsomia and hearing difficulties. The condition can be associated with colobomas of the eyelids (upper > lower eyelid) and with aural fistulae. In addition, scoliosis can develop secondary to incomplete development of the vertebrae. Corneal dermoids can occur independently of Goldenhar-Gorlin syndrome and are choristomas that result from faulty development of eyelid folds; thus, they are displaced embryonic tissue that was destined to become skin. Dermoids are composed of fibrous and fatty tissue and occasionally hair and sebaceous gland material. Limbal dermoids are covered by conjunctiva and often have an arcuslike deposition of lipid along their anterior corneal border. See Table 8-5 for additional clinical findings.

MANAGEMENT Corneal dermoids can lead to amblyopia if they induce significant corneal astigmatism. As the child grows, the dermoid enlarges with the eye; it has virtually no malignant potential. The elevated portion of the dermoids can be surgically shaved down to improve cosmetic appearance, but the lesions often extend deep into underlying tissues. Some corneal astigmatism might remain, but it can permit fitting of a rigid contact lens. LK can also improve the cosmetic appearance.

Al-Shamekh S, Traboulsi EI. Skeletal and connective tissue disorders with anterior segment manifestations. In: Mannis MJ, Holland EJ, eds. *Cornea.* Vol 1. 4th ed. Philadelphia: Elsevier; 2017:645–664.

Nutritional Disorder: Vitamin A Deficiency

Vitamin A deficiency is a leading cause of blindness in developing countries and is responsible for at least 20,000–100,000 new cases of blindness worldwide each year. The earliest manifestation of vision loss is night blindness, or nyctalopia. At greatest risk are malnourished infants and babies born to vitamin A–deficient mothers, especially infants who have another biological stressor, such as measles or diarrhea. Superficial concurrent infections due to herpes simplex virus, measles virus, or bacterial agents probably further predispose these children to keratomalacia and blindness. Although xerophthalmia usually results from low dietary intake of vitamin A, decreased absorption of vitamin A may also be responsible. In cases of vitamin A deficiency and xerophthalmia occurring in countries with a low rate of malnutrition, the condition is usually caused by unusual self-imposed dietary practices, chronic alcoholism, or lipid malabsorption (seen in cystic fibrosis, biliary cirrhosis, and bowel resection). The increase in gastric bypass surgical procedures may lead to an increased incidence of vitamin A deficiency.

PATHOGENESIS Vitamin A deficiency causes blindness by inhibiting the production of rhodopsin. Xerosis (abnormal dryness) of the conjunctiva and cornea due to vitamin A deficiency is associated with loss of mucus production by the goblet cells. Similar changes can occur in epithelial cells of the gastrointestinal, genitourinary, and respiratory tracts.

CLINICAL PRESENTATION One ocular consequence is the Bitôt spot (Fig 8-13), a superficial foamy, gray, triangular lesion on the bulbar conjunctiva that appears in the palpebral aperture. This spot consists of keratinized epithelium, inflammatory cells, debris, and *Corynebacterium xerosis.* *Corynebacterium* bacilli metabolize the debris, producing the foamy

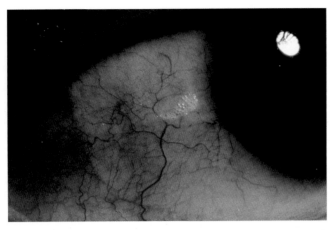

Figure 8-13 Clinical photograph showing a foamy Bitôt spot in the bulbar conjunctiva, close to the limbus, in a patient with anorexia. *(Courtesy of Stephen E. Orlin, MD.)*

appearance. Prolonged vitamin A deficiency may lead to corneal ulcers and scars and eventually cause diffuse corneal necrosis (keratomalacia). The World Health Organization classifies the ocular surface changes into 3 stages:

1. conjunctival xerosis, without (X1A) or with (X1B) Bitôt spots
2. corneal xerosis (X2)
3. corneal ulceration, with keratomalacia involving less than one-third (X3A) or more than one-third (X3B) of the corneal surface

MANAGEMENT Systemic vitamin A deficiency, best characterized by keratomalacia, is a medical emergency with a mortality rate of 50% if untreated. Although the administration of oral vitamin A will address the acute manifestations of keratomalacia, patients with this condition are usually affected by much broader protein-energy malnutrition and should be treated with both vitamin and protein-calorie supplements. Malabsorption may render oral administration ineffective in patients with acute vitamin A deficiency. Maintenance of adequate corneal lubrication and prevention of secondary infection and corneal melting are essential steps in treating keratomalacia, but identification and proper treatment of the underlying causes are vital to successful clinical management of the ocular complications.

Mannis T, Mannis MJ, Paranjpe DR, Kirkness CM. Nutritional disorders. In: Mannis MJ, Holland EJ, eds. *Cornea*. Vol 1. 4th ed. Philadelphia: Elsevier; 2017:676–687.

Sommer A. Vitamin A deficiency and clinical disease: an historical overview. *J Nutr.* 2008; 138(10):1835–1839.

Hematologic Disorders

The excess synthesis of immunoglobulins by plasma cells in multiple myeloma, Waldenström macroglobulinemia, and benign monoclonal gammopathy may be associated with crystalline corneal deposits (Fig 8-14).

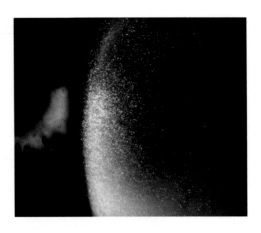

Figure 8-14 Slit-lamp photograph from a patient with multiple myeloma, showing polychromatic stromal crystals. *(Courtesy of Stephen E. Orlin, MD.)*

PATHOGENESIS Monoclonal proliferation of plasma cells (B lymphocytes) leads to overproduction of both light (κ or λ) chains and heavy (α, γ, ε, δ, or μ) chains (collectively termed M proteins), overproduction of light chains with or without production of heavy chains (Bence Jones protein), or overproduction of heavy chains without light chains (heavy-chain disease). Pathogenesis is related either to direct tissue invasion, particularly of the bone marrow, or to hyperviscosity syndrome. Secondary hypercalcemia may occur. Deposition of paraproteins in the cornea is very rare and is related to diffusion of the proteins—probably from the limbal vessels or, alternatively, from the tears or aqueous humor—followed by precipitation that may be related to corneal temperature or local tissue factors.

CLINICAL PRESENTATION Ophthalmic findings may include the following:

- crystalline deposition in all layers of the cornea or in the conjunctiva
- copper deposition in the cornea
- "sludging" of blood flow in the conjunctiva and retina
- pars plana proteinaceous cysts
- infiltration of the sclera
- orbital bony invasion with proptosis

Corneal deposits are numerous, scintillating, and polychromatic. They are typical of immunoglobulin G κ-chain deposition and may be related to the size of the paraprotein and the chronicity of the disease.

Waldenström macroglobulinemia is characterized by malignant proliferation of plasma cells generating immunoglobulin M, causing hyperviscosity syndrome, principally in older men. It has been associated with needlelike crystals and amorphous deposits subepithelially and in deep stroma (Fig 8-15).

Benign monoclonal gammopathy is a frequent (up to 6%) finding in individuals older than 60 years. Results of the systemic evaluation in these cases are negative, but a mild increase in paraprotein (<3 g/dL) is detected. Slit-lamp findings of iridescent crystals resemble those of myeloma and are very infrequent (approximately 1%–2% of affected patients).

Cryoglobulins, proteins that precipitate upon exposure to cold, occur nonspecifically in autoimmune disorders, immunoproliferative disorders, and hepatitis B infection.

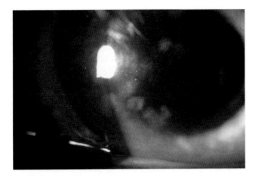

Figure 8-15 Clinical photograph from a patient with Waldenström macroglobulinemia, showing amorphous deposits in the stroma. *(Courtesy of Robert W. Weisenthal, MD.)*

Ophthalmic findings include signs of retinal hyperviscosity, occasional crystalline corneal deposits, amorphous limbal masses, and signs of autoimmune disease.

LABORATORY EVALUATION There are many causes of corneal crystalline deposits. The appearance and location of the deposits can help distinguish the underlying etiology.

Serum protein electrophoresis, complete blood count (CBC), and general screening for albumin/globulin and calcium levels are performed when clinical suspicion of immunoglobulin excess arises. Further testing for systemic evaluation depends on clinical suspicion and the initial findings.

MANAGEMENT No ophthalmic treatment is necessary unless the amorphous deposits interfere with vision and need to be removed with LK. Crystals resolve slowly after successful treatment of an underlying malignancy. See Table 8-2 for a list of other causes of corneal crystals.

Choulakian MY. Hematologic diseases and malignancies. In: Mannis MJ, Holland EJ, eds. *Cornea*. Vol 1. 4th ed. Philadelphia: Elsevier; 2017:688–695.

Endocrine Diseases

Diabetes Mellitus

The most common disorder of carbohydrate metabolism, diabetes mellitus (DM), has nonspecific corneal manifestations. See BCSC Section 1, *Update on General Medicine*, for detailed discussion of DM.

CLINICAL PRESENTATION Diabetic keratopathy includes superficial punctate epitheliopathy, epithelial erosions, hypoesthesia, persistent epithelial defects, and corneal edema. These changes occur with increasing severity and duration of the disease. Surgical removal of diabetic epithelium results in the loss of the basal cells and basement membrane, often leading to prolonged healing difficulties. Faint vertical folds in the Descemet membrane and deep stroma (Waite-Beetham lines) are not specific to DM but may represent early corneal endothelial dysfunction and increased stromal hydration.

LABORATORY EVALUATION An increase in glycosylated hemoglobin is related to poor control of DM and may correlate with poor corneal healing in addition to progressive retinopathy.

MANAGEMENT Diabetes mellitus is not a contraindication to PK or other corneal surgery. Measures that can improve diabetic epitheliopathy include the following:

- perioperative management of meibomian gland dysfunction (increased comorbidity with DM)
- minimizing epithelial debridement at surgery
- increasing lubrication
- avoiding toxic medications
- using therapeutic contact lenses, exercising caution because of the risk of infection

Srinivasan S, Shehadeh-Mashor R, Slomovic AR. Corneal manifestations of metabolic diseases. In: Mannis MJ, Holland EJ, eds. *Cornea*. Vol 1. 4th ed. Philadelphia: Elsevier; 2017:620–644.

Multiple Endocrine Neoplasia

Multiple endocrine neoplasia (MEN) is a group of disorders that affect the body's endocrine system. MEN typically involves tumors (neoplasia) in at least 2 endocrine glands. These growths can be benign or malignant. The condition is classified as MEN 1, MEN 2A, or MEN 2B, depending on the glands involved.

PATHOGENESIS MEN 2 results from a spontaneous mutation of the *RET* gene, or it is inherited in an autosomal dominant fashion.

CLINICAL PRESENTATION MEN 2B is characterized by medullary carcinoma of the thyroid gland, pheochromocytoma, and mucosal neuromas. Patients with MEN 2B have enlarged corneal nerves. In addition, they often have a marfanoid habitus. Conjunctival and eyelid neuromas and keratoconjunctivitis sicca may occur. Patients with MEN 2A also have been noted to have enlarged corneal nerves. Table 8-7 lists other causes of prominent corneal nerves (Fig 8-16) from either true enlargement or increased visibility.

Parathyroid Disease

Parathyroid hormone and calcitonin (one of the hormones produced by the thyroid gland) play key roles in regulating the amount of calcium in the blood and within the bones.

PATHOGENESIS Primary hyperparathyroidism is most commonly associated with benign proliferation of chief cells within a single parathyroid gland and, in rare cases, with

Table 8-7 Conditions Associated With Prominent Corneal Nerves

Enlarged Corneal Nerves	More Visible Corneal Nerves
Multiple endocrine neoplasia type 2B	Keratoconus
Phytanic acid storage disease (Refsum syndrome)	Ichthyosis
Hansen disease (leprosy, beading of nerves)	Fuchs endothelial corneal dystrophy
Familial dysautonomia (Riley-Day syndrome)	Corneal edema
Neurofibromatosis	Congenital glaucoma
Acanthamoeba perineuritis	—

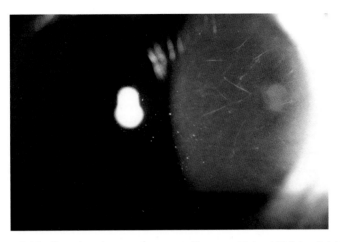

Figure 8-16 Prominent corneal nerves. *(Courtesy of Robert W. Weisenthal, MD.)*

MEN. Secondary hyperparathyroidism can be caused by renal disease in which excessive amounts of calcium are lost and the glands release a compensatory amount of parathyroid hormone. Parathyroid hyperplasia can occur in the presence of hypercalcemia and hypophosphatemia associated with milk-alkali syndrome, sarcoidosis, and excessive intake of vitamin D. Calcium deposition can occur despite normal parathyroid function and normal levels of systemic serum calcium. See Chapter 6 for further discussion.

CLINICAL PRESENTATION Calcium deposits within the interpalpebral area of the cornea are known as *band keratopathy*. The calcium is deposited in the superficial layers of the cornea and the Bowman layer.

MANAGEMENT If symptomatic with decreased vision or discomfort, the calcium can be removed with EDTA.

Darvish-Zargar M, Bartow RM. Endocrine disease and the cornea. In: Mannis MJ, Holland EJ, eds. *Cornea.* Vol 1. 4th ed. Philadelphia: Elsevier; 2017:696–704.

Dermatologic Diseases

Dermatologic disorders commonly have associated ophthalmic findings, particularly involving the eyelids.

Ichthyosis

Ichthyosis represents a diverse group of hereditary skin disorders characterized by excessively dry skin and accumulation of scales. These diseases are usually diagnosed during the first year of life.

    Ichthyosis vulgaris, an autosomal dominant trait, is the most common hereditary scaling disorder, affecting 1 in 250–300 people. Ocular involvement varies with this form of ichthyosis.

CLINICAL PRESENTATION Eyelid scaling, cicatricial ectropion, and conjunctival thickening are common in ichthyosis. Primary corneal opacities are noted in 50% of patients with X-linked ichthyosis but are rarely seen in patients with ichthyosis vulgaris. Dotlike or filament-shaped opacities appear diffusely in pre–Descemet membrane or in deep stroma and become more apparent with age without affecting vision. Nodular corneal degeneration and band keratopathy have been described. Secondary corneal changes such as vascularization and scarring from severe ectropion-related exposure can develop.

MANAGEMENT The goal of treatment in all ichthyosis disorders is to hydrate the skin and eyelids, remove scales, and slow the turnover of epidermis, when appropriate. These disorders are not responsive to corticosteroids.

Ectodermal Dysplasia

Ectodermal dysplasia is a heterogeneous group of conditions characterized by the following:

- presence of abnormalities at birth
- nonprogressive course
- diffuse involvement of the epidermis plus at least 1 of its appendages (hair, nails, teeth, sweat glands)
- various inheritance patterns

PATHOGENESIS Ectodermal dysplasia is a rare hereditary condition that displays variable defects in the morphogenesis of ectodermal structures, including hair, skin, nails, and teeth. It is a component of at least 150 distinct hereditary syndromes.

CLINICAL PRESENTATION Many ocular abnormalities have been described in the ectodermal dysplasias, including sparse eyelashes and eyebrows, blepharitis, ankyloblepharon, hypoplastic lacrimal ducts, diminished tear production, abnormal meibomian glands, dry conjunctivae, pterygia, corneal scarring and neovascularization, cataract, and glaucoma. The ocular surface changes may be due to limbal stem cell deficiency. Although the dermatologic manifestations are nonprogressive, the corneal conditions can worsen with time.

MANAGEMENT The ocular surface changes and blepharitis can be managed with tear replacement and preservation, together with eyelid hygiene. Keratolimbal autograft transplantation in combination with PK can be performed.

Xeroderma Pigmentosum

PATHOGENESIS Xeroderma pigmentosum is a rare, autosomal recessive disease characterized by extreme skin photosensitivity resulting from an impaired ability to repair sunlight-induced damage to DNA.

CLINICAL PRESENTATION During the first or second decade of life, the patient's sun-exposed skin develops areas of focal hyperpigmentation, atrophy, actinic keratosis, and telangiectasia—as though the patient received a heavy dose of radiation. Later, many cutaneous neoplasms appear; these include squamous cell carcinoma, basal cell carcinoma, and melanoma. Ophthalmic manifestations include photophobia, tearing, blepharospasm, and signs and symptoms of keratoconjunctivitis sicca. The conjunctiva is dry and inflamed with telangiectasia and hyperpigmentation. Pingueculae and pterygia often occur. Corneal complications include exposure keratitis, ulceration, neovascularization, scarring, and even perforation. Keratoconus and gelatinous droplike corneal dystrophy have also been reported. Ocular neoplasms occur in 11% of affected patients, most frequently at the limbus. Squamous cell carcinoma is the most frequent histologic type, followed by basal cell carcinoma and melanoma. The eyelids can be involved, with progressive atrophy, madarosis, trichiasis, scarring, symblepharon, entropion, ectropion, and sometimes even loss of the entire lower eyelid.

Other dermatologic disorders that have ocular manifestations include seborrhea, staphylococcal hypersensitivity, rosacea, and atopic disease. The cornea may show marginal ulceration, neovascularization, and pannus formation. These topics are discussed in depth in Chapter 3.

MANAGEMENT Skin protection from ultraviolet radiation, including use of sunscreen and protective clothing, is the mainstay of therapy. In addition, patients with xeroderma pigmentosum should be monitored for skin and eyelid malignancies.

Mannis MJ, Macsai MS, Huntley AC, eds. *Eye and Skin Disease.* Philadelphia: Lippincott-Raven; 1996.

Sadowsky AE. Dermatologic disorders and the cornea. In: Mannis MJ, Holland EJ, eds. *Cornea.* Vol 1. 4th ed. Philadelphia: Elsevier; 2017:705–718.

CHAPTER 9

Infectious Diseases of the External Eye: Basic Concepts and Viral Infections

Highlights

- Tetracaine provides better conjunctival anesthesia than proparacaine hydrochloride; however, it has antimicrobial properties that may interfere with organism recovery when cultures are performed.
- Most organisms are eventually cleared from the site of an acute infection, but some persist in the host indefinitely. For example, after primary infection, herpes simplex virus and varicella-zoster virus establish latency in trigeminal ganglion cells.
- Topical antivirals for herpes simplex keratitis are rarely needed for longer than 7–10 days. Persistent disease despite topical antiviral therapy suggests misdiagnosis, medication toxicity, or immune dysfunction.

Normal Ocular Flora

Bacterial colonization of the eyelid margin and conjunctiva is normal and can be beneficial as long as normal flora competitively inhibit pathogenic strains. The spectrum of normal ocular flora varies with the age and geographic locale of the host. In the eye of an infant delivered vaginally, multiple bacterial species predominate, including *Staphylococcus aureus*, *Staphylococcus epidermidis*, streptococci, and *Escherichia coli*; streptococci and pneumococci then predominate during the first 2 decades of life. Although gram-negative bacteria are more commonly isolated with age, *S epidermidis* and other coagulase-negative staphylococci, *S aureus*, and diphtheroids remain some of the most common species identified from the external eye (Table 9-1). Nonpathogenic colonization of the eyelid margin with *Demodex folliculorum* and *Demodex brevis* also becomes more common with age, and these parasites become almost ubiquitous over time. Any use of topical antibiotics or corticosteroids can alter the character and spectrum of eyelid and conjunctival flora.

Table 9-1 Relative Prevalence of the Normal Flora of the External Eye

Microorganisms	Normal Conjunctiva	Normal Eyelid Margin
Staphylococcus epidermidis	+ + +	+ + +
Staphylococcus aureus	+ +	+ +
Micrococcus spp	+	+ +
Corynebacterium spp (diphtheroids)	+ +	+ +
Propionibacterium acnes	+ +	+ +
Streptococcus spp*	+	±
Haemophilus influenzae*	±	−
Moraxella spp	±	−
Enteric gram-negative bacilli	±	−
Bacillus spp	±	−
Anaerobic bacteria	+	±
Yeasts (Malassezia furfur, Candida spp, etc)	−	+
Filamentous fungi	±	−
Demodex spp	−	+ +

*More common in children.

Fintelmann RE, Hoskins EN, Lietman TM, et al. Topical fluoroquinolone use as a risk factor for in vitro fluoroquinolone resistance in ocular cultures. *Arch Ophthalmol.* 2011;129(4): 399–402.

Graham JE, Moore JE, Jiru X, et al. Ocular pathogen or commensal: a PCR-based study of surface bacterial flora in normal and dry eyes. *Invest Ophthalmol Vis Sci.* 2007;48(12): 5616–5623.

Kemal M, Sümer Z, Toker MI, Erdoğan H, Topalkara A, Akbulut M. The prevalence of *Demodex folliculorum* in blepharitis patients and the normal population. *Ophthalmic Epidemiol.* 2005;12(4):287–290.

Pathogenesis of Ocular Infections

Ocular infection can occur via *exogenous inoculation* or *hematogenous seeding,* which is rare. The initiation, severity, and characteristics of subsequent infection are influenced by the interplay between the virulence of the pathogen, the inoculum size, and the competence and nature of host defense mechanisms. Microbial virulence factors represent evolutionary adaptations by each microorganism that increase the organism's odds of infection and survival. For example, highly virulent pathogens are more likely to cause infection than an equal number of less virulent pathogens; however, an infection may still result from either exposure, with the only difference being chance. The status of host defense mechanisms also determines the threshold of inoculum at which infection is more likely to occur. Compromised cells or organisms may not be able to avert infection as well as healthy cells or tissues (see Defense Mechanisms of the External Eye and Cornea in Chapter 1).

In ocular surface infections acquired via exogenous inoculation, adherence of organisms to ocular surface epithelium is the first step. Many microorganisms express *adhesins,* proteins that bind with high affinity to host cell surface molecules, for example:

- *Candida albicans* expresses surface proteins that mimic mammalian *integrins* (transmembrane proteins that mediate cell–cell and cell–extracellular matrix interactions).

- Viruses typically express surface proteins or glycoproteins that attach to constitutive cell surface molecules such as heparan sulfate (herpes simplex virus) or sialic acid (adenovirus).
- *Acanthamoeba* trophozoites express a mannose-binding protein that attaches to surface epithelial cells.

Few organisms can invade an intact epithelium. Those that can include

- *Neisseria gonorrhoeae*
- *Neisseria meningitidis*
- *Corynebacterium diphtheriae*
- *Shigella* species
- *Haemophilus influenzae* biotype III (formerly *Haemophilus aegyptius*)
- *Listeria monocytogenes*
- *Fusarium species*

Others must rely on a break in epithelial barrier function. For example, microbial proteases facilitate invasion by inducing cell lysis, degrading the extracellular matrix, and activating native corneal matrix–derived metalloproteinases (MMPs), triggering autodigestion. Bacterial exotoxins, such as those produced by streptococci, staphylococci, and *Pseudomonas aeruginosa,* can induce corneal cell necrosis. *Acanthamoeba* species and certain fungi secrete collagenases, whereas *P aeruginosa* elastase and alkaline protease destroy collagen and proteoglycan components of the cornea and degrade immunoglobulins, complement, interleukins, and other inflammatory cytokines. For viruses, adherence interactions facilitate invasion by the appropriation of host cell mechanisms.

Once adherent, some bacteria protect themselves from unfavorable elements of their physical environment, such as immunologic cells or antibacterial molecules in the tears, by the expression of exopolysaccharides organized into a *biofilm,* a 3-dimensional structure that allows interbacterial communication and signaling and interferes with phagocytosis. For viruses, evasion of the immune response involves multiple strategies.

Most organisms are eventually cleared from the site of an acute infection, but some persist in the host indefinitely. For example, following primary infection, herpes simplex virus and varicella-zoster virus establish latency in trigeminal ganglion cells. Chlamydial organisms survive and cause local chronic disease by persistence within intracellular phagosomes.

McDougald D, Rice SA, Barraud N, Steinberg PD, Kjelleberg S. Should we stay or should we go: mechanisms and ecological consequences for biofilm dispersal. *Nat Rev Microbiol.* 2011;10(1):39–50.

Momburg F, Hengel H. Corking the bottleneck: the transporter associated with antigen processing as a target for immune subversion by viruses. *Curr Top Microbiol Immunol.* 2002; 269:57–74.

Ocular Microbiology

Of the many potentially pathogenic microorganisms capable of causing infectious external eye disease, those encountered most often are listed in Table 9-2.

Diagnostic Laboratory Techniques

The recent rise in the number of atypical ocular infections and the emergence of antibiotic-resistant strains have significantly increased the importance of specific microbiologic diagnosis. Interpretation of diagnostic specimens requires an understanding of the normal flora and cytology of the ocular surface. For optimal specimen collection, the appropriate materials should be available (Tables 9-3, 9-4). See BCSC Section 4, *Ophthalmic Pathology and Intraocular Tumors,* for additional discussion of specimen collection and handling, as well as laboratory evaluation for individual disease entities.

> Thompson PP, Kowalski RP. A 13-year retrospective review of polymerase chain reaction testing for infectious agents from ocular samples. *Ophthalmology.* 2011;118(7):1449–1453.

Specimen collection

Eyelid specimens Eyelid vesicles or pustules may be opened with a sharp-pointed surgical blade or small-gauge needle. Material for cytology is smeared onto a glass slide and

Table 9-2 Principal Causes of External Ocular Infections

Condition	Viruses	Bacteria	Fungi	Parasites
Dermatoblepharitis	Herpes simplex	*Staphylococcus aureus*	—	—
	Varicella-zoster	*Streptococcus* spp		
Blepharitis	Herpes simplex	*Staphylococcus* spp	—	*Phthirus pubis*
	Molluscum contagiosum	*Moraxella* spp		*Demodex* spp
Conjunctivitis	Adenovirus	*Chlamydia trachomatis*	—	—
	Herpes simplex	*Staphylococcus aureus*		
	Picornavirus	*Streptococcus* spp		
		Neisseria gonorrhoeae		
		Haemophilus influenzae		
		Moraxella spp		
Keratitis	Herpes simplex	*Pseudomonas aeruginosa*	*Fusarium* spp	*Acanthamoeba* spp
		Staphylococcus aureus	*Aspergillus* spp	
		Staphylococcus epidermidis	*Candida albicans*	
		Streptococcus pneumoniae		
		Moraxella spp		
Dacryoadenitis	Epstein-Barr virus	*Staphylococcus aureus*	—	—
	Mumps	*Streptococcus pneumoniae*		
Canaliculitis	Herpes simplex	Actinomycetes	*Candida* sp,	—
		Streptococcus spp	*Aspergillus* sp	
		Staphylococcus spp		
Dacryocystitis		*Staphylococcus* spp	*Candida* (rare)	—
		Streptococcus spp		

Table 9-3 Materials for Collecting Eyelid, Conjunctival, and Corneal Specimens for Ocular Microbiology

Viral Infections	Chlamydial Infections	Microbial Infections
Topical anesthetic (proparacaine hydrochloride 0.5%)	Topical anesthetic (proparacaine hydrochloride 0.5%)	Topical anesthetic (proparacaine hydrochloride 0.5%)
Dacron swabs	Dacron swabs	Calcium alginate or Dacron swabs
Spatula	Spatula	Spatula
Glass slides	Glass slides	Glass slides
Acetone fixative	Methanol or acetone fixative	Methanol fixative
Viral transport medium	Chlamydial transport medium	Blood agar plate
Ice	Ice	Chocolate agar plate
		Sabouraud dextrose agar plate or brain–heart infusion agar
		Nonnutrient agar plate with *Enterobacter aerogenes* overlay
		Thioglycollate or meat broth

Table 9-4 Commonly Used Stains and Culture Media for Microbial Keratitis

Suspected Organism	Stain	Media
Aerobic bacteria	Gram	Blood agar
	Acridine orange	Chocolate agar
		Thioglycollate broth
Anaerobic bacteria	Gram	Anaerobic blood agar
	Acridine orange	Phenylethyl alcohol agar in anaerobic chamber
		Thioglycollate or chopped meat broth
Mycobacteria	Gram	Blood agar
	Acid-fast	Lowenstein-Jensen agar
	Lectin	
Fungi	Gram	Blood agar (25°C)
	Acridine orange	Sabouraud agar (25°C)
	Calcofluor white	Brain–heart infusion agar (25°C)
Acanthamoeba	Acridine orange	Nonnutrient agar with bacterial overlay *(Enterobacter aerogenes, Escherichia coli)*
	Calcofluor white	
	Gram	
	Giemsa	Blood agar
	Indirect immunofluorescence antibody	Buffered charcoal–yeast extract agar

fixed in methanol or acetone for immunofluorescent staining. Collected vesicular fluid can be inoculated into a chilled viral transport medium for culture isolation in the laboratory. Microbial cultures are obtained by wiping the abnormal area with a broth-moistened swab, followed by direct inoculation of culture media. Culture of epilated eyelashes may be helpful in cases of chronic infection.

Conjunctival specimens To minimize contamination of and inhibitory effects on organisms recovered, conjunctival swabbing for microbial specimens should be performed without topical anesthetic. For specimen collection, the clinician must debride enough conjunctival epithelial cells so that intracellular microbes can be seen on chemical stains. Calcium alginate or sterile Dacron swabs slightly moistened with thioglycollate broth are preferable to cotton-tipped swabs because the latter contain fatty acids, which may inhibit bacterial and viral growth. The swabbed material should be plated directly onto warmed solid media (blood, chocolate, and Sabouraud dextrose agar). The "nonhandled" distal end of the swab may then be broken off and placed directly into the remaining thioglycollate broth tube. If these media are not available, the specimens may be harvested with any standard culturette tube system that contains appropriate transport media.

When more conjunctival epithelial cells are desired, conjunctival scraping is the preferred method and reduces contamination from debris on the ocular surface. A local anesthetic is applied topically to the everted eyelid. Use of proparacaine hydrochloride 0.5% minimizes inhibition of organism recovery compared with tetracaine. A sterile spatula is scraped firmly across the tarsus; this should cause blanching but minimal bleeding. Alternatively, a cytobrush may be used to rub the conjunctiva, after which it is placed in a buffer solution to release the epithelial cells onto a Millipore filter. The cells are then fixed.

Appropriate instrumentation and proper handling are critical for specimens destined for polymerase chain reaction (PCR) testing, because any residual foreign DNA in the specimen may be detected by PCR. Conjunctival biopsy can be performed to help in the diagnosis of conditions such as Parinaud oculoglandular syndrome, mucous membrane pemphigoid, and human papillomavirus infection. See Chapter 13 for a more detailed description of conjunctival biopsy.

Corneal specimens A corneal culture is important to determine the etiology of large or sight-threatening ulcers, ulcers in which an atypical organism is suspected, or any ulcer that is not responding to therapy. A microbial specimen can be collected from a corneal ulcer by scraping the lesion with any of the following (with similar yields): platinum Kimura spatula, sterile needle, surgical blade, or thioglycollate-moistened calcium alginate or Dacron swab. For larger corneal ulcers (>2 mm), samples should be taken from several regions. A blade or spatula is preferable for preparing smears for chemical staining, but either a spatula or swab is acceptable for inoculation of culture media.

Specimens are best inoculated immediately onto microbiologic media that have been warmed to room temperature in anticipation of the culture procedure; microscopic slides should be prepared for Gram, Giemsa, or other special stains. To avoid contamination and false positives, care must be taken to avoid touching the blade or swab to the eyelids, fingers, or other nonsterile surface; in addition, a sterile instrument or swab should be used for each separate row of C-shaped streaks on each agar plate (Fig 9-1) and for each type of broth culture. For a viral culture, a Dacron swab is used to obtain virus-infected corneal or conjunctival cells; the swab is agitated in a chilled viral transport medium and then discarded. Calcium alginate and cotton swabs should be avoided, as both may inhibit viral recovery.

Corneal biopsy may be necessary in cases of apparent and significant microbial infection when repeated cultures from corneal scrapings are negative. See Chapter 13.

In vivo confocal microscopy may be a helpful diagnostic and management tool with reasonable sensitivity and specificity for larger microorganisms such as *Acanthamoeba* and fungi.

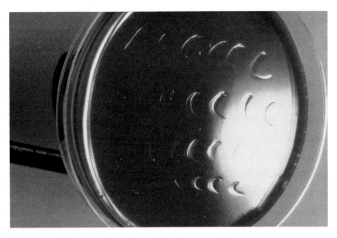

Figure 9-1 "C" streaks on a chocolate blood agar plate. *(Courtesy of James Chodosh, MD.)*

Alexandrakis G, Haimovici R, Miller D, Alfonso EC. Corneal biopsy in the management of progressive microbial keratitis. *Am J Ophthalmol.* 2000;129(5):571–576.

Kumar RL, Cruzat A, Hamrah P. Current state of in vivo confocal microscopy in management of microbial keratitis. *Semin Ophthalmol.* 2010;25(5–6):166–170.

Younger JR, Johnson RD, Holland GN, et al. Microbiologic and histopathologic assessment of corneal biopsies in the evaluation of microbial keratitis. *Am J Ophthalmol.* 2012;154(3): 512–519.e2.

Isolation techniques For viral, chlamydial, and microsporidial infections, an appropriate tissue-culture cell line is selected for inoculation and examined for the development of cytopathic effects (CPEs) and cellular inclusions. For bacterial and fungal infections, directly inoculated blood, chocolate, and Sabouraud agars and thioglycollate broth are examined daily to detect visible growth. Microorganisms are studied by chemical staining, chemical reactions, and antimicrobial sensitivity testing. *Acanthamoeba* may be identified by the trails left by trophozoites on blood agar, but nonnutrient agar with an overlay of killed *Enterobacter aerogenes* is the optimal isolation medium.

Staining methods
See Table 9-4 for recommended stains and culture media in the setting of suspected microbial keratitis.

Virology and Viral Infections

Viruses are small (10–400 nm in diameter) infectious units consisting of a single-stranded or double-stranded nucleic acid genome and a protein shell, or *capsid*, with or without an external lipid envelope. Viral nucleic acid consists of either RNA or DNA. RNA viral genome may be either single-stranded or double-stranded. Antiviral medications typically target viral gene transcription. Therefore, the clinical significance of the nucleic acid type lies principally in differences in susceptibility to antiviral medications.

The viral capsid interacts internally with the genome to stabilize it, protects the genome from the external environment, and, in the case of nonenveloped viruses, expresses on its surface the ligand for virus–host cell binding.

In some virus families, a host cell–derived lipid bilayer, or envelope, surrounds the protein capsid. Viral genome–encoded glycoproteins bound to the membrane act as ligands (antigens) for neutralizing antibodies directed against the virus. The lipid envelope is vulnerable to damage by ultraviolet (UV) light, detergents, alcohols, and general-use antiseptics. Because of this vulnerability, *enveloped viruses,* such as herpes simplex virus and human immunodeficiency virus (HIV), are intrinsically susceptible to the external environment, and their infectivity is short-lived outside the host. Enveloped viruses are difficult to transmit via fomites or medical instruments, and alcohol treatment of medical instrumentation is generally sufficient to prevent iatrogenic infection.

In contrast, *nonenveloped viruses,* such as adenoviruses, are relatively resistant to environmental insult and, in some cases, can persist for weeks outside the human host. To reduce the spread of such viruses in an office practice, the Centers for Disease Control and Prevention recommends the application of dilute bleach (1 part household bleach [containing 5.25%–6.15% sodium hypochlorite] and 9 parts water) to tonometer tips for at least 10 minutes; however, care must be taken to clean residual bleach from the tonometer tip before use to prevent corneal toxicity. Alcohol sterilization is ineffective in this setting. For further discussion of infectious diseases, see BCSC Section 1, *Update on General Medicine.*

King AMQ, Lefkowitz E, Adams MJ, Carstens EB. *Virus Taxonomy: Ninth Report of the International Committee on Taxonomy of Viruses.* Oxford, UK: Elsevier; 2012.

Rutala WA, Weber DJ; Healthcare Infection Control Practices Advisory Committee (HICPAC). Guideline for disinfection and sterilization in healthcare facilities, 2008. Centers for Disease Control and Prevention website. www.cdc.gov/infectioncontrol /guidelines/disinfection/index.html. Updated December 29, 2009. Accessed November 20, 2017.

DNA Viruses: Herpesviruses

The structure of all herpesviruses includes a core of linear double-stranded DNA genome, surrounded by an icosahedral protein capsid, which is contained in an envelope studded with viral glycoproteins. Of the 8 known human herpesviruses, those that affect the eye include herpes simplex virus types 1 and 2 (HSV-1, HSV-2), varicella-zoster virus (VZV), Epstein-Barr virus (EBV), cytomegalovirus (CMV), and Kaposi sarcoma–associated herpesvirus (KSHV). All herpesviruses establish latency in their natural hosts, but the site of latency varies. For example, whereas HSV-1, HSV-2, and VZV establish latent infections in neurons of the sensory ganglia such as the trigeminal ganglion, EBV latency occurs in B lymphocytes.

Herpes Simplex Eye Diseases

Herpes simplex virus infection is ubiquitous in humans; at autopsy, nearly 100% of persons older than 60 years are found to harbor HSV. Worldwide, most primary exposure to HSV occurs early in life, but in developing countries, primary exposure is increasingly delayed. It has been estimated that one-third of the world population experiences recurrent infection. HSV infections are, therefore, a large and worldwide public health problem.

PATHOGENESIS HSV-1 and HSV-2 are antigenically related. HSV-1 more commonly causes infection above the waist (orofacial and ocular infection) and HSV-2, below the waist (genital infection); but either virus can cause disease in either location. Primary infection with HSV-1 frequently manifests as a nonspecific upper respiratory tract infection and is recognized as HSV less than 5% of the time. In industrialized societies, 40%–80% of adults have serum antibodies to HSV-1, which represents a decline in infection from previous decades, and the age at which individuals undergo serologic conversion is increasing; HSV is now more commonly acquired in adolescence than in childhood. HSV infection is spread by direct contact with infected lesions or their secretions, most commonly as a result of exposure to viruses shed without clinical symptoms. HSV can be transmitted to the neonate during passage through the birth canal of a mother with active genital infection. In the newborn, HSV can cause systemic infection, including encephalitis, or disease confined to the skin and mucous membranes. BCSC Section 6, *Pediatric Ophthalmology and Strabismus,* discusses neonatal herpes infection in greater detail.

HSV spreads from infected skin and mucosal epithelium via sensory nerve axons to establish latent infection in associated sensory nerve ganglia, most commonly the trigeminal ganglion. Latent infection of the trigeminal ganglion may occur in the absence of recognized primary infection, and reactivation of the virus may follow in any of the 3 branches of cranial nerve V (ophthalmic nerve [V_1], maxillary nerve [V_2], and mandibular nerve [V_3]), despite primary disease in the area of innervation of 1 particular branch. Approximately 0.15% of the US population has a history of external ocular HSV infection, and in approximately one-fifth of these individuals, stromal keratitis, the most common blinding manifestation of infection, develops.

Liesegang TJ. Herpes simplex virus epidemiology and ocular importance. *Cornea.* 2001;20(1): 1–13.

Pepose JS, Keadle TL, Morrison LA. Ocular herpes simplex: changing epidemiology, emerging disease patterns, and the potential of vaccine prevention and therapy. *Am J Ophthalmol.* 2006;141(3):547–557.

Primary ocular infection

CLINICAL PRESENTATION Primary ocular HSV infection typically manifests as a blepharoconjunctivitis. The conjunctival inflammatory response is follicular and accompanied by a palpable preauricular lymph node. Vesicles on the skin (Fig 9-2) or eyelid margin (Fig 9-3) are important for diagnosis. Patients with primary ocular HSV infection can develop epithelial keratitis (Fig 9-4), but stromal keratitis and uveitis are uncommon.

Signs that can help the clinician distinguish acute primary ocular HSV infection from acute primary infection associated with adenovirus include the following:

- vesicles on the skin or eyelid margin or ulcers on the bulbar conjunctiva (HSV)
- dendritic epithelial keratitis (HSV)
- conjunctival membranes or pseudomembranes (adenovirus)

Laterality is not a reliable distinguishing feature. Although adenoviral infections are more commonly bilateral, they can be unilateral, bilateral but asymmetric, or bilateral with

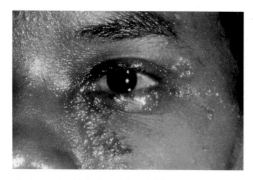

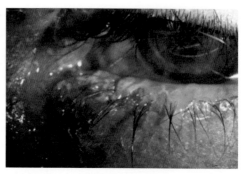

Figure 9-2 Skin vesicles of herpes simplex virus (HSV) dermatoblepharitis. *(Courtesy of James Chodosh, MD.)*

Figure 9-3 Eyelid margin ulcers characteristic of primary ocular HSV infection after vesicular rupture. *(Courtesy of Cornea Service, Paulista School of Medicine, Federal University of São Paulo.)*

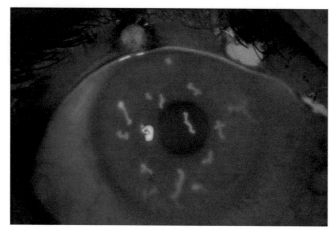

Figure 9-4 Fluorescein staining of an eye with primary HSV infection demonstrates characteristic upper eyelid margin ulcers and a coarse dendritic epithelial keratitis. *(Courtesy of James Chodosh, MD.)*

delayed involvement of the second eye. Similarly, primary HSV infection may be either unilateral (most common) or bilateral.

LABORATORY EVALUATION Demonstration of HSV is possible in productive epithelial infection with viral culture or antigen- or DNA-detection methodologies. Results of serologic tests for neutralizing or complement-fixing immunoglobulins may show a rising antibody titer during primary infection, but these tests are of no diagnostic assistance during recurrent episodes. As most adults are latently infected with HSV, serologic testing generally is helpful only when the results are negative.

Laboratory tests are indicated in complicated cases when the clinical diagnosis is uncertain and in all cases of suspected neonatal herpes infection. Vesicles can be opened with a needle, and vesicular fluid cultured. Scrapings from the vesicle base can be tested by cytology or for the presence of HSV antigen. Conjunctival scrapings or impression cytology specimens can be similarly analyzed by culture, antigen detection, or PCR.

MANAGEMENT Primary ocular HSV infection is a self-limited condition. Oral antiviral therapy speeds resolution of signs and symptoms. Table 9-5 summarizes the antiviral agents that are effective against ocular HSV infections. For discussion about their use, see the respective clinical syndromes below.

Recurrent ocular infection

PATHOGENESIS Recurrent HSV infection is caused by reactivation of the virus in a latently infected sensory ganglion, transport of the virus down the nerve axon to sensory nerve endings, and subsequent infection of ocular surface epithelia. HSV latency locally, in the cornea, as a cause of recurrent disease remains a controversial concept.

Table 9-5 Antiviral Agents in External/Corneal Infections With Herpes Simplex Virus

Agent	Mechanism of Action	Administration	Dosage for Acute Disease
Vidarabine	Purine analogue Inhibits DNA polymerase	3% ophthalmic ointment*	5×/day for 10 days
Trifluridine	Pyrimidine analogue Blocks DNA synthesis	1% ophthalmic solution	8×/day for 10 days
Acyclovir	Activated by HSV thymidine kinase to inhibit viral DNA polymerase	3% ophthalmic ointment[†]	5×/day for 10 days
		200, 400, 800 mg; 200 mg/ 5 mL suspension	400 mg 5×/day for 10 days
		5% dermatologic ointment[‡]	6×/day for 7 days
Famciclovir[§]	Prodrug of penciclovir	125, 250, 500 mg	250 mg 3×/day for 10 days
Valacyclovir[§]	L-valyl ester of acyclovir	500, 1000 mg	1000 mg 2×/day for 10 days
Valganciclovir	L-valyl ester of ganciclovir	450 mg	Induction: 900 mg (two 450-mg tablets) 2×/day for 21 days Maintenance: 900 mg (two 450-mg tablets) 1×/day
Penciclovir	Inhibits viral DNA polymerase	1% dermatologic cream[‡]	8×/day for 4 days
Ganciclovir	Cytomegalovirus nucleoside analogue Inhibits DNA polymerase	0.15% topical ophthalmic gel	5×/day until epithelium heals; then 3×/day for 7 days

* No longer manufactured; can be obtained through compounding pharmacies.
† Not commercially available in the United States.
‡ Not for ophthalmic use.
§ Optimal dose for ocular disease not determined.

The concept of environmental factors (psychological stress, systemic infection, sunlight exposure, menstrual cycle, and contact lens wear) acting as triggers for the recurrence of HSV ocular disease was not confirmed by the Herpetic Eye Disease Study (HEDS), despite reports of UV light–induced reactivation of herpes labialis and keratitis. HSV keratitis recurs more frequently in patients with HIV infection, but the severity of the keratitis is equal to that occurring in immunocompetent persons.

> Herpetic Eye Disease Study Group. Psychological stress and other potential triggers for recurrences of herpes simplex virus eye infections. *Arch Ophthalmol.* 2000;118(12): 1617–1625.

CLINICAL PRESENTATION Recurrent HSV infection can affect almost any ocular tissue, including the eyelid, conjunctiva, cornea, iris, uveal tract, trabecular meshwork, retina, and optic nerve, and it is typically unilateral, with only 3% of patients demonstrating bilateral disease (see Table 9-7). The presence of bilateral disease should raise the possibility of immune dysfunction (eg, atopic dermatitis).

Blepharoconjunctivitis Eyelid and/or conjunctival involvement can occur in patients with recurrent ocular HSV infection, although it may be clinically indistinguishable from primary infection. The condition is self-limited, but it can be treated with antiviral agents to shorten the course of illness and thus reduce the cornea's exposure to infectious virus.

Epithelial keratitis One of the most common presentations of clinically recognizable recurrent ocular HSV infection is epithelial keratitis.

CLINICAL PRESENTATION Patients with epithelial keratitis report foreign-body sensation, light sensitivity, redness, and blurred vision. HSV infection of human corneal epithelium manifests as areas of punctate epithelial keratitis (Fig 9-5) that may coalesce into 1 or more arborizing dendritic epithelial ulcers whose branches have terminal bulbs. The cytopathic swollen corneal epithelium at the edge of a herpetic ulcer stains with rose bengal (Fig 9-6) or lissamine green because of loss of cell membrane glycoproteins and subsequent lack of mucin binding by the cells. The bed of the ulcer stains with fluorescein (Fig 9-7) because of loss of cellular integrity and absence of intercellular tight junctions.

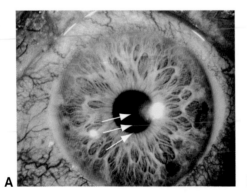
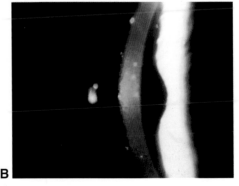

A **B**

Figure 9-5 **A,** Punctate epithelial keratitis *(arrows)*; the lesion was culture-positive for HSV. **B,** Note the atypical raised edges and depressed center. *(Courtesy of Woodford S. Van Meter, MD.)*

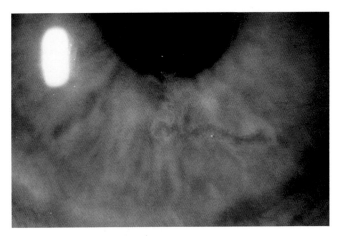

Figure 9-6   Rose bengal staining of herpetic epithelial keratitis outlines a typical dendrite. *(Courtesy of James Chodosh, MD.)*

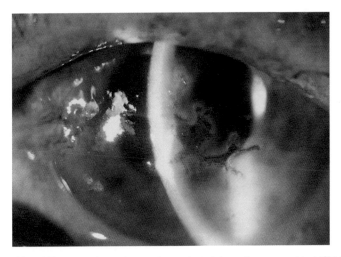

Figure 9-7   Combined fluorescein and rose bengal staining of geographic HSV keratitis. *(Courtesy of Cornea Service, Paulista School of Medicine, Federal University of São Paulo.)*

Areas of dendritic keratitis may coalesce further, enlarging into a more expansive geographic epithelial ulcer (Fig 9-8; see also Fig 9-7), particularly when topical corticosteroids are used.

Patients with HSV epithelial keratitis exhibit a ciliary flush and mild conjunctival injection. Mild stromal edema and subepithelial white blood cell infiltration may occur beneath the epithelial keratitis. Following resolution of dendritic epithelial keratitis, nonsuppurative subepithelial infiltration and scarring may be seen just beneath the area of prior epithelial ulceration, resulting in a ghost image, or ghost dendrite (Fig 9-9), which reflects the position and shape of the prior epithelial involvement.

Focal or diffuse reduction in corneal sensation occurs following HSV epithelial keratitis. The distribution of corneal hypoesthesia is related to the extent, duration, severity,

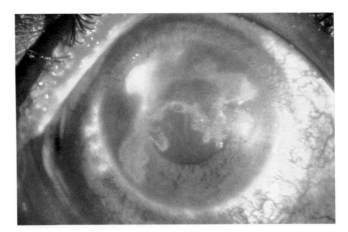

Figure 9-8 Herpetic geographic epithelial keratitis. *(Reprinted with permission from Chodosh J. Viral keratitis. In: Parrish RK, ed. The University of Miami Bascom Palmer Eye Institute Atlas of Ophthalmology. Boston: Current Medicine; 1999.)*

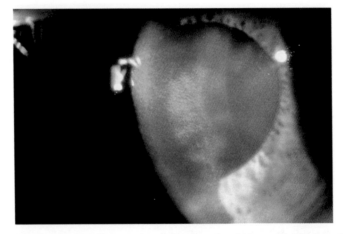

Figure 9-9 Residual stromal inflammation following dendritic epithelial keratitis may leave the impression of a ghost image of the dendrite. *(Reprinted with permission from Chodosh J. Viral keratitis. In: Parrish RK, ed. The University of Miami Bascom Palmer Eye Institute Atlas of Ophthalmology. Boston: Current Medicine; 1999.)*

and number of recurrences of herpetic keratitis. See Chapter 4 for a more detailed description of neurotrophic keratopathy.

Dendritiform epithelial lesions may develop in various settings, including

- VZV (see the discussion later in the chapter)
- adenovirus (uncommon)
- EBV (rare)
- epithelial regeneration line
- neurotrophic keratopathy (postherpetic, diabetes mellitus)
- soft contact lens wear (due to solutions containing thimerosal)
- topical medication use (antivirals, beta-blockers)

- *Acanthamoeba* epithelial keratitis
- epithelial deposits (eg, iron lines, Fabry disease, tyrosinemia type II, systemic drug use)

LABORATORY EVALUATION A specific clinical diagnosis of HSV as the cause of dendritic keratitis can usually be made based on the presence of characteristic clinical features. Multinucleated giant cells (nonspecific) and intranuclear inclusions (more specific of herpesviruses) may be seen on corneal scrapings. Tissue culture, antigen detection techniques (ELISA), and PCR may be helpful in establishing the diagnosis in atypical cases.

MANAGEMENT Most cases of HSV epithelial keratitis resolve spontaneously, and there is no clinical evidence to suggest that antiviral therapy influences the subsequent development of stromal keratitis or recurrent epithelial disease. However, treatment shortens the clinical course and might conceivably reduce the magnitude of any associated herpetic neuropathy, subepithelial scarring, or the potential risk of immune-mediated diseases of the cornea. Antiviral therapy can be used alone or in combination with epithelial debridement. Trifluridine 1% solution 8 times daily is efficacious for both dendritic and geographic epithelial keratitis. Ganciclovir 0.15% gel seems to have similar efficacy to topical acyclovir but is less toxic to the ocular surface than is trifluridine. Acyclovir 3% ophthalmic ointment has been reported to be as effective as and less toxic than trifluridine and vidarabine, but the ophthalmic form is not available in the United States at this time except through specialty compounding pharmacies. Treatment of the disease with topical antivirals generally should be discontinued within 10–14 days to avoid unnecessary toxicity to the ocular surface. Gentle epithelial debridement with a dry cotton-tipped applicator or cellulose sponge speeds resolution and may be helpful as adjunctive therapy in drug-resistant HSV keratitis.

Oral acyclovir has been reported to be as effective as topical antivirals for the treatment of epithelial keratitis and does not cause ocular toxicity. For this reason, oral therapy is preferred by an increasing number of physicians. Valacyclovir, a prodrug of acyclovir, is just as effective for ocular HSV disease but can cause thrombotic thrombocytopenic purpura/hemolytic uremic syndrome in severely immunocompromised patients such as those with AIDS; thus, it must be used with caution if the patient's liver function is compromised or the immune status is unknown. Alternative systemic antiviral drugs are listed in Table 9-5.

As previously noted, topical corticosteroids are contraindicated in the presence of active herpetic epithelial keratitis; patients with this disease who are using systemic corticosteroids for other indications should be treated aggressively with systemic antiviral therapy.

Stromal keratitis HSV stromal keratitis is the most common cause of infectious corneal blindness in the United States, and it is the form of recurrent herpetic external disease associated with the greatest visual morbidity. Stromal involvement results from immunologic activity generated by the host against the virus. Each episode of active stromal keratitis increases the risk of future episodes.

CLINICAL PRESENTATION *Herpetic stromal keratitis* can be nonnecrotizing (interstitial or disciform) or necrotizing, and different forms may present simultaneously. *Herpetic interstitial keratitis* presents as unifocal or multifocal interstitial haze or whitening of the stroma

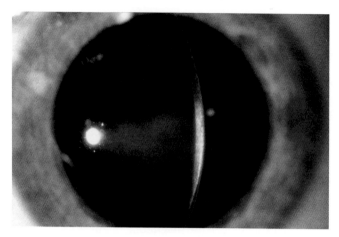

Figure 9-10 Herpetic interstitial keratitis (nonnecrotizing). *(Reprinted with permission from Chodosh J. Viral keratitis. In: Parrish RK, ed.* The University of Miami Bascom Palmer Eye Institute Atlas of Ophthalmology. *Boston: Current Medicine; 1999.)*

in the absence of epithelial ulceration (Fig 9-10). Mild stromal edema may accompany the haze, but epithelial edema is not typical. In the absence of significant extracorneal inflammatory signs such as conjunctival injection or anterior chamber cells, it may be difficult to identify active disease in an area of previous scarring and thinning. Long-standing or recurrent HSV interstitial keratitis may be associated with corneal vascularization. The differential diagnosis of herpetic interstitial keratitis includes

- VZV keratitis
- *Acanthamoeba* keratitis
- syphilis
- EBV keratitis
- mumps keratitis
- Lyme disease
- sarcoidosis
- Cogan syndrome
- atopic keratitis
- vernal keratitis

Herpetic disciform keratitis is a primary endotheliitis, which presents as corneal stromal and epithelial edema in a round or oval distribution, associated with keratic precipitates underlying the zone of edema (Fig 9-11). Iridocyclitis can be associated, and the disciform keratitis may be confused with uveitis with secondary corneal endothelial decompensation. However, in disciform keratitis, disc-shaped stromal edema and keratic precipitates appear out of proportion to the degree of anterior chamber reaction. Disciform keratitis due to HSV and that due to VZV are clinically indistinguishable.

Necrotizing herpetic keratitis appears as suppurative corneal inflammation (Fig 9-12). It may be severe, progress rapidly, and appear clinically indistinguishable from fulminant bacterial or fungal keratitis. Overlying epithelial ulceration is common, but the epithelial defect may occur somewhat eccentric to the infiltrate, and the edges of the epithelial ulcer

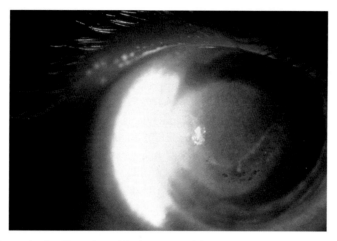

Figure 9-11 Herpetic disciform keratitis (nonnecrotizing). *(Reprinted with permission from Chodosh J. Viral keratitis. In: Parrish RK, ed.* The University of Miami Bascom Palmer Eye Institute Atlas of Ophthalmology. *Boston: Current Medicine; 1999.)*

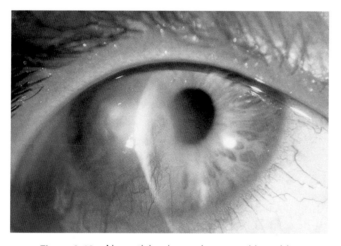

Figure 9-12 Necrotizing herpetic stromal keratitis.

do not stain with rose bengal dye. Corneal stromal vascularization is common. The differential diagnosis for necrotizing herpetic keratitis includes microbial keratitis due to bacteria, fungi, or *acanthamoebae;* retained foreign body; and topical anesthetic abuse.

Farooq AV, Shukla D. Corneal latency and transmission of herpes simplex virus-1. *Future Virol.* 2011;6(1):101–108.

Kip KE, Cohen F, Cole SR, et al; Herpetic Eye Disease Study Group. Recall bias in a prospective cohort study of acute time-varying exposures: example from the Herpetic Eye Disease Study. *J Clin Epidemiol.* 2001;54(5):482–487.

Liesegang TJ. Herpes simplex virus epidemiology and ocular importance. *Cornea.* 2001;20(1):1–13.

Young RC, Hodge DO, Liesegang TJ, Baratz KH. Incidence, recurrence, and outcomes of herpes simplex virus eye disease in Olmsted County, Minnesota, 1976–2007: the effect of oral antiviral prophylaxis. *Arch Ophthalmol.* 2010;128(9):1178–1183.

MANAGEMENT Many past controversies regarding the optimal management of HSV stromal keratitis have been resolved by the landmark HEDS (Table 9-6). Most important, HEDS findings showed that topical corticosteroids given with a prophylactic antiviral reduce persistence or progression of stromal inflammation and shorten the duration of HSV stromal keratitis; in addition, long-term suppressive oral acyclovir therapy reduces the rate of recurrent HSV keratitis and helps preserve vision. Lifelong antiviral prophylaxis is recommended for patients with multiple recurrences of HSV stromal keratitis.

The experimental protocol applied by HEDS investigators for patients with herpetic stromal keratitis is a useful starting point for a treatment algorithm. Visually significant herpetic interstitial keratitis is treated initially with prednisolone 1% drops every 2 hours, accompanied by a prophylactic antiviral drug, either topical trifluridine 4 times daily or an oral agent such as acyclovir 400 mg twice daily or valacyclovir 500 mg once a day. The prednisolone drops are tapered every 1–2 weeks depending on the degree of clinical improvement. The antiviral is given to prevent severe epithelial keratitis should the patient shed HSV while using corticosteroid drops, and it is generally continued until the patient has completely stopped the corticosteroids or is using less than 1 drop of prednisolone 1% per day. The corticosteroid should be tapered to the lowest possible dosage that controls the patient's inflammation.

Currently available topical antiviral medications are not absorbed by the cornea through an intact epithelium, but orally administered acyclovir penetrates an intact cornea and anterior chamber. In this context, anecdotal evidence suggests that oral acyclovir might benefit the deep corneal inflammation of disciform keratitis. The HEDS showed no additional benefit when acyclovir was added to trifluridine and prednisolone for the treatment of herpetic stromal keratitis, but disciform keratitis was not analyzed as a separate group. Some cornea specialists routinely substitute oral acyclovir for topical trifluridine in treating disciform keratitis.

Necrotizing stromal keratitis is probably the least common but most destructive form of herpetic keratitis. The diagnosis is frequently one of exclusion following negative cultures for fungal and bacterial pathogens, but it is suggested by a history of facial, conjunctival, and/or corneal HSV infection. The toxicity of topical antiviral agents may be undesirable in patients with necrotizing inflammation and can confuse the clinical picture. Therefore, an oral antiviral such as acyclovir is preferred. Fortunately, necrotizing herpetic keratitis seems to be very sensitive to topical corticosteroids, and twice-a-day dosing may be sufficient to control inflammation in many patients.

Iridocyclitis Granulomatous or nongranulomatous iridocyclitis may accompany necrotizing stromal keratitis or occur independently of corneal disease. Elevated intraocular pressure (IOP) caused by trabeculitis and/or patchy iris transillumination defects may be found in patients with HSV iridocyclitis. Infectious virus has been cultured from the anterior chamber of such patients and its presence positively correlated with ocular hypertension. Therefore, the diagnosis of HSV iridocyclitis is suggested by a unilateral presentation associated with an elevated IOP with or without focal iris transillumination defects. A history or clinical evidence of prior HSV ocular disease is suggestive. One HEDS trial suggested a statistical trend toward the benefit of oral acyclovir (400 mg, 5 times daily) in

Table 9-6 The Herpetic Eye Disease Study

No.	Question	Study Design	Findings	Comment
1	Do topical corticosteroids treat stromal keratitis?	106 patients with stromal keratitis randomized to topical corticosteroids or placebo for 10 weeks. Treatment started with prednisolone 1% 8×/day and tapered to prednisolone 1/8 % once a day. Both groups received topical trifluridine.	Yes. Topical corticosteroids significantly decreased stromal inflammation and shortened duration of keratitis.	The optimal corticosteroid regimen was not evaluated. Some patients respond to less corticosteroid and some may need a shorter/longer taper. Delaying corticosteroids for several weeks had no detrimental effect on vision.
2	Is oral acyclovir (in addition to treatment with trifluridine and corticosteroids) helpful in treating stromal keratitis?	104 patients with stromal keratitis randomized to oral acyclovir (400 mg 5×/day) or placebo for a 10-week course. Both groups also received topical prednisolone and trifluridine.	No. Treatment of nonnecrotizing stromal keratitis with oral acyclovir was not beneficial.	Insufficient patients with necrotizing stromal keratitis to comment on effectiveness of acyclovir.
3	Is treatment-dose oral acyclovir helpful in treating HSV iritis?	50 patients with iritis treated with oral acyclovir (400 mg 5×/day) vs placebo for 10-week course.	Too few patients. A nonstatistically significant trend favoring the use of oral acyclovir.	Many clinicians favor use of oral acyclovir for treatment of HSV iridocyclitis.
4	Does oral acyclovir prevent stromal keratitis and iritis from developing in patients with epithelial keratitis?	287 patients with epithelial keratitis received 3-week oral acyclovir (400 mg 5×/day) vs placebo; followed for 12 months.	No. No difference in development of stromal keratitis or iritis.	Best predictor for stromal keratitis is history of previous stromal keratitis.
5	Does acyclovir prophylaxis minimize HSV recurrences?	703 patients with inactive disease and off medications randomized to oral acyclovir (400 mg 2×/day) vs placebo for 12 months; followed for 18 months.	Recurrent ocular disease was less (about 50%) in acyclovir prophylaxis group, especially in patients with recurrent stromal keratitis.	Long-term prophylaxis recommended for patients with recurrent HSV stromal keratitis.
6	What triggers HSV recurrences?	308 patients kept weekly log of stress, systemic infections, sunlight exposure, menstruation, CL wear, and eye injury.	No factors confirmed as triggers for recurrence.*	

*With 33 valid recurrences, none of these factors was associated with a recurrence of ocular HSV infection. When the 26 recurrences excluded for being reported late were examined, high stress and systemic infection were found to have been reported significantly more frequently than in the 33 valid responses. (Kip KE, Cohen F, Cole SR, et al; Herpetic Eye Disease Study Group. Recall bias in a prospective cohort study of acute time-varying exposures: example from the Herpetic Eye Disease Study. *J Clin Epidemiol.* 2001;54(5):482–487).

treating HSV iridocyclitis in patients also receiving topical corticosteroids, but the number of patients recruited was too small to achieve statistically conclusive results.

See BCSC Section 1, *Update on General Medicine,* for additional discussion of viral therapeutics, and Section 2, *Fundamentals and Principles of Ophthalmology,* for discussion of specific antiviral agents.

Barron BA, Gee L, Hauck WW, et al. Herpetic Eye Disease Study. A controlled trial of oral acyclovir for herpes simplex stromal keratitis. *Ophthalmology.* 1994;101(12):1871–1882.

Herpetic Eye Disease Study Group. A controlled trial of oral acyclovir for iridocyclitis caused by herpes simplex virus. *Arch Ophthalmol.* 1996;114(9):1065–1072.

Herpetic Eye Disease Study Group. A controlled trial of oral acyclovir for the prevention of stromal keratitis or iritis in patients with herpes simplex virus epithelial keratitis. The Epithelial Keratitis Trial. *Arch Ophthalmol.* 1997;115(6):703–712.

Herpetic Eye Disease Study Group. Acyclovir for the prevention of recurrent herpes simplex virus eye disease. *N Engl J Med.* 1998;339(5):300–306.

Herpetic Eye Disease Study Group. Oral acyclovir for herpes simplex virus eye disease: effect on prevention of epithelial keratitis and stromal keratitis. *Arch Ophthalmol.* 2000;118(8):1030–1036.

Wilhelmus KR, Gee L, Hauck WW, et al. Herpetic Eye Disease Study. A controlled trial of topical corticosteroids for herpes simplex stromal keratitis. *Ophthalmology.* 1994;101(12):1883–1895.

Complications of herpetic eye disease

Complications of herpetic eye disease affect all layers of the cornea. *Epitheliopathy* is common when topical antiviral treatment is prolonged, and its severity and duration are directly related to the duration of antiviral use. Topical antiviral toxicity presents most commonly as diffuse punctate corneal epithelial erosions with conjunctival injection. Limbal stem cell deficiency may result either from recurrent infection and inflammation or from the frequent use of many of the topical antiviral drugs. *Neurotrophic keratopathy* may develop in patients with reduced corneal sensation secondary to previous herpetic infection. (See the section Neurotrophic Keratopathy and Persistent Corneal Epithelial Defects in Chapter 4.) Punctate epithelial erosions, sometimes with a vortex pattern of punctate fluorescein staining, chronic epithelial regeneration lines, and frank neurotrophic ulcers, characterize neurotrophic keratopathy. These ulcers can be distinguished from herpetic epithelial keratitis by a relative absence of rose bengal staining. Neurotrophic ulcers (see Chapter 4, Fig 4-1) are typically round or oval and located in the central, inferior, or inferonasal cornea. Corneal epithelium at the edges of a neurotrophic ulcer may appear to roll under itself and typically has a gray, elevated appearance. Liberal use of nonpreserved lubricating drops, gels, and ointments; autologous serum; and punctal occlusion are the mainstays of therapy. To prevent progressive stromal thinning and perforation, tarsorrhaphy and/or amniotic membrane application, either surgical or self-retaining, is indicated for neurotrophic ulcers that fail to respond to conservative therapy. On occasion, active or resolving interstitial stromal keratitis due to HSV is associated with a chronic epithelial defect that does not stain with rose bengal. This so-called *metaherpetic ulcer* probably results from neurotrophic mechanisms or a devitalized corneal stroma.

Severe or long-standing disciform keratitis can result in *persistent bullous keratopathy*. Stromal inflammation in general, whether interstitial or necrotizing, commonly leads to permanent corneal scarring and irregular astigmatism. Both scarring and astigmatism may improve with time in some patients. Fitting with a gas-permeable contact lens usually improves vision beyond that achieved with spectacle refraction. In patients with deep corneal stromal vascularization due to prior necrotizing herpetic inflammation, secondary lipid keratopathy may further impair the vision. Topical corticosteroids may suppress new vessel growth and halt additional lipid deposition.

Surgical treatment

Penetrating keratoplasty (PK) or deep anterior lamellar keratoplasty (DALK) is indicated in selected patients with visually significant stromal scarring not correctable with a spectacle or contact lens. Oral antiviral therapy may improve graft survival by reducing the risk of HSV recurrence and allow more liberal use of topical corticosteroids. Oral antiviral agents are not toxic to the corneal epithelium and are therefore generally preferable to topical antivirals in patients after PK. Optical PK is successful in nearly 80% of cases when performed in eyes without signs of active inflammation for at least 6 months prior to surgery. See Chapter 15 for additional discussion of PK and DALK. Tectonic surgery is indicated in eyes with impending or frank corneal perforation due to necrotizing or neurotrophic ulcers, although stromal inflammation and ulceration may develop and graft failure may occur in inflamed herpetic eyes. Therefore, small descemetoceles and perforations in inflamed eyes may best be treated by applying therapeutic tissue adhesive and a bandage contact lens and delaying surgery until inflammation can be controlled. Amniotic membrane transplantation or conjunctival flaps may also be used for persistent epithelial defects with and without corneal thinning. Keratoprostheses may have an important role because of the risk of rejection and recurrence in HSV corneal disease.

Varicella-Zoster Virus Dermatoblepharitis, Conjunctivitis, and Keratitis

As with other herpesviruses, VZV causes a primary infection (varicella, or chickenpox) and establishes a subsequent latent infection, occasionally followed later by recurrent disease (zoster, or shingles, discussed later). VZV infection of childhood, now uncommon in countries with widespread HZV vaccination programs, is usually a self-limited infection rarely associated with long-term sequelae. However, infection of adults or immunosuppressed individuals can be fatal. In children, VZV infection manifests with fever, malaise, and a vesicular dermatitis that lasts 7–10 days. Except for eyelid vesicles and follicular conjunctivitis, ocular involvement is uncommon during primary infection. VZV infection, whether primary or recurrent, can usually be distinguished from HSV infection through a careful history and examination. Distinguishing features of each infection are listed in Table 9-7.

PATHOGENESIS Primary VZV infection occurs upon direct contact with VZV skin lesions or respiratory secretions via airborne droplets and is highly contagious for naive individuals. As with HSV, the site of VZV latency is the sensory ganglia and, in approximately 20% of infected individuals, the virus reactivates later. Of all cases with zoster, 15% involve the

Table 9-7 Differentiating Features of Eye Disease Caused by Herpes Simplex Virus and Reactivation of Varicella-Zoster Virus

	Herpes Simplex Virus	Varicella-Zoster Virus
Dermatomal distribution	Incomplete	Complete
Pain	Moderate	Severe
Dendrite morphology	Central epithelial ulceration with terminal bulbs; geographic in presence of corticosteroids	Smaller without central ulceration or terminal bulbs; dendritiform mucous plaques occur later
Skin scarring	No	Common
Postherpetic neuralgia	No	Common
Iris atrophy	Patchy	Sectoral
Bilateral involvement	Uncommon	No
Recurrent epithelial keratitis	Common	Rare
Corneal hypoesthesia	Focal or diffuse	May be severe

cranial nerve (CN) V, or the trigeminal nerve; see "Herpes zoster ophthalmicus" later in this chapter.

CLINICAL PRESENTATION The rash of chickenpox begins as macules and progresses to papules, vesicles, and then pustules that dry, crust over, and may leave individual scars. Ocular involvement may include follicular conjunctivitis, occasionally associated with a vesicular lesion on the bulbar conjunctiva or eyelid margins. Punctate or dendritic epithelial keratitis is uncommon. Although subepithelial infiltrates, microdendritic keratitis, stromal keratitis, disciform keratitis, uveitis, and elevated IOP are rare, recurrent varicella keratouveitis may cause significant morbidity in some patients.

LABORATORY EVALUATION Laboratory confirmation of acute or recurrent VZV infection is possible by immunodiagnostic methods, viral culture, and PCR. Serologic testing is used primarily to identify varicella-naive adults who might benefit from prophylactic vaccination. As with HSV, scrapings from the base of a vesicle can be tested by cytology, PCR, or culture, or for the presence of VZV antigen. Conjunctival scrapings or corneal impression cytology specimens can be similarly analyzed by culture, antigen detection, or PCR.

MANAGEMENT Because infected individuals shed the virus in respiratory secretions before the onset of the characteristic rash, avoiding infected persons is not always possible. Vaccination against varicella is recommended for anyone older than 12 months without a history of chickenpox or with a negative serologic test result. The severity of signs and symptoms may be reduced in clinically ill patients by the administration of oral acyclovir. Significant keratitis or uveitis can be treated with topical corticosteroids.

Herpes zoster ophthalmicus

PATHOGENESIS Following primary infection, VZV establishes latency in sensory ganglia. Zoster (shingles) represents endogenous reactivation of latent virus in individuals with a waning level of immunity to infection. Most patients with zoster are in their sixth to ninth decades of life, and the majority are healthy, with no specific predisposing factors.

However, zoster is more common in patients on immunosuppressive therapy; in those with a systemic malignancy, a debilitating disease, or HIV infection; and after major surgery, trauma, or radiation therapy. Herpes zoster in otherwise healthy children has been described in the literature.

CLINICAL PRESENTATION Zoster manifests as a painful vesicular dermatitis typically localized to a single dermatome on the thorax or face. Initially, affected patients may report fever and malaise and experience warmth, redness, and increased sensation in the affected dermatome. The most commonly affected dermatomes are on the thorax (T3 through L3) and those supplied by CN V. The ophthalmic division of the trigeminal nerve is affected more often than the maxillary and mandibular branches, and its involvement is referred to as *herpes zoster ophthalmicus (HZO)* (Fig 9-13). A maculopapular rash, followed by vesicles and then pustules, is characteristic. Zoster dermatitis may result in large scabs that resolve slowly and leave significant scarring. Neurotrophic keratopathy and sectoral iris atrophy are characteristic. Inflammation of almost any ocular tissue can occur and recur in HZO.

Zoster dermatitis is accompanied by pain and dysesthesia. The pain usually decreases as lesions resolve; however, neuralgia in the affected dermatome can continue for months to years. The severity of pain ranges from mild to incapacitating. Ocular involvement occurs in more than 70% of patients with zoster of the first division of CN V and may appear in association with any branch, including the nasociliary, frontal, or lacrimal branches. Ophthalmic complications also may occur with zoster of the second (maxillary) division of CN V. In immunosuppressed patients, zoster may involve more than 1 branch of the trigeminal nerve at the same time; after reactivation, disease may be chronic, and there may be multiple recurrences. See BCSC Section 2, *Fundamentals and Principles of Ophthalmology,* for discussion of the innervation of the eye and face.

Eyelid vesicular eruption can lead to secondary bacterial infection, eyelid scarring, marginal notching, loss of cilia, trichiasis, and cicatricial entropion or ectropion. Scarring and occlusion of the lacrimal puncta or canaliculi may occur. Episcleritis or scleritis associated with zoster may be nodular, zonal, or diffuse.

Both punctate and dendritic epithelial keratitis caused by viral replication in corneal epithelium are common manifestations of ophthalmic zoster. Herpes zoster pseudodendrites (distinguished from the true dendrites of HSV corneal disease, which have a central

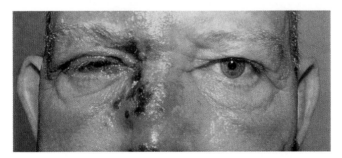

Figure 9-13 Herpes zoster ophthalmicus (HZO). *(Courtesy of Vincent P. deLuise, MD.)*

epithelial ulceration) form branching or "medusa-like" lesions that resemble raised mucous plaques, stain minimally with fluorescein and rose bengal, and have blunt rather than bulbous ends. The elevated dendritiform mucous plaques may occur on the cornea weeks to months after resolution of the skin lesions. These may be chronically culture-positive for VZV in patients with AIDS. Diminished corneal sensation occurs in up to 50% of patients. Nummular corneal infiltrates are said to be characteristic of zoster stromal keratitis (Fig 9-14), but the interstitial keratitis, disciform keratitis, and anterior uveitis with increased IOP in HZO are clinically indistinguishable from those caused by HSV infection. Chronic corneal stromal inflammation can lead to corneal vascularization, lipid keratopathy (Fig 9-15), and corneal opacity. Corneal anesthesia may be profound, and neurotrophic keratopathy due to HZO can be extremely difficult to manage.

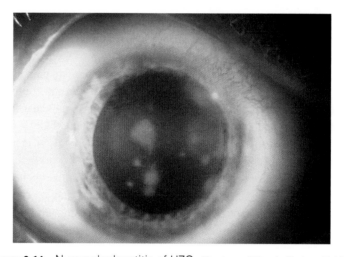

Figure 9-14 Nummular keratitis of HZO. *(Courtesy of Rhea L. Siatkowski, MD.)*

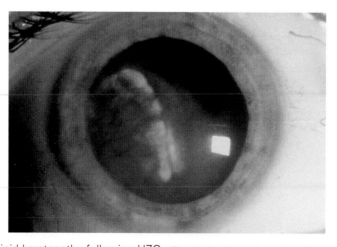

Figure 9-15 Lipid keratopathy following HZO. *(Reprinted with permission from Chodosh J. Viral keratitis. In: Parrish RK, ed. The University of Miami Bascom Palmer Eye Institute Atlas of Ophthalmology. Boston: Current Medicine; 1999.)*

Focal choroiditis, occlusive retinal vasculitis, and retinal detachment have been reported. Ipsilateral acute retinal necrosis (ARN) temporally associated with HZO is uncommon.

Orbital or central nervous system involvement as a result of an occlusive arteritis may lead to eyelid ptosis, orbital edema, and proptosis. Papillitis or retrobulbar optic neuritis may also develop. Cranial nerve palsies, when meticulously investigated, have been reported to occur in up to one-third of cases of HZO, with CN III (oculomotor) most commonly affected. Cranial nerve involvement may occur within the orbit or the cavernous sinus. Systemic dissemination is unusual in immunocompetent patients but can occur in up to 25% of those who are immunocompromised.

MANAGEMENT A varicella-zoster vaccine was approved by the US Food and Drug Administration (FDA) after testing in 38,000 patients showed a 50% reduction in incidence of zoster and a 66% reduction in postherpetic neuralgia (PHN). This live, attenuated vaccine is similar to the childhood vaccine but contains a higher dose of the vaccine virus. In the United States, the vaccine is recommended for immunocompetent individuals aged 60 years and older but was recently made available to those aged 50 years and older. Recent studies indicate, however, that the incidence of herpes zoster rises with increasing age, starting from age 50 years, suggesting that the vaccine should be recommended for persons younger than 60 years. There is concern that the average age at infection with herpes zoster will become significantly lower with the widespread use of both vaccines and the consequential reduction in exposure to virus-shedding individuals, who inadvertently boost community immunity. This would most likely affect persons aged 20–50 years—those not currently covered by the vaccines—and could eventually lead to a change in age indications. There are currently no clear recommendations concerning the use of the adult vaccine in patients with previous HZO, but the potential to reactivate or exacerbate HZO-related inflammation exists, as such cases have been reported. It is suggested that vaccinations be administered during an extensive quiet period.

Oral antiviral therapy for HZO was found in randomized clinical trials to reduce viral shedding from vesicular skin lesions, reduce the chance of systemic dissemination of the virus, and decrease the incidence and severity of the most common ocular complications. Oral antiviral therapy may reduce the duration and severity if not the incidence of PHN, if begun within 72 hours of the onset of symptoms. There are also reports to suggest that initiating antiviral therapy after 72 hours, especially in the presence of new vesicles, is beneficial.

The current recommendation for HZO is oral famciclovir 500 mg 3 times per day, valacyclovir 1 g 3 times per day, or acyclovir 800 mg 5 times per day for 7–10 days, best if started within 72 hours of the onset of skin lesions. Topical antiviral medications are not effective, except in the treatment of corneal epithelial mucoid plaques or more chronic epithelial disease. Intravenous acyclovir therapy (10 mg/kg every 8 hours) is indicated in patients at risk for disseminated zoster due to immunosuppression. Cutaneous lesions may be treated with moist warm compresses and topical antibiotic ointment. Topical corticosteroids and cycloplegics are indicated for keratouveitis. Oral corticosteroids, used with a tapering dosage, are recommended by some for treating patients older than 60 years with HZO to reduce the pain associated with early zoster and facilitate a rapid return to a normal quality of life. However, the use of oral corticosteroids is controversial; their use does not seem to affect the incidence or duration of PHN.

Postherpetic neuralgia may respond to capsaicin cream applied to the involved skin, but low doses of amitriptyline, desipramine, clomipramine, or carbamazepine may be necessary to control severe symptoms. Gabapentin and pregabalin have been shown to be efficacious in managing PHN. Aggressive lubrication with nonpreserved artificial tears, gels, or ointments, combined with punctal occlusion and tarsorrhaphy as necessary, may be indicated for neurotrophic keratopathy. For a patient with significant pain, early referral to a pain management specialist should be considered.

Liesegang TJ. Herpes zoster ophthalmicus: natural history, risk factors, clinical presentation, and morbidity. *Ophthalmology.* 2008;115(2 Suppl):S3–S12.

Liesegang TJ. Varicella-zoster virus vaccines: effective, but concerns linger. *Can J Ophthalmol.* 2009;44(4):379–384.

Oxman MN, Levin MJ, Johnson GR, et al; Shingles Prevention Study Group. A vaccine to prevent herpes zoster and postherpetic neuralgia in older adults. *N Engl J Med.* 2005; 352(22):2271–2284.

Schmader KE, Levin MJ, Gnann JW Jr, et al. Efficacy, safety, and tolerability of herpes zoster vaccine in persons aged 50–59 years. *Clin Infect Dis.* 2012;54(7):922–928.

Epstein-Barr Virus Dacryoadenitis, Conjunctivitis, and Keratitis

PATHOGENESIS Epstein-Barr virus (EBV) is a ubiquitous herpesvirus that infects most humans by early adulthood. Spread of EBV occurs by the sharing of saliva, and the virus results in subclinical infection in the first decade of life; if acquired later in life, it causes infectious mononucleosis. The virus remains latent in B lymphocytes and pharyngeal mucosal epithelial cells throughout life. Ocular disease is uncommon.

CLINICAL PRESENTATION Epstein-Barr virus is the most common cause of acute dacryoadenitis, characterized by inflammatory enlargement of 1 or both lacrimal glands. Acute follicular conjunctivitis, Parinaud oculoglandular syndrome, and bulbar conjunctival nodules have been reported in patients with acute infectious mononucleosis and may be the result of EBV infection. There are 3 principal forms of EBV stromal keratitis; the diagnosis is made on the basis of a history of recent infectious mononucleosis and/or persistently high EBV serologic titers:

- Type 1: multifocal subepithelial infiltrates that resemble adenoviral keratitis
- Type 2: multifocal, blotchy, pleomorphic infiltrates with active inflammation (Fig 9-16) or granular ring-shaped opacities (inactive form) in anterior to midstroma
- Type 3: multifocal deep or full-thickness peripheral infiltrates, with or without vascularization, that resemble interstitial keratitis due to syphilis

EBV-associated keratitis may be unilateral or bilateral and may, in select cases, appear similar to the interstitial keratitis induced by HSV, VZV, Lyme disease, adenovirus, or syphilis. As EBV is rare, clinical suspicion for it is usually low; EBV should be considered in patients with disease refractory to conventional antiviral treatment.

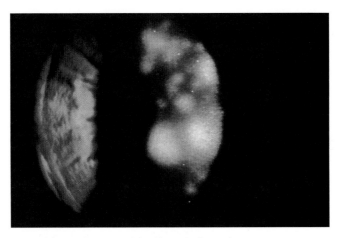

Figure 9-16 Interstitial keratitis caused by Epstein-Barr virus. *(Reprinted with permission from Chodosh J. Viral keratitis. In: Parrish RK, ed.* The University of Miami Bascom Palmer Eye Institute Atlas of Ophthalmology. *Boston: Current Medicine; 1999.)*

DIAGNOSIS AND MANAGEMENT Because it is difficult to isolate the virus, the diagnosis of EBV infection depends on the detection of antibodies to various viral components. During acute infection, first immunoglobulin (Ig) M and then IgG antibodies to viral capsid antigens (VCAs) appear. Anti-VCA IgG may persist for the life of the patient. There is an increase in the level of antibodies to early antigens during the acute phases of the disease and a subsequent decrease to low or undetectable levels in most individuals. Antibodies to EBV nuclear antigens appear weeks to months later, providing serologic evidence of past infection. Acyclovir is not an effective treatment for the clinical signs and symptoms of infectious mononucleosis, but the impact of antiviral therapy on the corneal manifestations of EBV infection remains unknown. Corticosteroids may be effective in patients with reduced vision due to apparent EBV stromal keratitis, but they should not be administered without a prophylactic antiviral if HSV infection is a possibility.

Chodosh J. Epstein-Barr virus stromal keratitis. *Ophthalmol Clin North Am.* 1994;7(4): 549–556.

Cytomegalovirus Keratitis and Anterior Uveitis

PATHOGENESIS Cytomegalovirus (CMV) is a ubiquitous herpesvirus that infects over 90% of humans by 80 years of age. Spread of CMV occurs through the sharing of saliva, ingestion of breast milk, or sexual contact. CMV causes subclinical infection in children and a nonspecific febrile illness lasting 1–3 weeks in adults. A viremia transmits the virus to the bone marrow, where it becomes latent in CD34+ myeloid progenitor cells until these cells are activated, which allows expression and shedding of the virus.

CLINICAL PRESENTATION Cytomegalovirus has been most commonly associated with a sectoral, necrotizing retinitis that is seen almost exclusively in AIDS and other immunocompromised states. Few anterior segment complications were previously associated with

CMV retinitis, with the exception of thin stellate keratic precipitates. In rare cases, epithelial and stromal CMV keratitis have been described, usually when CMV infection was undiagnosed prior to keratoplasty. However, CMV has been increasingly identified as a significant cause of anterior uveitis and corneal endotheliitis (Fig 9-17). This is probably due, in part, to improved diagnostic acumen. The anterior uveitis is characterized by an acute or chronic iritis, with moderate to severe rises in IOP that are variably responsive to topical corticosteroids. The addition of keratic precipitates, endothelial cell loss, and diffuse or local corneal edema suggests CMV endotheliitis. These presentations are often misdiagnosed as HSV-related endotheliitis, trabeculitis, or Posner-Schlossman syndrome and can be distinguished only by their response to therapy and by results of laboratory investigation.

LABORATORY EVALUATION Laboratory confirmation of CMV-associated anterior segment disease is usually accomplished through PCR testing of aqueous humor for CMV. Aqueous humor is obtained by an anterior chamber tap, which must be performed during an episode of active disease for greatest yield. Concurrent serum testing should also be performed to rule out a systemic viremia as a cause of intraocular detection. In addition, concomitant testing for other herpesviruses can be performed. CMV-associated anterior segment disease may also be diagnosed through histologic examination of corneal biopsy or surgical specimens.

MANAGEMENT Cytomegalovirus-associated anterior segment disease is treated with ganciclovir and is not responsive to famciclovir, acyclovir, or its derivatives. Resistance of a presumed HSV infection to these agents should raise suspicion for CMV. The optimal treatment of CMV-associated anterior segment disease is unknown, but treatment with oral valganciclovir 900 mg twice daily (with the possibility of lower maintenance dosing) is effective. Valganciclovir may be poorly tolerated and, unfortunately, recurrence of disease with withdrawal of the medication is common. Alternatives include ganciclovir implants and topical ganciclovir, which has demonstrated therapeutic effects when used as an adjunct to systemic therapy and when used in a maintenance role. Recurrence is possible after keratoplasty. The role of corticosteroids is unclear, as there is some suggestion that corticosteroid use may prolong or worsen CMV-associated anterior segment disease. Corticosteroids should therefore be used judiciously in this setting.

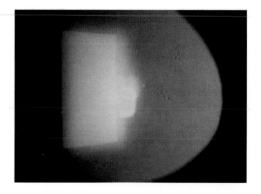

Figure 9-17 Clusters of keratic precipitates in cytomegalovirus corneal endotheliitis. *(Courtesy of Cornea Service, Paulista School of Medicine, Federal University of São Paulo.)*

Carmichael A. Cytomegalovirus and the eye. *Eye (Lond).* 2012;26(2):237–240.

Chan AS, Mehta JS, Al Jajeh I, Iqbal J, Anshu A, Tan DT. Histological features of Cytomegalovirus-related corneal graft infections, its associated features and clinical significance. *Br J Ophthalmol.* 2016;100(5):601–606. Epub 2015 Aug 20.

Chee SP, Bacsal K, Jap A, Se-Thoe SY, Cheng CL, Tan BH. Corneal endotheliitis associated with evidence of cytomegalovirus infection. *Ophthalmology.* 2007;114(4):798–803.

Koizumi N, Suzuki T, Uno T, et al. Cytomegalovirus as an etiologic factor in corneal endotheliitis. *Ophthalmology.* 2008;115(2):292–297.

DNA Viruses: Adenoviruses

The Adenoviridae are nonenveloped double-stranded DNA viruses. Originally isolated in 1953 from surgically removed human adenoids, adenoviruses cause a broad spectrum of diseases, including infections of the upper respiratory tract and ocular surface, meningoencephalitis, acute hemorrhagic cystitis in young boys, diarrhea in children, acute respiratory disease in children and military recruits, and respiratory and hepatic failure in an immunocompromised host. There are 49 serotypes, which are divided into 6 distinct subgroups (labeled A–F) on the basis of genetic sequencing. Adenovirus subgroups associate broadly with specific clinical syndromes. For instance, subgroup D adenoviruses are strongly associated with epidemic keratoconjunctivitis (EKC). The nonenveloped protein capsid of all the adenovirus subgroups forms a regular icosahedron. For most adenovirus subgroups, a projecting capsid protein on a cell surface serves as the ligand for the adenovirus receptor, and the interaction of an adjacent cell surface capsid protein with cell surface integrins mediates internalization of the virus.

Knipe DM, Howley PM, eds. *Fields' Virology.* 5th ed. Philadelphia: Lippincott Williams & Wilkins; 2006.

PATHOGENESIS Adenoviruses are transmitted by close contact with ocular or respiratory secretions, contaminated fomites, or contaminated swimming pools. Transmission occurs more readily in populations living in close quarters, such as schools, nursing homes, military housing, and summer camps. Transmission of adenoviruses by contaminated instruments or eyedrops in physicians' offices may also occur. For this reason, IOP measurements should be taken with an instrument that has a disposable cover.

CLINICAL PRESENTATION Each subgroup (A–F) of adenoviruses and, to a lesser degree, each serotype possess unique tissue tropisms that reveal the association of specific adenoviruses with distinct clinical syndromes. Most adenoviral eye disease presents clinically as 1 of 3 classic syndromes:

- simple follicular conjunctivitis (multiple serotypes)
- pharyngoconjunctival fever (most commonly serotype 3 or 7)
- EKC (usually serotype 8, 19, or 37, subgroup D)

The different adenoviral syndromes are indistinguishable early in infection and may be unilateral or bilateral.

Adenoviral follicular conjunctivitis is self-limited, not associated with systemic disease, and often so transient that patients do not seek care. Epithelial keratitis, if present, is mild and fleeting. *Pharyngoconjunctival fever* is characterized by fever, headache, pharyngitis, follicular conjunctivitis, and preauricular adenopathy. The systemic signs and symptoms may mimic those of influenza. Any associated epithelial keratitis is mild.

Epidemic keratoconjunctivitis is the only adenoviral syndrome with significant corneal involvement and may be preceded by an upper respiratory tract infection. EKC is bilateral in most patients. One week to 10 days after inoculation, severe follicular conjunctivitis develops, associated with a punctate epithelial keratitis. The conjunctival morphology is follicular but may be obscured by chemosis. Petechial conjunctival hemorrhages and, occasionally, larger subconjunctival hemorrhages can occur. Preauricular adenopathy is prominent. Pseudomembranes or true membranes (Fig 9-18) occur predominantly on the tarsal conjunctiva and may be missed on cursory examination. Patients report tearing, light sensitivity, and foreign-body sensation. Large central geographic corneal erosions can develop and may persist for several days despite patching and lubrication. Within 7–14 days after onset of ocular symptoms, multifocal subepithelial (stromal) corneal infiltrates become apparent on slit-lamp examination (Fig 9-19).

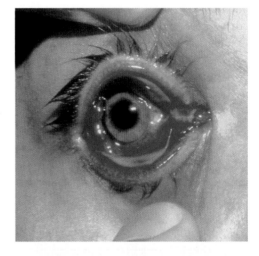

Figure 9-18 Conjunctival membranes in a patient with epidemic keratoconjunctivitis (EKC). *(Courtesy of James Chodosh, MD.)*

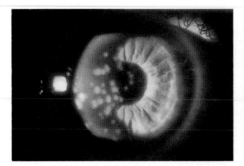
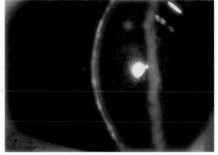

Figure 9-19 Subepithelial corneal infiltrates in a patient with EKC. *(Courtesy of Vincent P. deLuise, MD.)*

Photophobia and reduced vision from adenoviral subepithelial infiltrates may persist for months to years.

Epithelial keratitis occurs because of adenovirus replication within the corneal epithelium. Subepithelial infiltrates are likely caused by an immunopathologic response to viral infection of keratocytes in the superficial corneal stroma. The evolution of keratitis in EKC is summarized in Figure 9-20. Chronic complications of conjunctival membranes include subepithelial conjunctival scarring, symblepharon formation, and dry eye due to alterations within the lacrimal glands or lacrimal ducts.

LABORATORY EVALUATION The diagnosis of EKC is suggested in the setting of bilateral follicular conjunctivitis associated with petechial conjunctival hemorrhages, conjunctival pseudomembrane or frank membrane formation, or, later in the clinical course, the presence of bilateral subepithelial infiltrates. Other adenoviral ocular syndromes have less specific signs, but laboratory diagnosis is only rarely indicated. Although viral cultures

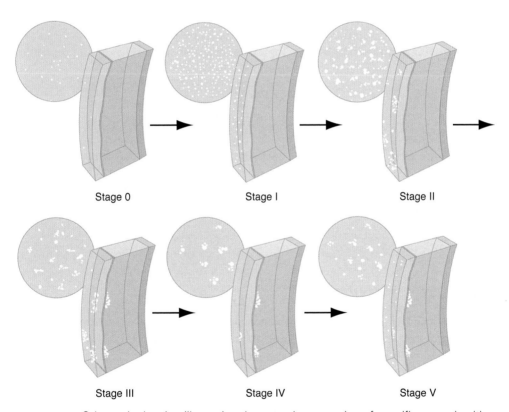

Stage 0   Stage I   Stage II

Stage III   Stage IV   Stage V

Figure 9-20 Schematic drawing illustrating the natural progression of specific corneal epithelial and stromal pathology in EKC. *Stage 0,* Poorly staining, minute punctate opacities within the corneal epithelium. *Stage I,* Fine punctate epithelial keratitis (PEK). *Stage II,* Fine and coarse PEK. Stains brightly with rose bengal. *Stage III,* Coarse granular infiltrates within deep epithelium, early subepithelial infiltrates, diminished PEK. *Stage IV,* Classic subepithelial infiltrates without PEK. *Stage V,* Punctate epithelial granularity adjacent to and distinct from the subepithelial infiltrates. *(Adapted from Jones DB, Matoba AY, Wilhelmus KR. Problem solving in corneal and external diseases. Course 626, presented at the American Academy of Ophthalmology. Atlanta, GA; 1995.)*

readily differentiate adenovirus from HSV infection, the clinical disease typically subsides or resolves before results become available. A rapid immunodetection assay to detect adenovirus antigens in the conjunctiva is available.

MANAGEMENT Therapy for adenoviral ocular infection is primarily supportive. Cool compresses and artificial tears may provide symptomatic relief. Topical combination antibiotic-corticosteroid drops may be indicated only when the clinical signs, such as mucopurulent discharge, suggest an associated bacterial infection or when a viral cause is less certain.

Topical corticosteroids also reduce photophobia and improve vision impaired by adenoviral subepithelial infiltrates. Because corticosteroids may prolong viral shedding from adenovirus-infected patients and can lead to worsening of HSV infections, their use should be reserved for patients with clinical signs of adenovirus infection who present with specific indications for treatment, including conjunctival membranes and reduced vision due to bilateral subepithelial infiltrates. Topical corticosteroids will produce rapid resolution of the infiltrates, but it may be difficult to wean patients from them, prolonging the course of the disease. Nonsteroidal anti-inflammatory drugs are ineffective therapy for adenoviral subepithelial infiltrates, but they may be helpful in preventing recurrence following tapering of the corticosteroids. Topical cyclosporine 1% or other immunomodulatory agents may be considered when other therapies fail.

Actively infected persons readily transmit adenoviruses. Viral shedding may persist for 10–14 days after the onset of clinical signs and symptoms. Transmission can be prevented by personal hygiene measures, including frequent hand washing; cleaning of towels, pillowcases, and handkerchiefs; and disposal of contaminated facial tissues. Individuals who work with the public, in schools, or in health care facilities in particular should consider a temporary leave of absence from work to prevent infecting others, especially those who are already ill. Patients should be considered infectious if they are still hyperemic and tearing. It is more difficult to assess transmissibility in patients treated with topical corticosteroids, who may still shed the virus even though the disease appears to be in a quiet period.

DNA Viruses: Poxviruses

The Poxviridae are a large family of enveloped, double-stranded DNA viruses, with a distinctive brick or ovoid shape and a complex capsid structure. The best-known poxviruses are molluscum contagiosum, vaccinia, and smallpox (variola) virus.

Molluscum Contagiosum

PATHOGENESIS Molluscum contagiosum virus is spread by direct contact with infected individuals. Infection produces 1 or more umbilicated nodules on the skin and eyelid margin and, less commonly, on the conjunctiva. Eyelid nodules release viral particles into the tear film.

CLINICAL PRESENTATION A molluscum nodule is smooth, with an umbilicated central core. It is smaller and associated with less inflammation than a keratoacanthoma. Punctate

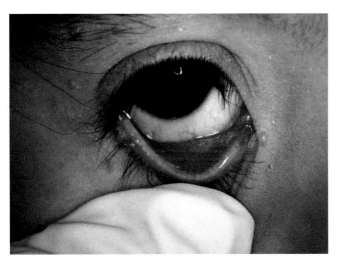

Figure 9-21 Multiple molluscum contagiosum nodules, associated with a follicular conjunctivitis in an immunocompetent child. *(Reprinted with permission from Tu EY. Conjunctivitis. In: Schlossberg D, ed. Clinical Infectious Disease. 3rd ed. New York: Cambridge University Press; 2008.)*

epithelial erosions and, in rare cases, a corneal pannus may occur. Any chronic follicular conjunctivitis should instigate a careful search for eyelid margin molluscum lesions (Fig 9-21).

LABORATORY EVALUATION AND MANAGEMENT The molluscum contagiosum virus cannot be cultured using standard techniques. Histologic examination of an expressed or excised nodule shows eosinophilic, intracytoplasmic inclusions (Henderson-Patterson bodies) within epidermal cells. The diagnosis is based on detection of the characteristic eyelid lesions in the presence of a follicular conjunctivitis. Extensive facial and eyelid molluscum lesions may occur in association with AIDS (Fig 9-22). Spontaneous resolution occurs but can take months to years. Treatment options include complete excision, cryotherapy, or incision of the central portion of the lesion.

Vaccinia

Discussion of vaccinia, the cause of smallpox, was previously removed from the BCSC series because of the worldwide eradication of smallpox. More recently, however, concern that smallpox virus might be used as a biological weapon has prompted the reinstitution of a smallpox vaccination program, especially for military personnel. Ocular complications from self-inoculation have been reported, including potentially severe periorbital pustules, conjunctivitis, and keratitis. Treatment includes topical trifluridine. Use of vaccinia-immune globulin (VIG) is controversial but is indicated for severe ocular disease. Concern about the use of VIG stems from limited rabbit studies that have demonstrated a possible increase in corneal scarring. Individuals who are immunosuppressed, atopic, pregnant, breastfeeding, allergic to the vaccine, or living with a high-risk household contact should not receive the vaccine because of the risk of the possibly fatal, progressive vaccinia.

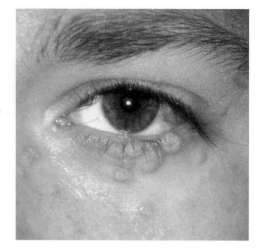

Figure 9-22 Multiple molluscum contagiosum lesions on the eyelid of a patient with AIDS. *(Courtesy of James Chodosh, MD.)*

Fillmore GL, Ward TP, Bower KS, et al. Ocular complications in the Department of Defense Smallpox Vaccination Program. *Ophthalmology.* 2004;111(11):2086–2093.

Neff JM, Lane JM, Fulginiti VA, Henderson DA. Contact vaccinia—transmission of vaccinia from smallpox vaccination. *JAMA.* 2002;288(15):1901–1905.

DNA Viruses: Papovaviruses

Human papovaviruses, also called papillomaviruses (HPV), are small, nonenveloped, double-stranded DNA viruses with an icosahedral capsid. Persistent viral infection of susceptible epithelial cells induces cellular proliferation and can lead to malignant transformation. Papillomavirus proteins can induce transformation of the cell and loss of senescence. HPV subtypes 6 and 11 are maintained in a latent state within basal epithelial cells as circular episomes with very limited viral gene transcription and low copy number. Early viral gene products stimulate cell growth and lead to a skin wart or a conjunctival papilloma. As HPV-containing basal epithelial cells mature and differentiate into superficial epithelial cells, they become permissive for complete viral gene expression and produce infectious virus. Neoplastic transformation due to HPV 6 or 11 is very rare. In contrast, HPV 16 and 18 stereotypically integrate their viral genome into host chromosomal DNA, and this in turn is associated with malignant transformation and squamous cell carcinoma. Recently implemented immunization strategies specifically targeted against HPV oncogenes may result in a decreased incidence of these tumors in the future.

Verrucae and *papillomas* are caused by papillomavirus infection of the skin and conjunctival epithelium (Fig 9-23). Papillomavirus-associated conjunctival intraepithelial neoplasia and squamous cell carcinoma share many histologic features with similar lesions in the uterine cervix. Treatment of conjunctival papillomas can be frustrating. Medical therapeutic options include systemic cimetidine 30 mg/kg/day in 3 divided doses for 3 months or more, or topical interferon alfa-2b three times a day for the same treatment

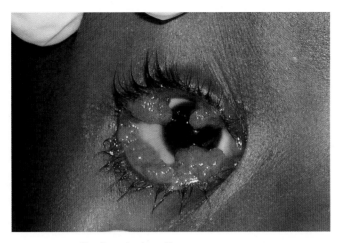

Figure 9-23 Conjunctival papillomas. *(Courtesy of Elmer Y. Tu, MD.)*

period. "No-touch" surgical excision with adjuvant cryotherapy is the preferred surgical option and is followed by administration of oral cimetidine or topical interferon, as described above. Seeding of adjacent conjunctiva may occur following surgical excision, resulting in spread. Another neoplasm, Kaposi sarcoma of the skin or conjunctiva, is associated with infection with human herpesvirus 8, not HPV. These entities are discussed in greater detail in Chapter 12.

Kaliki S, Arepalli S, Shields CL, et al. Conjunctival papilloma: features and outcomes based on age at initial examination. *JAMA Ophthalmol.* 2013;131(5):585–593.

RNA Viruses

Patients with eye infections due to RNA viruses present to the ophthalmologist less often than those with infection due to DNA viruses, and these infections most commonly manifest as follicular conjunctivitis associated with an upper respiratory tract infection (Table 9-8). However, certain RNA virus infections may cause pathologic changes in virtually any ocular tissue. For example, influenza virus can induce inflammation in the lacrimal gland, cornea, iris, retina, optic nerve, and other cranial nerves.

The Paramyxoviridae are a family of single-stranded, enveloped RNA viruses that cause numerous human diseases. The most-recognized paramyxoviruses are measles and mumps. The classic triad of postnatally acquired measles (rubeola) consists of cough, coryza, and follicular conjunctivitis. Mild epithelial keratitis may be present. Optic neuritis, retinal vascular occlusion, and pigmentary retinopathy occur less commonly. Measles keratopathy, a major source of blindness in the developing world, typically presents as corneal ulceration in malnourished, vitamin A–deficient children. (For further information on the ocular effects of vitamin A deficiency, see Chapter 8.) A rare and fatal complication of infection with the measles virus, subacute sclerosing panencephalitis (SSPE), occurs in approximately 1 per 100,000 cases, often years after clinically apparent measles.

Table 9-8 RNA Viruses Known to Cause Ocular Surface Disease

Virus Family	Virus	Clinical Syndrome
Retroviridae	Human immunodeficiency virus	Seroconversion conjunctivitis
Orthomyxovirus	Influenza	Follicular conjunctivitis
		Inflammation of the lacrimal gland, cornea, iris, retina, optic nerve, and other cranial nerves
Paramyxoviridae	Avulavirus	Newcastle disease
	Measles (rubeola)	Follicular conjunctivitis, measles keratopathy
	Mumps	Follicular conjunctivitis
Togavirus	Rubella	Congenital rubella syndrome: salt-and-pepper retinopathy, microphthalmos, cataract, deafness, congenital heart disease, other systemic abnormalities
Rhabdoviridae	Rabies	Transmission via corneal transplant
Picornaviridae	Rhinovirus	Common cold
		Follicular conjunctivitis
	Enterovirus 70	Acute hemorrhagic conjunctivitis
	Coxsackievirus A24	Acute hemorrhagic conjunctivitis

Infection with the mumps virus may result in dacryoadenitis, sometimes concurrent with parotid gland involvement. Follicular conjunctivitis, epithelial and stromal keratitis, iritis, trabeculitis, and scleritis have all been reported within the first 2 weeks after onset of parotitis.

Rubella virus (a togavirus), when acquired in utero, may cause microphthalmos, corneal haze, cataracts, iris hypoplasia, iridocyclitis, glaucoma, and salt-and-pepper pigmentary retinopathy. Congenital ocular abnormalities due to rubella are much worse when maternal infection ensues early in pregnancy. Measles, mumps, and rubella are all uncommon in places where childhood vaccination is regularly performed.

Rabies virus (Rhabdoviridae) is an enveloped virus and can be transmitted via corneal transplant. Corneal biopsy and impression cytology have been useful in the early diagnosis of rabies virus infection.

Acute hemorrhagic conjunctivitis (AHC), caused by enterovirus 70 and coxsackievirus A24 variant, and, less commonly, adenovirus 11, is one of the most dramatic ocular viral syndromes. Sudden onset of follicular conjunctivitis associated with multiple petechial hemorrhages of bulbar and tarsal conjunctiva characterizes AHC. The hemorrhages may become confluent and resemble those associated with trauma. Eyelid edema, preauricular adenopathy, chemosis, and punctate epithelial keratitis may be associated with infection. AHC is highly contagious and occurs in large and rapidly spreading epidemics. In approximately 1 out of 10,000 cases due to enterovirus 70, a polio-like paralysis follows; neurologic deficits are permanent in up to one-third of affected individuals.

Retroviruses are positive-sense, single-stranded, enveloped RNA viruses that encode a viral enzyme, reverse transcriptase, that assists in conversion of the single-stranded RNA genome into a circular double-stranded DNA molecule.

The retrovirus of greatest medical importance is human immunodeficiency virus (HIV), the etiologic agent of AIDS. HIV enters the human host via sexual contact at mucosal surfaces, through breastfeeding, or via blood-contaminated needles. Sexually transmitted infection is facilitated by uptake of HIV by dendritic cells at mucosal surfaces. $CD4^+$ T lymphocytes are a primary target of the virus, as are dendritic cells and monocyte-macrophages. Infection of these cell types induces predictable defects of innate and acquired (both humoral and cellular) immunity. Primary viremia results in an infectious mononucleosis-like HIV prodrome, followed by seeding of the peripheral lymphoid organs and development of a measurable immune response. Conjunctivitis may occur during this seroconversion prodrome in a small number of patients and is self-limited. Infected patients may remain otherwise asymptomatic for several years, but $CD4^+$ T lymphocytes are progressively depleted. Clinical immunodeficiency eventually develops.

AIDS-related ocular disorders include HZO, molluscum contagiosum, keratoconjunctivitis sicca, microsporidial keratoconjunctivitis, HIV neuropathy, cryptococcal optic neuritis, retinal microvasculopathy, choroiditis and retinitis due to syphilis, mycobacteria, pneumocystosis, toxoplasmosis, CMV, HSV, and VZV. For more information regarding HIV, see BCSC Section 1, *Update on General Medicine,* and Section 9, *Intraocular Inflammation and Uveitis.*

Cunningham ET Jr, Margolis TP. Ocular manifestations of HIV infection. *N Engl J Med.* 1998; 339(4):236–244.

Lai TY, Wong RL, Luk FO, Chow VW, Chan CK, Lam DS. Ophthalmic manifestations and risk factors for mortality of HIV patients in the post-highly active anti-retroviral therapy era. *Clin Experiment Ophthalmol.* 2011;39(2):99–104.

Zaidman GW, Billingsley A. Corneal impression test for the diagnosis of acute rabies encephalitis. *Ophthalmology.* 1998;105(2):249–251.

CHAPTER 10

Infectious Diseases of the External Eye: Microbial and Parasitic Infections

Highlights

- In children, the number of bacterial conjunctivitis cases is similar to that of viral conjunctivitis cases, but in adults, 80% of cases of infectious conjunctivitis are viral in origin.
- Most cases of acute bacterial conjunctivitis resolve in 2 to 7 days without treatment. Some prospective studies suggest that delaying treatment until day 3 or 4 would significantly reduce the unnecessary use of antibiotics without affecting outcomes. However, treatment may be necessary in cases with persistent or worsening signs.
- American Academy of Ophthalmology (AAO) practice guidelines recommend that initial cultures be obtained for patients with central, deep stromal, or large (>2 mm) corneal infiltrates and for patients whose history or clinical features suggest fungal, amebic, mycobacterial, or drug-resistant organisms as the causative agents.

Bacteriology

Bacteria are prokaryotes, organisms in which the genetic material is not separated from the cytoplasm by a nuclear membrane. Most bacterial genes exist as part of a single circular chromosome, but some are present on smaller extrachromosomal circles called *plasmids*, which typically determine inheritance of 1 or a few characteristics. Plasmid DNA is passed between bacterial strains and species more easily than is chromosomal DNA and represents an important mechanism in the rapid proliferation of mutations such as antibiotic resistance.

The prokaryote cell wall imparts shape and rigidity to the cell and also mediates interactions with other bacteria, bacterial viruses, and the environment, including therapeutic drugs. Bacteria are broadly characterized by their microscopic shape as either cocci (round) or bacilli (elongated, or rodlike), with some being indeterminate. Bacteria are further characterized as either gram-positive or gram-negative, according to the reaction of the cell wall (blue or red, respectively) to the Gram stain. This characteristic provides critical information on the structure and biochemical composition of the cell wall that can

243

Table 10-1 Bacterial Classification for Gram Staining

	Gram-Positive	Gram-Negative
Cocci	*Staphylococcus* spp *Streptococcus* spp *Enterococcus* spp	*Neisseria* spp
Rods	*Corynebacterium* spp *Propionibacterium* spp *Bacillus* spp (or gram-variable)	*Pseudomonas* spp *Enterobacter* spp *Haemophilus* spp *Bartonella henselae*
Filaments	*Mycobacterium* spp *Nocardia* spp (or gram-variable) *Actinomyces* spp	

be predictive of the bacteria's antibiotic susceptibility (Table 10-1). The cell wall of gram-positive bacteria consists of a thick layer of peptidoglycan, the primary target of penicillin, and teichoic acid, whereas the cell wall of gram-negative bacteria is composed of a thin layer that is covered by an external lipopolysaccharide membrane (endotoxin), which excludes certain antibiotics. Some bacteria stain poorly with Gram stain, including *Mycobacteria* and *Nocardia asteroides,* visualized best with acid-fast stain.

Structures external to the cell wall facilitate bacterial interactions, including *flagella* (motility), *pili* (bacterial conjugation [transfer of bacterial DNA from one bacterial cell to another]), *fimbriae* (bacterial adherence), and *adhesins* (mucosal surface adhesion). The rapid replication times of bacteria, combined with plasmid-mediated and chromosome-mediated mutations as well as biofilm formation, favor bacterial survival and make it largely inevitable that bacteria will develop resistance to antibiotics.

Gram-positive Cocci

Staphylococcus *species*

Staphylococci inhabit the skin, skin glands, and mucous membranes of healthy mammals. They grow in grapelike clusters in culture but may be seen singly, in pairs, or in short chains in smears from ocular specimens. Staphylococci produce an external biofilm that interferes with phagocytosis and secrete a variety of extracellular proteins—including toxins, enzymes, and enzyme activators—that facilitate both colonization and disease induction. These bacteria adapt quickly and effectively to administered antibacterial agents and may develop resistance to β-lactams, macrolides, tetracyclines, and quinolones. Ocular and nonocular infections due to methicillin-resistant *Staphylococcus aureus* (MRSA) are an increasing problem, leading to the common use of vancomycin, which continues to provide reliable gram-positive coverage for ocular pathogens. Resistance to vancomycin is emerging, however, requiring the development and introduction of newer drugs.

Streptococcus *species*

Streptococci inhabit the mucous membranes of the normal upper respiratory tract and female genital tract (Fig 10-1) and grow in pairs and chains. The historical classification of streptococci was based on serologic grouping of their cell wall carbohydrates (Lancefield

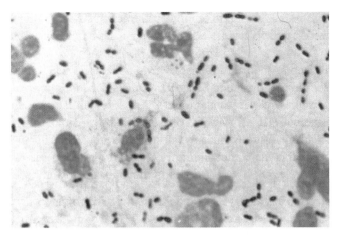

Figure 10-1 Gram-positive cocci *(Streptococcus pneumoniae).* (Gram stain, original magnification ×1000.) *(Courtesy of James Chodosh, MD.)*

groups) and their ability to hemolyze blood-containing agar media, which is useful for initial recognition of clinical isolates. These methods are used less often today, given the availability of genetic sequence data.

Streptococcus pneumoniae appear in smears as lancet-shaped diplococci and express a polysaccharide capsule that resists phagocytosis by macrophages and neutrophils. The toxin pneumolysin is liberated by autolysis and inhibits neutrophil chemotaxis, phagocytosis, lymphocyte proliferation, and antibody synthesis.

Enterococcus *species*

Enterococci, seen in either pairs or short chains, are a common source of antibiotic resistance such as vancomycin-resistant enterococci (VRE). *Enterococcus faecalis* is an important cause of endophthalmitis.

Gram-negative Cocci

Neisseria *species*

Neisseria gonorrhoeae causes urogenital, rectal, and pharyngeal infections, as well as hyperacute conjunctivitis, and can invade intact corneal epithelium, induce keratolysis of the corneal stroma, and perforate the cornea. *N gonorrhoeae* is always a pathogen, whereas the closely related species *Neisseria meningitidis* may be commensal in the pharynx without causing disease. *N gonorrhoeae* is a bean-shaped, gram-negative diplococcus usually seen within neutrophils on a clinical smear taken from ocular or genital sites (Fig 10-2).

Gram-positive Rods

Corynebacterium *species*

Corynebacterium species are pleomorphic bacilli that display palisading or cuneiform patterns in smears. *Corynebacterium diphtheriae* is an exotoxin-producing agent and cause of acute membranous conjunctivitis. Other *Corynebacterium* species, referred to

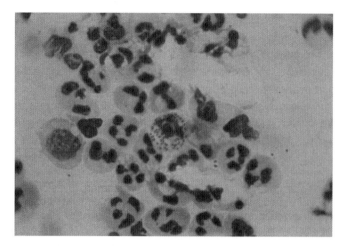

Figure 10-2 Gram-negative cocci *(Neisseria gonorrhoeae)*. (Gram stain, original magnification ×1000.)

as diphtheroids, are routinely isolated from the external eye in the absence of clinical infection. *Corynebacterium xerosis* is commonly seen on histologic sections of vitamin A deficiency–associated conjunctival Bitôt spots, but its significance in conjunctival xerosis is unknown.

Propionibacterium *species*

Propionibacterium acnes and related species are normal inhabitants of human skin. They are aerotolerant but prefer an anaerobic environment. These slender, slightly curved gram-positive rods sometimes have a beaded appearance (Fig 10-3). *P acnes* is a major cause of chronic postoperative endophthalmitis and can cause microbial keratitis.

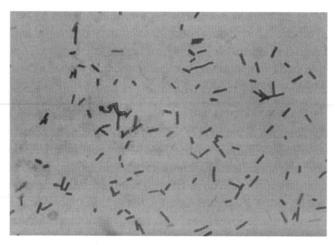

Figure 10-3 Gram-positive rods *(Propionibacterium acnes)*. (Gram stain, original magnification ×1000.)

Bacillus *species*

Bacillus species are ubiquitous gram-positive or gram-variable rods commonly found in soil and characterized by the production of spores, a form of the bacteria that allows survival for extended periods under extremely harsh conditions. *Bacillus* species are typically motile, and this feature may play a role in the explosive character of *Bacillus cereus–*induced posttraumatic endophthalmitis. *B cereus* produces a number of toxins that may rapidly damage ocular tissues. The closely related genus *Clostridium* is anaerobic; *Bacillus* species are aerobes or facultative anaerobes.

Gram-negative Rods

Pseudomonas *species*

Pseudomonas aeruginosa comprises slender gram-negative rods (Fig 10-4) commonly found as contaminants of water. *P aeruginosa* ocular infections are among the most fulminant. Permanent tissue damage and scarring are the rule following corneal infection. Structural virulence factors of *P aeruginosa* include polar flagella, adhesins, and surface pili. *P aeruginosa* organisms secrete a number of toxins that disrupt protein synthesis and damage cell membranes of ocular cells, as well as proteases that degrade the corneal stromal extracellular matrix.

Enterobacteriaceae

The family Enterobacteriaceae includes multiple genera of enteric non–spore-forming gram-negative rods, including *Escherichia, Klebsiella, Enterobacter, Citrobacter, Serratia, Salmonella, Shigella,* and *Proteus*. In particular, the genera *Klebsiella, Enterobacter, Citrobacter, Serratia,* and *Proteus* include species that are important causes of keratitis. Pathogenetic factors include pili, adhesins, cytolysins, and toxins. Enteropathogenic *Escherichia coli* expresses a protein similar to cholera toxin.

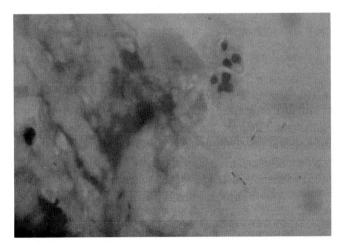

Figure 10-4 Gram-negative rods *(Pseudomonas aeruginosa)*. (Gram stain, original magnification ×1000.)

Haemophilus *species*

Haemophilus species vary in morphology from oval (coccobacilli) to short rods. Culture isolation requires enriched media such as chocolate agar. Along with streptococci, *Haemophilus* species are important etiologic agents of bleb infections following glaucoma filtering surgery. *Haemophilus influenzae* can be divided into biotypes based on biochemical reactions; capsulated strains are further divided into serotypes based on their capsular polysaccharides. *H influenzae* type b (Hib) is the primary human pathogen, and its capsule is a major virulence factor.

Bartonella henselae

Bartonella henselae, the etiologic agent of cat-scratch disease, is a gram-negative aerobic rod best seen with Warthin-Starry staining of a biopsy specimen. *B henselae* infection can be confirmed by culture, polymerase chain reaction (PCR), immunocytologic staining (of histologic specimens), and serologic testing. Cats, especially young cats, are a natural reservoir of *B henselae,* and despite the disease's association with a history of cat scratch or contact with fleas, infection may be transmitted by any contact with an infected cat. (See Parinaud Oculoglandular Syndrome later in the chapter.)

Gram-positive Filaments

Mycobacterium *species*

Mycobacteria are nonmotile, aerobic, weakly gram-positive, but acid-fast; in smears, they appear as straight or slightly curved rods. Löwenstein-Jensen medium is most commonly used for culture isolation. Mycobacteria are obligate intracellular pathogens and are divided into 2 main groups based on their growth rate. *Mycobacterium tuberculosis* and *Mycobacterium leprae* are slow growers. Ocular infection by *M tuberculosis* is uncommon, but it can manifest as a scleritis or posterior uveitis. The fast-growing atypical mycobacteria, including *Mycobacterium fortuitum* and *Mycobacterium cheloneae*, are a more common cause of ulcerative keratitis in the setting of an immunocompromised ocular surface or refractive surgery. Although their importance as a cause of keratitis following refractive surgery remains, atypical mycobacteria have been supplanted by MRSA as the predominant causative agent in this setting.

Nocardia *species*

Nocardia asteroides and related filamentous bacilli are gram-variable or gram-positive, weakly acid-fast bacteria. They may cause keratitis that is clinically similar to one caused by the atypical mycobacteria.

Actinomyces *species*

Actinomycetes are gram-positive, non–acid-fast anaerobic bacteria that colonize the mouth, intestines, and genital tract. They are an important cause of canaliculitis.

Chlamydia Species

Chlamydiae are spherical or ovoid obligate intracellular parasites of mucosal epithelium with a dimorphic life cycle. The infectious form is the *elementary body (EB),* which develops within an infected host eukaryotic cell into the intracellular replicating form, the *reticulate body (RB)*. Only the EB survives outside the host, and only the EB is infectious. Reticulate bodies divide by binary fission to produce 1 or more EBs within a cytoplasmic vacuole, seen on light microscopy as a cellular inclusion.

Borrelia burgdorferi

Borrelia species are obligate parasites, best visualized with Giemsa stain. *B burgdorferi,* the etiologic agent of Lyme disease, is transmitted to humans by the deer tick. The clinical manifestations of Lyme disease are divided into 3 stages, with the most characteristic feature of stage 1 (local disease) being a macular rash, known as erythema chronicum migrans. The pathogenic factors of *B burgdorferi* include the expression of proteinases that facilitate tissue invasion, the induction of proinflammatory cytokines upon binding to phagocytes, and the activation of the complement cascade. Although the organism can be cultured from biopsy specimens taken from erythema migrans skin lesions, the diagnosis of Lyme disease is determined by the results of serologic testing and typical clinical findings. See BCSC Section 1, *Update on General Medicine,* and Section 9, *Intraocular Inflammation and Uveitis,* for further discussion.

Mycology

Fungi are eukaryotes that develop branching filaments. Their cell walls are rigid and contain chitin and polysaccharides. Fungi are classically divided into 2 groups: *yeasts,* round or oval fungi that reproduce by budding and sometimes form pseudohyphae by elongation during budding; and *molds,* multicellular fungi composed of tubular hyphae, either septate or nonseptate, that grow by branching and apical extension (Table 10-2). Yeasts may also form hyphae under certain circumstances. The branching hyphae of molds can form a *mycelium,* an interconnected network of hyphae. *Septate fungi* are distinguished by the presence of walls that divide the filaments into separate cells, each containing one or more nuclei (Fig 10-5). *Dimorphic fungi* grow in 2 distinct forms as a result of changes in cell wall synthesis in different environments and may often constitute highly virulent pathogens. Fungal cell walls stain with Gomori methenamine silver but, except for *Candida,* do not take up Gram stain. Classification of filamentous fungi is based on microscopic features of *conidia* (fungal elements that form asexually) and *conidiophores* (the specialized hyphae where conidia are formed). However, the histologic morphology of fungi varies significantly when they are isolated from tissue (corneal scraping/biopsy); fungi thus require laboratory isolation for definitive identification.

Table 10-2 Fungi

Yeasts	Molds (filamentous)	
	Septate	Nonseptate
Candida spp	*Fusarium* spp	*Mucor*
Cryptococcus neoformans	*Aspergillus*	*Rhizopus*
Rhinosporidium spp	*Curvularia*	*Absidia*

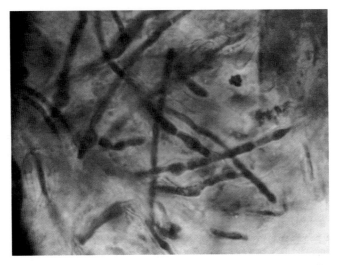

Figure 10-5 Septate hyphae of filamentous fungus *(Fusarium solani)*. (Diff-Quik stain, original magnification ×100.) *(Courtesy of Elmer Y. Tu, MD.)*

Most antifungal medications target the fungal cell wall either through direct toxicity or interference with cell wall synthesis.

Yeasts

The incidence of mycotic infections has increased significantly with the rise of immuno-suppressed states, both disease related and pharmacologically induced, as well as with the increase in long-term antibacterial use by immunocompromised patients and the general population. *Candida* species are ubiquitous in the environment and are ordinarily resident flora of, and recoverable from, the gastrointestinal and genitourinary tracts, the oropharynx, and the skin (with *Candida albicans* being the most common species at these sites; Fig 10-6).

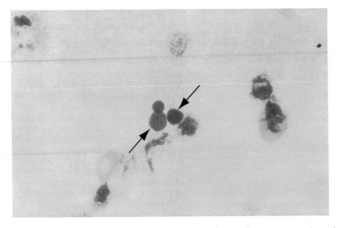

Figure 10-6 Yeasts *(Candida albicans)*. Budding yeast form *(lower arrow)* and solitary yeast *(upper arrow)*. (Gram stain, original magnification ×1000.) *(Courtesy of James Chodosh, MD.)*

Yeast is a disproportionate cause of fungal keratitis in cooler northern climes. The pathogenesis of this yeast in the cornea is enhanced by the formation of pseudohyphae, which express proteases and phospholipases, facilitating tissue penetration.

Cryptococcus neoformans infection is acquired through inhalation and causes clinical disease in the brain and optic nerve, eye, lung, skin, and prostate in immunosuppressed patients.

Rhinosporidium seeberi is present in soil and groundwater and presumably infects humans through contact with these sources. Ocular rhinosporidiosis manifests as sessile or pedunculated papillomatous or polypoid lesions in the conjunctiva, which may be associated with similar lesions in the nose and nasopharynx.

Molds

Septate filamentous fungi

The vast majority of external ocular mold infections are caused by septate fungi. *Fusarium* species (eg, *Fusarium solani* and *Fusarium oxysporum*) are common pathogens encountered in warm, humid environments as a cause of fulminant keratitis. Among the genera that have been isolated from the external eye are *Aspergillus, Alternaria, Curvularia, Paecilomyces, Scedosporium,* and *Phialophora*. Most cases of oculomycosis occur following trauma with soil or vegetable matter and, less frequently, with contact lens usage.

Nonseptate filamentous fungi

Nonseptate filamentous fungi include the *Mucor, Rhizopus,* and *Absidia* species in class Zygomycetes, order Mucorales, family Mucoraceae. These ubiquitous fungi are an uncommon cause of external ocular infections. They can also cause life-threatening infections of the paranasal sinuses, brain, and orbit in immunocompromised patients, particularly those with diabetes mellitus.

Thomas PA, Geraldine P. Oculomycosis. In: Merz WG, Hay RJ, eds. *Medical Mycology.* 10th ed. London: Hodder Arnold; 2005:273–344. *Topley & Wilson's Microbiology and Microbial Infections;* vol 5.

Other molds

Pythium insidiosum is an oomycete (water mold) unrelated to the fungal pathogens described previously. It is increasingly recognized as a corneal pathogen, primarily in Southeast Asia, but has also been reported worldwide. *P insidiosum* is more closely related to kelp or brown algae and is therefore resistant to currently available antifungals. Identification of *P insidiosum* is very difficult because of clinicians' unfamiliarity with this pathogen and because identification is based solely on morphology and evolving PCR techniques. Cure of associated keratitis is achieved mainly through early suspicion, recognition, and keratoplasty, with most keratitis cases progressing to either enucleation or evisceration, although reports of successful medical therapy have emerged.

Sharma S, Balne PK, Motukupally SR, et al. *Pythium insidiosum* keratitis: clinical profile and role of DNA sequencing and zoospore formation in diagnosis. *Cornea.* 2015;34(4): 438–442.

Parasitology

Protozoa

Acanthamoeba species are protozoa (unicellular eukaryotes) that can cause an isolated infection of the human cornea as their primary disease in humans. Other conditions have been described, such as disseminated dermatitis, visceral infestation, and encephalitis unrelated to ocular disease. The *Acanthamoeba* life cycle includes a motile trophozoite form (15–45 μm in diameter) and a dormant cyst form (10–25 μm in diameter) (Fig 10-7). The cysts are double-walled and very hardy, resistant to most environmental extremes and toxins, including chlorine. Classification of *Acanthamoeba* species has been based on morphology, but molecular methods are more accurate and increasingly utilized.

Microsporidia are obligate intracellular parasites and, recently, have also been linked to the Fungi kingdom. Of the phylum Microspora, the following genera have been implicated in human infection: *Nosema, Encephalitozoon, Pleistophora, Vittaforma, Trachipleistophora, Enterocytozoon,* and unclassified microsporida.

Leishmania *species*

Leishmania is a genus of flagellate protozoa. Cutaneous leishmaniasis is transmitted by the bite of its vector, the female sandfly, in endemic areas of tropical Asia, Africa, and Latin America. An infected eyelid ulcer may become granulomatous. Scrapings or biopsy material obtained from the ulcer can show intracellular parasites by Giemsa or immunofluorescent stains. The parasites can sometimes be isolated on blood agar or insect tissue culture medium.

Helminths

Onchocerciasis is caused by onchocercal filariae transmitted by the bite of the blackfly (genus *Simulium*), which lays its eggs on vegetation in fast-flowing rivers (hence the

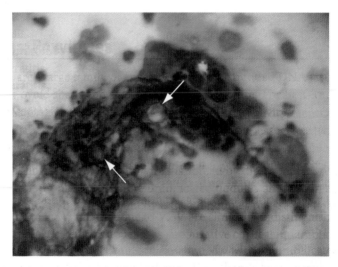

Figure 10-7 *Acanthamoeba* cyst *(arrows)*. (Diff-Quik stain, original magnification ×100.) *(Courtesy of Elmer Y. Tu, MD.)*

common name for the disease, *river blindness*) and is endemic in parts of sub-Saharan Africa, the Middle East, and Latin America. Microfilariae penetrate the skin and mature in subcutaneous nodules formed at the site of the bite for approximately 1 year, after which mating produces microfilariae offspring (≈300 μm in length)—up to 1500 a day per female (100 cm in length). These worms can live as long as 15 years in the human host; thus, diagnosis can be made with skin snips demonstrating the microfilariae.

Migration of microfilariae to the skin and eye results in clinical onchocerciasis, and subsequent blackfly bites can carry the organism to other individuals. Microfilariae enter the peripheral cornea, where they can be visualized by slit-lamp examination, and may reach the inner eye. Keratitis (including punctate keratitis and "snowflake" and sclerosing peripheral corneal opacities), anterior uveitis, and chorioretinitis occur upon death of the microfilariae. The intense, blinding inflammatory keratitis has been shown to be a reaction less to the microfilariae than to a bacterial endosymbiont, *Wolbachia,* which is essential to filariae reproduction. Antifilarial therapy can produce a systemic inflammatory response, but prior treatment with systemic doxycycline has been shown to reduce this response. Treatment by nodulectomy or with oral ivermectin (the discoverers of which were awarded the Nobel Prize in Physiology or Medicine 2015) and control of local blackfly populations have been successful in reducing the incidence of onchocerciasis in selected areas.

Loa loa larvae enter the skin at the bite of an infected deer fly (genus *Chrysops*). Adult worms may grow to 6 cm in length and migrate through the connective tissues, causing transient hypersensitivity reactions. *Loa loa* may also appear beneath the conjunctiva.

Visceral larval migrans is a multisystem disease in young children that is caused by the migrating larvae of *Toxocara canis* and *Toxocara cati,* natural residents of dogs and cats, respectively. *Toxocara* larvae develop and mate in the intestines of their natural host; human ingestion of fertilized eggs in pet feces results in infection. *Toxocara* larvae in the human intestine do not receive the proper environmental signals and consequently migrate throughout the body, invading and destroying tissues as they go. Ocular larval migrans occurs in older children, and the viscera are typically spared.

Arthropods

Phthirus pubis

Phthiriasis is a venereally acquired crab louse *(Phthirus pubis)* infestation of coarse hair in the pubic, axillary, chest, and facial regions. Adult female crab lice (Fig 10-8) and immature nits on the eyelashes are a cause of blepharoconjunctivitis.

Demodex *species*

Demodex folliculorum and *Demodex brevis* inhabit normal superficial hair and eyelash follicles and deeper sebaceous and meibomian glands, respectively. An increased number of these species in the facial glands is associated with rosacea (Fig 10-9). Eyelash colonization increases with age and may be associated with blepharoconjunctivitis.

Cox FEG, Wakelin D, Gillespie SH, Despommier DD, eds. *Parasitology.* 10th ed. London: Hodder Arnold; 2005. *Topley & Wilson's Microbiology and Microbial Infections;* vol 6.

Tu EY. *Acanthamoeba* and other parasitic corneal infections. In: Mannis MJ, Holland EJ, eds. *Cornea.* Vol 1. 4th ed. Philadelphia: Elsevier; 2017:976–985.

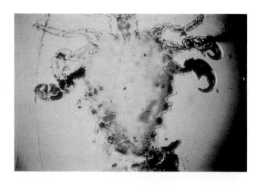

Figure 10-8 Crab louse *(Phthirus pubis).* (Wet mount, original magnification ×200.)

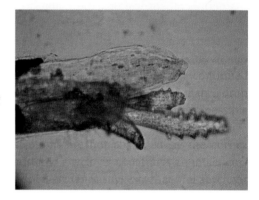

Figure 10-9 *Demodex* species. (Wet mount, original magnification ×100.) *(Courtesy of Elmer Y. Tu, MD.)*

Prions

Prions are altered proteins that cause lethal transmissible encephalopathies, including Creutzfeldt-Jakob disease, kuru, scrapie in sheep, and bovine spongiform encephalopathy ("mad cow" disease). Transmission of Creutzfeldt-Jakob disease following corneal transplantation has been reported. See also BCSC Section 5, *Neuro-Ophthalmology.*

> Prusiner SB. Shattuck Lecture: neurodegenerative diseases and prions. *N Engl J Med.* 2001; 344(20):1516–1526.

Microbial and Parasitic Infections of the Eyelid Margin and Conjunctiva

Staphylococcal Blepharitis

Staphylococcal bacteria on the anterior eyelid margin can cause blepharitis. This condition is not purely infectious, however; antimicrobial therapy is rarely curative because of a significant inflammatory component that may predispose to bacterial overgrowth and perpetuate a local immune deviation. This disorder is discussed in detail in Chapter 3.

Fungal and Parasitic Infections of the Eyelid Margin

Demodex is a genus of mites that are normal commensal acarian parasites of humans. On slit-lamp biomicroscopy, their presence is suggested as waxy "sleeves" around eyelashes

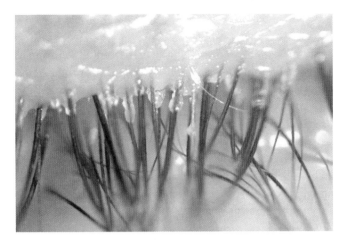

Figure 10-10 *Demodex*-associated "sleeves." *(Courtesy of Elmer Y. Tu, MD.)*

(Fig 10-10) or as "cylinders" extending from sebaceous glands of the eyelid margin. The role of these parasites in the pathogenesis of blepharitis is unclear, but some patients may experience an inflammatory response with infestation. The infestation may respond to diluted tea tree oil applied to the base of the eyelashes. Other organisms that survive on lipids of eyelid glands, such as *Malassezia furfur,* have also been implicated in certain types of blepharitis.

A focal granuloma or dermatitis affecting the eyelid or conjunctiva can be caused by very rare infections, including

- blastomycosis
- sporotrichosis
- rhinosporidiosis
- cryptococcosis
- leishmaniasis
- ophthalmomyiasis

Lice infestation of the eyelids and eyelashes, also known as *phthiriasis palpebrum,* is an uncommon form of conjunctivitis or blepharitis affecting adolescents and young adults and is caused by the pubic louse and its ova. In rare instances, pediculosis involves the ocular region by localized extension of head or body lice (*Pediculus humanus capitis* or *Pediculus humanus corporis,* respectively). Mechanical removal of the lice and nits (eggs) can be performed with jeweler's forceps, but pubic hairs are usually treated with a pediculicide. Any ointment can smother the lice and should be applied twice daily for at least 10 days, because the incubation period (of the nits) is 7–10 days. Periodic reexamination is recommended over 10–14 days to detect recurrence and remove any new nits. Bed linen, clothing, and any items of close contact should be washed and dried at the highest temperature setting (at least 50°C).

Bacterial Conjunctivitis in Children and Adults

PATHOGENESIS Overall, 80% of cases of infectious conjunctivitis in adults are viral in origin. While, in children, the number of bacterial conjunctivitis cases is similar to that of viral conjunctivitis cases, bacterial conjunctivitis is much less common than viral conjunctivitis in adults.

Bacterial conjunctivitis is characterized by bacterial overgrowth and infiltration of the conjunctival epithelial layer and sometimes the substantia propria. The source of infection is either direct contact with an infected individual's secretions (usually through eye–hand contact) or the spread of infection from the organisms colonizing the patient's own nasal and sinus mucosa. In an adult with unilateral bacterial conjunctivitis, the nasolacrimal system should be examined, as nasolacrimal duct obstruction, dacryocystitis, or canaliculitis may be the underlying cause.

Though usually self-limited, bacterial conjunctivitis can occasionally be severe and sight-threatening when caused by virulent bacterial species such as *N gonorrhoeae* or *Streptococcus pyogenes*. In rare cases, it may presage life-threatening systemic disease, as with conjunctivitis caused by *N meningitidis*.

CLINICAL PRESENTATION Bacterial conjunctivitis should be suspected in patients with conjunctival inflammation and a purulent discharge. The rapidity of onset and severity of conjunctival inflammation and discharge are suggestive of the possible causative organism. Table 10-3 outlines the clinical classification of bacterial conjunctivitis based on these parameters.

Acute purulent conjunctivitis

PATHOGENESIS Acute purulent conjunctivitis is a self-limited infection of the conjunctiva characterized by an acute inflammatory response with purulent discharge of less than 3 weeks' duration (definition of *acute*). Cases may occur spontaneously or in epidemics. The most common etiologic pathogens are *S pneumoniae, Streptococcus viridans, H influenzae,* and *S aureus,* with the relative frequency of each varying depending on patient age and geographic location.

CLINICAL PRESENTATION *Streptococcus pneumoniae* conjunctivitis is characterized by a moderate purulent discharge, eyelid edema, chemosis, conjunctival hemorrhages, and occasional inflammatory membranes on the tarsal conjunctiva. Corneal ulceration occurs in rare instances.

Haemophilus influenzae conjunctivitis occurs in young children, sometimes in association with otitis media, and in adults, particularly those chronically colonized with *H influenzae* (eg, smokers or patients with chronic bronchopulmonary disease). Acute purulent conjunctivitis caused by *H influenzae* biotype III (formerly *Haemophilus aegyptius*) resembles that caused by *S pneumoniae*; however, conjunctival membranes do not develop, and peripheral corneal epithelial ulcers and stromal infiltrates occur more commonly. *H influenzae* preseptal cellulitis may be associated with fulminant *Haemophilus* meningitis, in which up to 20% of patients who recover have long-term neurologic sequelae. The incidence of infection has been reduced by a vigorous program of vaccination against Hib.

Staphylococcus aureus may produce an acute blepharoconjunctivitis. The discharge tends to be somewhat less purulent than that seen in pneumococcal conjunctivitis, and the associated signs are generally less severe.

Table 10-3 Clinical Classification of Bacterial Conjunctivitis

Course of Onset	Severity	Common Organisms	Ophthalmia Neonatorum Postpartum Onset and Associated Findings
Slow (days to weeks)	Mild to moderate	*Staphylococcus aureus* *Moraxella lacunata* *Proteus* spp Enterobacteriaceae	Variable onset
		Pseudomonas aeruginosa	Rare Keratitis, corneal perforation
		Chlamydia trachomatis	Onset: day 5–14 Absence of conjunctival follicles Pneumonitis, otitis media (50% of cases)
		Herpes simplex (viral)	Onset: in the first 2 weeks of life Nonspecific conjunctivitis
Acute or subacute (hours to days)	Moderate to severe	*Haemophilus influenzae* biotype III* *Haemophilus influenzae*	Variable onset
		Streptococcus pneumoniae	Variable onset
		Streptococcus viridans	Variable onset
		Staphylococcus aureus	Variable onset
Hyperacute (<24 hours)	Severe	*Neisseria gonorrhoeae*	Onset: day 1–13 (commonly day 3–5) Keratitis, endophthalmitis, systemic infection
		Neisseria meningitidis	

*Previously referred to as *Haemophilus aegyptius.*

LABORATORY EVALUATION Gram-stained smears and culture of the conjunctiva are usually not necessary in uncomplicated, largely self-limited cases of suspected bacterial conjunctivitis but should be used for the following:

- certain compromised hosts, such as neonates or debilitated or immunocompromised individuals, to assess the risk of local and systemic complications
- severe cases of purulent conjunctivitis, to differentiate it from hyperpurulent conjunctivitis, which generally requires systemic therapy
- cases unresponsive to initial therapy

MANAGEMENT Most cases of acute bacterial conjunctivitis resolve in 2–7 days without treatment. Some prospective studies suggest that delaying treatment until day 3 or 4 would significantly reduce the unnecessary use of antibiotics without affecting outcomes. Initiating treatment at this time only for persistent or worsening signs would generally shorten the course and improve symptoms. If the conjunctivitis is improving on day 4, antibiotics may not be necessary at all, as these studies also indicate that initiation of antibiotics after day 4 provides limited benefit. Cases likely to represent a viral conjunctivitis should *not* be routinely treated with empiric antibiotics.

When the physician believes that further intervention is indicated, the initial treatment should be weighted toward the results of the Gram-stained morphology of the bacteria identified on the conjunctival smear. Definitive treatment should be based on the culture results, if available, as smear results may sometimes be inconclusive as to the predominant category of organism responsible for the infection. Cultures of the nose or throat may be obtained if an associated sinusitis or pharyngitis is present. Even if no overt sinusitis, rhinitis, or pharyngitis is present, nasal or throat swabs should be considered in cases of relapsing conjunctivitis, because organisms persisting in and colonizing the respiratory tract mucosa may be the source of infection.

Empiric therapy with polymyxin B-trimethoprim, aminoglycoside or fluoroquinolone drops, or bacitracin or ciprofloxacin ointment can be initiated before results of the Gram stain or culture have been received. The dosing schedule is 4–6 times daily for approximately 5–7 days unless otherwise indicated. Cases with gram-negative coccobacilli on Gram-stained smears are probably caused by *Haemophilus* species and should be treated with polymyxin B-trimethoprim. Supplemental oral antibiotics are recommended for patients with acute purulent conjunctivitis associated with pharyngitis, for those with conjunctivitis-otitis syndrome, and for children with *Haemophilus* conjunctivitis.

Hyperacute gonococcal conjunctivitis

PATHOGENESIS Gonococcal conjunctivitis presents with explosive onset and very rapid progression of severe purulent conjunctivitis: massive exudation; severe chemosis; eyelid edema; marked conjunctival hyperemia; and, in untreated cases, corneal infiltrates, melting, and perforation. The organism most commonly responsible for hyperpurulent conjunctivitis is *N gonorrhoeae* (Fig 10-11). Gonococcal conjunctivitis is a sexually transmitted disease resulting from direct transmission of the organism, for example, from the genitalia to the hands and then to the eyes or from the mother to the neonate during vaginal delivery.

CLINICAL PRESENTATION Gonococcal conjunctivitis is one of the few bacterial diseases associated with preauricular lymphadenopathy and the formation of conjunctival membranes. Keratitis, the principal cause of sight-threatening complications, has been reported to occur in 15%–40% of cases. Corneal involvement may consist of diffuse epithelial haze, epithelial defects, marginal infiltrates, and ulcerative keratitis that can rapidly progress to perforation.

LABORATORY EVALUATION *Neisseria gonorrhoeae* grows well on chocolate agar and Thayer-Martin media.

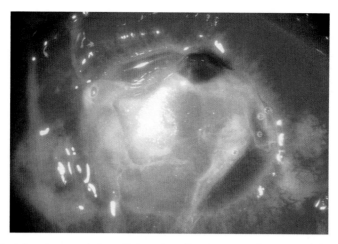

Figure 10-11 Peripheral corneal ulceration and perforation occurring several days after onset of hyperacute conjunctivitis caused by *N gonorrhoeae.*

MANAGEMENT Gonococcal conjunctivitis requires systemic antibiotic therapy, with topical ophthalmic antibiotics used as adjunctive therapy only. Current treatment regimens for gonococcal conjunctivitis reflect the increasing prevalence of *penicillin-resistant N gonor-rhoeae (PRNG)* in the United States. Ceftriaxone, a third-generation cephalosporin, is highly effective against PRNG. Patients with gonococcal conjunctivitis without corneal ulceration may be treated on an outpatient basis with 1 intramuscular (IM) ceftriaxone (1 g) injection; patients with corneal ulceration should be admitted to the hospital and treated with intrave-nous (IV) ceftriaxone (1 g IV every 12 hours) for 3 consecutive days. Patients with penicillin allergy can be given spectinomycin (2 g IM) or oral fluoroquinolones (ciprofloxacin 500 mg or ofloxacin 400 mg orally twice daily for 5 days). When possible, fluoroquinolones should be avoided in children because of potential adverse effects on joint cartilage.

Erythromycin ointment, bacitracin ointment, gentamicin ointment, and ciprofloxa-cin solution have been recommended for topical therapy. Treatment of severe cases should include copious, frequent (every 30–60 minutes) irrigation of the conjunctival sac with normal saline to remove inflammatory cells, proteases, and debris that may be toxic to the ocular surface and contribute to corneal melting.

Up to one-third of patients with gonococcal conjunctivitis have been reported to have concurrent chlamydial venereal disease. Because of this frequent association, it is advis-able to give patients supplemental oral antibiotics for treatment of chlamydial infection. Treatment regimens for chlamydia are discussed later in this chapter. Patients should be instructed to refer their sex partners for evaluation and treatment. Other sexually trans-mitted pathogens causing conjunctivitis include *Chlamydia trachomatis, Treponema palli-dum,* human immunodeficiency virus, and herpes simplex virus (Table 10-4). For further discussion of syphilis, see BCSC Section 1, *Update on General Medicine,* and Section 9, *Intraocular Inflammation and Uveitis.*

American Academy of Ophthalmology Cornea/External Disease Panel. Preferred Practice Pattern Guidelines. *Conjunctivitis.* San Francisco: American Academy of Ophthalmology; 2013. Available at www.aao.org/ppp.

Table 10-4 Sexually Transmitted Pathogens Associated With Conjunctivitis

Organism	Onset	Presentation
Neisseria gonorrhoeae	<24 hours	Hyperacute with copious discharge, conjunctival edema
Human immunodeficiency virus	Day 11–28	Conjunctival edema, watery discharge
Chlamydia trachomatis	Days to weeks	Follicular conjunctivitis
Treponema pallidum		Granulomatous conjunctivitis
Herpes simplex virus	2 weeks	Follicular conjunctivitis

Cortina MS, Tu EY. Antibiotic use in corneal and external eye infections. *Focal Points: Clinical Modules for Ophthalmologists.* San Francisco: American Academy of Ophthalmology; 2011, module 6.

Chlamydial conjunctivitis

PATHOGENESIS The bacterium *C trachomatis* causes several different conjunctivitis syndromes; each is associated with different serotypes of *C trachomatis*:

- trachoma: serotypes A–C
- adult and neonatal inclusion conjunctivitis: serotypes D–K
- lymphogranuloma venereum: serotypes L1, L2, and L3

There have been reports of rare cases of keratoconjunctivitis in humans caused by *Chlamydia* species that typically infect animals, such as *Chlamydophila psittaci* (formerly *Chlamydia psittaci*), an agent generally associated with disease in parrots, and the feline pneumonitis agent.

LABORATORY EVALUATION As an obligate intracellular pathogen, *C trachomatis* cannot be easily isolated using standard ophthalmic culture techniques, requiring either direct observation of the intracellular bacterium or cell culture. Direct visualization is possible with a Giemsa stain or direct fluorescent antibody staining. PCR probes are available and increasingly being used in place of other diagnostic methods.

CLINICAL PRESENTATION AND MANAGEMENT Trachoma and adult inclusion conjunctivitis are discussed individually in the following sections.

Trachoma Trachoma is an infectious disease that occurs in communities with poor hygiene and inadequate sanitation. It affects approximately 150 million individuals worldwide and is the leading cause of preventable blindness. Trachoma is currently endemic in the Middle East and in developing regions around the world. In the United States, it occurs sporadically among American Indians and in mountainous areas of the South. Most infections are transmitted from eye to eye. Transmission may also occur by flies and household fomites, which spread other bacteria as well, causing secondary bacterial infections in patients with trachoma.

Solomon AW, Holland MJ, Alexander ND, et al. Mass treatment with single-dose azithromycin for trachoma. *N Engl J Med.* 2004;351(19):1962–1971.

CLINICAL PRESENTATION The initial symptoms of trachoma include foreign-body sensation, redness, tearing, and mucopurulent discharge. A severe follicular reaction develops, most prominently in the superior tarsal conjunctiva, but sometimes in the superior and inferior fornices, inferior tarsal conjunctiva, semilunar fold, and limbus. In acute trachoma, follicles on the superior tarsus may be obscured by diffuse papillary hypertrophy and inflammatory cell infiltration. Large tarsal follicles in trachoma may become necrotic and eventually heal with significant scarring. Linear or stellate scarring of the superior tarsus *(Arlt line)* typically occurs (Fig 10-12). Involution and necrosis of follicles may result in limbal depressions known as *Herbert pits* (Fig 10-13). Corneal findings in trachoma include epithelial keratitis, focal and multifocal peripheral and central

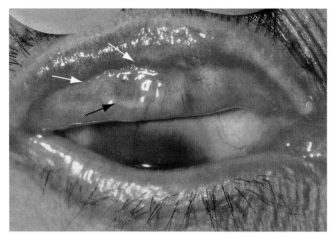

Figure 10-12 Linear scarring of the superior tarsal conjunctiva (Arlt line, *white arrows*) in a patient with old trachoma with subconjunctival fibrosis *(black arrow)*. *(Courtesy of Vincent P. deLuise, MD.)*

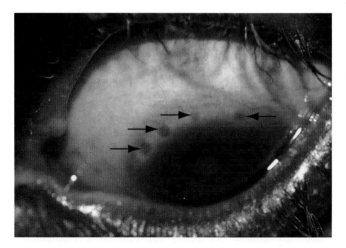

Figure 10-13 Trachoma exhibiting Herbert pits *(arrows)* of the superior limbus (round to oval, pigmented areas within pannus). *(Courtesy of Tom Lietman, MD.)*

stromal infiltrates, and a superficial fibrovascular pannus, which is most prominent in the superior third of the cornea but may extend centrally into the visual axis (Fig 10-14).

Clinical diagnosis of trachoma requires at least 2 of the following clinical features:

- follicles on the upper tarsal conjunctiva
- limbal follicles and their sequelae (Herbert pits)
- typical tarsal conjunctival scarring
- vascular pannus most marked on the superior limbus

Severe conjunctival and lacrimal gland duct scarring from chronic trachoma can result in aqueous tear deficiency, tear drainage obstruction, trichiasis, and entropion.

The World Health Organization (WHO) devised a simple severity-grading system for trachoma based on the presence or absence of 5 key signs:

1. follicular conjunctival inflammation
2. diffuse conjunctival inflammation
3. tarsal conjunctival scarring
4. aberrant lashes
5. corneal opacification

The WHO grading system was developed for use by trained personnel other than ophthalmologists to assess the prevalence and severity of trachoma in population-based surveys in endemic areas.

Thylefors B, Dawson CR, Jones BR, West SK, Taylor HR. A simple system for the assessment of trachoma and its complications. *Bull World Health Organ.* 1987;65(4):477–483.

MANAGEMENT Current recommendations for treatment of active trachoma are tetracycline 1% ophthalmic ointment, applied twice daily for 2 months, and oral azithromycin 1000 mg, given as a single dose. Although azithromycin is more effective and easier for patient adherence, cost and availability dictate the best therapy. Topical erythromycin,

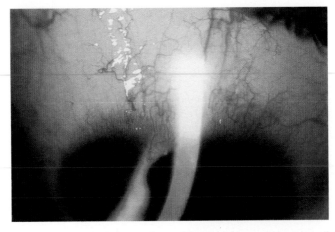

Figure 10-14 Superior micropannus in a patient with adult chlamydial conjunctivitis (trachoma).

given at the same frequency as topical tetracycline, and oral tetracycline 1.5–2.0 g daily in divided doses for 3 weeks are also effective. Oral erythromycin is recommended for treatment of rare tetracycline-resistant cases. Management of the vision-threatening complications of trachoma may include tear substitutes for dry eye and eyelid surgery for entropion or trichiasis.

Adult chlamydial conjunctivitis Adult chlamydial conjunctivitis is a sexually transmitted disease often found in conjunction with chlamydial urethritis or cervicitis. It is most prevalent in sexually active adolescents and young adults. Chlamydia is a systemic disease. The eye is usually infected by direct or indirect contact with infected genital secretions, but other modes of transmission may include shared eye cosmetics and inadequately chlorinated swimming pools. Onset of conjunctivitis is typically 1–2 weeks after ocular inoculation and is not as acute as with adenoviral keratoconjunctivitis. Often patients may report having had mild symptoms for weeks to months.

CLINICAL PRESENTATION External signs of adult inclusion conjunctivitis include a follicular conjunctival response that is most prominent in the lower palpebral conjunctiva and fornix, scant mucopurulent discharge, and palpable preauricular adenopathy. Follicles in the bulbar conjunctiva and semilunar fold are frequently present, and these are a helpful and specific sign in patients not using topical medications associated with the finding. Unlike with neonatal forms, inflammatory conjunctival membranes do not develop in adult chlamydial keratoconjunctivitis.

Corneal involvement may consist of fine or coarse epithelial infiltrates, occasionally associated with subepithelial infiltrates. The keratitis is more likely to be found in the superior cornea but may also occur centrally and resemble adenoviral keratitis. A micropannus, usually extending less than 3 mm from the superior cornea, may develop.

MANAGEMENT Left untreated, adult chlamydial conjunctivitis often resolves spontaneously in 6–18 months. Currently, one of the following oral antibiotic regimens is recommended:

- azithromycin 1000 mg single dose
- doxycycline 100 mg twice daily for 7 days
- tetracycline 250 mg 4 times daily for 7 days
- erythromycin 500 mg 4 times daily for 7 days

Patients with laboratory-confirmed chlamydial conjunctivitis and their sexual contacts should be evaluated for coinfection with other sexually transmitted diseases, such as syphilis or gonorrhea, before antibiotic treatment is started. Sexual partners should be concomitantly treated to avoid reinfection.

Centers for Disease Control and Prevention; Workowski KA, Berman SM. Sexually transmitted diseases treatment guidelines 2006. *MMWR Recomm Rep.* 2006;55(RR-11):1–94.

Bacterial conjunctivitis in neonates

Neisseria gonorrhoeae causes the most severe neonatal conjunctivitis. (*Neonatal* is defined as occurring within the first month of life.) In order of decreasing prevalence, the causes of neonatal bacterial conjunctivitis, reflective of the vaginal and nosocomial flora, are as follows (see Table 10-3):

- *C trachomatis*
- *S viridans*
- *S aureus*
- *H influenzae*
- group D *Streptococcus*
- *Moraxella catarrhalis*
- *E coli* and other gram-negative rods
- *N gonorrhoeae*

Ophthalmia neonatorum is discussed in more detail in BCSC Section 6, *Pediatric Ophthalmology and Strabismus.*

Neonatal gonococcal conjunctivitis Prenatal screening for maternal gonococcal genital infection and neonatal antibiotic prophylaxis have reduced the overall rate of neonatal gonococcal conjunctivitis, a bilateral conjunctival discharge that typically develops 3–5 days after parturition. The discharge may be serosanguineous during the first several days, with a copious purulent exudate, severe corneal complications, and endophthalmitis developing later (see "Hyperacute gonococcal conjunctivitis" earlier in the chapter). Infected infants may also have other localized gonococcal infections, including rhinitis and proctitis. Disseminated gonococcal infection with arthritis, meningitis, pneumonia, and sepsis resulting in death of the infant is a rare complication.

MANAGEMENT Because of the developing resistance of *N gonorrhoeae* to various antibiotics—including penicillin (PRNG), fluoroquinolones (QRNG), and tetracycline—the currently recommended first-line treatment for neonatal gonococcal conjunctivitis is ceftriaxone. For *nondisseminated* infections, a single IM or IV ceftriaxone injection (up to 125 mg or a dose of 25–50 mg/kg) or cefotaxime at a single dose of 100 mg/kg IV or IM is recommended. For *disseminated* infection, treatment should be augmented according to consultation with a specialist in infectious diseases. Either of these regimens should be combined with hourly saline irrigation of the conjunctiva until discharge is eliminated. If corneal involvement is suspected, application of topical erythromycin or gentamicin ointment or frequent application of a topical fluoroquinolone should be considered. Topical cycloplegia may also prove beneficial. Systemic treatment is advised for infants born to mothers with active gonorrhea, even in the absence of conjunctivitis.

American Academy of Pediatrics. Gonococcal infections. In: Pickering LK, Baker CJ, Kimberlin DW, Long SS, eds. *2009 Red Book: Report of the Committee on Infectious Diseases.* 28th ed. Elk Grove Village, IL: American Academy of Pediatrics; 2009:305–313.

Centers for Disease Control and Prevention; Workowski KA, Berman SM. Sexually transmitted diseases treatment guidelines 2006. *MMWR Recomm Rep.* 2006;55(RR-11):1–94.

Cortina MS, Tu EY. Antibiotic use in corneal and external eye infections. *Focal Points: Clinical Modules for Ophthalmologists.* San Francisco: American Academy of Ophthalmology; 2011, module 6.

Neonatal chlamydial conjunctivitis Chlamydial conjunctivitis in neonates differs clinically from that in adults in the following ways:

- There is no follicular response in newborns.
- The amount of mucopurulent discharge is greater in newborns.
- Pseudomembranes can develop on the tarsal conjunctiva in newborns.
- Intracytoplasmic inclusions are seen in a greater percentage of Giemsa-stained conjunctival specimens in newborns.
- The infection in newborns is more likely to respond to topical medications.

Both Gram and Giemsa stains of conjunctival scrapings are recommended in neonates with conjunctivitis to identify *C trachomatis* and *N gonorrhoeae,* as well as other bacteria, as causative agents. Other *Chlamydia*-associated infections, such as pneumonitis and otitis media, can accompany inclusion conjunctivitis in the newborn. Therefore, systemic erythromycin (12.5 mg/kg oral or IV 4 times daily for 14 days) is recommended, even though inclusion conjunctivitis in the newborn usually responds to topical erythromycin or sulfacetamide.

Parinaud Oculoglandular Syndrome

Granulomatous conjunctivitis with regional lymphadenopathy is an uncommon condition called *Parinaud oculoglandular syndrome. Cat-scratch disease (CSD),* which causes most cases of the syndrome, is estimated to affect 22,000 people annually in the United States, with conjunctivitis developing in approximately 10%. The primary causative agent is *B henselae.* Other, infrequent causes of Parinaud oculoglandular syndrome include

- *Afipia felis*
- other *Bartonella* species
- coccidioidomycosis
- sporotrichosis
- syphilis
- tuberculosis
- tularemia

PATHOGENESIS *Bartonella henselae* causes a transient infection in kittens and their fleas but may enter a carrier state. Despite the name "cat-scratch" disease, infection may be transmitted to humans by a cat bite or lick or by contact with a cat's fleas. Human-to-human transmission is not known to occur. Local infection causes a granulomatous reaction.

CLINICAL PRESENTATION Unilateral granulomatous conjunctivitis with one or more raised or flat gelatinous, hyperemic, granulomatous lesions develops on the superior or inferior tarsal conjunctiva, fornix, or bulbar conjunctiva about 3–10 days after inoculation. Either concurrently or 1–2 weeks later, ipsilateral regional preauricular and submandibular lymph nodes, and occasionally cervical nodes, become firm and tender. Approximately 10%–40% of the nodes enlarge and become suppurative. Mild systemic symptoms of fever, malaise, headache, and anorexia develop in about 10%–30% of patients, with severe, disseminated complications—including encephalopathy, encephalitis, thrombocytopenic purpura, osteolysis, hepatitis, and splenitis—occurring in approximately 2% of CSD patients. Optic neuritis and neuroretinitis have been reported.

LABORATORY EVALUATION Serologic testing is the most cost-effective means of diagnosing typical CSD. Antibodies to *B henselae* can be detected by indirect fluorescent antibody testing or by enzyme immunoassay. The enzyme immunoassay for *B henselae* is more sensitive than the indirect fluorescent antibody test and is available from specialty laboratories. The skin test antigen for CSD is neither commercially available nor standardized. Atypical CSD is best approached by combining serologic testing with culture or PCR.

MANAGEMENT The ideal treatment has not yet been determined. Various antibacterial treatment regimens have reported success. Suggested agents generally include azithromycin, erythromycin, or doxycycline. Rifampin is often used as an adjuvant. Responses to trimethoprim-sulfamethoxazole and fluoroquinolones have also been reported but appear to be inconsistent.

> Birnbaum AD, Tu EY. Parinaud's oculoglandular syndrome. In: Tasman W, Jaeger EA, eds. *Duane's Clinical Ophthalmology.* Vol 4. Philadelphia: Lippincott Williams & Wilkins; 2011.

Microbial and Parasitic Infections of the Cornea and Sclera

Primary Infectious Keratitis

Contact lens–related infectious keratitis

In the United States, the most frequent risk factor for bacterial keratitis is contact lens wear, which has been identified in 19%–42% of patients with culture-proven microbial keratitis and accounts for up to one-third of emergency department visits for corneal infection. Epidemiologic studies in Australia have estimated the annual incidence of cosmetic contact lens–related ulcerative keratitis at 0.21% for individuals using extended-wear soft lenses and 0.02% for patients using daily-wear soft lenses; this incidence is unaltered by the use of newer lens materials or variation in hygiene practices. The risk of corneal infection is increased nearly tenfold in contact lens wearers; it is even higher in patients who wear their contact lenses overnight, and it is positively correlated with the number of consecutive days that lenses are worn without removal.

PATHOGENESIS Contact lens wear predisposes the cornea to infection through a number of mechanisms, including introduction of a contaminated foreign body to the corneal surface; interruption of the normal tear flow, which is essential to corneal immunity; induction of corneal epithelial microtrauma; alteration of ocular surface immunity; and induction of corneal hypoxia. Various hygiene-related factors increase the risk of both infectious and noninfectious corneal inflammatory events. See BCSC Section 3, *Clinical Optics,* for further discussion of noninfectious contact lens–related disease.

MANAGEMENT Eliciting a history of contact lens wear is critical in the evaluation of corneal inflammation, and a history of lens wear should raise the suspicion of corneal infection.

Bacteria are both the most common pathogen and the most immediate threat to vision. Therefore, unless otherwise indicated, initial management should provide coverage for the most common bacterial pathogen in contact lens–related keratitis, *P aeruginosa*, as is done in empiric therapy for bacterial keratitis unrelated to contact lens wear. *Acanthamoeba* and fungal pathogens should be suspected if the clinical presentation or clinical course is atypical.

> Cortina MS, Tu EY. Antibiotic use in corneal and external eye infections. *Focal Points: Clinical Modules for Ophthalmologists.* San Francisco: American Academy of Ophthalmology; 2011, module 6.

Bacterial keratitis

Bacterial infection of the eye is a common sight-threatening condition. Some cases have explosive onset and rapidly progressive stromal inflammation. Untreated, it often leads to progressive tissue destruction with corneal perforation or extension of infection to adjacent tissue. Bacterial keratitis is frequently associated with risk factors that disturb the corneal epithelial integrity. Common predisposing factors include

- contact lens wear (see the section "Contact lens–related infectious keratitis")
- trauma
- contaminated ocular medications
- impaired defense mechanisms
- altered structure of the corneal surface

PATHOGENESIS Although bacterial keratitis restricted to the epithelial layer only has been reported, corneal pathogens generally must first adhere to the cornea and then invade and proliferate in the corneal stroma. Certain risk factors will often select for specific pathogens, based on their particular mechanism of adherence. For example, *P aeruginosa* becomes more pathogenic in lens-related biofilms, in turn enabling enhanced binding to molecular receptors exposed on injured epithelial cells. Once adherent, bacteria will proliferate and invade the corneal stroma, often with the aid of bacteria-specific proteases. Reactive host inflammation begins with the expression of various cytokines and chemokines, recruitment of inflammatory cells from the tears and limbal vessels, and subsequent secretion of matrix metalloproteinases leading to characteristic corneal necrosis. Reduction of bacterial loads and, potentially, direct control of the inflammatory response may reduce keratolysis. See BCSC Section 1, *Update on General Medicine,* for further discussion of bacteriology.

CLINICAL PRESENTATION Rapid onset of pain is accompanied by conjunctival injection, photophobia, and decreased vision in patients with bacterial corneal ulcers. The rate of progression of these symptoms depends on the virulence of the infecting organism. Bacterial corneal ulcers are typically a single infiltrate and show a sharp epithelial demarcation with underlying dense, suppurative stromal inflammation that has indistinct edges and is surrounded by edema. *P aeruginosa* typically causes stromal necrosis with a shaggy surface and adherent mucopurulent exudate (Fig 10-15). An endothelial inflammatory plaque, marked anterior chamber reaction, and hypopyon frequently occur.

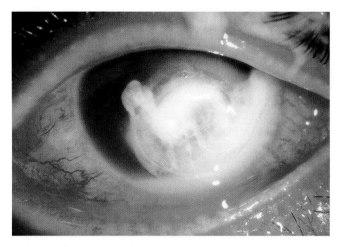

Figure 10-15 Suppurative ulcerative keratitis caused by *P aeruginosa*.

Patients with infections caused by slow-growing, fastidious organisms such as myco-bacteria or anaerobes may have a nonsuppurative infiltrate and intact epithelium. *Infectious crystalline keratopathy,* for example, presents as densely packed, white, branching aggregates of organisms in the virtual absence of a host inflammatory response, shielded by the bacte-rial biofilm coating. Risk factors include corticosteroid use, contact lens wear, and previ-ous corneal surgery. Infectious crystalline keratopathy has been reported with a number of bacterial and fungal species, most commonly α-hemolytic *Streptococcus* species (Fig 10-16).

LABORATORY EVALUATION The prevalence of a particular causative organism depends on the geographic location and risk factors for the infection. Causative organisms in bacterial keratitis are listed in Table 10-5.

Studies indicate that for bacterial keratitis, clinical appearance of the infection is an unreliable guide in determining the causative pathogen. The successful use of topical

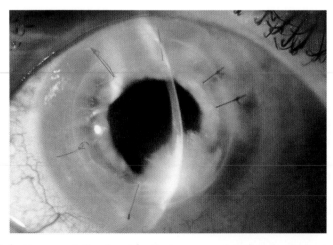

Figure 10-16 Infectious crystalline keratopathy in a corneal graft caused by α-hemolytic *Strep-tococcus* species.

Table 10-5 Causes of Bacterial Keratitis

Common Organisms	Uncommon Organisms
Staphylococcus aureus	Neisseria spp
Staphylococcus epidermidis	Moraxella spp
Streptococcus pneumoniae and other Streptococcus spp	Mycobacterium spp
Pseudomonas aeruginosa (most common organism in soft contact lens wearers)	Nocardia spp
	Non–spore-forming anaerobes
Enterobacteriaceae (Proteus spp, Enterobacter spp, Serratia spp)	Corynebacterium spp

fluoroquinolones in the 1990s led to a reduction in the number of cultures performed for cases of presumed infectious keratitis. The American Academy of Ophthalmology practice guidelines continue to recommend that initial cultures be obtained for infiltrates extending to the middle of the cornea, into deep stroma, or across a large area (>2 mm), as well as for patients whose history or clinical features suggest fungal, amebic, mycobacterial, or drug-resistant organisms as the causative agents. In addition to corneal culture, it may be helpful to culture contact lenses, contact lens cases and solutions, and any other potential sources of contamination, such as inflamed eyelids. Some correlation has been shown between cultures of such sources and corneal scrapings.

The yield for corneal cultures and smears is significantly higher before the initiation of antibiotic treatment, but cases unresponsive to such therapy should still be cultured, with some suggesting discontinuation of antibiotics for 12–24 hours to encourage yield. However, a positive smear result at any point does not obviate the need for broad-spectrum coverage, although it may cause coverage to be weighted toward a different class of microorganism and/or provide guidance for later treatment in the absence of a positive culture. (See Chapter 9 in this volume and BCSC Section 4, *Ophthalmic Pathology and Intraocular Tumors*, for discussion of specimen collection, culturing, staining, and interpretation.)

MANAGEMENT In any keratitis, the primary goal of therapy is preservation of sight and corneal clarity. Bacterial pathogens can produce irreversible corneal scarring over a period of hours because of their rapid growth, keratolytic enzymes, and stimulation of destructive host immune responses. Therefore, therapy must be initiated before definitive diagnosis is obtained in order to rapidly reduce the bacterial load and minimize later visual disability.

Initial therapy consists of empiric, broad-spectrum topical antibiotics. In routine corneal ulcers, monotherapy with topical fluoroquinolones provides outcomes equivalent to those of combination therapy, because of the excellent penetration achieved with commercially available concentrations of fluoroquinolones. These antibiotics should initially be given every 30–60 minutes and then tapered in frequency according to the clinical response. In severe cases, administration of antibiotics every 5 minutes for 30 minutes as a loading dose can more rapidly achieve therapeutic concentrations in the corneal stroma. Second-generation fluoroquinolones (ciprofloxacin, ofloxacin) continue to have excellent *Pseudomonas* coverage but lack useful gram-positive activity. Third- and fourth-generation fluoroquinolones (eg, moxifloxacin, gatifloxacin, levofloxacin, and besifloxacin) have improved gram-positive and atypical mycobacterial coverage but limited activity against MRSA.

Alternatively, topical combination therapy with an agent active against gram-positive bacteria and another agent active against gram-negative bacteria can be used as initial therapy (Table 10-6). Although "fortified" antibiotics (compounded at increased

Table 10-6 Initial Therapy for Bacterial Keratitis

Organism	Antibiotic	Topical Dose	Subconjunctival Dose
Gram-positive cocci	Cefazolin	50 mg/mL	100 mg in 0.5 mL
	Vancomycin*	25–50 mg/mL	25 mg in 0.5 mL
	Moxifloxacin, gatifloxacin, levofloxacin, besifloxacin	5–6 mg/mL	Not available
Gram-negative rods	Tobramycin	9–14 mg/mL	20 mg in 0.5 mL
	Ceftazidime	50 mg/mL	100 mg in 0.5 mL
	Ciprofloxacin, ofloxacin, moxifloxacin, gatifloxacin, levofloxacin, besifloxacin	3–6 mg/mL	Not available
No organism or multiple types of organisms	Cefazolin with	50 mg/mL	100 mg in 0.5 mL
	Tobramycin or	9–14 mg/mL	20 mg in 0.5 mL
	Fluoroquinolones	3–6 mg/mL	Not available
Gram-negative cocci	Ceftriaxone	50 mg/mL	100 mg in 0.5 mL
	Ceftazidime	50 mg/mL	100 mg in 0.5 mL
	Ciprofloxacin, ofloxacin, moxifloxacin, gatifloxacin, levofloxacin, besifloxacin	3–6 mg/mL	Not available
Mycobacteria	Clarithromycin	10 mg/mL 0.03%	
	Moxifloxacin, gatifloxacin, besifloxacin	5–6 mg/mL	Not available
	Amikacin	20–40 mg/mL	20 mg in 0.5 mL

*For resistant *Staphylococcus* species.

Notes for Table 10-6: Preparation of topical antibiotics
Cefazolin 50 mg/mL
1. Add 9.2 mL of artificial tears to a vial of cefazolin in 1 g (powder for injection).
2. Dissolve. Take 5 mL of this solution and add it to 5 mL of artificial tears.
3. Refrigerate and shake well before instillation.

Vancomycin 50 mg/mL (Dilution can be extrapolated to a 15–25 mg/mL concentration by a compounding pharmacy.)
1. Add 10 mL of 0.9% sodium chloride for injection USP (no preservatives) or artificial tears to a 500-mg vial of vancomycin to produce a solution of 50 mg/mL.
2. Refrigerate and shake well before instillation.

Ceftazidime 50 mg/mL
1. Add 9.2 mL of artificial tears to a vial of ceftazidime 1 g (powder for injection).
2. Dissolve. Take 5 mL of this solution and add it to 5 mL of artificial tears.
3. Refrigerate and shake well before instillation.

Tobramycin 14 mg/mL
1. Withdraw 2 mL of tobramycin injectable from vial (40 mg/mL).
2. Add 2 mL to a tobramycin ophthalmic solution (5 mL) to give a 14 mg/mL solution.
3. Refrigerate and shake well before instillation.

concentrations compared with their commercial formulations in order to achieve therapeutic levels in the corneal stroma) are more difficult to obtain and may have a greater toxic effect on the ocular surface, the clinician should consider using them, especially in combination with vancomycin for gram-positive coverage when MRSA is suspected, with large or vision-threatening ulcers, or with prior antibiotic failure. Effectively treated, most infectious keratitis is culture negative after 48–72 hours. Once the offending microbe is identified or the clinical response shows improvement, appropriate monotherapy may be considered (see Table 10-6) to maintain coverage and reduce toxicity. However, laboratory sensitivities are based on antibiotic tissue levels achievable by systemic administration, and the levels achieved by topical administration are much higher. Often, a bacterial keratitis will respond in vivo even when in vitro data suggest resistance. Any changes in medical therapy should therefore be based primarily on clinical response. Several clinical parameters are useful for monitoring clinical response to antibiotic therapy:

- blunting of the perimeter of the stromal infiltrate
- decreased density of the stromal infiltrate
- reduction of stromal edema and endothelial inflammatory plaque
- reduction in anterior chamber inflammation
- reepithelialization
- cessation of corneal thinning

Systemic antibiotics—especially the fluoroquinolones, which have excellent ocular penetration—and intensive topical antibiotics are indicated in cases with suspected scleral and/or intraocular extension of infection.

The role of corticosteroid therapy for bacterial keratitis remains controversial. Tissue destruction results from a combination of the direct effects of the bacteria and an exuberant host inflammatory response consisting of polymorphonuclear leukocytes and proteolytic enzymes, which predominate even after corneal sterilization. Corticosteroids are effective at modifying this response, but they also inhibit the host response to infection. The literature strongly suggests that corticosteroid therapy administered *prior to* appropriate antibiotic therapy worsens prognosis. The literature is inconclusive, though, about steroid therapy used concomitantly with antibiotic therapy or after it is initiated, as demonstrated in a randomized clinical trial in which topical corticosteroids were given 48 hours after initiation of topical antibiotics for bacterial keratitis. At 3 months, no effect on final visual outcome or complication rate was seen, but a trend toward improved outcomes was noted in those patients with the worst initial vision who received corticosteroids and for the corticosteroid group at 1-year follow-up. Notably in this study, *Nocardia* keratitis, which is uncommon in the United States, fared worse with corticosteroid treatment.

The indiscriminate or universal use of corticosteroids is, therefore, unsupported but does not appear to increase the general risk of poor outcomes or complications in treated bacterial keratitis. In fact, certain patients may benefit from the addition of corticosteroids to antibiotic therapy. Future study of the appropriate timing and dosage may further refine the indications for corticosteroid use. As there is still significant risk associated with corticosteroid use in patients with bacterial or other forms of infectious keratitis not appropriately treated, following are recommended criteria for instituting corticosteroid therapy for bacterial keratitis:

- Corticosteroids should not be used in the absence of appropriate antibiotic therapy.
- The patient must be able to return for frequent follow-up examinations and demonstrate adherence to appropriate antibiotic therapy.
- No other associated virulent or difficult-to-eradicate organism is found or suspected.

Corticosteroid drops may be started in moderate dosages (prednisolone acetate or phosphate 1% every 6 hours), and the patient should be monitored at 24 and 48 hours after initiation of therapy. If the patient shows no adverse effects, the frequency of administration may be adjusted based on clinical response. Collagen crosslinking is increasingly used as an adjunctive therapy for bacterial keratitis, with anecdotal success; as this technology becomes more available in the United States, its precise role and application are evolving.

Penetrating keratoplasty (PK) for treatment of bacterial keratitis is indicated if the disease progresses despite therapy, descemetocele formation or perforation occurs, or the keratitis is unresponsive to antimicrobial therapy. The involved area should be identified preoperatively and an attempt made to circumscribe all areas of infection. Peripheral iridectomies are indicated, because seclusion of the pupil may develop from inflammatory pupillary membranes. Interrupted sutures are recommended. The patient should be treated with appropriate antibiotics, cycloplegics, and intense topical corticosteroids postoperatively. See Chapter 15 in this volume for a more detailed discussion of PK and BCSC Section 2, *Fundamentals and Principles of Ophthalmology*, for an in-depth discussion of ocular pharmacology.

American Academy of Ophthalmology Cornea/External Disease Panel. Preferred Practice Pattern Guidelines. *Bacterial Keratitis.* San Francisco: American Academy of Ophthalmology; 2013. Available at www.aao.org/ppp.

Price MO, Tenkman LR, Schrier A, Fairchild KM, Trokel SL, Price FW Jr. Photoactivated riboflavin treatment of infectious keratitis using collagen cross-linking technology. *J Refract Surg.* 2012;28(10):706–713.

Schein OD, Glynn RJ, Poggio EC, Seddon JM, Kenyon KR. The relative risk of ulcerative keratitis among users of daily-wear and extended-wear soft contact lenses. A case-control study. Microbial Keratitis Study Group. *N Engl J Med.* 1989;321(12):773–778.

Srinivasan M, Mascarenhas J, Rajaraman R; Steroids for Corneal Ulcers Trial Group. Corticosteroids for bacterial keratitis: the Steroids for Corneal Ulcers Trial (SCUT). *Arch Ophthalmol.* 2012;130(2):143–150.

Srinivasan M, Mascarenhas J, Rajaraman R; Steroids for Corneal Ulcers Trial Group. The steroids for corneal ulcers trial (SCUT): secondary 12-month clinical outcomes of a randomized controlled trial. *Am J Ophthalmol.* 2014;157(2):327–333.

Atypical mycobacteria

Atypical mycobacteria are important pathogens in infections following laser in situ keratomileusis (LASIK) (Fig 10-17). The most common pathogens are *Mycobacterium fortuitum* and *Mycobacterium chelonae,* which may be found in soil and water. These organisms should be suspected in delayed-onset postrefractive infections, classically with

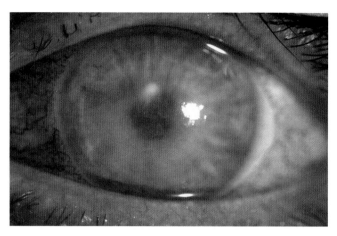

Figure 10-17 Atypical mycobacterial infection following laser in situ keratomileusis (LASIK). *(Courtesy of Elmer Y. Tu, MD.)*

recalcitrant, nonsuppurative infiltrates. The diagnosis may be confirmed with acid-fast stain or culture on Löwenstein-Jensen medium. Medical treatment options include oral and topical clarithromycin, amikacin, linezolid, and the fluoroquinolones with antimyco-bacterial activity, including moxifloxacin, besifloxacin, and gatifloxacin.

> Chang MA, Jain S, Azar DT. Infections following laser in situ keratomileusis: an integration of the published literature. *Surv Ophthalmol.* 2004;49(3):269–280.
>
> Hyon JY, Joo MJ, Hose S, Sinha D, Dick JD, O'Brien TP. Comparative efficacy of topical gati-floxacin with ciprofloxacin, amikacin, and clarithromycin in the treatment of experimental *Mycobacterium chelonae* keratitis. *Arch Ophthalmol.* 2004;122(8):1166–1169.

Fungal keratitis

PATHOGENESIS Fungal keratitis is less common than bacterial keratitis, generally represent-ing less than 5%–10% of corneal infections in reported clinical series in the United States. Filamentous fungal keratitis occurs more frequently in warmer, more humid parts of the United States than in other regions of the country. Trauma to the cornea with plant or vegetable material is the leading risk factor for fungal keratitis. Contact lens wear has emerged as another risk factor for the development of fungal keratitis. Topical corticoste-roids are a major risk factor as well, as they appear to activate and increase the virulence of fungal organisms in part by reducing the cornea's resistance to infection. *Candida* spe-cies cause ocular infections in immunocompromised hosts and in corneas with chronic erosions/ulceration from other causes. Systemic corticosteroid and immunosuppressant use in these patients may suppress the host immune response, thereby predisposing to fungal keratitis. Other common risk factors include corneal surgery (eg, PK, radial kera-totomy) and chronic keratitis (eg, herpes simplex virus, herpes zoster, or vernal/allergic conjunctivitis).

In early 2006, an outbreak of contact lens–associated *Fusarium* keratitis was ob-served, first in Singapore and the Pacific Rim and then in the United States. The epidemic occurred in association with the use of Renu with MoistureLoc solution (Bausch + Lomb, Rochester, NY). Bausch + Lomb withdrew the solution from the world market on May 15, 2006, with a subsequent steep decline in *Fusarium* cases across the United States.

Chang DC, Grant GB, O'Donnell K, et al; Fusarium Keratitis Investigation Team. Multistate outbreak of *Fusarium* keratitis associated with use of a contact lens solution. *JAMA.* 2006; 296(8):953–963.

CLINICAL PRESENTATION Patients with fungal keratitis tend to have fewer inflammatory signs and symptoms during the initial period than those with bacterial keratitis and may have little or no conjunctival injection upon initial presentation. On the other hand, pain in fungal keratitis can be out of proportion to the relatively uninflamed cornea. Filamentous fungal keratitis frequently manifests as a gray-white, dry-appearing infiltrate that has irregular feathery or filamentous margins (Fig 10-18). Superficial lesions may appear gray-white; elevate the surface of the cornea; and have a dry, rough, or gritty texture detectable at the time of diagnostic corneal scraping. Occasionally, multifocal or satellite infiltrates may be present, although these are less common than previously reported. In addition, a deep stromal infiltrate may occur in the presence of an intact epithelium. An endothelial plaque and/or hypopyon may also occur if the fungal infiltrate(s) is sufficiently deep or large or has penetrated into the anterior chamber.

As the keratitis progresses, intense suppuration may develop, and the lesions may resemble those of bacterial keratitis. At this point, rapidly progressive hypopyon and anterior chamber inflammatory membranes may develop. Extension of fungal infection into the anterior chamber is often a cause of rapidly progressive anterior chamber inflammation. Occasionally, fungus may invade the iris or posterior chamber, and angle-closure glaucoma may develop from inflammatory pupillary block.

Yeast keratitis is most frequently caused by *Candida* species. This form of fungal keratitis frequently presents with superficial white, raised colonies in a structurally altered eye.

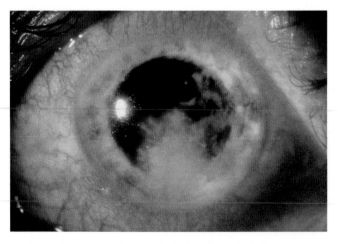

Figure 10-18 Fungal keratitis caused by *F solani* with characteristic dry-appearing, white stromal infiltrate with feathery edges.

Although most cases tend to remain superficial, deep invasion may occur with suppuration resembling keratitis induced by gram-positive bacteria.

LABORATORY EVALUATION The fungal cell wall stains with Gomori methenamine silver but, except for *Candida,* does not take up Gram stain. Blood agar, Sabouraud dextrose agar, and brain–heart infusion agar are the preferred media for fungal culture. Because of progressive enhancements to in vitro antifungal sensitivity testing, these tests are better correlated with clinical outcomes for fungal keratitis and should be pursued. Confocal microscopy is very useful in detecting branching filaments in the cornea, as well as the individual septa found in the majority of corneal mold pathogens.

MANAGEMENT Natamycin 5% suspension is recommended for the treatment of most cases of filamentous fungal keratitis, particularly those caused by *Fusarium* species, which are the most common causative agents for exogenous fungal keratitis occurring in the humid areas of the southern United States. Most clinical and experimental evidence suggests that topical amphotericin B (0.15%–0.30%) is the most efficacious agent available to treat yeast keratitis; most corneal yeast infections respond readily to the drug. Amphotericin B is also recommended for filamentous keratitis caused by *Aspergillus* species. Topical voriconazole 1% is increasingly utilized and has been effective in treating some cases of fungal keratitis unresponsive to other therapy; however, significant resistance has been reported, and a recent prospective, randomized clinical trial concluded that this agent is inferior to natamycin for empiric therapy, especially for *F solani.*

Systemic administration may be considered for treatment of more severe keratitis or keratitis with intracameral extension. The use of older azoles, including ketoconazole (200–600 mg/day), fluconazole (200–400 mg/day), and itraconazole (200 mg/day), for this purpose has been described. Oral voriconazole (200–400 mg/day) and posaconazole (800 mg/day) are rapidly replacing other oral antifungals because of their excellent intraocular penetration and broader spectrum of coverage. Alternatively, intrastromal administration of aqueous-soluble amphotericin B (5–10 µg/0.1 cc) or voriconazole (50–100 µg/0.1 cc) as primary or secondary treatment of deep fungal keratitis, and intracameral injection of either agent for intraocular extension are becoming more widely validated. Unresponsive cases of culture-proven or histologically proven fungal keratitis require definitive speciation of the pathogen as well as antifungal sensitivity testing. As classic morphologic identification is often inaccurate, a look-alike species or *P insidiosum* (discussed earlier) can be suspected in these cases. Collagen crosslinking has been investigated as an adjunctive therapy for fungal keratitis; it appears to have no role in deeper stromal disease and achieves mixed results in superficial fungal infections.

When the smear result is negative and fungal infection is suspected, repeated scrapings or biopsy may be necessary to identify fungal material. Furthermore, mechanical debridement may be beneficial for cases of superficial fungal keratitis. Fungal infiltration of the deep corneal stroma may not respond to topical antifungal therapy, because the penetration of these agents is reduced in the presence of an intact epithelium. Penetration of natamycin or amphotericin B has been shown to be significantly enhanced by debridement of the corneal epithelium, and animal experiments indicate that frequent topical application (every 5 min) for 1 hour can readily achieve therapeutic levels. Cases with progressive disease despite maximal topical and/or oral antifungal therapy may require therapeutic PK to prevent scleral or intraocular extension of the fungal infection. Both of these latter conditions carry a very poor prognosis for salvaging the eye.

Bunya VY, Hammersmith KM, Rapuano CJ, Ayres BD, Cohen EJ. Topical and oral voriconazole in the treatment of fungal keratitis. *Am J Ophthalmol.* 2007;143(1):151–153.

Loh AR, Hong K, Lee S, Mannis M, Acharya NR. Practice patterns in the management of fungal corneal ulcers. *Cornea.* 2009;28(8):856–859.

Prajna NV, Krishnan T, Mascarenhas J; Mycotic Ulcer Treatment Trial Group. The mycotic ulcer treatment trial: a randomized trial comparing natamycin vs voriconazole. *JAMA Ophthalmol.* 2013;131(4):422–429.

Acanthamoeba *keratitis*

PATHOGENESIS *Acanthamoeba* is a genus of free-living ubiquitous protozoa found in freshwater and soil. These organisms are resistant to killing by freezing; desiccation; and the levels of chlorine routinely used in municipal water supplies, swimming pools, and hot tubs. They may exist as motile trophozoites or dormant cysts. Initial corneal epithelial adherence is thought to be mediated by a mannose-binding protein, with subsequent stromal invasion promoted by the expression of a mannose-induced protein (MIP-133) and various collagenases. In Western countries, the majority ($\approx$90%) of reported cases of amebic keratitis have been associated with contact lens use, with the remainder associated with various other risk factors. Historically, episodic outbreaks of disease have been associated with water contamination, as for example, homemade saline contact lens solutions that were inappropriately made, groundwater contaminated because of river flooding (United States), or contaminated rooftop cisterns (United Kingdom).

Since 2003, an increased number of *Acanthamoeba* cases have occurred in the United States, particularly on the East Coast and in the Midwest. Two initial case-control studies found an association between *Acanthamoeba* keratitis and the use of Complete MoisturePlus multipurpose cleaning solution (Advanced Medical Optics, Santa Ana, CA) for soft contact lens care, resulting in the voluntary recall of the product from the market in May 2007. Unfortunately, the outbreak has persisted, prompting a second multistate case-control study in 2011, led by the Centers for Disease Control and Prevention, which, to date, has not identified a definitive source for the outbreak.

Joslin CE, Tu EY, McMahon TT, Passaro DJ, Stayner LT, Sugar J. Epidemiological characteristics of a Chicago-area *Acanthamoeba* keratitis outbreak. *Am J Ophthalmol.* 2006;142(2): 212–217.

Joslin CE, Tu EY, Shoff ME, et al. The association of contact lens solution use and *Acanthamoeba* keratitis. *Am J Ophthalmol.* 2007;144(2):169–180.

CLINICAL PRESENTATION Patients with amebic keratitis are classically described as having severe ocular pain; photophobia; and a protracted, progressive course. The disease is bilateral in 7%–11% of patients. Frequently, they have shown no therapeutic response to a variety of topical antimicrobial agents. In early cases, however, *Acanthamoeba* infection is localized to the corneal epithelium and may manifest as a mildly symptomatic, diffuse punctate epitheliopathy or dendritic epithelial lesion. Epithelial pseudodendrites are often misdiagnosed as herpetic keratitis and treated with antiviral agents and/or corticosteroids. Stromal infection typically manifests in the central cornea, and early cases have a gray-white superficial, nonsuppurative infiltrate. As the disease progresses, a centered, partial or complete ring infiltrate in the central cornea is frequently observed (Fig 10-19). When noted, inflamed corneal nerves, called *radial perineuritis* or *radial keratoneuritis,* are nearly pathognomonic of amebic keratitis; limbitis, scleritis (focal, nodular, or diffuse), or even dacryoadenitis may be seen as well. Although intraocular extension may occur, consecutive encephalitis has not been reported.

LABORATORY EVALUATION Diagnosis of *Acanthamoeba* keratitis is made by visualizing amebae in stained smears or by culturing organisms obtained from corneal scrapings. However, culture yield is laboratory dependent, with larger studies reporting only 35%–50% positivity for *Acanthamoeba;* a significant number of cases are treated based on clinical presentation and/or confocal microscopy findings. Lamellar corneal biopsy may be required to establish the diagnosis in some cases. Contact lenses and related paraphernalia can be examined, but amebic contamination is not uncommon, even in patients without disease.

Amebae are seen in smears stained with Giemsa or with periodic acid–Schiff (PAS), calcofluor white, or acridine orange stains. Nonnutrient agar with *E coli* or *Enterobacter aerogenes* overlay is the preferred medium for culturing amebae, but the organisms also grow well on buffered charcoal–yeast extract agar. Characteristic trails form as the motile trophozoites travel across the surface of the culture plate. In vivo confocal microscopy can also be used to show organisms, particularly the cyst forms (Fig 10-20).

MANAGEMENT Early diagnosis of *Acanthamoeba* keratitis is the most important prognostic indicator of a successful treatment outcome. Diagnostic delay is common, however, because of the nonspecific presentation of the disease and the need for special microbiological

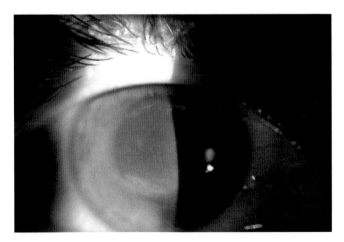

Figure 10-19 Ring infiltrate in *Acanthamoeba* keratitis. *(Courtesy of Elmer Y. Tu, MD.)*

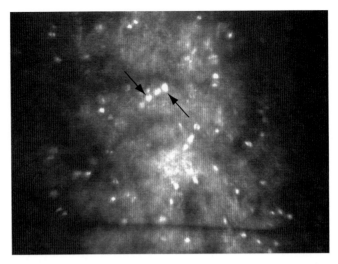

Figure 10-20 In vivo confocal microscopy image of *Acanthamoeba* cysts *(arrows)*. *(Courtesy of Elmer Y. Tu, MD.)*

diagnostic methods. Clinical features that suggest a diagnosis of *Acanthamoeba* keratitis rather than herpes simplex virus (HSV) keratitis include

- noncontiguous or multifocal pattern of granular epitheliopathy and subepithelial opacities (unlike the contiguous, dendritic pattern in HSV keratitis)
- disproportionately severe ocular pain (unlike disproportionately mild pain secondary to trigeminal nerve involvement in HSV)
- presence of epidemiologic risk factors such as contact lens use or exposure to possibly contaminated freshwater
- failure to respond to initial antiviral therapy

Cases identified early, defined as epithelial or anterior stromal, have an excellent visual prognosis and generally respond well to epithelial debridement, followed by an extended (3–4-month) course of antiamebic therapy. The presence of deep stromal inflammation, a ring infiltrate, or extracorneal manifestations significantly worsens the prognosis because of the development of stromal scarring and often necessitates longer treatment (up to a year or more), other adjunctive therapy, or therapeutic keratoplasty.

A number of antimicrobial agents have been recommended for medical treatment of *Acanthamoeba* keratitis based on their in vitro amebicidal effects as well as their clinical effectiveness. Agents used for topical administration include

- *diamidines:* propamidine, hexamidine
- *biguanides:* polyhexamethylene biguanide (polyhexanide), chlorhexidine
- *aminoglycosides:* neomycin, paromomycin
- *imidazoles/triazoles:* voriconazole, miconazole, clotrimazole, ketoconazole, itraconazole

Of these, only the biguanides have been shown to have consistent in vitro and clinical efficacy against both cysts and trophozoites; the others are effective primarily against trophozoites. Therefore, the mainstay of pharmacologic treatment is a biguanide, with a diamidine sometimes used early in the course of therapy, although successful resolution can be achieved with a biguanide alone. A comparison of biguanides did not detect a difference between chlorhexidine 0.02% and polyhexamethylene biguanide (PHMB) 0.02%. Single-agent systemic treatment with voriconazole has been shown to be efficacious in some recalcitrant cases.

Corticosteroid exposure incites acanthamoebal excystment in vitro and may worsen clinical outcomes when used prior to effective antiacanthamoebal therapy. Much of the morbidity of *Acanthamoeba* keratitis is from the exuberant host response, however, which causes noninfectious corneal and extracorneal complications, including scleritis, glaucoma, and cataracts. The judicious use of topical and systemic immunosuppressants in selected cases is valuable after the patient has been treated for a period of at least 2 weeks.

Traditionally, keratoplasty has been reserved for vision rehabilitation after completion of treatment or for cases that are progressing despite maximal medical therapy and leading to possible perforation. However, recent reports find that with effective antiacanthamoebal agents used as adjunctive therapy, lamellar and penetrating keratoplasty may now have a lower rate of recurrent infection, have a successful visual outcome, and avoid the primary risk factor for graft failure, late inflammatory sequelae, including glaucoma. Medical treatment is preferred, however, in the vast majority of cases. Because late recurrences can occur when medical therapy is stopped before completion, it is advisable to perform any optical keratoplasties only after a full course of amebicidal therapy. Collagen crosslinking is increasingly described as an adjunctive therapy for *Acanthamoeba* keratitis; its mechanism of action is unclear, however, and this treatment is unlikely to be beneficial in advanced disease.

Dart JK, Saw VP, Kilvington S. *Acanthamoeba* keratitis: diagnosis and treatment update 2009. *Am J Ophthalmol.* 2009;148(4):487–499.e2.

Robaei D, Carnt N, Minassian DC, Dart JK. The impact of topical corticosteroid use before diagnosis on the outcome of *Acanthamoeba* keratitis. *Ophthalmology.* 2014;121(7):1383–1388.

Robaei D, Carnt N, Minassian DC, Dart JK. Therapeutic and optical keratoplasty in the management of *Acanthamoeba* keratitis: risk factors, outcomes, and summary of the literature. *Ophthalmology.* 2015;122(1):17–24.

Tu EY. *Acanthamoeba* and other parasitic corneal infections. In: Mannis MJ, Holland EJ, eds. *Cornea.* Vol 1. 4th ed. Philadelphia: Elsevier; 2017:976–985.

Tu EY, Joslin CE, Sugar J, Shoff ME, Booton GC. Prognostic factors affecting visual outcome in *Acanthamoeba* keratitis. *Ophthalmology.* 2008;115(11):1998–2003.

Corneal Stromal Inflammation Associated With Systemic Infections

Nonsuppurative stromal keratitis can be caused by the following:

- reactive arthritis
- congenital or acquired syphilis
- Lyme disease
- tuberculosis
- leprosy (Hansen disease)
- onchocerciasis

Many of these conditions are discussed in BCSC Section 9, *Intraocular Inflammation and Uveitis.*

Microsporidiosis

PATHOGENESIS Microsporidia are intracellular protozoa known to cause ocular infection. Initially recognized as an opportunistic pathogen in individuals with AIDS and those with other forms of immunosuppression, this organism is increasingly reported as the cause of infection in immunocompetent persons in Southeast Asia.

CLINICAL PRESENTATION AND EVALUATION There are 2 distinct clinical presentations of microsporidial infections, depending on the immune status of the patient. In immunocompetent individuals, a corneal stromal keratitis may develop, and in patients with AIDS, conjunctivitis and an epithelial keratopathy may occur (Fig 10-21). The latter group may also have disseminated microsporidiosis involving the sinuses, respiratory tract, or gastrointestinal tract.

Patients present with symptoms that include ocular irritation, photophobia, decreased vision, and bilateral conjunctival injection with little or no associated inflammation. Stromal keratitis is caused by agents of the genus *Nosema*, whereas the genera *Encephalitozoon* and *Septata* have been associated with keratoconjunctivitis. In the keratoconjunctivitis variant, corneal findings include superficial nonstaining opacities described as "mucoid" in appearance, along with dense areas of fine punctate fluorescein staining. The corneal stroma remains clear, with minimal or no iritis.

With light microscopy using the Brown and Hopps stain, small gram-positive microsporidial spores may be identified in conjunctival epithelial cells (Fig 10-22). Transmission electron microscopy (Fig 10-23), immunofluorescence antibody techniques, or elaborate tissue culture techniques may also be used.

MANAGEMENT Restoration of immune function can lead to resolution of microsporidial keratitis. Although there is no definitive treatment, topical fumagillin has been used to successfully treat microsporidial keratoconjunctivitis, with little toxic effect. In severe cases of *Vittaforma corneae* (formerly *Nosema corneum*) infection, granulomatous inflammation

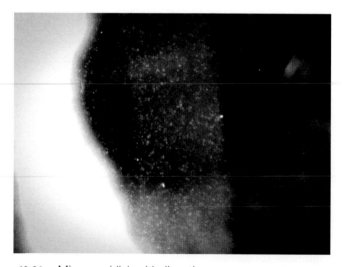

Figure 10-21 Microsporidial epitheliopathy. *(Courtesy of Woodford S. Van Meter.)*

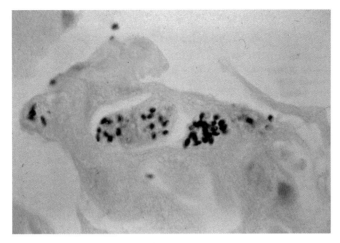

Figure 10-22 Light microscopy shows the intracellular spores of microsporidia. *(Courtesy of Woodford S. Van Meter.)*

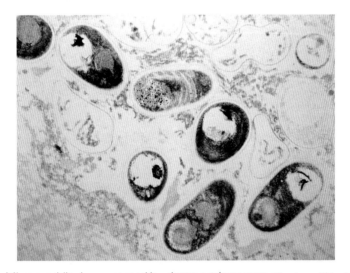

Figure 10-23 Microsporidia demonstrated by electron microscopy. *(Courtesy of Woodford S. Van Meter.)*

may lead to necrotic thinning and perforation. PK may then become the only available treatment for severe stromal thinning. In general, medical regimens require long-term use, and recurrence is common after treatment discontinuation. More recent cases have been reported to be self-limited or responsive to a wide array of commercially available topical ophthalmic antibiotics.

Joseph J, Sridhar MS, Murthy S, Sharma S. Clinical and microbiological profile of microsporidial keratoconjunctivitis in southern India. *Ophthalmology.* 2006;113(4):531–537.

Loh RS, Chan CM, Ti SE, Lim L, Chan KS, Tan DT. Emerging prevalence of microsporidial keratitis in Singapore: epidemiology, clinical features, and management. *Ophthalmology.* 2009;116(12):2348–2353.

Loiasis

Infection with *Loa loa* (loiasis) and other filarial nematodes can cause conjunctivitis; these infections also have dermatologic manifestations. After the bite of an infected vector, such parasites can burrow subcutaneously to reach the eye area. The microfilarial stage is transmitted from human to human by the bite of an infected female deer fly (genus *Chrysops*) indigenous to West and Central Africa. A migrating worm moves under the skin at about 1 cm/min but is most conspicuous when it is seen or felt wriggling under the periocular skin or bulbar conjunctiva (Fig 10-24). Extraction of the filarial worm cures the conjunctivitis; antiparasitic treatment for disseminated infestation follows. Diethylcarbamazine is generally given 2 mg/kg 3 times a day for 3 weeks and repeated as necessary. Ivermectin 150 mg/kg may also be effective, but significant adverse effects have been reported in patients with prominent intravascular loiasis. Concurrent administration of corticosteroids and/or antihistamines may be necessary to minimize allergic reactions.

Microbial Scleritis

PATHOGENESIS Bacterial and fungal infections of the sclera are very rare. Most cases result from the extension of microbial keratitis involving the peripheral cornea. Trauma and contaminated foreign bodies (including scleral buckles) are possible risk factors. Bacterial scleritis has also occurred in sclera damaged by previous pterygium surgery, especially when beta irradiation or mitomycin has been used (Fig 10-25). Bacteria and fungi can also invade tissue of the eye wall surrounding a scleral surgical wound, but endophthalmitis is more likely in this setting. Scleral inflammation can also be a feature of syphilis, tuberculosis, or leprosy, or infection with *Acanthamoeba* species, *Nocardia* species, or atypical mycobacteria. Tuberculous scleritis should be considered in chronic steroid-dependent scleritis or in the setting of surgically induced necrotizing scleritis (SINS). Diffuse or nodular scleritis is an occasional complication of varicella-zoster virus eye disease.

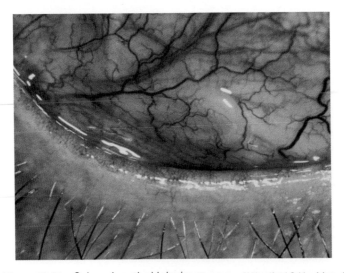

Figure 10-24 Subconjunctival loiasis. *(Courtesy of Woodford S. Van Meter.)*

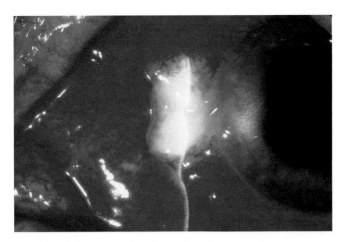

Figure 10-25 Bacterial scleritis occurring 2 weeks after pterygium surgery. *(Courtesy of Kirk R. Wilhelmus, MD.)*

LABORATORY EVALUATION Evaluating suppurative scleritis is similar to evaluating microbial keratitis. Smears and cultures are obtained before antimicrobial therapy is begun. If the overlying epithelium is intact, a scleral or episcleral biopsy should be performed to obtain specimens for culture, histologic examination, and molecular diagnostic testing. The workup of nonsuppurative scleritis is guided by the history and findings from the physical examination, as described in Chapter 11.

MANAGEMENT Topical antimicrobial therapy is begun just as for microbial keratitis. Because of the difficulty in controlling microbial scleritis, subconjunctival injections and intravenous antibiotics may also be used. Long-term oral therapy shows promise.

Diagnosis and Management of Immune-Related Disorders of the External Eye

Highlights

- In the acute phase of Stevens-Johnson syndrome or toxic epidermal necrolysis, early intervention in severe cases with an amniotic membrane transplant of the entire ocular surface, including the eyelid margins, is very helpful.
- Signs of mucous membrane pemphigoid include trichiasis and subepithelial conjunctival fibrosis, indicated by the presence of gray-white linear scarring of the forniceal conjunctiva. Conjunctival biopsy may be helpful to confirm the diagnosis.
- Early recognition of the signs and symptoms of Cogan syndrome and timely systemic treatment may prevent irreversible hearing loss and death.
- Patients with necrotizing keratitis, scleritis, and/or peripheral ulcerative keratitis have a significant risk of underlying collagen vascular disease; thus, systemic evaluation and workup are important.

See BCSC Section 9, *Intraocular Inflammation and Uveitis,* for discussion of the principles of immunology.

Immune-Mediated Diseases of the Eyelid

Contact Dermatoblepharitis

PATHOGENESIS Topical ophthalmic medications, cosmetics, and environmental substances can occasionally trigger a local allergic reaction. Hypersensitivity reactions are divided into 4 types in the Gell and Coombs classification. Type I reactions are immunoglobulin (Ig) E mediated, and type IV reactions are T-cell mediated; see BCSC Section 9, *Intraocular Inflammation and Uveitis,* for further details.

CLINICAL PRESENTATION Type I (immediate hypersensitivity) reactions typically occur within minutes after exposure to an allergen. Ocular reactions are associated with itching, eyelid erythema and swelling, and conjunctival hyperemia and chemosis (Fig 11-1). In rare cases, signs of systemic anaphylaxis may develop in the patient.

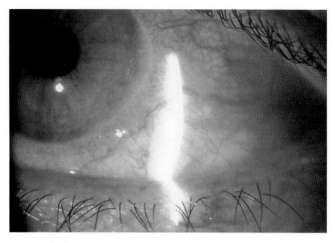

Figure 11-1 Acute anaphylactic reaction to a topical ophthalmic medication with conjunctival hyperemia and chemosis.

A type IV (delayed) hypersensitivity reaction usually begins 24–72 hours following instillation of a topical agent. Patients are often sensitized by previous exposure to the offending drug or preservative. An acute eczematous reaction develops with erythema, leathery thickening, and scaling of the eyelid (Fig 11-2). Sequelae of chronic contact blepharoconjunctivitis include hyperpigmentation, dermal scarring, and lower eyelid ectropion. A papillary conjunctivitis and a mucoid or mucopurulent discharge may develop. Punctate epithelial erosions may be noted on the inferior cornea. Medications and preservatives that are commonly associated with contact blepharoconjunctivitis include

- cycloplegics such as atropine and homatropine
- aminoglycosides such as neomycin, gentamicin, and tobramycin
- antiviral agents such as idoxuridine and trifluridine
- preservatives such as thimerosal and EDTA

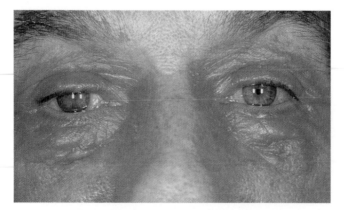

Figure 11-2 Delayed allergic contact dermatitis secondary to use of a topical ophthalmic medication.

MANAGEMENT Treatment of hypersensitivity reactions requires the identification and discontinuation of the offending agent. Usually, the history provides the necessary clues, but sometimes a "challenge test" is necessary to confirm a suspicion. Such tests should never be done in patients with a known systemic allergy to a drug.

Initial management of type I hypersensitivity reactions includes allergen avoidance or discontinuation of the causative agent. Adjunctive therapy may involve the use of cold compresses, artificial lubricants, topical antihistamines, mast-cell stabilizers, and/or nonsteroidal anti-inflammatory drugs (NSAIDs) for pain. Topical vasoconstrictors, either alone or in combination with antihistamines, may provide acute symptomatic relief but should not be used long term.

Type IV hypersensitivity reactions are also treated with allergen withdrawal. In severe cases, a brief (several-day) course of mild topical corticosteroids or tacrolimus ointment (0.03% or 0.1%) applied to the eyelids and periocular skin may speed resolution of eyelid and conjunctival inflammation.

Atopic Dermatitis

PATHOGENESIS Atopic dermatitis is a chronic condition in genetically susceptible individuals that usually begins in infancy or childhood and may or may not involve the external eye. The pathogenesis of atopic dermatitis involves a type IV hypersensitivity reaction, increased IgE hypersensitivity, an increase in histamine released from mast cells and basophils, and impaired cell-mediated immunity.

CLINICAL PRESENTATION Diagnostic criteria for atopic dermatitis include pruritus, lesions on the eyelid and other sites (eg, joint flexures in adolescents and adults, face and extensor surfaces in infants and young children), and a personal or family history of other atopic disorders, such as asthma, allergic rhinitis, nasal polyps, and aspirin hypersensitivity. Other ocular findings include periorbital darkening, exaggerated eyelid folds, meibomianitis, ectropion, and chronic papillary conjunctivitis. The appearance of the skin lesions varies depending on the age of the patient. Infants typically have an erythematous rash, children tend to have eczematous dermatitis with secondary lichenification from scratching, and adults have scaly patches with thickened and wrinkled dry skin.

MANAGEMENT Allergens in the environment and in foods should be identified and minimized whenever possible. In general, the services of an allergist should be sought. Moisturizing lotions and petrolatum gels can be useful for skin hydration. Acute lesions can be controlled with a topical corticosteroid cream or ointment (clobetasone butyrate 0.05%), but long-term use of such medications is strongly discouraged to avoid skin thinning and ocular complications of corticosteroids (eg, cataract, glaucoma). Topical tacrolimus ointment 0.03% or 0.1% is also effective and has fewer adverse effects. Oral antipruritic agents such as antihistamines and mast-cell stabilizers can alleviate itching but may exacerbate dry eye with their anticholinergic activity.

Guglielmetti S, Dart JK, Calder V. Atopic keratoconjunctivitis and atopic dermatitis. *Curr Opin Allergy Clin Immunol.* 2010;10(5):478–485.

Immune-Mediated Disorders of the Conjunctiva

Hay Fever Conjunctivitis and Perennial Allergic Conjunctivitis

PATHOGENESIS Hay fever (seasonal) conjunctivitis and perennial allergic conjunctivitis are largely type I hypersensitivity reactions. The allergen, which is typically airborne, enters the tear film and comes into contact with conjunctival mast cells that bear allergen-specific IgE antibodies. Degranulation of mast cells releases histamine and a variety of other inflammatory mediators that promote vasodilation, edema, and recruitment of other inflammatory cells, such as eosinophils. In a presensitized individual, the activation and degranulation of mast cells can be triggered within minutes of allergen exposure.

CLINICAL PRESENTATION Patients with hay fever conjunctivitis often have other atopic conditions, such as allergic rhinitis or asthma. Symptoms develop rapidly after allergen exposure and consist of itching, eyelid swelling, conjunctival hyperemia, chemosis, and mucoid discharge. Intense itching is a hallmark symptom. Attacks are usually short lived and episodic.

LABORATORY EVALUATION The diagnosis of hay fever conjunctivitis is generally made clinically. Conjunctival scrapings reveal the characteristic eosinophils, which are not normally present on the ocular surface. Challenge testing with a panel of allergens can be performed.

MANAGEMENT Efforts should first be directed at avoidance or abatement of allergen exposure. Thorough cleaning (or changing) of unclean or old carpets, linens, and bedding can be effective in removing accumulated allergens such as animal dander and house dust mites. Contributing factors, including contact lenses and dry eye, should be identified, as they can play an important role in facilitating allergen contact with the ocular surface. Glasses or goggles can also serve as physical barriers. Treatment should be based on the severity of patient symptoms and includes one or more of the following:

Supportive

- cold compresses
- artificial tears

Topical

- topical antihistamines and mast-cell stabilizers
- topical NSAIDs
- judicious, selective use of topical corticosteroids
- topical vasoconstrictors

Systemic

- oral antihistamines (may be effective for the short term but may be associated with increased dry eye)

Artificial tears are beneficial in diluting and flushing away allergens and other inflammatory mediators. Topical vasoconstrictors, alone or in combination with antihistamines, may provide acute symptom relief. However, their use for more than 5–7 consecutive days may predispose to compensatory chronic vascular dilation. Topical mast cell–stabilizing agents such as cromolyn sodium and lodoxamide tromethamine may be useful for treating seasonal allergic conjunctivitis. Treatment effects usually require continued use over 7 or more days; hence, these drugs are generally ineffective in the acute phase of hay fever conjunctivitis. Topical cyclosporine and oral antihistamines may provide symptom relief in some patients. Hyposensitization injections (immunotherapy) can be beneficial if the offending allergen has been identified. Certain topical NSAIDs have been approved by the US Food and Drug Administration for use in ocular atopy, but their efficacy varies greatly. Reports of corneal perforations with the use of NSAIDs, especially the generic forms, suggest the need for careful monitoring. Refills should be limited, and follow-up appointments need to be maintained. Topical corticosteroids are very effective in managing ocular allergy; however, they should be reserved for cases unresponsive to other treatments and must be used with caution. If corticosteroids are prescribed, patients must be clearly informed of the risks and closely monitored for adverse effects. Topical tacrolimus can be used to treat the associated dermatitis. See BCSC Section 2, *Fundamentals and Principles of Ophthalmology,* for a discussion of topical antihistamines and mast-cell stabilizers.

Mantelli F, Lambiase A, Bonini S, Bonini S. Clinical trials in allergic conjunctivitis: a systematic review. *Allergy.* 2011;66(7):919–924.

Mishra GP, Tamboli V, Jwala J, Mitra AK. Recent patents and emerging therapeutics in the treatment of allergic conjunctivitis. *Recent Pat Inflamm Allergy Drug Discov.* 2011;5(1): 26–36.

Ueta M, Kinoshita S. Ocular surface inflammation is regulated by innate immunity. *Prog Retin Eye Res.* 2012;31(6):551–575.

Vernal Keratoconjunctivitis

PATHOGENESIS Vernal keratoconjunctivitis (VKC) is a seasonally recurring, bilateral inflammation of the cornea and conjunctiva that occurs predominantly in young males, who frequently, but not invariably, have a personal or family history of atopy. The disease may persist year-round in tropical climates. The immunopathogenesis seems to involve both types I and IV hypersensitivity reactions. The conjunctival inflammatory infiltrate in VKC consists of eosinophils, lymphocytes, plasma cells, and monocytes.

Abu El-Asrar AM, Al-Mansouri S, Tabbara KF, Missotten L, Geboes K. Immunopathogenesis of conjunctival remodeling in vernal keratoconjunctivitis. *Eye (Lond).* 2006;20(1):71–79.

CLINICAL PRESENTATION Symptoms consist of itching, blepharospasm, photophobia, blurred vision, and copious mucoid discharge. Clinically, 2 forms of VKC may be seen: palpebral and limbal.

The inflammation in palpebral VKC is located predominantly on the palpebral conjunctiva, where a diffuse papillary hypertrophy develops, usually more prominently in the upper region. Bulbar conjunctival hyperemia and chemosis may also occur. In more severe cases, giant papillae resembling cobblestones may develop on the upper tarsus (Fig 11-3).

Limbal VKC may develop alone or in association with palpebral VKC. It occurs predominantly in patients of African or Asian descent and is more prevalent in hot climates. The limbus has a thickened, gelatinous appearance, with scattered opalescent mounds and vascular injection. Horner-Trantas dots, whitish macroaggregates of degenerated

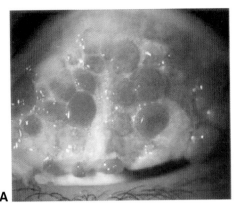 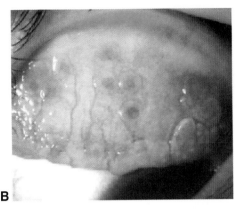

Figure 11-3 Palpebral vernal keratoconjunctivitis before **(A)** and after treatment **(B)** with tacrolimus. *(Reproduced with permission from Ohashi Y, Ebihara N, Fujishima H, et al. A randomized, placebo-controlled clinical trial of tacrolimus ophthalmic suspension 0.1% in severe allergic conjunctivitis. J Ocul Pharmacol Ther. 2010;26(2):165–174.)*

eosinophils and epithelial cells, may be seen in the hypertrophied limbus of patients with limbal VKC (Fig 11-4).

Several types of corneal changes associated with upper-tarsal lesions may also develop in VKC. Punctate epithelial erosions in the superior and central cornea are frequently noted. Pannus occurs most commonly in the superior cornea, but occasionally 360° corneal vascularization may develop. Oval or shield-shaped noninfectious epithelial ulcers (the so-called shield ulcer) with underlying stromal opacification may develop in the superior or central cornea (Fig 11-5). An association between VKC and keratoconus has been reported. Stem cell deficiency may also occur in severe cases.

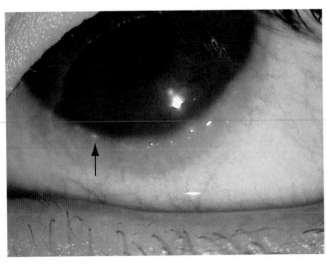

Figure 11-4 Limbal vernal keratoconjunctivitis. Note the Horner-Trantas dots *(arrow). (Courtesy of Charles S. Bouchard, MD.)*

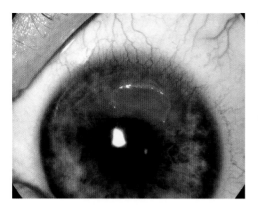

Figure 11-5 Shield ulcer in vernal keratocon-junctivitis. *(Courtesy of Stephen Tuft, MD.)*

MANAGEMENT Therapy should be based on the severity of the patient's symptoms and the ocular surface disease. Mild cases may be successfully managed with topical anti-histamines. Climatotherapy, such as the use of home air-conditioning or relocation to a cooler environment, can be helpful. Patients with mild to moderate disease may respond to topical mast-cell stabilizers. In patients with seasonal exacerbations, these drops are typically started at least 2 weeks before symptoms usually begin. In patients with year-round disease, long-term maintenance dosing can be used. Severe cases may require the use of topical corticosteroids. Because of the likely development of corticosteroid-related complications from long-term administration, however, these drugs should be reserved for exacerbations that result in moderate to severe discomfort and/or decreased vision. During these exacerbations, intermittent (pulse) therapy is very effective. Topical cortico-steroids can be used relatively frequently (eg, every 2 hours) for 5–7 days and then rapidly tapered. Because of the propensity of particles of suspended corticosteroid (eg, predniso-lone acetate) to lodge between papillae, the use of less potent but soluble corticosteroids such as dexamethasone phosphate is generally preferred. Low-dose steroids can be useful in some cases for maintenance treatment of VKC. Whenever steroids are prescribed, the potential dangers of long-term topical corticosteroid use are critical to review to empha-size the importance of close follow-up and monitoring for adverse effects.

Cooperative patients can be offered an alternative to topical delivery that avoids the problem of continuing self-medication: supratarsal injection of corticosteroid. The su-pratarsal subconjunctival space is located superior to the upper border of the superior tarsus and is most easily reached by everting the upper eyelid. After the upper eyelid is everted and the supratarsal conjunctiva has been anesthetized, supratarsal injection of 0.5–1.0 mL of either a relatively short-acting corticosteroid such as dexamethasone phosphate (4 mg/mL) or a longer-acting corticosteroid such as triamcinolone acetonide (40 mg/mL) can be performed. Monitoring of intraocular pressure is mandatory, as corti-costeroid spikes are possible. The importance of close follow-up with an eye care provider is essential to monitor for cataract formation or permanent vision loss.

Steroid-sparing agents have been shown to be effective. Topical cyclosporine 0.5%–2.0% applied 2–4 times daily, topical tacrolimus ointment 0.03%–0.10% applied twice daily, or tacrolimus suspension 0.10% can also be used to treat refractory cases of VKC. Reported adverse effects of cyclosporine include punctate epithelial keratopathy and ocular surface irritation. Systemic anti-inflammatory therapy should be reserved for very severe cases.

Harada N, Inada N, Ishimori A, Shoji J, Sawa M. Follow-up study on patients with vernal keratoconjunctivitis undergoing topical 0.1% tacrolimus treatment. *Nippon Ganka Gakkai Zasshi.* 2014;118(4):378–384.

Hazarika AK, Singh PK. Efficacy of topical application of 0.03% tacrolimus eye ointment in the management of allergic conjunctivitis. *J Nat Sci Biol Med.* 2015;6(Suppl 1):S10–S12.

Labcharoenwongs P, Jirapongsananuruk O, Visitsunthorn N, Kosrirukvongs P, Saengin P, Vichyanond P. A double-masked comparison of 0.1% tacrolimus ointment and 2% cyclosporine eye drops in the treatment of vernal keratoconjunctivitis in children. *Asian Pac J Allergy Immunol.* 2012;30(3):177–184.

Pucci N, Caputo R, di Grande L, et al. Tacrolimus vs. cyclosporine eyedrops in severe cyclosporine-resistant vernal keratoconjunctivitis: A randomized, comparative, double-blind, crossover study. *Pediatr Allergy Immunol.* 2015;26(3):256–261.

Sangwan VS, Jain V, Vemuganti GK, Murthy SI. Vernal keratoconjunctivitis with limbal stem cell deficiency. *Cornea.* 2011;30(5):491–496.

Atopic Keratoconjunctivitis

PATHOGENESIS One or more manifestations of atopic keratoconjunctivitis (AKC) develop in approximately one-third of patients with atopic dermatitis. Atopic individuals show signs of type I hypersensitivity responses as well as depressed systemic cell-mediated immunity. As a consequence of this altered immunity, they are susceptible to herpes simplex virus keratitis and colonization of the eyelids with *Staphylococcus aureus*. Complications related to this predisposition to infection may contribute to, or compound, the primary immunopathogenic manifestations. AKC is primarily a type IV reaction; therefore, the use of mast-cell therapy may not be effective.

CLINICAL PRESENTATION The ocular findings of AKC are similar to those of VKC (discussed earlier in the chapter), with the following differences:

- Patients with AKC frequently have disease year-round, with minimal seasonal exacerbation.
- Patients with AKC are older.
- The papillae are more apt to be small or medium-sized than giant.
- The papillae occur in the upper and lower palpebral conjunctiva.
- Milky conjunctival edema, with variable subepithelial fibrosis, is often present (Fig 11-6).
- Extensive corneal vascularization and opacification secondary to chronic epithelial disease (likely due to some degree of direct trauma from eyelid changes and/or limbal stem cell dysfunction) can occur (Fig 11-7).
- Eosinophils in conjunctival cytology specimens are less numerous and are less often degranulated.
- Conjunctival scarring often occurs, with occasional symblepharon formation.
- Posterior subcapsular and/or multifaceted or shield-shaped anterior subcapsular lens opacities may develop.

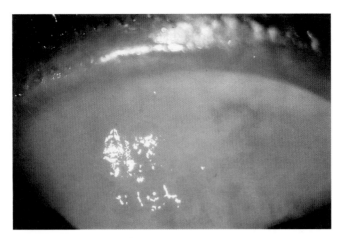

Figure 11-6 Atopic keratoconjunctivitis demonstrating small papillae, edema, and subepithelial fibrosis.

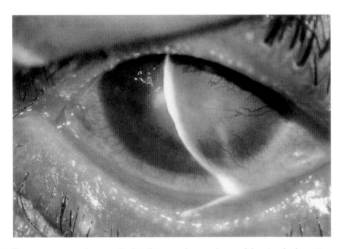

Figure 11-7 Severe corneal vascularization and scarring with atopic keratoconjunctivitis.

- Corneal findings include persistent epithelial defects, an increased incidence of ectatic corneal diseases such as keratoconus and pellucid marginal degeneration (possible association with eye rubbing), and an increased incidence of staphylococcal and herpes simplex infections.

MANAGEMENT Treatment of AKC involves allergen avoidance and the use of pharmacotherapeutic agents similar to those used in the treatment of VKC. Cold compresses may also be of benefit. In addition, patients should be carefully monitored for complications of infectious diseases that may warrant specific therapy, such as secondary staphylococcal infections and herpes simplex keratitis, which is more common and more likely to be bilateral in patients with AKC (see Chapter 9).

In severe cases, the indications for systemic therapy include chronic ocular surface inflammation unresponsive to topical treatment, ocular discomfort, progressive cicatrization, and peripheral ulcerative keratopathy. Systemic immunosuppression (eg, cyclosporine or tacrolimus) should be monitored in coordination with an internist or rheumatologist. Systemic treatment of AKC may be beneficial in suppressing the interleukin-2 (IL)-2 response, which promotes lymphocyte proliferation.

Akova YA, Rodriguez A, Foster CS. Atopic keratoconjunctivitis. *Ocul Immunol Inflamm.* 1994; 2(3):125–144.

Anzaar F, Gallagher MJ, Bhat P, Arif M, Farooqui S, Foster CS. Use of systemic T-lymphocyte signal transduction inhibitors in the treatment of atopic keratoconjunctivitis. *Cornea.* 2008; (8):884–888.

Erdinest N, Solomon A. Topical immunomodulators in the management of allergic eye disease. *Cur Opin Allergy Clin Immunol.* 2014;14(5):457–463.

García DP, Alperte JI, Cristóbal JA, et al. Topical tacrolimus ointment for treatment of intractable atopic keratoconjunctivitis: a case report and review of the literature. *Cornea.* 2011; 30(4):462–465.

Ligneous Conjunctivitis

Ligneous conjunctivitis is a rare, chronic autosomal recessive disorder characterized by the formation of firm ("woody"), yellowish fibrinous pseudomembranes on the conjunctival surface (Fig 11-8). These membranes are composed of an admixture of fibrin, fibrin-bound tissue plasminogen activator (tPA), epithelial cells, and mixed inflammatory cells that adhere to the conjunctival surface. Latent and activated forms of matrix metalloproteinase-9 have also been identified.

PATHOGENESIS The cause of ligneous conjunctivitis has been linked to severe type I plasminogen deficiency, with hypofibrinolysis as the primary defect. More than 12% of patients have severe hypoplasminogenemia. The genetic defect in the plasminogen gene *(PLG)* is located at band 6q26.

CLINICAL PRESENTATION Ligneous conjunctivitis can affect patients of all ages. Patients present with symptoms of ocular irritation and foreign-body sensation. The cardinal finding consists of yellowish, platelike masses that overlie one or more of the palpebral surfaces and are readily visible with eversion of the eyelid (see Fig 11-8). Ligneous conjunctivitis is generally bilateral and frequently recurs after excision.

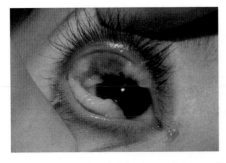
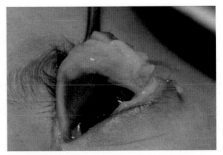

Figure 11-8 Firm yellowish lesions of the eyelids characteristic of ligneous conjunctivitis. *(Courtesy of John Dart, MD.)*

MANAGEMENT Cultures can be taken at initial diagnosis to exclude a bacterial pseudo-membranous or membranous conjunctivitis. Surgical excision with or without adjunctive cryotherapy has been advocated. However, recurrences are frequent. Use of purified plasminogen, fresh frozen plasma, heparin, corticosteroids, azathioprine, and amniotic membrane has been reported. No single treatment has been shown to be consistently effective or superior. Many cases of ligneous conjunctivitis eventually resolve spontaneously after several months to a few years.

Heidemann DG, Williams GA, Hartzer M, Ohanian A, Citron ME. Treatment of ligneous conjunctivitis with topical plasmin and topical plasminogen. *Cornea.* 2003;22(8):760–762.

Hiremath M, Elder J, Newall F, Mitchell S, Dyas R, Monagle P. Heparin in the long-term management of ligneous conjunctivitis: a case report and review of literature. *Blood Coagul Fibrinolysis.* 2011;22(7):606–609.

Rodríguez-Ares MT, Abdulkader I, Blanco A, et al. Ligneous conjunctivitis: a clinicopathological, immunohistochemical, and genetic study including the treatment of two sisters with multiorgan involvement. *Virchows Arch.* 2007;451(4):815–821.

Schuster V, Seregard S. Ligneous conjunctivitis. *Surv Ophthalmol.* 2003;48(4):369–388.

Stevens-Johnson Syndrome, Stevens-Johnson Syndrome/Toxic Epidermal Necrolysis Overlap, and Toxic Epidermal Necrolysis

Stevens-Johnson syndrome (SJS), SJS/toxic epidermal necrolysis (SJS/TEN) overlap, and TEN are acute inflammatory vesiculobullous reactions involving the skin and at least 2 mucous membranes. The current nomenclature is based on the amount of skin involvement:

- less than 10%: SJS
- 10%–30%: SJS/TEN overlap
- more than 30%: TEN

In this book, the term SJS–TEN is used to refer collectively to SJS, SJS/TEN overlap, and TEN.

A recent review by Jain et al discusses the incidence of SJS and TEN. The reported incidence of SJS ranges from 1.2 to 6 per million patient-years, and the reported incidence of TEN ranges from 0.4 to 1.2 per million patient-years. The incidence increases with advancing age, and patients with human immunodeficiency virus infection seem to be at higher risk. Jain et al also review the reported mortality rates, which are significant, ranging from 1% to 5% in SJS and 25% to 35% in TEN.

Jain R, Sharma N, Basu S, et al. Stevens Johnson syndrome: the role of an ophthalmologist. *Surv Ophthalmol.* 2016;61(4):369–399. Epub 2016 Jan 30.

PATHOGENESIS SJS and TEN are hypersensitivity reactions to infectious diseases (eg, due to herpes simplex virus, adenovirus, or streptococcal bacteria) or, predominantly, to drugs. Approximately 80% of TEN and 50%–80% of SJS cases are thought to be drug induced; the conjunctiva and oropharynx are the tissues most frequently involved. Although more than 100 drugs of various classes have been found to be associated with SJS–TEN, sulfonamides, anticonvulsants, NSAIDs, and allopurinol are frequently implicated.

Although the pathogenesis of the disease is not completely understood, in cases of drug-induced SJS and TEN, the keratinocyte apoptosis is thought to be triggered by drug-specific cytotoxic T lymphocytes via the perforin–granzyme pathway. As granzyme enters a target cell through the perforin channels, it leads to keratinocyte apoptosis. If Fas is the death receptor protein on the target cell membrane, extension of the apoptosis can result. Granule-mediated exocytosis, mainly of perforin and granzyme B or Fas-Fas ligand (FasL, or CD95L) interactions, is thought to play a role. One report demonstrated that blister cells from skin lesions of patients with SJS or TEN consisted mainly of cytotoxic T lymphocytes and natural killer cells and that both the blister fluid and the cells were cytotoxic. Gene expression profiling identified granulysin as the most highly expressed cytotoxic molecule. Results of studies investigating the association between HLA class I and II antigens and SJS–TEN suggest that there are strong ethnic differences in the HLA–SJS associations.

Borchers AT, Lee JL, Naguwa SM, Cheema GS, Gershwin ME. Stevens-Johnson syndrome and toxic epidermal necrolysis. *Autoimmun Rev.* 2008;7(8):598–605.

Chung WH, Hung SI, Yang JY, et al. Granulysin is a key mediator for disseminated keratinocyte death in Stevens-Johnson syndrome and toxic epidermal necrolysis. *Nat Med.* 2008;14(12):1343–1350.

Ueta M, Tokunaga K, Sotozono C, et al. HLA class I and II gene polymorphisms in Stevens-Johnson syndrome with ocular complications in Japanese. *Mol Vis.* 2008;14:550–555.

CLINICAL PRESENTATION Fever, arthralgia, malaise, and upper or lower respiratory tract symptoms are usually sudden in onset. Skin eruption follows within a few days, with a classic "target" lesion consisting of a red center surrounded by a pale ring and then a red ring, although maculopapular or bullous lesions are also common. The mucous membranes of the eyes, mouth, and genitalia may be affected by bullous lesions with membrane or pseudomembrane formation. New lesions may appear over 4–6 weeks, with approximately 2-week cycles for each crop of lesions.

The primary ocular finding is a mucopurulent conjunctivitis and episcleritis. Conjunctival and corneal epithelial sloughing and necrosis with severe inflammation and scarring may develop (Fig 11-9). Patients are at risk of infection because of loss of the

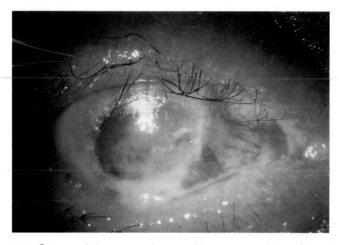

Figure 11-9 Stevens-Johnson syndrome with severe ocular surface disease.

epithelial barrier. Ocular surface cicatrization results in long-term ocular complications such as conjunctival shrinkage, eyelid margin keratinization, trichiasis, and tear deficiency. Eyelid margin keratinization and scarring are important risk factors for poor long-term outcomes in these patients.

Gerull R, Nelle M, Schaible T. Toxic epidermal necrolysis and Stevens-Johnson syndrome: a review. *Crit Care Med.* 2011;39(6):1521–1532.

Jain R, Sharma N, Basu S, et al. Stevens Johnson syndrome: the role of an ophthalmologist. *Surv Ophthalmol.* 2016;61(4):369–399. Epub 2016 Jan 30.

MANAGEMENT Management of acute and chronic disease should be distinguished.

Acute phase. Acute SJS, SJS/TEN overlap, and TEN are medical emergencies with significant risk of morbidity and mortality. Management requires a team-based approach, similar to that used for thermal burn victims, and includes intensive care providers, anesthesiologists, surgeons who specialize in the treatment of burns, and ophthalmologists. The offending agent must be immediately discontinued. Systemic therapy is mainly supportive and is aimed at managing dehydration and superinfection. Systemic treatment with immunosuppressive or immunomodulatory agents remains controversial.

The mainstay of acute ocular therapy is lubrication with preservative-free artificial tears and ointments and vigilant surveillance for the early manifestations of ocular infections. Topical antibiotics are sometimes used as prophylaxis. The efficacy of topical corticosteroids for the ocular manifestations of this condition remains controversial. Symblepharon may form during the acute phase because the raw, necrotic palpebral and bulbar conjunctival surfaces can adhere to one another (Fig 11-10). Repeated conjunctival lysis of the symblepharon may exacerbate inflammation and surface morbidity. Significant long-term benefit has been demonstrated with early amniotic membrane transplantation covering the entire ocular surface, including the eyelid margins. This is one of the few potentially

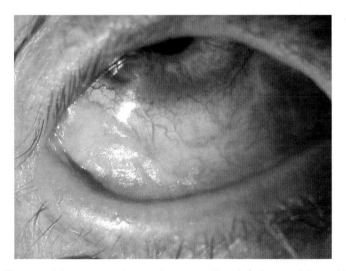

Figure 11-10 Stevens-Johnson syndrome demonstrating inferior eyelid symblepharon and ocular surface keratinization. *(Courtesy of Charles S. Bouchard, MD.)*

beneficial therapeutic interventions for this devastating disease. Amniotic membrane grafting should be performed very early in the course of this disease to prevent serious sequelae. Various techniques can be used, and the procedure can be done in the operating room or at the bedside for patients who cannot be taken to the operating room immediately.

Chronic phase. Management of chronic SJS, SJS/TEN overlap, and TEN, as summarized by Jain et al, is targeted at treating dry eye and mechanical abnormalities of the eyelids and eyelashes (which cause ocular surface trauma and inflammation), as well as rehabilitation of vision.

Dry eye is a significant problem secondary to scarring of the ocular surface and damage to the meibomian glands. Chronic dryness contributes to the development of further ocular surface damage, epithelial defects, symblephara, and limbal stem cell deficiency. Eyelid sequelae such as entropion, trichiasis, and keratinization, which result from cicatrizing conjunctivitis, cause chronic ocular surface irritation and inflammation. Treatment of dry eye includes lubrication (preservative free), punctal occlusion, and eyelid hygiene. Topical and systemic corticosteroids have been reported to help reduce active inflammation but must be used with caution and under close monitoring. Depending on the extent of the chronic disease, other treatment options include debridement of keratin from eyelid margins, use of scleral lenses, salivary gland transplantation, and mucous membrane grafting.

Vision rehabilitation in patients with chronic disease is challenging and high risk. Prosthetic replacement of the ocular surface ecosystem (PROSE; BostonSight, Needham, MA), a custom-designed prosthetic device to support impaired ocular surface system functions, may improve patient comfort and vision and help certain patients avoid surgery. Surgical treatments should be avoided unless there are no other options, as they carry significant risks and limitations, which must be fully explained to the patient. Limbal stem cell transplantation and cultivated oral mucosal epithelial transplantation have been reported. Penetrating keratoplasty in patients with chronic disease is associated with an extremely poor prognosis and is generally reserved for eyes with progressive thinning or perforation. In desperate cases, rare favorable results have been achieved with a keratoprosthesis. Unfortunately, many patients with chronic SJS, SJS/TEN overlap, or TEN are young and left with lifelong ocular morbidity. Rehabilitation is hindered not only by sequelae of the acute disease, but also by ongoing, chronic immune deviation of the ocular surface.

Ciralsky JB, Sippel KC, Gregory DG. Current ophthalmologic treatment strategies for acute and chronic Stevens-Johnson syndrome and toxic epidermal necrolysis. *Curr Opin Ophthalmol.* 2013;24(4):321–328.

Gregory, DG. New grading system and treatment guidelines for the acute ocular manifestations of Stevens-Johnson syndrome. *Ophthalmology.* 2016;123(8):1653–1658.

Iyer G, Srinivasan B, Agarwal S, Pillai V, Ahuja A. Treatment modalities and clinical outcomes in ocular sequelae of Stevens-Johnson Syndrome over 25 years—a paradigm shift. *Cornea.* 2016;35(1):46–50.

Jain R, Sharma N, Basu S, et al. Stevens Johnson syndrome: the role of an ophthalmologist. *Surv Ophthalmol.* 2016;61(4):369–399. Epub 2016 Jan 30.

Kohanim S, Palioura S, Saeed HN, et al. Stevens-Johnson syndrome/toxic epidermal necrolysis—a comprehensive review and guide to therapy. I. Systemic disease. *Ocul Surf.* 2016;14(1):2–19. Epub 2015 Nov 5.

Mucous Membrane Pemphigoid

PATHOGENESIS The exact mechanism of mucous membrane pemphigoid (MMP), formerly called *ocular cicatricial pemphigoid,* remains unknown, although MMP may represent a cytotoxic (type II) hypersensitivity, in which cell injury results from the action of autoantibodies directed against a cell surface antigen in the basement membrane zone (BMZ). Bullous pemphigoid antigen II (BP180) and its soluble extracellular domains have been identified as possible autoantigens. Antibody activates complement, with a subsequent breakdown of the conjunctival membrane. A number of proinflammatory cytokines, such as IL-1 and tumor necrosis factor α (TNF-α), are overexpressed. TNF-α has been shown to induce the expression of migration inhibition factor, a cytokine found to have elevated levels in the conjunctival tissues of patients with MMP. Macrophage colony-stimulating factor has also been shown to have an increased expression in the conjunctival tissue of patients with active MMP.

Cellular immunity may also play a role. HLA-DR4, a special genetic locus in the major histocompatibility complex (MHC), has been associated with this condition, but not all affected individuals are positive for this background; hence, HLA typing is not useful for diagnosis.

Pseudopemphigoid, which has a clinical picture similar to that of pemphigoid, has been associated with the long-term use of certain topical ophthalmic medications. Case reports have implicated pilocarpine, epinephrine, timolol, idoxuridine, echothiophate iodide, and demecarium bromide. The main difference between pseudopemphigoid and true pemphigoid is that in the former, disease progression generally ceases once the offending agent is recognized and removed. The clinical findings of pseudopemphigoid are similar to those of ocular MMP, and immunohistologic evaluation of biopsied tissue can be helpful.

CLINICAL PRESENTATION Mucous membrane pemphigoid is a chronic cicatrizing conjunctivitis of autoimmune etiology. Although it is a vesiculobullous disease primarily involving the conjunctiva, it frequently affects other mucous membranes, including those of the mouth and oropharynx, genitalia, and anus. Difficulty swallowing may be an important early symptom. Skin involvement can occur in some cases.

Patients with MMP are usually older than 60 years at the time of diagnosis. They often present with recurrent attacks of mild and nonspecific conjunctival inflammation with an occasional mucopurulent discharge. Patients with early MMP may present with conjunctival hyperemia, edema, ulceration, and tear dysfunction.

According to the Foster staging system, close examination of the conjunctiva in the early stages of the disease (stage I) reveals subepithelial fibrosis (Fig 11-11). Fine gray-white linear opacities, best seen with an intense but thin slit beam, appear in the deep conjunctiva. However, in many cases, the disease in its early stages produces nonspecific symptoms with minimal overt physical findings, such as chronic red eye. Oral mucosal lesions may be a clue that can lead to early diagnosis.

Transient bullae of the conjunctiva rupture, leading to subepithelial fibrosis. Loss of goblet cells, shortening of the inferior fornices (stage II), symblepharon formation (stage III; Fig 11-12), and, on occasion, restricted ocular motility with extensive adhesions between the eyelid and the globe (stage IV) can follow. Ophthalmologists should attempt to diagnose this condition in its early stages and watch for an inferior fornix depth of less than

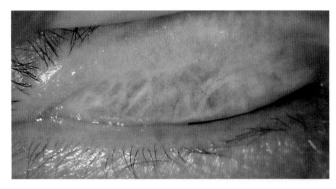

Figure 11-11 Ocular mucous membrane pemphigoid (MMP) showing subepithelial fibrosis. *(Courtesy of Charles S. Bouchard, MD.)*

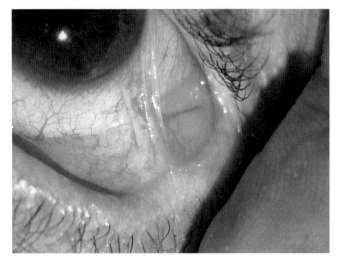

Figure 11-12 Subepithelial fibrosis, symblepharon, and shortening of the inferior fornix in MMP are demonstrated. *(Courtesy of Charles S. Bouchard, MD.)*

8 mm, which is abnormal and should prompt further evaluation. A subtle inferior symblepharon can be detected when the lower eyelid is pulled down while the patient looks up.

Recurrent attacks of conjunctival inflammation can lead to destruction of goblet cells and eventually obstruction of the lacrimal gland ductules. The resultant aqueous and mucous tear deficiency leads to keratinization of the already thickened conjunctiva. Entropion and trichiasis may develop as scarring progresses, leading to abrasions, corneal vascularization, further scarring, ulceration, and epidermalization of the ocular surface. Corneal abrasions in these patients are emergencies and must be treated immediately to minimize progression to perforation, scarring, and ankyloblepharon formation. Although the clinical course varies, progressive deterioration usually occurs in untreated cases. Remissions and exacerbations are common. Surgical intervention can incite further scarring but may be essential in managing entropion and trichiasis.

The differential diagnosis of cicatrizing conjunctivitis includes 4 major categories, which are listed in Table 11-1. The diagnosis of unilateral MMP should be made with

Table 11-1 Differential Diagnosis of Cicatricial Conjunctivitis

Infectious	Allergic	Autoimmune	Miscellaneous
Adenovirus	Atopic	Lichen planus	Chemical burns
Skin infections due to	keratoconjunctivitis	Lupus	Medicamentosa
Corynebacterium	Stevens-Johnson	Mucous membrane	Neoplasia (para-neoplastic)
diphtheriae	syndrome	pemphigoid	Ocular rosacea
Trachoma		Sarcoidosis	Radiation
		Scleroderma	Trauma

caution because other diseases, including many of those listed in Table 11-1, may masquerade as MMP. Also, linear IgA dermatosis, a rare dermatologic condition, can result in an ocular syndrome that is clinically identical to MMP and requires similar treatment.

In patients with unexplained persistent epithelial defects (ie, after cataract surgery), MMP should be considered in the differential diagnosis and the patient carefully examined for any other signs of the disease.

> Williams GP, Radford C, Nightingale P, Dart JK, Rauz S. Evaluation of early and late presentation of patients with ocular mucous membrane pemphigoid to two major tertiary referral hospitals in the United Kingdom. *Eye (Lond)*. 2011;25(9):1207–1218.

LABORATORY EVALUATION Although MMP is a bilateral disease, one eye may be more severely involved than the other. Pathologic support for a diagnosis of pemphigoid can be obtained from direct immunofluorescence or immunoperoxidase staining of conjunctival biopsy specimens. False-negative results are not uncommon, however.

Biopsy specimens should be obtained from an actively affected area of the conjunctiva or, if involvement is diffuse, from the inferior conjunctival fornix. Oral mucosal biopsies may be useful, especially in the presence of an active lesion. In pseudopemphigoid, conjunctival biopsies may or may not be positive for immunoreactants. Immunohistochemical staining techniques can demonstrate complement 3, IgG, IgM, and/or IgA localized in the epithelial BMZ of the conjunctiva in pemphigoid (Fig 11-13). Circulating anti–basement

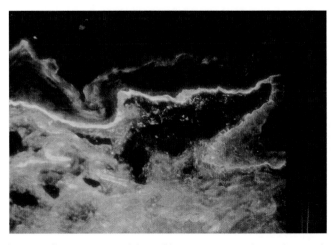

Figure 11-13 Immunofluorescent staining of basement membrane in a patient with MMP.

membrane antibody has been identified in some patients with pemphigoid. End-stage disease may produce negative results because of the destruction of basement membrane. (See also BCSC Section 4, *Ophthalmic Pathology and Intraocular Tumors.*)

Radford CF, Rauz S, Williams GP, Saw VP, Dart JK. Incidence, presenting features, and diagnosis of cicatrizing conjunctivitis in the United Kingdom. *Eye (Lond).* 2012;26(9):1199–1208.

MANAGEMENT A multidisciplinary approach is required in the management of MMP. It is helpful to involve an ophthalmologist who specializes in the treatment of this disease, and collaboration with other providers who have experience using systemic treatment is recommended to maximize patient outcome. Classifying patients according to their risk for disease progression (low or high) is valuable when appropriate therapy is being determined. Because progression is often slow, careful clinical staging of the disease and photo documentation (with the patient in differing positions of gaze) are generally recommended in evaluation of the disease course and response to therapy. Different staging systems to determine disease severity have been developed. Mondino and Brown staged MMP by the amount of inferior fornix depth lost. The Foster staging system is based on the presence or absence of specific clinical findings. Tauber proposed a modification to these staging systems (Table 11-2).

Table 11-2 Staging Systems for Mucous Membrane Pemphigoid

Previously Published Staging Systems	
System	**Characteristics**
Foster stages	
I	Subconjunctival scarring and fibrosis
II	Fornix foreshortening of any degree
III	Presence of symblepharon, any degree
IV	Ankyloblepharon, frozen globe
Mondino stages	
I	0%–25% loss of inferior fornix depth
II	25%–50% loss of inferior fornix depth
III	50%–75% loss of inferior fornix depth
IV	75%–100% loss of inferior fornix depth
Staging System Proposed by Tauber*	
Staging†	**Description**
To describe degrees within stages II and III	
a	0%–25%
b	25%–50%
c	50%–75%
d	75%–100%
For stage II	
a–d	Describes % loss of inferior fornix depth
For stage III	
a–d	Describes % of horizontal involvement by
(n)	Describes number of symblephara countable

*Utilizes Foster stages I–IV.
† For example, IIbIIIb(2), 50% fornix loss, 50% horizontal involvement by 2 discrete symblephara.

Modified with permission from Tauber J, Jabbur N, Foster CS. Improved detection of disease progression in ocular cicatricial pemphigoid. *Cornea.* 1992;11(5):447.

It is important to remember that MMP is a systemic disease. Topical treatments (steroids, cyclosporine A, tacrolimus) may help alleviate symptoms but will not prevent disease progression. Systemic therapy is required. Several systemic therapies have been reported for the treatment of MMP, with regimens varying depending on the severity of the disease and the presence or absence of sight-threatening complications. Cyclophosphamide remains a mainstay of therapy for severe disease when sight is threatened. The use of intravenous immunoglobulin, anti-TNF-α medications, and rituximab has been reported in patients who were unresponsive to or who experienced complications from conventional treatments.

These systemic treatments have significant adverse effects, including death; thus, it is critical for the ophthalmologist to partner with providers who are experienced in the administration and management of these treatments (ie, rheumatologists, hematologists, oncologists).

Any procedure or surgery (eyelid, intraocular) can cause disease flare, so adequate immunosuppression therapy is necessary. Also, surgical correction of eyelid deformities or treatment of trichiasis is important. In severe cases, hard palate and buccal mucosal grafting can be useful techniques in fornix reconstruction. Punctal occlusion, which may have already resulted from cicatrization, can be useful in the management of any associated dry eye condition. In general, patients with cicatrizing conjunctivitis have a higher rate of spontaneous extrusion of silicone punctal plugs; thus, permanent punctal occlusion with cautery is often required. Standard penetrating keratoplasty in MMP patients with severe corneal disease is generally associated with a very guarded prognosis. In patients who become blind due to MMP, keratoprosthesis surgery, performed as a last resort, has achieved some success. It is often difficult to distinguish sequelae of uncontrolled disease from inflammation secondary to structural and mechanical problems related to prior active disease. Careful examination is critical to determine whether there is active disease requiring further control.

Foster CS, Chang PY, Ahmed AR. Combination of rituximab and intravenous immunoglobulin for recalcitrant ocular cicatricial pemphigoid: a preliminary report. *Ophthalmology.* 2010;117(5):861–869.

Queisi M, Zein M, Lamba N, Meese H, Foster CS. Update on ocular cicatricial pemphigoid and emerging treatments. *Surv Ophthalmol.* 2016;61(3):314–317. Epub 2015 Dec 19.

Saw VP, Dart JK, Rauz S, et al. Immunosuppressive therapy for ocular mucous membrane pemphigoid: strategies and outcomes. *Ophthalmology.* 2008;115(2):253–261.

Srikumaran D, Tzu JH, Akpek EK. Cicatrizing conjunctivitis. *Focal Points: Clinical Modules for Ophthalmologists.* San Francisco: American Academy of Ophthalmology; 2011, module 1.

Valenzuela FA, Perez VL. Mucous membrane pemphigoid. In: Mannis MJ, Holland EJ, eds. *Cornea.* Vol 1. 4th ed. Philadelphia: Elsevier; 2017:549–557.

Ocular Graft-vs-Host Disease

PATHOGENESIS The pathogenesis of ocular surface disease in graft-vs-host disease (GVHD) is multifactorial but has 2 main components: (1) conjunctival inflammation with or without subepithelial fibrosis and (2) severe keratoconjunctivitis sicca (KCS) from lacrimal gland infiltration. KCS occurs in 40%–60% of patients with chronic GVHD (cGVHD).

GVHD is a relatively common complication of allogeneic bone marrow transplantation, which is performed most commonly for hematopoietic malignancies. In this condition, the grafted cells can attack the patient's tissues, including the skin, gut, lungs, liver, gastrointestinal tract, and eyes. GVHD can be acute or chronic (developing more than 3 months after a bone marrow transplant), with most ocular complications occurring as a manifestation of cGVHD.

Jabs DA, Wingard J, Green WR, Farmer ER, Vogelsang G, Saral R. The eye in bone marrow transplantation. III. Conjunctival graft-vs-host disease. *Arch Ophthalmol.* 1989;107(9): 1343–1348.

CLINICAL PRESENTATION The clinical features of ocular GVHD (eg, KCS, cicatricial conjunctivitis, scleritis) mirror those of other ocular inflammatory conditions associated with autoimmune and collagen-vascular diseases. Conjunctival inflammation in GVHD, which can be severe, may be associated with limbal stem cell deficiency and secondary corneal scarring, although fortunately, this inflammation is rare.

Inamoto Y, Chai X, Kurland BF, et al. Validation of measurement scales in ocular graft-versus-host disease. *Ophthalmology.* 2012;119(3):487–493.

Lin X, Cavanagh HD. Ocular manifestations of graft-versus-host disease: 10 years' experience. *Clin Ophthalmol.* 2015;9:1209–1213.

Ogawa Y, Shimmura S, Dogru M, Tsubota K. Immune processes and pathogenic fibrosis in ocular chronic graft-versus-host disease and clinical manifestations after allogeneic hematopoietic stem cell transplantation. *Cornea.* 2010;29(11):S68–S77.

MANAGEMENT These patients should be approached in a stepwise, multimodal fashion in consultation with their hematologist and/or oncologist. Aggressive ocular lubrication and punctal occlusion are the mainstays of local therapy. Punctal fibrosis is common and must be monitored closely because it can lead to plug extrusion. Severe filamentary keratitis can be treated with mucolytic agents (acetylcysteine 10%) or bandage contact lenses. Topical cyclosporine or tacrolimus may also be useful in controlling ocular GVHD. Visual disturbances are more commonly due to surface irregularity, but these patients also have a high rate of posterior subcapsular cataracts, which contribute to decreased vision. Autologous serum tears may also be considered. Gas-permeable scleral contact lenses, therapeutic soft contact lenses (Fig 11-14), and the PROSE treatment (discussed earlier in the chapter) can be important management tools for patients with severe ocular surface disease. Keratoprosthesis may be a last-resort option for patients with end-stage ocular surface disease who are not candidates for other conventional corneal procedures. Severe GVHD may require systemic therapy.

DeLoss KS, Le HG, Gire A, Chiu GB, Jacobs DS, Carrasquillo KG. PROSE treatment for ocular chronic graft-versus-host disease as a clinical network expands. *Eye Contact Lens.* 2016; 42(4):262–266.

Dietrich-Ntoukas T, Steven P. Ocular graft-versus-host disease. *Ophthalmologe.* 2015;112(12): 1027–1040.

Jung JW, Lee YJ, Yoon SC, Kim TI, Kim EK, Seo KY. Long-term result of maintenance treatment with tacrolimus ointment in chronic ocular graft-versus-host disease. *Am J Ophthalmol.* 2015;159(3):519–527.

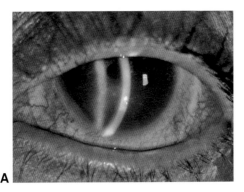 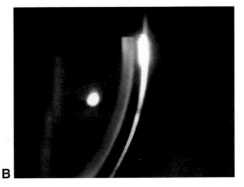

Figure 11-14 **A,** Patient with graft-vs-host disease fitted with a therapeutic scleral contact lens. The inferior paracentral cornea demonstrates subepithelial scarring. **B,** High magnification shows the space between the contact lens and cornea. *(Courtesy of Charles S. Bouchard, MD.)*

Liu C, Okera S, Tandon R, Herold J, Hull C, Thorp S. Visual rehabilitation in end-stage inflammatory ocular surface disease with the osteo-odonto-keratoprosthesis: results from the UK. *Br J Ophthalmol.* 2008;92(9):1211–1217.

Malta JB, Soong HK, Shtein RM, et al. Treatment of ocular graft-versus-host disease with topical cyclosporine 0.05%. *Cornea.* 2010;29(12):1392–1396.

Conjunctivitis/Episcleritis Associated With Reactive Arthritis

Reactive arthritis (formerly called *Reiter syndrome*) is a systemic disorder characterized by the classic triad of ocular (conjunctivitis/episcleritis, iridocyclitis, or keratitis), urethral, and joint inflammation. The joint inflammation is often highly asymmetric and involves a few joints (oligoarticular). These manifestations can appear simultaneously or separately, in any sequence. Less common manifestations include keratoderma blennorrhagicum (a scaling skin eruption), balanitis, aphthous stomatitis, fever, lymphadenopathy, pneumonitis, pericarditis, and myocarditis. Attacks are self-limited, lasting from 2 to several months, but they may recur periodically over the course of several years.

PATHOGENESIS Reactive arthritis may occur after dysentery due to gram-negative bacteria (most frequently *Salmonella, Shigella,* and *Yersinia* species) or after nongonococcal urethritis caused by *Chlamydia trachomatis.* More than 75% of patients with reactive arthritis are HLA-B27–positive. See BCSC Section 9, *Intraocular Inflammation and Uveitis,* for discussion of HLA-B27–related diseases and illustrations of nonocular manifestations of reactive arthritis.

CLINICAL PRESENTATION The most common ocular finding in reactive arthritis is a bilateral papillary conjunctivitis with mucopurulent discharge, which has been reported in 30%–60% of patients. The conjunctivitis is self-limited, lasting for days to weeks. Some patients present more often with episcleritis rather than with conjunctivitis. Mild nongranulomatous anterior uveitis has been reported to occur in 3%–12% of patients. Various forms of keratitis—including diffuse punctate epithelial erosions, superficial or deep focal infiltrates, or superficial or deep vascularization—may occur in rare cases. Reactive arthritis should be considered in any case of chronic, nonfollicular, mucopurulent conjunctivitis with negative culture results.

MANAGEMENT Treatment is mainly palliative. Corneal infiltrates and vascularization often respond to topical corticosteroids. Systemic treatment of any related infection with oral antibiotics may be beneficial. Occasionally, the intraocular (uveitic) component of the disease can be very severe and require systemic immunosuppression (see BCSC Section 9, *Intraocular Inflammation and Uveitis*).

Other Immune-Mediated Diseases of the Skin and Mucous Membranes

Other immune-mediated disorders that can, in rare cases, affect the conjunctiva include linear IgA bullous dermatosis, dermatitis herpetiformis, epidermolysis bullosa, lichen planus, paraneoplastic pemphigus, pemphigus vulgaris, and pemphigus foliaceus.

Immune-Mediated Diseases of the Cornea

Thygeson Superficial Punctate Keratitis

PATHOGENESIS The etiology of Thygeson superficial punctate keratitis (SPK) is unknown. Although many of the clinical features resemble those of a viral infection of the corneal epithelium, attempts to confirm viral particles by electron microscopy or culture have been unsuccessful. No inflammatory cells are evident. The rapid response of the lesions to corticosteroid therapy suggests that Thygeson keratitis is largely immunopathogenically derived.

> Connell PP, O'Reilly J, Coughlan S, Collum LM, Power WJ. The role of common viral ocular pathogens in Thygeson's superficial punctate keratitis. *Br J Ophthalmol.* 2007;91(8): 1038–1041.

CLINICAL PRESENTATION This condition, first reported by Thygeson in 1950, is characterized by recurrent episodes of tearing, foreign-body sensation, photophobia, and reduced vision. It affects children to older adults and is typically bilateral, although it may develop initially in 1 eye or may be markedly asymmetric in some cases. The hallmark finding is multiple (up to 40 but as few as 2–3) slightly elevated corneal epithelial lesions with "negative staining," which are noted during exacerbations. The epithelial lesions are round or oval conglomerates of gray, granular, or "crumblike" opacities associated with minimal conjunctival reaction, in contrast to adenoviral keratoconjunctivitis. High magnification reveals each opacity to be a cluster of multiple smaller pinpoint opacities (Fig 11-15). A characteristic feature is the waxing and waning appearance of individual epithelial opacities, which change in location and number over time. The greatest density of these lesions is typically found in the central cornea. The raised punctate epithelial lesions themselves stain faintly with fluorescein and rose bengal.

No conjunctival inflammatory reaction is noted during exacerbations, but occasionally patients have mild bulbar conjunctival hyperemia. In rare cases, a mild subepithelial opacity may develop under the epithelial lesion—more commonly in patients who have

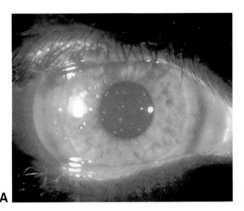 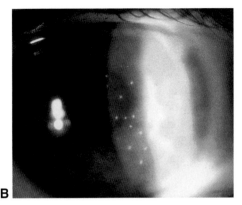

Figure 11-15 **A,** Thygeson superficial punctate keratitis. **B,** At higher magnification, each lesion is seen to consist of raised, granular opacities.

received topical antiviral therapy. The important facet of this condition is that the patient's symptoms may far exceed the apparent signs; frequently, patients report severe photophobia and foreign-body sensation in the setting of only a few central epithelial lesions.

MANAGEMENT Supportive therapy with artificial tears is often adequate in mild cases. Treatment alternatives for persistently symptomatic cases include low-dose topical corticosteroids and bandage contact lenses. Currently, antiviral therapy is not the standard of care, as there are no firm data to associate this condition with an active replicative viral infection.

If a topical corticosteroid is prescribed, a very mild preparation may be effective (eg, fluorometholone 0.1%). Because the lesions are quite responsive to corticosteroids, treatment will hasten their resolution, but they frequently recur in the same or different locations on the cornea after the topical corticosteroids are stopped. Overall, corticosteroid use should be minimized in these cases and monitored closely because of their associated risks. Topical cyclosporine or tacrolimus ophthalmic preparations may also be effective in causing regression of the lesions. It is important to remember to treat the symptoms, not the clinical findings, in patients with Thygeson SPK.

Marquezan MC, Nascimento H, Vieira LA, et al. Effect of topical tacrolimus in the treatment of Thygeson's superficial punctate keratitis. *Am J Ophthalmol.* 2015;160(4):663–668.

Vieira AC, Schwab IR. Superficial punctate keratitis of Thygeson. In: Mannis MJ, Holland EJ, eds. *Cornea.* Vol 1. 4th ed. Philadelphia: Elsevier; 2017:1030–1034.

Interstitial Keratitis Associated With Infectious Diseases

PATHOGENESIS Interstitial keratitis (IK) is a nonsuppurative inflammation of the corneal stroma that features cellular infiltration and usually vascularization without primary involvement of the epithelium or endothelium. Most cases result from a type IV hypersensitivity response to infectious microorganisms or other antigens in the corneal stroma. The topographic distribution (diffuse versus focal or multifocal) and depth of the stromal infiltration, in addition to associated systemic signs, are useful in determining the cause of IK.

Congenital syphilis was the first infection to be linked with IK. Herpes simplex virus, which accounts for most cases of stromal keratitis, and varicella-zoster virus keratitis are discussed earlier in this volume. Many other microorganisms are much rarer causes of IK; these include

- *Mycobacterium tuberculosis*
- *Mycobacterium leprae*
- *Borrelia burgdorferi* (Lyme disease)
- measles virus
- Epstein-Barr virus (infectious mononucleosis)
- *C trachomatis* (lymphogranuloma venereum)
- *Leishmania* species
- *Onchocerca volvulus* (onchocerciasis)

Syphilitic interstitial keratitis

Syphilitic eye disease is discussed further in BCSC Section 6, *Pediatric Ophthalmology and Strabismus,* and Section 9, *Intraocular Inflammation and Uveitis.* Systemic aspects of syphilis are discussed in Section 1, *Update on General Medicine.*

CLINICAL PRESENTATION Keratitis may be caused by either congenital or acquired syphilis, although most cases are associated with congenital syphilis. Manifestations of congenital syphilis that occur early in life (within the first 2 years) are infectious. However, IK is a later, immune-mediated manifestation of congenital syphilis. Affected children typically show no evidence of corneal disease in their first years; stromal keratitis lasting for several weeks develops late in the first decade of life (or even later). These patients may also have nonocular signs of congenital syphilis:

- dental deformities: notched incisors and mulberry molars
- bone and cartilage abnormalities: saddle nose, palatal perforation, saber shins, and frontal bossing
- cranial nerve VIII (vestibulocochlear) deafness
- rhagades (circumoral radiating scars)
- cognitive impairment

Widely spaced, peg-shaped teeth; eighth nerve deafness; and interstitial keratitis constitute the Hutchinson triad. Congenital syphilitic keratitis is bilateral in 80% of cases, although both eyes may not be affected simultaneously or to the same degree. Initial symptoms are pain, tearing, photophobia, and perilimbal injection. The inflammation may last for weeks if left untreated. Sectoral superior stromal inflammation and keratic precipitates are typically seen early in the disease course. As the disease progresses, deep stromal neovascularization develops. Eventually, the inflammation spreads centrally, and corneal opacification and edema may develop. In some cases, the deep corneal vascularization becomes so intense that the cornea appears pink—hence the term *salmon patch* (Fig 11-16). Sequelae of stromal keratitis include corneal scarring, corneal thinning, and ghost vessels in the deep layers of the stroma. Vision may be reduced because of irregular astigmatism and stromal opacification.

Stromal keratitis develops only rarely in acquired (as opposed to congenital) syphilis and, if it does, is unilateral in 60% of cases. The ocular findings are similar to those seen

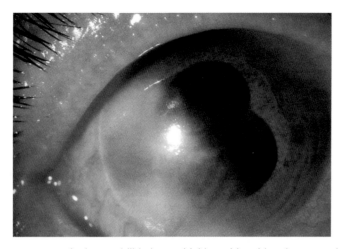

Figure 11-16 Active syphilitic interstitial keratitis with salmon patch.

in congenital syphilitic keratitis. In general, uveitis and retinitis are much more common manifestations of acquired syphilis than keratitis.

LABORATORY EVALUATION AND MANAGEMENT A diagnosis of congenital syphilis is confirmed by identification of *Treponema pallidum* by dark-field microscopy or fluorescent antibody. The detection of specific IgM is currently the most sensitive serologic method. During the acute phase, ocular inflammation should be treated with cycloplegic drugs and topical corticosteroids to limit stromal inflammation and late scarring. The corneal disease can be suppressed with topical corticosteroids. If untreated, the disease can "burn out" over time; because it can lead to severe corneal opacification, earlier treatment can be beneficial in preventing ophthalmic sequelae. Patients with findings of IK should have a workup for syphilis. Systemic syphilis (or neuroretinal manifestations) should be treated with penicillin or an appropriate alternative antibiotic in accordance with the protocol for either congenital or acquired syphilis. The necessity of lumbar puncture in syphilitic IK is uncertain, and any patient with suspected syphilis should be referred for immediate consultation with a specialist in infectious diseases.

Cogan Syndrome

PATHOGENESIS Cogan syndrome is a rare autoimmune disorder, the etiology of which is obscure. However, the disease shares some clinicopathologic features with polyarteritis nodosa. Progressive ocular and audiovestibular symptoms—which can lead to blindness, deafness, and even death from systemic vasculitits—develop in affected patients.

CLINICAL PRESENTATION Cogan syndrome typically occurs in young adults and produces stromal keratitis, vertigo, and hearing loss. The history may reveal a recent upper respiratory tract infection, bout of diarrhea, dental infection, or immunization. The earliest corneal findings are bilateral faint, white subepithelial infiltrates resembling those occurring in viral keratoconjunctivitis but located in the peripheral cornea. Multifocal nodular infiltrates may develop in the posterior cornea later. A systemic vasculitis that presents as polyarteritis nodosa occurs in some patients.

LABORATORY EVALUATION When the cause of stromal keratitis is not apparent, a VDRL or rapid plasma reagin (RPR) test and FTA-ABS or microhemagglutination assay for *T pallidum* are performed (VDRL and RPR tests may become nonreactive in congenital syphilis). Other infectious syndromes should also be considered. Antibodies to chlamydia have been reported in cases of Cogan syndrome. The presence of autoantibodies against the inner ear and endothelial antigens has been reported in some patients with Cogan syndrome. Hearing testing should be performed when Cogan syndrome is being considered. The erythrocyte sedimentation rate (ESR) and/or the C-reactive protein (CRP) level may be elevated. Fifty percent of patients with Cogan syndrome may test positive for anti–heat shock protein antibodies. Also, case reports have noted that affected patients test positive for antineutrophil cytoplasmic antibody (ANCA), rheumatoid factor (RF), antinuclear antibody (ANA), and anticardiolipin antibodies. However, laboratory findings are not consistent in Cogan syndrome, and there is no definitive test. This syndrome thus remains a diagnosis of exclusion, and it must be considered early on in the differential diagnosis of any patient who has the symptoms and clinical findings mentioned earlier.

> Tirelli G, Tomietto P, Quatela E, et al. Sudden hearing loss and Crohn disease: when Cogan syndrome must be suspected. *Am J Otolaryngol.* 2015;36(4):590–597.

MANAGEMENT The acute keratitis of Cogan syndrome is treated with frequent topical corticosteroids. Oral corticosteroids are recommended for the vestibular and auditory symptoms because this treatment improves the long-term prognosis. Cytotoxic agents may also have a therapeutic role but are reserved for severe or unresponsive cases. Early recognition and treatment of Cogan syndrome is critical to prevent the rapid progression to vision loss, blindness, deafness, and death from systemic vasculitis. Early consultation with an otolaryngologist and rheumatologist for management is recommended.

> Espinoza GM, Prost A. Cogan's syndrome and other ocular vasculitides. *Curr Rheumatol Rep.* 2015;17(4):24.
>
> Gluth MB, Baratz KH, Matteson EL, Driscoll CL. Cogan syndrome: a retrospective review of 60 patients throughout a half century. *Mayo Clin Proc.* 2006;81(4):483–488.

Marginal Corneal Infiltrates

PATHOGENESIS The limbus plays an important role in immune-mediated corneal disorders. The limbus has a population of antigen-presenting cells (APCs) that constitutively express MHC class II antigens and are capable of efficient mobilization and induction of T-cell responses. Therefore, immune-related corneal changes often occur in a peripheral location adjacent to the limbus. In addition, because the peripheral cornea is adjacent to the vascularized (posterior) limbus, circulating immune cells, immune complexes, and complement factors tend to deposit adjacent to the terminal capillary loops of the limbal vascular arcades, thereby producing a variety of immune phenomena that manifest in the corneal periphery. Predisposing factors include

- blepharoconjunctivitis (see Chapter 3)
- contact lens wear
- trauma
- endophthalmitis

CLINICAL PRESENTATION Marginal infiltrates (also referred to as *catarrhal infiltrates*) are creamy white elliptical opacities typically separated from the limbus by a relatively lucent zone. They most often occur near the point of intersection of the eyelid margin and the limbus, that is, at 10, 2, 4 and 8 o'clock (see Chapter 3, Fig 3-19). In chronic disease, superficial blood vessels may cross the clear interval into the area of corneal infiltration. The epithelium overlying marginal infiltrates may be intact, show punctate epithelial erosions, or be ulcerated. Stromal opacification, peripheral corneal thinning, and/or pannus may develop following resolution of the acute marginal infiltrates. The management of marginal infiltrates is discussed in Chapter 3.

> Ozcura F. Successful treatment of *Staphylococcus*-associated marginal keratitis with topical cyclosporine. *Graefes Arch Clin Exp Ophthalmol.* 2010;248(7):1049–1050.

Peripheral Ulcerative Keratitis Associated With Systemic Immune-Mediated Diseases

PATHOGENESIS Autoimmune peripheral keratitis may develop in patients who have systemic immune-mediated and rheumatic diseases. Peripheral ulcerative keratitis (PUK) occurs most often in association with rheumatoid arthritis but may also be seen in other conditions (Table 11-3). Biopsy of conjunctival tissue adjacent to marginal corneal disease—though not a standard diagnostic procedure—typically shows evidence of immune-mediated vaso-occlusive disease.

Central corneal melting in the setting of systemic collagen-vascular disease may be due to a different mechanism associated with a T-lymphocyte infiltration.

Table 11-3 Differential Diagnosis of Peripheral Ulcerative Keratitis

Ocular Conditions and Diseases	Systemic Conditions and Diseases
Microbial	Microbial
Bacterial *(Staphylococcus, Streptococcus, Gonococcus, Moraxella, Haemophilus)*	Bacterial (tuberculosis, syphilis, gonorrhea, borreliosis, bacillary dysentery)
Viral (herpes simplex, herpes zoster)	Viral (herpes zoster, AIDS, hepatitis C)
Acanthamoeba	Helminthiasis
Fungal	Rheumatoid arthritis
Mooren ulcer	Systemic lupus erythematosus
Traumatic or postsurgical	Granulomatosis with polyangiitis (Wegener granulomatosis)
Terrien marginal degeneration	Polyarteritis nodosa
Exposure keratopathy	Relapsing polychondritis
Rosacea	Progressive systemic sclerosis and scleroderma
	Sjögren syndrome
	Behçet disease
	Sarcoidosis
	Inflammatory bowel disease
	α_1-Antitrypsin deficiency
	Malignancy

Modified with permission from Dana MR, Qian Y, Hamrah P. Twenty-five-year panorama of corneal immunology: emerging concepts in the immunopathogenesis of microbial keratitis, peripheral ulcerative keratitis, and corneal transplant rejection. *Cornea.* 2000;19(5):630.

CLINICAL PRESENTATION A history of connective tissue disease is often (but not invariably) present, although in some patients the ocular finding of peripheral corneal infiltration or frank stromal melting may be the first sign of the underlying systemic illness. Autoimmune PUK generally correlates with exacerbations of systemic disease activity. Follow-up of patients with autoimmune PUK reveals that if they are treated inadequately, severe disease-related morbidity may occur in a high number of these patients. The term *keratolysis* refers to the significant (and often rapid) stromal melting seen in some cases of immune-mediated PUK associated with systemic autoimmunity.

Although autoimmune PUK can be bilateral and extensive, it is usually unilateral and limited to 1 sector of the peripheral cornea (Fig 11-17). The initial lesions appear in a zone within 2 mm of the limbus and are accompanied by varying degrees of vaso-occlusion of the adjacent limbal vascular networks. In most cases, the epithelium is absent in the affected area and the underlying stroma thinned; however, if the disease is detected early, epithelial involvement may be patchy and the stroma still of near-normal thickness. Ulceration may or may not be associated with a significant cellular infiltrate in the corneal stroma, and the adjacent conjunctiva can be minimally or severely inflamed. The sclera can be involved in patients with systemic immune-mediated diseases (eg, necrotizing scleritis in patients with rheumatoid arthritis); careful, complete examination must be performed.

Foster CS. Ocular manifestations of the potentially lethal rheumatologic and vasculitic disorders. *J Fr Ophthalmol.* 2013;36(6):526–532.

MANAGEMENT The goal of therapy is to provide local supportive measures to decrease melting. This is achieved through maneuvers intended to promote epithelialization, improve wetting, and suppress immune-mediated inflammation both locally and systemically.

Maintaining enhanced lubrication of the ocular surface is very important, as many patients with rheumatoid arthritis have KCS as a manifestation of their secondary Sjögren syndrome and because lubrication may help diminish the effect of inflammatory cytokines

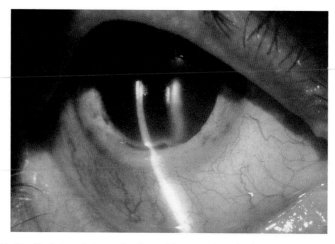

Figure 11-17 Peripheral ulcerative keratitis associated with rheumatoid disease.

in the tear film. Melting will stop or slow appreciably if the epithelium can be made to heal by means of lubricants, patching, or a bandage contact lens. A number of topical collagenase inhibitors (eg, sodium citrate 10%, acetylcysteine solution 20%, medroxyprogesterone 1%) and systemic collagenase inhibitors such as tetracyclines (eg, doxycycline) are of potential value. Topical cyclosporine has been shown to be effective in patients with central melting that is likely due to a T-cell–mediated process rather than occlusive vasculitis.

Topical corticosteroids, which also inhibit collagenase function, can have variable effects. In general, when considering steroids, the clinician must weigh the benefits of treating inflammation against the risks of impaired healing. Excision or recession of adjacent limbal conjunctiva (as has been advocated for Mooren ulcer; see the following section) is often followed by healing of the ulcer, presumably because the procedure eliminates a source of inflammatory cells and collagenolytic enzymes.

Definitive management often cannot be achieved by local measures alone and requires institution or escalation of systemic treatment, including immunosuppression therapy with oral prednisone, cytotoxic agents such as cyclophosphamide, or immunomodulatory agents such as methotrexate or cyclosporine. Biologic agents such as infliximab have reportedly been used with some success in more severe cases. Patients with severe, rapid melting may require intravenous therapy with high-dose cyclophosphamide, with or without corticosteroid therapy. Threatened perforation should be treated with temporizing measures such as cyanoacrylate glue and bandage contact lens placement until systemic therapy has been initiated, because lamellar and penetrating grafts are also susceptible to melting. Sometimes multiple tectonic grafts are required to preserve the globe while the systemic therapy is being adjusted. Once the underlying disease process has been controlled, keratoplasty for visual restoration can be performed (see Chapter 15). Although conjunctival flaps can be very helpful in controlling the stromal melting in difficult-to-manage microbial keratitis, they are probably best avoided in immune-mediated disease. Bringing the conjunctival vasculature even closer to the area of corneal disease could accelerate melting. It is very important to partner with a rheumatologist in caring for patients with immune-mediated disease, as their risk of morbidity and death is significant.

Bhat P, Birnbaum AD. Diagnosis and management of noninfectious corneal ulceration and melting. *Focal Points: Clinical Modules for Ophthalmologists.* San Francisco: American Academy of Ophthalmology; 2015, module 3.

Huerva V, Sanchez MC, Traveset A, Jurjo C, Ruiz A. Rituximab for peripheral ulcerative keratitis with Wegener granulomatosis. *Cornea.* 2010;29(6):708–710.

Kaçmaz RO, Kempen JH, Newcomb C, et al. Cyclosporine for ocular inflammatory diseases. *Ophthalmology.* 2010;117(3):576–584.

Pham M, Chow CC, Badawi D, Tu EY. Use of infliximab in the treatment of peripheral ulcerative keratitis in Crohn disease. *Am J Ophthalmol.* 2011;152(2):183–188.e2.

Mooren Ulcer

PATHOGENESIS By definition, Mooren ulcer is of unknown cause. PUK due to known local (eg, rosacea) or systemic (eg, rheumatoid arthritis) diseases should not be called Mooren ulcer. Evidence is mounting that autoimmunity plays a key role in the pathogenesis of Mooren ulcer, as the following have been found in patients with this condition:

- abnormal function of T-suppressor cells
- increased level of IgA
- increased concentration of plasma cells and lymphocytes in the conjunctiva adjacent to the ulcerated areas
- increased CD4$^+$-to-CD8$^+$ and B7-2$^+$-to-APC ratios as well as increased vascular cell adhesion molecule 1, very late antigen 4, and intercellular adhesion molecule 1 in the vascular endothelium of conjunctival vessels
- tissue-fixed immunoglobulins and complement in the conjunctival epithelium and peripheral cornea

A significant number of resident cells in Mooren ulcer specimens express MHC class II antigens, a reflection of the degree of immune-mediated inflammation in the tissue. It has been suggested that autoreactivity to a cornea-specific antigen may play a role in the pathogenesis of this disorder, and humoral and cell-mediated immune mechanisms may be involved in the initiation and perpetuation of corneal destruction. The proximity of the ulcerative lesion to the limbus probably has pathophysiologic importance (as discussed earlier, in the section on PUK), because resection or recession of the limbal conjunctiva can often have a beneficial therapeutic effect.

Although the cause of Mooren ulcer is unknown, precipitating factors include accidental trauma, surgery, or exposure to parasitic infection. The latter is of considerable importance, as the incidence of Mooren ulcer is particularly high in areas where parasitic (eg, helminthic) infections are endemic. The principal hypotheses are that inflammation associated with previous injury or infection may alter the expression of corneal or conjunctival antigens (to which autoantibodies are then produced) or that cross-reactivity occurs between the immune effectors generated in response to infection and corneal autoantigens. The simultaneous presence of multiple types of inflammatory cells, adhesion molecules, and costimulatory molecules in Mooren ulcer conjunctiva suggests that their interaction may contribute to a sustained immune activation as at least part of the pathogenic mechanism of this disorder.

Kafkala C, Choi J, Zafirakis P, et al. Mooren ulcer: an immunopathologic study. *Cornea*. 2006; 25(6):667–673.

CLINICAL PRESENTATION Mooren ulcer is a chronic, painful, progressive ulceration of the peripheral corneal stroma and epithelium. Typically, the ulcer starts in the periphery of the cornea and spreads circumferentially and then centripetally, with a leading undermined edge of deepithelialized tissue (Fig 11-18). Slower ulceration proceeds toward the sclera. The eye is inflamed and pain can be intense, with photophobia and tearing. Perforation may occur with minor trauma or during secondary infection. Extensive vascularization and fibrosis of the cornea may occur.

In some patients, it may be very difficult to differentiate Mooren ulcer from idiopathic PUK. An important distinguishing feature is the purely corneal involvement of Mooren ulcer; in PUK, the sclera is often involved.

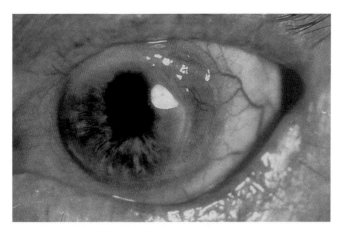

Figure 11-18 Mooren ulcer. *(Courtesy of Vincent P. deLuise, MD.)*

Two clinical types of Mooren ulcer have been described. Unilateral Mooren ulcer typically occurs in an older patient population. Sex distribution is equal in this form, which is slowly progressive. A second type of Mooren ulcer is more common in Africa. This form is usually bilateral, rapidly progressive, and poorly responsive to medical or surgical intervention. Corneal ulceration (Fig 11-19) and perforation are frequent. Many patients with this form of Mooren ulcer also have coexisting parasitemia. It is possible that in this subgroup of West African males, Mooren ulcer may be triggered by antigen–antibody reaction to helminthic toxins or antigens deposited in the limbal cornea during the bloodborne phase of parasitic infection. Hepatitis C should be considered in patients who present with Mooren ulcer–like findings.

MANAGEMENT The multitude of therapeutic strategies used against Mooren ulcer underscores the relative lack of effective treatment. Topical corticosteroids (including difluprednate), contact lenses, acetylcysteine 10% and L-cysteine (0.2 molar), topical cyclosporine,

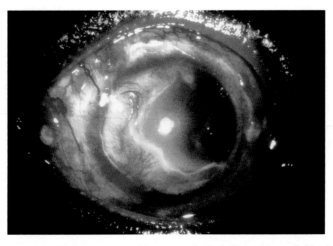

Figure 11-19 Mooren ulcer with severe limbal ulceration and thinning.

limbal conjunctival excision, and lamellar keratoplasty have all reportedly been used with variable success. Topical interferon-α_{2a} (IFN-α_{2a}) and topical cyclosporine 2%, as well as infliximab, have been reported as effective alternatives. Systemic immunosuppressive treatment of Mooren ulcer with agents such as oral corticosteroids, cyclophosphamide, methotrexate, cyclosporine, and TNF-α inhibitors has been described. Hepatitis C–associated cases of Mooren ulcer–type PUK have responded to interferon therapy.

Alhassan MB, Rabiu M, Agbabiaka IO. Interventions for Mooren's ulcer. *Cochrane Database Syst Rev.* 2014;(1):CD006131.

Cordero-Coma M, Benito MF, Fuertes CL, Antolín SC, García Ruíz JM. Adalimumab for Mooren's ulcer. *Ophthalmology.* 2009;116(8):1589, 1589.e1.

Garg P, Reddy JC, Sangwan VS. Mooren ulcer. In: Mannis MJ, Holland EJ, eds. *Cornea.* Vol 1. 4th ed. Philadelphia: Elsevier; 2017:1082–1087.

Wilson SE, Lee WM, Murakami C, Weng J, Moninger GA. Mooren-type hepatitis C virus-associated corneal ulceration. *Ophthalmology.* 1994;101(4):736–745.

Corneal Transplant Rejection

The cornea was the first successfully transplanted solid tissue. After other tissues had been transplanted, it was observed that corneas were rejected less frequently than other transplanted tissues. The concept that the cornea was a site of "immunologic privilege" and that corneal grafts were somehow protected from immunologic destruction subsequently emerged. Early immunologists attributed ocular immune privilege to "immunologic ignorance" due to the absence of lymphatics draining the anterior segment. It was later recognized that corneal grafts are not different from other tissue grafts and that the allogeneic cells of the transplant elicit an immune response, but the response is aberrant. There is a profound antigen-specific suppression of cell-mediated immunity, especially T-cell–mediated inflammation, such as delayed hypersensitivity and a concomitant induction of antibody responses.

Tolerance of a corneal graft is recognized as an active process, based on several features:

- absence of blood and lymphatic channels in the graft and its bed
- absence of MHC class II$^+$ APCs in the graft
- reduced expression of MHC-encoded alloantigens on graft cells replaced with minor peptides (nonclassical MHC-Ib molecules) to avoid lysis by natural killer cells
- expression of T-cell–deleting CD95 ligand (Fas ligand, or FasL) on endothelium, which can induce apoptosis in killer T cells
- immunosuppressive microenvironment of the aqueous humor, including transforming growth factor β_2, α-melanocyte-stimulating hormone, vasoactive intestinal peptide, and calcitonin gene–related peptide
- anterior chamber–associated immune deviation (ACAID) involving the development of suppressor T cells (ACAID is a downregulation of delayed-type cellular immunity. Antigens released into the aqueous humor are, presumably, recognized by dendritic cells of the iris and ciliary body. These APCs can then enter venous circulation and induce regulatory T cells in the spleen, bypassing the lymphatic system.)

For an immune response to occur, an antigenic substance is introduced and "recognized" (afferent arm; sensitization), resulting in the synthesis of specific antibody molecules and the appearance of effector lymphocytes that react specifically with the immunizing antigen (efferent arm; rejection). Although antibodies to foreign tissues are formed during graft rejection, they are not believed to be important in the usual type of allograft rejection. Rather, extensive evidence indicates that allograft rejection is associated with cellular immune mechanisms. Such T-lymphocyte–mediated responses are delayed hypersensitivity reactions. Other mechanisms are also probably involved. For the endothelial cells to be rejected, they must express MHC class II antigens.

See also the discussion of clinical signs of corneal transplant rejection in Chapter 15 of this volume. BCSC Section 9, *Intraocular Inflammation and Uveitis*, discusses and illustrates the principles of immunology in greater detail.

Angiogenesis and Lymphangiogenesis in the Cornea

Though not normally present in the cornea, blood vessels and lymphatic vessels may extend into the cornea—as sprouts of the vascular endothelium from the limbal tissue—after inflammatory, infectious, traumatic, chemical, or toxic insults. Inflammatory cells infiltrate tissue at local sites of vascular remodeling, where they secrete proangiogenic factors and metalloproteinases. Vascular endothelial growth factor (VEGF) is upregulated in inflamed and vascularized corneas in humans and in animal models.

Targeting angiogenesis in order to modulate immune responses after corneal transplant has been the primary area of interest for many researchers. Treatment of corneal neovascularization after corneal transplant may limit both the afferent and efferent arms of alloimmunity and thus reduce the tendency toward inflammatory reactions, which can jeopardize graft survival. VEGF inhibitors, including ranibizumab, bevacizumab, and aflibercept, are used to treat neovascular age-related macular degeneration. The efficacy of these antiangiogenic therapies, which are administered topically and subconjunctivally after transplantation, has been demonstrated. Novel antiangiogenic "t" molecules, which target the intracellular pathways of angiogenesis (small interfering RNA, antisense oligonucleotides), have been reported to provide a promising alternative.

VEGF-C induces lymphangiogenesis in various animal models. Lymphatics transport APCs to regional lymphoid tissue, where the APCs initiate the T-cell response. The growth of new lymphatic vessels thus facilitates access of donor and host APCs and antigenic material to regional lymph nodes, accelerating sensitization to graft antigens. Recently, the targeting of lymphangiogenesis has also become a focused area of research. There is evidence that blocking lymphatic vessels may play a key role in the prevention and treatment of corneal graft rejection.

Abudou M, Wu T, Evans JR, Chen X. Immunosuppressants for the prophylaxis of corneal graft rejection after penetrating keratoplasty. *Cochrane Database Syst Rev.* 2015;(8):CD007603. Epub 2015 Aug 27.

Albuquerque RJC, Hayashi T, Cho WG, et al. Alternatively spliced vascular endothelial growth factor receptor-2 is an essential endogenous inhibitor of lymphatic vessel growth. *Nat Med.* 2009;15(9):1023–1030.

Bachmann B, Taylor RS, Cursiefen C. Corneal neovascularization as a risk factor for graft failure and rejection after keratoplasty: an evidence-based meta-analysis. *Ophthalmology.* 2010;117(7):1300–1305.e7.

Benayoun Y, Petellat F, Leclerc O, et al. Current treatments for corneal neovascularization. *J Fr Ophtalmol.* 2015;38(10):996–1008.

Bourghardt Peebo B, Fagerholm P, Traneus-Röckert C, Lagali N. Time-lapse in vivo imaging of corneal angiogenesis: the role of inflammatory cells in capillary sprouting. *Invest Ophthalmol Vis Sci.* 2011;52(6):3060–3068.

Maruyama K, Ii M, Cursiefen C, et al. Inflammation-induced lymphangiogenesis in the cornea arises from CD11b-positive macrophages. *J Clin Invest.* 2005;115(9):2363–2372.

Skobe M, Dana R. Blocking the path of lymphatic vessels. *Nat Med.* 2009;15(9):993–994.

Immune-Mediated Diseases of the Episclera and Sclera

Episcleritis

PATHOGENESIS Episcleritis is a generally benign inflammation of the episcleral tissues. An underlying systemic cause is found in only a minority of patients.

CLINICAL PRESENTATION Episcleritis is typically a transient (usually days to weeks), self-limited disease of sudden onset affecting adults aged 20–50 years, with most cases occurring in women. The patient's chief concern is usually ocular redness with irritation or pain. Slight tenderness may occur. The disease occurs most often in the exposed interpalpebral zone of the eye, in the area of a pinguecula. It may recur in the same or different locations. About one-third of patients have bilateral disease at one time or another.

Episcleritis is classified as simple (diffuse injection) or nodular. In simple episcleritis, the inflammation is localized to a sector of the globe in 70% of cases and to the entire episclera in 30% of cases. A localized mobile nodule develops in nodular episcleritis (Fig 11-20). Small peripheral corneal opacities can be observed adjacent to an area of episcleral inflammation in 10% of patients.

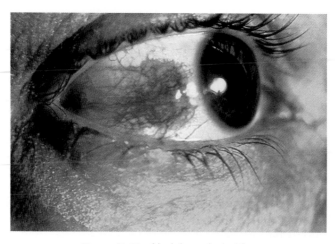

Figure 11-20 Nodular episcleritis.

Episcleral inflammation is superficial and will blanch with application of topical phenylephrine 2.5%. Episcleritis must be differentiated from the deeper inflammation seen in scleritis (often with associated scleral edema clearly discernible on slit-lamp examination). The inflamed episclera is characteristically bright red or salmon pink in natural light, unlike the violaceous hue seen in most forms of scleritis.

Sainz de la Maza M, Molina N, Gonzalez-Gonzalez LA, Doctor PP, Tauber J, Foster CS. Clinical characteristics of a large cohort of patients with scleritis and episcleritis. *Ophthalmology.* 2012;119(1):43–50.

MANAGEMENT A workup for underlying causes (eg, autoimmune connective tissue disease such as Sjögren syndrome or rheumatoid arthritis; other conditions such as gout, herpes zoster, syphilis, tuberculosis, Lyme disease, or rosacea) is rarely indicated except after multiple recurrences. Episcleritis generally clears without treatment, but topical or oral NSAIDs may be prescribed for patients bothered by the pain. Most patients simply need reassurance that their condition is not sight threatening and can be treated with lubricants alone. Topical corticosteroid use should be kept to a minimum in this benign, self-limited condition. In cases that do not respond to lubricants and NSAIDs, a course of topical corticosteroids may be necessary and beneficial.

Scleritis

PATHOGENESIS A much more severe ocular inflammatory condition than episcleritis, scleritis is caused by an immune-mediated (typically immune-complex) vasculitis that frequently leads to destruction of the sclera. Scleritis is often associated with an underlying systemic immunologic disease; about one-third of patients with diffuse or nodular scleritis and two-thirds of patients with necrotizing scleritis have a detectable connective tissue or autoimmune disease; the different forms of scleritis are discussed in the following subsections.

CLINICAL PRESENTATION Scleritis occurs most often in the fourth to sixth decades of life, is more common in women, and is exceedingly rare in children. About one-half of scleritis cases are bilateral at some time in their course. The onset of scleritis is usually gradual, extending over several days. Most patients with scleritis experience severe boring ocular pain, which may worsen at night and occasionally awaken them from sleep. The pain may be referred to other regions of the head or face on the involved side, and the globe is often tender. The inflamed sclera has a violaceous hue, which is best seen in sunlight. Inflamed scleral vessels have a crisscross pattern, adhere to the sclera, and cannot be moved with a cotton-tipped applicator. Scleral edema, often with overlying episcleral edema, is noted by slit-lamp examination. Scleritis may lead to structural alterations of the globe, with attendant visual morbidity. Scleritis can be classified clinically based on the anatomical location (anterior versus posterior sclera) and appearance of the scleral inflammation (Table 11-4). See BCSC Section 4, *Ophthalmic Pathology and Intraocular Tumors,* for histologic correlation.

Sainz de la Maza M, Molina N, Gonzalez-Gonzalez LA, Doctor PP, Tauber J, Foster CS. Clinical characteristics of a large cohort of patients with scleritis and episcleritis. *Ophthalmology.* 2012;119(1):43–50.

Table 11-4 Subtypes and Prevalence of Scleritis

Location	Subtype	Prevalence, %
Anterior sclera	Diffuse scleritis	75
	Nodular scleritis	14
	Necrotizing scleritis	5
	With inflammation	(4)
	Without inflammation (*scleromalacia perforans*)	(1)
Posterior sclera	Posterior scleritis	6

Information from Sainz de la Maza M, Molina N, Gonzalez-Gonzalez LA, et al. Clinical characteristics of a large cohort of patients with scleritis and episcleritis. *Ophthalmology*. 2012;119(1):43–50.

Diffuse versus nodular anterior scleritis

Diffuse anterior scleritis is characterized by a zone of scleral edema and redness. A part of the anterior sclera (<50%) is involved in 60% of cases; the entire anterior segment, in 40% (Fig 11-21). In *nodular anterior scleritis,* the scleral nodule is a deep violaceous color, immobile, and separated from the overlying episcleral tissue, which is raised by the nodule (Fig 11-22).

Necrotizing scleritis

Necrotizing scleritis is the most destructive form of scleritis. Ocular and systemic complications develop in 60% of affected patients, vision loss occurs in 40%, and a significant minority may die prematurely because of complications of vasculitis.

Necrotizing scleritis with inflammation Patients with necrotizing scleritis with inflammation typically present with severe pain. Most commonly, a localized patch of inflammation is noted initially, with the edges of the lesion more inflamed than the center. In more advanced disease (25% of cases), an avascular edematous patch of sclera is seen (Fig 11-23). Untreated, necrotizing scleritis may spread posteriorly to the equator and circumferentially until the entire anterior globe is involved. Severe tissue loss may result if treatment is not intensive and prompt. The sclera may develop a blue-gray appearance

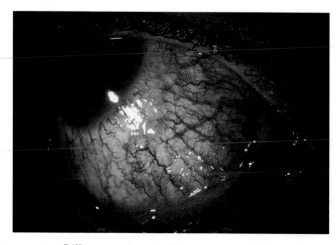

Figure 11-21 Diffuse anterior scleritis. *(Courtesy of Charles S. Bouchard, MD.)*

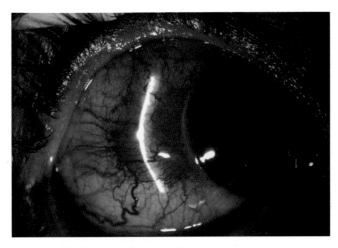

Figure 11-22 Nodular anterior scleritis. *(Courtesy of Charles S. Bouchard, MD.)*

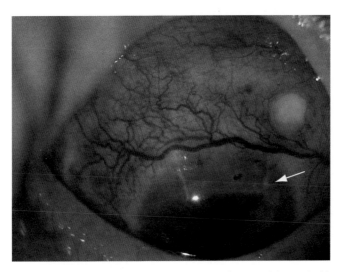

Figure 11-23 Diffuse anterior scleritis with a small area of necrotizing scleritis. Note also the partially resolved sclerokeratitis *(arrow)*. *(Courtesy of Charles S. Bouchard, MD.)*

(due to thinning, which allows the underlying choroid to show) and reveal an altered deep episcleral blood vessel pattern (large anastomotic blood vessels that may circumscribe the involved area) after the inflammation subsides.

Necrotizing scleritis without inflammation Though undoubtedly due to inflammation, this form of scleritis (also known as *scleromalacia perforans*) is said to be "without inflammation" because its clinical presentation is distinct from that of other forms of anterior scleritis, in which typical signs (redness, edema) and symptoms (pain) of inflammation are readily apparent.

Scleromalacia perforans typically occurs in patients with long-standing rheumatoid arthritis. Signs of inflammation are minimal, and this type of scleritis is generally painless. As the disease progresses, the sclera thins and the underlying dark uveal tissue becomes

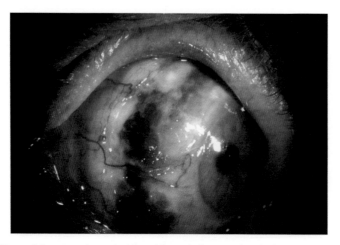

Figure 11-24 Necrotizing anterior scleritis without inflammation (scleromalacia perforans) in a patient with rheumatoid arthritis. *(Courtesy of Charles S. Bouchard, MD.)*

visible (Fig 11-24). In many cases, the uvea is covered with only thin connective tissue and conjunctiva. Large abnormal blood vessels surround and cross the areas of scleral loss. A bulging staphyloma develops if intraocular pressure is elevated; spontaneous perforation is rare, although these eyes may rupture with minimal trauma.

Posterior scleritis

Posterior scleritis can occur in isolation or concomitantly with anterior scleritis. Some investigators include posterior scleritis as an anterior variant of inflammatory pseudotumor. Patients present with pain, tenderness, proptosis, vision loss, and, occasionally, restricted motility. Choroidal folds, exudative retinal detachment, papilledema, and angle-closure glaucoma secondary to choroidal thickening may develop. Retraction of the lower eyelid may occur in upgaze, presumably caused by infiltration of muscles in the region of the posterior scleritis. The pain may be referred to other parts of the head, and the diagnosis can be missed in the absence of associated anterior scleritis. Demonstration of thickened posterior sclera by echography (Fig 11-25), computed tomography, or magnetic resonance

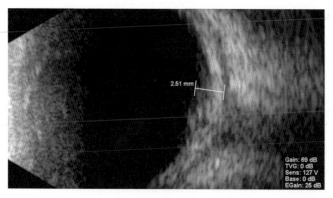

Figure 11-25 B-scan ultrasound image from a patient with posterior scleritis showing localized posterior scleral thickening (⊢⊣). *(Courtesy of James J. Reidy, MD.)*

imaging may be helpful in establishing the diagnosis. Often, no related systemic disease can be found in patients with posterior scleritis.

Complications of scleritis

Complications of scleritis are frequent and include peripheral keratitis (occurring in 37% of cases), scleral thinning (33%), uveitis (30%), glaucoma (18%), and cataract (7%). In sclerokeratitis, the peripheral cornea becomes opacified by fibrosis and lipid deposition in conjunction with neighboring scleritis (which may be severe or very mild; Fig 11-26). With progression, the central cornea becomes involved, resulting in opacification of a large segment of cornea. This type of keratitis commonly accompanies herpes zoster scleritis but may also occur in rheumatic diseases.

Anterior uveitis may occur as a spillover phenomenon in eyes with anterior scleritis. Some degree of posterior uveitis occurs in all patients with posterior scleritis and may also occur in anterior scleritis. Although one-third of patients with scleritis have evidence of scleral translucency and/or thinning, frank scleral defects are seen only in the most severe forms of necrotizing disease and in the late stages of scleromalacia perforans.

LABORATORY EVALUATION Scleritis can occur in association with various systemic infectious diseases, including syphilis, tuberculosis, herpes zoster, Lyme disease, "cat-scratch" disease, and leprosy (Hansen disease). It is most frequently seen, however, in association with autoimmune or connective tissue diseases such as rheumatoid arthritis, systemic lupus erythematosus, and seronegative spondyloarthropathies (eg, ankylosing spondylitis) or secondary to vasculitides such as granulomatosis with polyangiitis (Wegener granulomatosis), polyarteritis nodosa, and giant cell arteritis. Metabolic diseases such as gout may also, in rare instances, be associated with scleritis. More than 50% of patients with scleritis have an identifiable associated systemic disease. The differential diagnosis of scleritis is similar to that of PUK (see Table 11-3).

The workup of scleritis should therefore include a complete physical examination, with attention to the joints, skin, and cardiovascular and respiratory systems. It is recommended that the ophthalmologist consult with a rheumatologist or other internist with

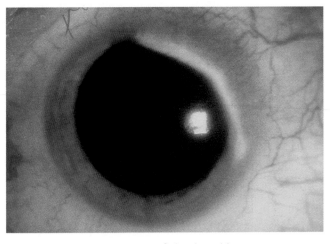

Figure 11-26 Sclerokeratitis.

Table 11-5 **Initial Laboratory Workup for Scleritis**

Chest x-ray
Complete blood cell count (CBC) with differential
Erythrocyte sedimentation rate (ESR) or C-reactive protein (CRP)
Serum angiotensin-converting enzyme and lysozyme, as appropriate (ie, sarcoidosis screening)
Serum autoantibody screening (antinuclear antibody [ANA], anti-DNA antibody, rheumatoid factor
  [RF], antineutrophil cytoplasmic antibody [ANCA])
Serum uric acid test
Syphilis serologic test
Urinalysis

experience in diagnosing and managing these conditions. Laboratory studies should always be guided by the history and findings of the physical examination. However, the laboratory tests listed in Table 11-5 are generally recommended as an initial screening.

MANAGEMENT Although topical corticosteroids can be used to alleviate symptoms, the treatment of scleritis is systemic. A guideline for the treatment of patients with scleritis has been proposed by Sainz de la Maza et al and is shown in Figure 11-27. It is important to clearly define treatment goals: treatment failure may be defined as progression of disease to a more severe form (eg, nodular to necrotizing) or failure to achieve response to treatment after 2–3 weeks of therapy, in which case an alternate therapeutic strategy will need to be instituted. Idiopathic diffuse and nodular forms of scleritis, which have no ocular complications and little scleral inflammation, may be responsive to treatment with oral NSAIDs (eg, ibuprofen, indomethacin). If one NSAID is not effective, another may be tried; only one NSAID should be prescribed at a time. Systemic corticosteroid treatment may be used if the patient is unresponsive to NSAIDs or inflammation is more severe; NSAIDs and steroids should not be given simultaneously. Prednisone may be started at 1 mg/kg daily and then tapered within the first 2 weeks of treatment. Remission may be maintained with NSAIDs. Gastroprotective medication should be given to patients prescribed NSAIDs or steroids.

If corticosteroid treatment fails or the patient relapses after tapering the steroid, immunosuppression therapy may be considered. These cases often respond to antimetabolites (eg, methotrexate, azathioprine, mycophenolate mofetil). Immunosuppression treatment (eg, antimetabolites; T-cell inhibitors such as cyclosporin A or tacrolimus; alkylating agents such as cyclophosphamide) or biologic response modifiers (eg, anti-TNF-α medications such as infliximab; anti-CD20 agents such as rituximab) are usually necessary in patients with associated systemic disease, necrotizing scleritis, and/or progressive destructive ocular lesions.

Patients receiving systemic treatment must be monitored closely by a physician specially trained in the administration of these medications and in the early detection and management of their complications. In addition, they should be informed that close follow-up with the ophthalmologist and partnering providers is necessary to monitor their disease status and treatment. Antituberculosis and anti-*Pneumocystis* coverage may be necessary for at-risk patients. In patients whose systemic evaluation is initially negative, it is important to repeat the workup annually.

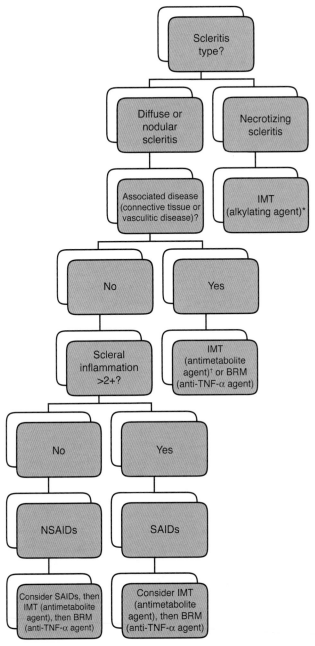

Figure 11-27 Suggested guideline for the treatment of patients with scleritis. BRM = biologic response modifier; IMT = immunomodulatory therapy; NSAIDs = nonsteroidal anti-inflammatory drugs; SAIDs = steroidal anti-inflammatory drugs; TNF = tumor necrosis factor; >2+ = grading of level of scleral inflammation (by authors of this figure). *Consider BRM such as rituximab for ovarian protection. †Consider first IMT (antimetabolite agent). If therapeutic failure, consider BRM (anti-TNF-α agent). If potentially lethal disease: alkylating agent IMT. *(Reproduced with permission from Sainz de la Maza M, Molina N, Gonzalez-Gonzalez LA, Doctor PP, Tauber J, Foster CS. Scleritis therapy. Ophthalmology. 2012;119(1):57.)*

Levy-Clarke G, Jabs DA, Read RW, Rosenbaum JT, Vitale A, Van Gelder RN. Expert panel recommendations for the use of anti-tumor necrosis factor biologic agents in patients with ocular inflammatory disorders. *Ophthalmology.* 2014;121(3):785–796.e3.

Ragam A, Kolomeyer AM, Fang C, Xu Y, Chu DS. Treatment of chronic, noninfectious, non-necrotizing scleritis with tumor necrosis factor alpha inhibitors. *Ocul Immunol Inflamm.* 2014;22(6):469–477.

Sainz de la Maza M, Molina N, Gonzalez-Gonzalez LA, Doctor PP, Tauber J, Foster CS. Scleritis therapy. *Ophthalmology.* 2012;119(1):51–58.

Singh J, Sallam A, Lightman S, Taylor S. Episcleritis and scleritis in rheumatic disease. *Curr Rheumatol Rev.* 2011;7(1):15–23.

Watson PG, Young RD. Scleral structure, organization and disease: a review. *Exp Eye Res.* 2004; 78(3):609–623.

CHAPTER 12

Clinical Approach to Neoplastic Disorders of the Conjunctiva and Cornea

Highlights

- Topical interferon-α_{2b}, mitomycin C, or 5-fluorouracil can be used to treat ocular surface squamous neoplasia.
- Sebaceous gland carcinoma is initially misdiagnosed in more than 50% of cases, often masquerading as chalazia or chronic unilateral blepharoconjunctivitis.
- Primary acquired melanosis (PAM) with moderate to severe atypia has a high risk of progression to melanoma. Biopsy is therefore important for suspicious-appearing PAM lesions.
- Lymphoid hyperplasia is clinically indistinguishable from lymphoma; biopsy is required in order to differentiate these conditions.

Introduction

In the United States, approximately 1 person in 2500 seeks ophthalmic care for a tumor of the eyelid or ocular surface each year, or about 100,000 per year. Benign neoplasms of the eyelid and ocular surface are at least 3 times more common than malignant lesions. Most of these tumors arise from the eyelid skin; they are discussed in BCSC Section 4, *Ophthalmic Pathology and Intraocular Tumors,* and Section 7, *Orbit, Eyelids, and Lacrimal System.*

Tumors of the conjunctiva and cornea are considered together because the lesions can affect both tissues concurrently. These lesions are classified by cell type: epithelium, melanocytes and nevus cells, vascular endothelium, mesenchymal cells, and lymphocytes. Many are analogous to lesions affecting the eyelid.

Shields CL, Alset AE, Boal NS, et al. Conjunctival tumors in 5002 cases. Comparative analysis of benign versus malignant counterparts. The 2016 James D. Allen Lecture. *Am J Ophthalmol.* 2017;173:106–133. Epub 2016 Oct 8.

Shields JA, Shields CL. *Eyelid, Conjunctival, and Orbital Tumors: An Atlas and Textbook.* 3rd ed. Philadelphia: Wolters Kluwer; 2016.

Approach to the Patient With a Neoplastic Ocular Surface Lesion

During the initial evaluation of a patient with a conjunctival or corneal neoplasm, the clinician should obtain a detailed history, including extensive sun exposure, skin cancer, or immunosuppression. The clinician should inquire about the length of time the patient has had the lesion and whether there has been any change in the lesion's appearance. The racial or ethnic background of the patient is relevant, as conjunctival pigmentation may be normal in some patients (eg, darker-skinned persons) but worrisome in others.

A complete eye examination, including a dilated fundus examination, should be performed during the initial evaluation of the patient with a suspicious ocular surface lesion. The entire ocular surface should be examined, including the superior fornix, which requires eyelid eversion. Palpation for lymphadenopathy in the neck and preauricular region is an important part of the examination of tumor patients—especially when malignancy is suspected—because malignant lesions, especially conjunctival melanoma, can spread to regional lymph nodes. The clinical characteristics of the lesion should be noted, with the following considered:

- Is there a single lesion, or is it multifocal?
- Is the lesion pigmented or amelanotic?
- Where is it located—on the bulbar conjunctiva, at the limbus, in the fornix, on the palpebral conjunctiva?
- Does the lesion extend onto the cornea?
- Is the lesion solid or cystic?
- Is it flat or elevated?
- Is the lesion fixed to underlying tissues, or is it mobile?
- Is there a feeder vessel?

The clinician should document the appearance and extent of the lesion, using either photographs or a detailed diagram. This aids in surgical planning if the lesion is to be removed or in following the lesion if observation is recommended.

Management of Patients With Ocular Surface Tumors

An experienced clinician often has an opinion about the nature of a conjunctival or corneal lesion after completing the history and physical examination. Many lesions are not worrisome for malignancy (eg, inclusion cysts); others will be indeterminate based on the history and results of the clinical examination. For these cases, observation may be a reasonable option. If observation is elected, regular ophthalmic examinations are essential. If growth or worrisome changes in the characteristics of the lesion are documented, surgery or topical chemotherapy is usually indicated. Tissue for histologic evaluation may be required for definitive diagnosis. Lesions that cause concern for possible malignancy

- are elevated
- are extensive, pigmented, even if flat

- are fixed to underlying tissues
- have a large feeder vessel

The next 2 sections, Surgical Treatment and Topical Chemotherapy, provide a paradigm for/general approach to the management of suspicious conjunctival and corneal neoplasms. Following these sections, the various types of ocular surface neoplastic disorders are discussed and additional comments on management are provided for specific lesions as appropriate.

Surgical Treatment

The standard surgical treatment of a suspicious conjunctival lesion is complete removal of the tumor, including a 2-mm margin of uninvolved tissue surrounding the lesion, when possible. The surgeon attempts to avoid touching the tumor during removal ("no touch" technique) in order to prevent inadvertent seeding of the remaining conjunctiva with tumor cells. Incisional biopsies should be avoided for the same reason, especially in pigmented lesions of the conjunctiva. Involvement of the corneal epithelium is managed with absolute alcohol–assisted epithelial curettage with a surgical blade or blunt-edged instrument such as a Kimura spatula; the surgeon takes care to avoid violating the Bowman layer, which is a natural barrier to tumor extension into the corneal stroma. Some lesions may require lamellar sclerectomy for complete removal. Cryotherapy at the time of ocular surface surgery has been shown to improve the prognosis.

Once the tumor is removed, additional manipulations should be performed with clean surgical instruments to reduce the risk of tumor seeding. Primary conjunctival closure or a conjunctival autograft may be considered if the conjunctival defect is small. Ocular surface reconstruction with amniotic membrane transplantation is useful in the management of conjunctival lesions and allows for wider tumor margins with less risk of postoperative scarring. Amniotic membrane also facilitates reepithelialization and reduces postoperative inflammation. The graft should be cut slightly larger than the defect and may be attached with fibrin tissue adhesive. If tissue adhesive is not available, either absorbable (9-0 or 10-0 polyglactin) or nonabsorbable (10-0 nylon) suture may be used to fixate the graft. If more than two-thirds of the limbal epithelium is removed, chronic epitheliopathy may result. Stem cell transplantation using tissue harvested from the fellow eye of the patient or an allograft may eventually be required.

Once removed from the ocular surface, the lesion can be placed on filter paper and the edges labeled with ink or suture to indicate the orientation of the lesion and facilitate histologic diagnosis. The surgeon should take care to avoid damage to the specimen during removal, as any damage could make the lesion more difficult to interpret. The clinical history is relevant to the pathologist's interpretation of the lesion; thus, the label should include the following information: the age and race or ethnicity of the patient, the duration of the lesion, and whether the lesion has changed clinically. Diagnosis of conjunctival tumors can be challenging, especially for general pathologists. If possible, a conjunctival tumor should be evaluated by an ophthalmic pathologist. Immunostaining can help in distinguishing benign from malignant lesions. See BCSC Section 4, *Ophthalmic Pathology and Intraocular Tumors,* for further discussion of specimen handling and histologic examination of various ocular surface tumors.

Shields JA, Shields CL, De Potter P. Surgical management of conjunctival tumors. The 1994 Lynn B. McMahan Lecture. *Arch Ophthalmol.* 1997;115(6):808–815.

Sivaraman KR, Karp CL. Medical and surgical management of ocular surface squamous neoplasia. In: Mannis MJ, Holland EJ, eds. *Cornea.* Vol 1. 4th ed. Philadelphia: Elsevier; 2017:427–433.

Topical Chemotherapy

Topical chemotherapy may be used as an alternative to surgical excision for primary treatment of ocular surface tumors or as adjunctive therapy preceding or following surgical excision. Some authors advocate using topical treatment prior to surgical removal, the purpose being to reduce the size of large ocular surface tumors. Topical chemotherapy has the advantage of treating beyond areas of clinically visible involvement, but unlike surgical excision, it does not lead to histologic diagnosis or enable determination of clear margins. Further, since the appearance of some tumors is similar (eg, amelanotic conjunctival melanoma may resemble squamous cell carcinoma), there is concern that if chemotherapy is elected and the tumor does not respond, valuable time in the management of a potentially deadly lesion may have been lost.

Options for first-line therapy for squamous lesions are topical interferon-α_{2b} or topical mitomycin C (MMC), or wide-margin surgical excision with cryotherapy (Figs 12-1,

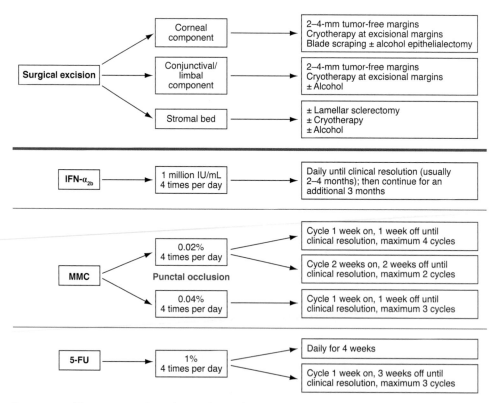

Figure 12-1 Treatment options for ocular surface squamous neoplasia. 5-FU = 5-fluorouracil; IFN-α_{2b} = interferon-α_{2b}; MMC = mitomycin C.

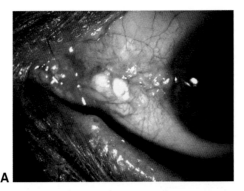 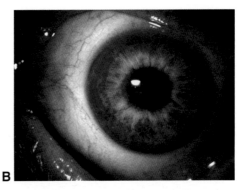

A   **B**

Figure 12-2 **A,** Ocular surface squamous neoplasia. **B,** The same eye 7 weeks after topical treatment with interferon-α_{2b} 1 million IU/mL 4 times daily. *(Courtesy of David D. Verdier, MD.)*

12-2). Interferon-α_{2b} is used most often as it has fewer adverse effects than MMC (ocular surface toxicity and potential stem cell deficiency); however, MMC can be used for a shorter duration—typically weeks rather than months—and may be more effective for melanocytic tumors. The antineoplastic 5-fluorouracil (5-FU) is less commonly used but may be considered for squamous lesions if other agents are unaffordable, ineffective, or poorly tolerated.

The optimal topical chemotherapy regimen has not been determined in controlled studies. Topical interferon-α_{2b} 1 million IU/mL is typically given 4 times daily until clinical resolution, usually within 2 to 4 months. It is not unusual for tumors to appear unresponsive during the first 3 months of treatment and then show abrupt regression. In fact, several additional months of treatment may be beneficial, given recent evidence, obtained with ultrahigh-resolution optical coherence tomography (OCT), that residual tumor may be present for up to 3 months following clinical resolution. Subconjunctival/perilesional injection of interferon-α_{2b} (3 million IU in 0.5 mL) can be given weekly in addition to, or as an alternative to, topical drops, especially if patient adherence is an issue. Subconjunctival interferon-α_{2b} is associated with flulike symptoms in 10% of patients. Topical MMC 0.02% or 0.04%, because of its potential toxicity, is typically administered 4 times daily for 1 week, followed by a 1-week structured treatment interruption (drug holiday), for a maximum of 3 or 4 treatment cycles. If residual tumor persists, alternative treatment should be considered to avoid potential MMC toxicity. 5-Fluorouracil 1% may be given 4 times daily for 1 month, with a structured treatment interruption of at least several months if treatment is repeated; alternatively, it may be given 4 times daily for 1 week, followed by a 3-week structured treatment interruption, until resolution (maximum of 3 treatment cycles). Application of topical corticosteroids may help with the surface toxicity. Placement of punctal plugs reduces the likelihood of systemic absorption and helps prevent punctal stenosis.

Once a tumor has been managed, long-term, regular follow-up is essential because malignant conjunctival tumors can recur. Complete examination of the ocular surface and palpation of regional lymph nodes should be performed at each visit. Patients with malignant ocular surface tumors should be referred to a dermatologist for a complete skin evaluation.

Fraunfelder FT, Wingfield D. Management of intraepithelial conjunctival tumors and squamous cell carcinomas. *Am J Ophthalmol.* 1983;95(3):359–363.

Nanji AA, Moon CS, Galor A, Sein J, Oellers P, Karp CL. Surgical versus medical treatment of ocular surface squamous neoplasia: a comparison of recurrences and complications. *Ophthalmology.* 2014;121(5):994–1000.

Parrozzani R, Lazzarini D, Alemany-Rubio E, Urban F, Midena E. Topical 1% 5-fluorouracil in ocular surface squamous neoplasia: a long-term safety study. *Br J Ophthalmol.* 2011;95: 355–359.

Thomas BJ, Galor A, Nanji AA, et al. Ultra high-resolution anterior segment optical coherence tomography in the diagnosis and management of ocular surface squamous neoplasia. *Ocul Surf.* 2014;12(1):46–58.

Tumors of Epithelial Origin

Table 12-1 lists the epithelial tumors of the conjunctiva and cornea.

Warner MA, Stagner AM, Jakobiec FA. Epithelial tumors of the conjunctiva. In: Mannis MJ, Holland EJ, eds. *Cornea.* Vol 1. 4th ed. Philadelphia: Elsevier; 2017:410–426.

Benign Epithelial Tumors

Conjunctival papilloma

There are 2 forms of conjunctival papilloma, sessile and pedunculated, and they differ etiologically, histologically, and clinically. See BCSC Section 4, *Ophthalmic Pathology and Intraocular Tumors,* for discussion of the histologic findings.

PATHOGENESIS *Human papillomavirus (HPV),* subtypes 6 and 11 (in children) or 16 (in adults), initiates a neoplastic growth of epithelial cells with vascular proliferation that gives rise to a pedunculated papilloma of the conjunctiva. A sessile conjunctival lesion, though also usually benign, may represent a dysplastic or carcinomatous lesion, especially when caused by HPV subtypes 16, 18, or 33.

CLINICAL PRESENTATION A pedunculated conjunctival papilloma is a fleshy, exophytic growth with a fibrovascular core (Fig 12-3A). It often arises in the inferior fornix but can also present on the tarsal or bulbar conjunctiva or along the plica semilunaris. The lesion emanates from a stalk and has a multilobulated appearance with smooth, clear epithelium and

Table 12-1 Tumors of Ocular Surface Epithelium

Benign	Preinvasive	Malignant
Papilloma	Conjunctival and corneal intraepithelial neoplasia	Squamous cell carcinoma
Pseudoepitheliomatous hyperplasia		Mucoepidermoid carcinoma
Benign hereditary intraepithelial dyskeratosis		

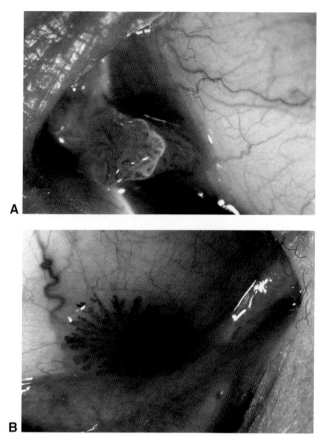

Figure 12-3 Conjunctival squamous papilloma. **A,** Pedunculated. **B,** Sessile. *(Reproduced with permission from Mannis MJ, Holland EJ, eds.* Cornea. *Vol 1. 4th ed. Philadelphia: Elsevier; 2017:412.)*

numerous underlying small corkscrew blood vessels. Multiple lesions sometimes occur, and the lesion may be extensive in patients with compromised immunity.

A sessile papilloma is typically found at the limbus and has a flat base (Fig 12-3B). With its glistening surface and numerous red dots, this form of papilloma resembles a strawberry. The lesion may spread onto the cornea. Signs of dysplasia include leukoplakia (indicative of keratinization), symblepharon formation, inflammation, and invasion. A very rare variant is an inverted papilloma.

MANAGEMENT A pedunculated papilloma that is small, cosmetically acceptable, and nonirritating may be observed. Spontaneous resolution can occur over many months to years. Surgical excision with cryotherapy or cautery to the base of the lesion is curative in approximately 90% of cases. An incomplete excision, however, can stimulate growth and lead to a worse cosmetic outcome. Surgical manipulation should be minimized to reduce the risk of dissemination of the virus to uninvolved healthy conjunctiva. Adjunctive treatment with topical interferon-α_{2b} or oral cimetidine may be of benefit for extensive or recalcitrant lesions.

A sessile limbal papilloma must be observed closely or excised. If the lesion enlarges or shows clinical features suggesting dysplastic or carcinomatous growth, excisional biopsy with adjunctive cryotherapy is indicated.

Kaliki S, Arepalli S, Shields CL, et al. Conjunctival papilloma: features and outcomes based on age at initial examination. *JAMA Ophthalmol.* 2013;131(5):585–593.

Ocular Surface Squamous Neoplasia

Ocular surface squamous neoplasia (OSSN) is an inclusive term used to describe a wide spectrum of conjunctival and corneal squamous tumors that may have similar clinical findings and require biopsy to differentiate. The traditional categorization of OSSN lesions as conjunctival or corneal intraepithelial neoplasia (CIN) or squamous cell carcinoma (SCC) is defined by histologic criteria. See also BCSC Section 4, *Ophthalmic Pathology and Intraocular Tumors.*

PATHOGENESIS Ultraviolet light exposure, aging, HPV infection, smoking, fair complexion, and immunosuppression play a role in the development of OSSN. Rapid growth may occur when the lesion is present in a person with AIDS. Systemic immunosuppression seems to potentiate squamous neoplasia. In a young adult, OSSN should prompt consideration of a serologic test for human immunodeficiency virus (HIV) infection.

Kamal S, Kaliki S, Mishra D, Batra J, Naik MN. Ocular Surface Squamous Neoplasia in 200 Patients. A case-control study of immunosuppression resulting from human immunodeficiency virus versus immunocompetency. *Ophthalmology.* 2015;122(8): 1688–1694.

Shields CL, Ramasubramanian A, Mellen PL, Shields JA. Conjunctival squamous cell carcinoma arising in immunosuppressed patients (organ transplant, human immunodeficiency virus infection). *Ophthalmology.* 2011;118(11):2133–2137.

Noninvasive OSSN: conjunctival or corneal intraepithelial neoplasia

Conjunctival or corneal intraepithelial neoplasia (CIN), or *dysplasia,* is analogous to actinic keratosis of the skin. In CIN, the dysplastic process does not involve the underlying basement membrane. CIN is considered a premalignant condition, at risk of transforming into squamous cell carcinoma. Related terms include *squamous dysplasia,* which is used when atypical cells invade only part of the epithelium, and *squamous carcinoma in situ,* used when cellular atypia involves the entire thickness of the epithelial layer.

CLINICAL PRESENTATION There are 3 principal clinical variants of conjunctival disease (Fig 12-4):

1. papilliform, in which a sessile papilloma harbors dysplastic cells
2. gelatinous, which occurs as a result of acanthosis and dysplasia
3. leukoplakic, which is caused by hyperkeratosis, parakeratosis, and dyskeratosis

CIN lesions are slow-growing tumors that are nearly always centered at the limbus but able to spread to other areas of the ocular surface. Mild inflammation and various degrees of abnormal vascularization may accompany CIN lesions; large feeder blood vessels indicate an increased probability of invasion beneath the epithelial basement membrane.

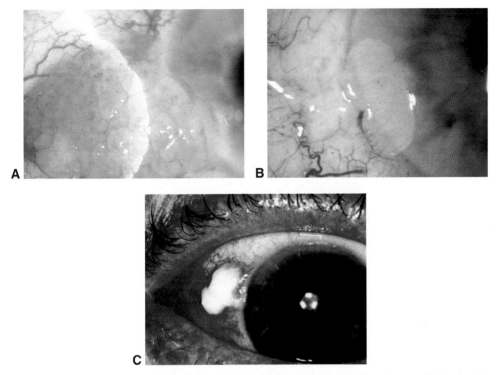

Figure 12-4 Conjunctival intraepithelial neoplasia. **A,** Papilliform. **B,** Gelatinous. **C,** Leukoplakic. *(Part A courtesy of James Chodosh, MD; parts B and C courtesy of James J. Reidy, MD.)*

Corneal involvement may present as a translucent, sometimes granular, gray epithelial sheet that is based at the limbus and extends onto the cornea. The edges of corneal lesions have characteristic fimbriated margins and pseudopodia-like extensions (Fig 12-5). Rose bengal and lissamine green staining help define the edges of the lesion. In some cases, the conjunctival or limbal component is not clinically apparent. Occasionally, free islands of corneal involvement are present.

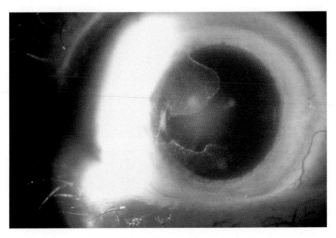

Figure 12-5 Corneal intraepithelial neoplasia. *(Courtesy of James Chodosh, MD.)*

Invasive OSSN: squamous cell carcinoma

In squamous cell carcinoma (SCC), involvement extends beyond the basement membrane into stroma, with metastatic potential. SCC is more common and aggressive in patients with compromised immunity and in those with xeroderma pigmentosum.

CLINICAL PRESENTATION A plaquelike, gelatinous, or papilliform growth occurs in limbal and bulbar conjunctiva, usually in the interpalpebral fissure zone. A broad base is often present along the limbus. The lesion tends to grow outward and have sharp borders; it may appear leukoplakic (Fig 12-6). Although histologic invasion beneath the epithelial basement membrane is present, growth usually remains superficial, with neoplastic cells infrequently penetrating the sclera or Bowman layer. Pigmentation can occur in dark-skinned patients. Engorged conjunctival vessels suggest malignancy. Note that the clinical appearance of CIN and invasive SCC may be similar (compare Figures 12-4C and 12-6).

Variants of squamous cell carcinoma *Mucoepidermoid carcinoma* is an aggressive variant of SCC that is more likely to invade the globe or orbit. It arises primarily in the salivary glands and rarely occurs in the conjunctiva. In addition to neoplastic epithelial cells, malignant goblet cells can be shown with mucin stains. Treatment is wide surgical excision; adjuvant therapy may include cryotherapy and radiotherapy.

Spindle cell carcinoma, another variant, is a rare, highly malignant SCC of the bulbar or limbal conjunctiva in which the anaplastic cells appear spindle shaped, like fibroblasts.

Shields JA, Shields CL. Premalignant and malignant lesions of the conjunctival epithelium. In: *Eyelid, Conjunctival, and Orbital Tumors: An Atlas and Textbook.* 3rd ed. Philadelphia: Wolters Kluwer; 2016:283–306.

Management of OSSN

All OSSN lesions should be treated as possible carcinoma with metastatic potential because it may be difficult to distinguish dysplasia from invasive squamous cell carcinoma clinically. See Figure 12-1, which summarizes the various treatment options for OSSN, as well as the section Management of Patients With Ocular Surface Tumors, earlier in the chapter.

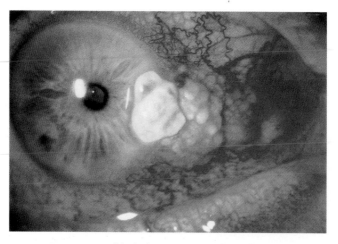

Figure 12-6 Limbal squamous cell carcinoma.

With the benefit of topical chemotherapy and modern surgical techniques, recurrence rates for OSSN range from less than 5% to 15%, compared with historical rates of up to 56%.

SCC can grow into the iris or trabecular meshwork or the orbit, providing a portal to the systemic circulation and metastasis. Orbital invasion may require orbital exenteration. Radiation therapy may be indicated as adjunctive therapy in select cases.

Glandular Tumors of the Conjunctiva

Oncocytoma

A slow-growing cystadenoma, an oncocytoma is a benign tumor arising from ductal and acinar cells of main and accessory lacrimal glands. Oncocytoma most commonly occurs in older persons and may present as a reddish-brown nodule on the surface of the caruncle.

Sebaceous Gland Carcinoma

Sebaceous gland carcinoma accounts for approximately 1% of all eyelid tumors and 5% of eyelid malignancies. It usually occurs in older individuals but may be seen in younger persons after radiation therapy. These tumors may masquerade as chalazia or as chronic unilateral blepharoconjunctivitis (Fig 12-7). Consequently, more than 50% of cases are initially misdiagnosed. Epithelial invasion of the conjunctiva occurs in almost 50% of

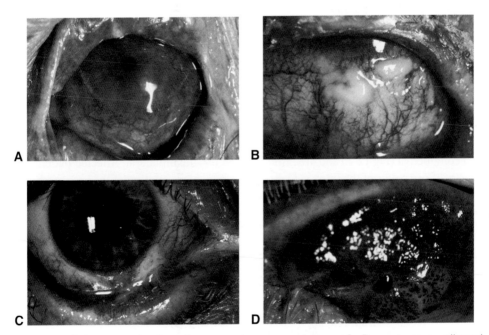

Figure 12-7 Sebaceous gland carcinoma: various presentations. **A,** Presents as a unilateral blepharoconjunctivitis with injection, pannus, thickened eyelid margin, and eyelash loss. **B,** White nodules composed of neoplastic sebaceous cells may be present near the limbus. **C,** Neoplastic symblepharon is present nasally. **D,** Upper palpebral conjunctival thickening. Papillary fronding may be present. *(Reproduced with permission from Mannis MJ, Holland EJ, eds.* Cornea. *Vol 1. 4th ed. Philadelphia: Elsevier; 2017:422.)*

cases and extends onto the cornea in more than 25% of cases. For further discussion, see BCSC Section 7, *Orbit, Eyelids, and Lacrimal System*.

Shields JA, Demirci H, Marr BP, Eagle RC Jr, Shields CL. Sebaceous carcinoma of the eyelids: personal experience with 60 cases. *Ophthalmology.* 2004;111(12):2151–2157.

Tumors of Neuroectodermal Origin

Table 12-2 lists the ocular surface tumors that arise from melanocytes, nevus cells, and other neuroectodermal cells. Some pigmented lesions of the globe are normal. For example, a *pigment spot of the sclera* is a collection of melanocytes associated with an intrascleral nerve loop or perforating anterior ciliary vessel. The term *melanosis* refers to excessive pigmentation without an elevated mass that may be congenital (whether epithelial or subepithelial) or acquired (whether primary or secondary). Conjunctival pigmentation can also occur because of long-term exposure to epinephrine compounds, minocycline, silver, or mascara (see Chapter 6, Fig 6-20).

Cameron JD, Maltry AC. Melanocytic neoplasms of the conjunctiva. In: Mannis MJ, Holland EJ, eds. *Cornea.* Vol 1. 4th ed. Philadelphia: Elsevier; 2017:434–441.

Shields CL, Demirci H, Karatza E, Shields JA. Clinical survey of 1643 melanocytic and non-melanocytic conjunctival tumors. *Ophthalmology.* 2004;111(9):1747–1754.

Benign Pigmented Lesions

Ocular melanocytosis

Congenital melanosis of the episclera occurs in approximately 1 in every 2500 individuals and is more common in black, Hispanic, and Asian populations.

PATHOGENESIS Ocular melanocytosis represents a focal proliferation of subepithelial melanocytes.

CLINICAL PRESENTATION Patches of episcleral pigmentation appear slate gray through the normal conjunctiva (Fig 12-8) and are immobile and usually unilateral. Affected patients may have a diffuse nevus of the uvea, evident as increased pigmentation of the iris and choroid.

Table 12-2 Tumors and Related Conditions of Neuroectodermal Cells of the Ocular Surface

Cell of Origin	Benign	Preinvasive/Malignant
Epithelial melanocytes	Freckle Complexion-associated melanosis	Primary acquired melanosis Melanoma
Subepithelial melanocytes	Ocular melanocytosis Melanocytoma	Melanoma
Nevus cells	Intraepithelial (junctional) nevus Compound nevus Subepithelial nevus	Melanoma
Neural and other cells	Neurofibroma	Leiomyosarcoma

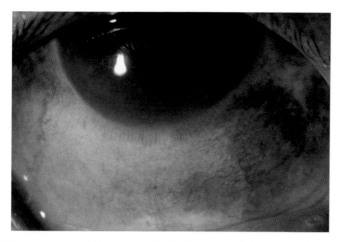

Figure 12-8 Episcleral pigmentation in a patient with congenital ocular melanocytosis. *(Courtesy of Kathryn Colby, MD, PhD.)*

In approximately 50% of patients with ocular melanocytosis, there is ipsilateral dermal melanocytosis and a proliferation of dermal melanocytes in the periocular skin of the first and second dermatomes of cranial nerve V. The combined ocular and cutaneous pigmentations are referred to as *oculodermal melanocytosis (nevus of Ota).* Approximately 5% of cases are bilateral. Table 12-3 compares the various pigmented lesions of the conjunctiva.

In 10% of patients with ocular melanocytosis, secondary glaucoma occurs in the affected eye. Malignant transformation is possible but rare and seems to occur only in patients

Table 12-3 Clinical Comparison of Conjunctival Pigmented Lesions

Lesion	Onset	Characteristics	Location	Malignant Potential
Nevus	First or second decade of life	Discrete, light tan to brown or amelanotic; may be flat or elevated. 50% contain epithelial inclusion cysts	Conjunctival epithelium and/or stroma	<1%
Complexion-associated melanosis (CAM)	Adulthood	Bilateral, flat, patchy, brown. Occurs in dark-skinned persons	Conjunctival epithelium	None to low
Ocular and oculodermal melanocytosis	Congenital	Usually unilateral; flat, slate gray	Episclera	<1%, uveal melanoma
Primary acquired melanosis (PAM)	Middle age	Unilateral, flat, patchy or diffuse, tan to brown. Occurs most often in light-skinned adults	Conjunctival epithelium	High risk with moderate to severe atypia
Malignant melanoma	Middle to late adulthood	Brown or amelanotic, often nodular, often vascular	Conjunctival stroma	Overall mortality rate 25%

with fair complexions. Malignant melanoma can develop in the skin, conjunctiva, uvea, or orbit. The lifetime risk of uveal melanoma in a patient with ocular melanocytosis is about 1 in 400—significantly greater than the approximate 6-per-million risk of the general population.

Nevus

Nevocellular nevi of the conjunctiva consist of nests or more diffuse infiltrations of benign melanocytes. They arise during the first or second decade of life. Conjunctival nevi are classified as junctional (confined to the epithelial–stromal junction); subepithelial, or stromal (confined to the stroma); or compound (combines junctional and stromal components). Pure intraepithelial nevi are rare except in children.

On histologic examination, nevi can occasionally be very difficult to differentiate from melanoma. Junctional nevi may be difficult to distinguish from primary acquired melanosis (see the section "Primary acquired melanosis" later in the chapter).

CLINICAL PRESENTATION A nevus near the limbus is usually almost flat. Nevi appearing elsewhere on the bulbar conjunctiva, plica semilunaris, caruncle, or eyelid margin tend to be elevated. Pigmentation of conjunctival nevi is variable: they may be light tan to brown or amelanotic (15% of cases; Fig 12-9). A subepithelial nevus often has a cobblestone appearance.

Small epithelial inclusion cysts occur within approximately half of all conjunctival nevi, particularly the compound or subepithelial varieties. Secretion of mucin by goblet cells in the inclusion cysts can cause a nevus to enlarge, giving a false impression of malignant change. Cellular proliferation may induce secondary lymphocytic inflammation. Rapid enlargement can occur at puberty, giving rise to a clinical impression of conjunctival melanoma. An amelanotic, vascularized nevus, when inflamed, may resemble an angioma, or it may be misdiagnosed as chronic conjunctivitis. See Table 12-3 for a clinical comparison of the various pigmented lesions of the conjunctiva.

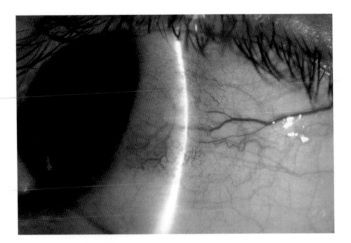

Figure 12-9 Amelanotic conjunctival nevus. *(Courtesy of Kathryn Colby, MD, PhD.)*

Jakobiec FA, Sandhu H, Bhat P, Colby K. Bilateral conjunctival melanocytic nevi of simultaneous onset simulating conjunctivitis in a child. *Cornea.* 2010;29(8):937–940.

Shields CL, Fasiuddin AF, Mashayekhi A, Shields JA. Conjunctival nevi: clinical features and natural course in 410 consecutive patients. *Arch Ophthalmol.* 2004;122(2):167–175.

MANAGEMENT Conjunctival nevi rarely become malignant and can be followed with an examination every 6–12 months that includes serial photography or detailed slit-lamp drawings incorporating dimensional measurements. Excisional biopsy should be performed on lesions that show suspicious change or growth. A biopsy should also be performed for pigmented lesions on the palpebral conjunctiva or cornea or in the fornix, as nevi are rare in these locations.

Complexion-associated melanosis

Complexion-associated melanosis (CAM; also called racial melanosis) is more commonly seen in individuals with darker complexions, but it occurs in all races (approximately 95% of blacks, 35% of Asians, 30% of Hispanics, and 5% of whites). CAM appears as flat, light- to dark-brown conjunctival patches with irregular margins that are most apparent at the limbus and less prominent as it extends into the fornix (Fig 12-10). The pigmentation can also involve the caruncle and palpebral conjunctiva as well as extend into the cornea with streaks or whorls (striate melanokeratosis). Histologic findings consist of hyperpigmentation of the conjunctival basal epithelial cells without atypia or hyperplasia. CAM is bilateral, fairly symmetric, and benign, with little risk of progression to melanoma. It is important to differentiate CAM from primary acquired melanosis (discussed in the following section), which seldom occurs in individuals with darker skin, is usually unilateral or highly asymmetric, and can transform to melanoma.

Shields JA, Shields CL. Conjunctival melanocytic lesions. In: *Eyelid, Conjunctival, and Orbital Tumors: An Atlas and Textbook.* 3rd ed. Philadelphia: Wolters Kluwer; 2016:307–348.

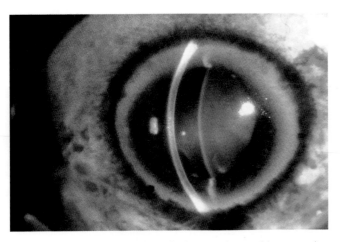

Figure 12-10 Complexion-associated melanosis in a patient with corneal arcus. *(Courtesy of James Chodosh, MD.)*

Preinvasive Pigmented Lesions

Primary acquired melanosis

CLINICAL PRESENTATION Primary acquired melanosis (PAM) is an acquired noncystic, flat, patchy or diffuse, tan to brown pigmentation of the conjunctival epithelium. The condition is usually unilateral or asymmetric if bilateral and is most often seen in light-skinned individuals (Fig 12-11). Secondary acquired melanosis has a similar appearance but is associated with systemic disease (eg, Addison disease), previous radiation, or pregnancy or is secondary to another conjunctival lesion (eg, squamous papilloma or carcinoma). Table 12-3 compares the various pigmented lesions of the conjunctiva.

Changes in the size of PAM may be associated with inflammation or may be the result of hormonal influences. Complete examination of the ocular surface (including double eversion of the upper eyelid) is essential in any patient with conjunctival pigmentation; see the following section for management of these lesions.

Folberg R, McLean IW, Zimmerman LE. Conjunctival melanosis and melanoma. *Ophthalmology.* 1984;91(6):673–678.

Shields JA, Shields CL. Conjunctival melanocytic lesions. In: *Eyelid, Conjunctival, and Orbital Tumors: An Atlas and Textbook.* 3rd ed. Philadelphia: Wolters Kluwer; 2016: 307–348.

MANAGEMENT Most cases of PAM are benign, but a substantial minority of cases may progress to melanoma. It is difficult to predict which lesions may progress, but clinical findings such as larger size (3 clock-hours or more) and caruncular, forniceal, or palpebral location portend a worse prognosis. Two clock-hours or less of conjunctival involvement is associated with a lower risk of malignant transformation; involvement of more than 2 clock-hours is an indication to remove the lesion for histologic diagnosis. Other worrisome signs include progressive enlargement, a nodular component, feeder vessels, and thickening.

The most important finding in predicting progression is the presence of cellular atypia, which can be determined only by excisional biopsy. As such, suspicious lesions should be removed and sent for histologic examination and immunohistochemistry. See

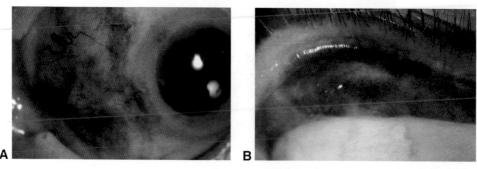

Figure 12-11 **A,** Diffuse primary acquired melanosis of the bulbar conjunctiva. **B,** Primary acquired melanosis of the palpebral conjunctiva. *(Courtesy of Kathryn Colby, MD, PhD.)*

BCSC Section 4, *Ophthalmic Pathology and Intraocular Tumors,* for a more detailed discussion of the evolving histologic classification of intraepithelial melanosis.

As PAM without atypia has little malignant potential, it may be followed (with examination every 6–12 months). PAM with mild atypia has a minimal risk of malignant transformation but should be followed more closely. However, PAM with moderate to severe atypia carriers a significant risk of progression to melanoma; thus, every effort should be made to eliminate all conjunctival pigment in patients with moderate to severe atypia. If the pigmentation is diffuse and not amenable to complete excision, adjuvant topical chemotherapy with mitomycin C may be useful to treat the entire ocular surface. The surgeon should exercise care in performing intraocular surgery in a patient with untreated ocular surface neoplasia, as violation of the Bowman layer may lead to tumor seeding within the corneal stroma and internal structures of the eye. Secondary acquired melanosis has no significant risk of progression to melanoma.

Cameron JD, Maltry AC. Melanocytic neoplasms of the conjunctiva. In: Mannis MJ, Holland EJ, eds. *Cornea.* Vol 1. 4th ed. Philadelphia: Elsevier; 2017:434–441.

Colby K, Bhat P, Novais G, Jakobiec FA. Recurrent primary acquired melanosis with atypia involving a clear corneal phacoemulsification wound. *Cornea.* 2011;30(1):114–116.

Jakobiec FA. Conjunctival primary acquired melanosis: is it time for a new terminology? *Am J Ophthalmol.* 2016;162:3–19.

Shields JA, Shields CL, Mashayekhi A, et al. Primary acquired melanosis of the conjunctiva: risks for progression to melanoma in 311 eyes. *Ophthalmology.* 2008;115(3):511–519.

Sugiura M, Colby KA, Mihm MC Jr, Zembowicz A. Low-risk and high-risk histologic features in conjunctival primary acquired melanosis with atypia: clinicopathologic analysis of 29 cases. *Am J Surg Pathol.* 2007;31(2):185–192.

Malignant Pigmented Lesions

Melanoma

With a prevalence of approximately 1 per 2 million in the population with European ancestry, conjunctival melanomas make up less than 1% of ocular malignancies in this group. Conjunctival melanomas are rare in black and Asian populations. Although malignant melanoma of the conjunctiva has a better prognosis than cutaneous melanoma, the overall mortality rate is 25%. The ONE Network on the American Academy of Ophthalmology website contains additional information on this topic, including video.

PATHOGENESIS Conjunctival melanomas may arise from PAM (70%) or nevi (5%) or may arise de novo (25%). Intralymphatic spread increases the risk of metastasis. In rare cases, an underlying ciliary body melanoma can extend through the sclera and mimic a conjunctival melanoma.

CLINICAL PRESENTATION Although conjunctival melanomas can arise in palpebral conjunctiva, they are most commonly found in the bulbar conjunctiva or at the limbus (Fig 12-12A). The degree of pigmentation is variable; approximately 25% of conjunctival melanomas are amelanotic. Recurrent melanomas are often amelanotic, even if the primary tumor was pigmented (Fig 12-12B). Because heavy vascularization is common,

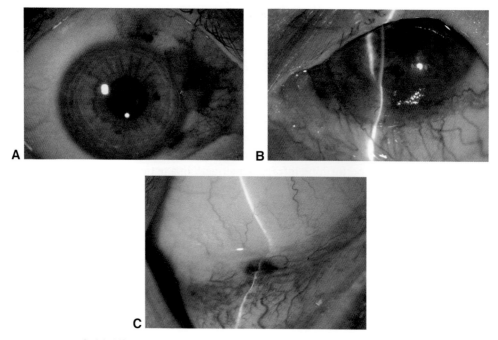

Figure 12-12 **A,** Multifocal, partially pigmented malignant melanoma of the limbal conjunctiva. **B,** Recurrent amelanotic conjunctival melanoma. The primary tumor was pigmented. **C,** Small conjunctival melanoma in the inferior fornix. *(Courtesy of Kathryn Colby, MD, PhD.)*

these tumors may bleed easily. They grow in a nodular fashion and can invade the globe or orbit. Poor prognostic indicators include

- location in the palpebral conjunctiva, caruncle, or fornix (Fig 12-12C)
- invasion into deeper tissues
- thickness >1.8 mm
- involvement of the eyelid margin
- pagetoid or full-thickness intraepithelial spread
- lymphatic invasion
- mixed cell type

Conjunctival melanomas may metastasize to regional lymph nodes, the brain, lungs, liver, and bone.

MANAGEMENT Ocular surface lesions worrisome for melanoma should be treated expeditiously using the paradigm described at the beginning of the chapter. Sentinel lymph node biopsy has been advocated by some authors but has not been widely adopted. Orbital exenteration is occasionally performed for advanced disease when local excision or enucleation cannot completely excise the tumor (when metastases have been excluded) or as palliative treatment for advanced, aggressive tumors that cannot be controlled locally. The role of adjunctive radiotherapy has not been determined.

Conjunctival melanoma has a high rate of recurrence (more than 50%). Patients with a history of conjunctival melanoma thus require lifelong, close ophthalmic follow-up and should be counseled to contact their physician immediately should they notice any changes in the involved eye. Conjunctival melanomas are potentially deadly tumors. In one study, metastasis was detected in 26% of patients, and death occurred in 13% of patients 10 years after surgical excision. Melanomas arising de novo (ie, not from preexisting nevi or PAM), tumors not involving the limbus, and residual involvement at the surgical margins are factors associated with an especially poor prognosis.

Manjandavida FP, Lally SE, Shields JA, Shields CL. *Conjunctival melanoma: what you should know.* [American Academy of Ophthalmology Annual Meeting Video]. San Francisco: American Academy of Ophthalmology; 2013. Available at www.aao.org.

Savar A, Ross MI, Prieto VG, Ivan D, Kim S, Esmaeli B. Sentinel lymph node biopsy for ocular adnexal melanoma: experience in 30 patients. *Ophthalmology.* 2009;116(11): 2217–2223.

Shields CL, Markowitz JS, Belinsky I, et al. Conjunctival melanoma. Outcomes based on tumor origin in 382 consecutive cases. *Ophthalmology.* 2011;118(2):389–395.

Shields JA, Shields CL. Conjunctival melanocytic lesions. In: *Eyelid, Conjunctival, and Orbital Tumors: An Atlas and Textbook.* 3rd ed. Philadelphia: Wolters Kluwer; 2016:307–348.

Neurogenic and Smooth-Muscle Tumors

Subconjunctival peripheral nerve sheath tumors such as *neurofibromas, schwannomas,* and *neuromas* have been reported, especially in multiple endocrine neoplasia (MEN). A neurofibroma of the conjunctiva or eyelid is almost always a manifestation of neurofibromatosis, an autosomal dominant phakomatosis (see BCSC Section 6, *Pediatric Ophthalmology and Strabismus*). A *neurilemoma* is a very rare tumor of the conjunctiva that originates from Schwann cells of a peripheral nerve sheath. A *leiomyosarcoma* is a very rare limbal lesion with the potential for orbital invasion.

Vascular and Mesenchymal Tumors

Vascular lesions of the eyelid margin or conjunctiva generally are benign hamartomas or secondary reactions to infection or other stimuli (Table 12-4).

Benign Tumors

Hemangioma

A capillary hemangioma is usually present at birth and may enlarge slowly. Isolated capillary and cavernous hemangiomas of the bulbar conjunctiva are rare and are more likely to represent extension from adjacent structures. The palpebral conjunctiva is frequently involved with a capillary hemangioma of the eyelid. The presence of diffuse hemangiomatosis of the

Table 12-4 Vascular Tumors of the Eyelid and Conjunctiva*

Hamartomatous	Reactive	Malignant
Nevus flammeus	Pyogenic granuloma	Kaposi sarcoma
Capillary hemangioma	Glomus tumor	Angiosarcoma
Cavernous hemangioma	Intravascular papillary endothelial hyperplasia	

*Tumors are not listed in any particular order, and lesions in one column do not necessarily correspond to those in parallel columns.

palpebral conjunctiva or conjunctival fornix indicates an orbital capillary hemangioma. A cavernous hemangioma of the orbit may present initially under the conjunctiva.

Nevus flammeus, a congenital lesion described as a port-wine stain, may occur alone or as part of Sturge-Weber syndrome, associated with vascular hamartomas, secondary glaucoma, and/or leptomeningeal angiomatosis. Some cases result from a mutation in the gene coding for the vascular endothelial protein receptor for angiopoietin 1, which controls the assembly of perivascular smooth muscle.

Ataxia-telangiectasia (also called Louis-Bar syndrome) is a syndrome of epibulbar telangiectasis, cerebellar abnormalities, and immune alterations. In this autosomal recessive disease, the epibulbar and interpalpebral telangiectasia of the arteries lacks an associated lymphatic component. The epibulbar vascular lesions of ataxia-telangiectasia can grow with the patient and the eyeball, but episodes of hemorrhage or swelling do not occur. See BCSC Section 6, *Pediatric Ophthalmology and Strabismus,* for additional discussion of ataxia-telangiectasia, including illustrations.

Inflammatory vascular tumors

Inflammatory conjunctival lesions often show vascular proliferation. *Pyogenic granuloma,* a common type of reactive hemangioma, is misnamed because it is not suppurative and does not contain giant cells. The lesion may occur over a chalazion or when minor trauma or surgery stimulates exuberant healing tissue with fibroblasts (granulation tissue) and proliferating capillaries that grow in a radiating pattern. This rapidly growing lesion is red, pedunculated, and smooth (Fig 12-13); it bleeds easily and stains with fluorescein dye. Topical or intralesional corticosteroids may be curative. Excision with cauterization to the base and generous postoperative topical corticosteroids may minimize recurrences.

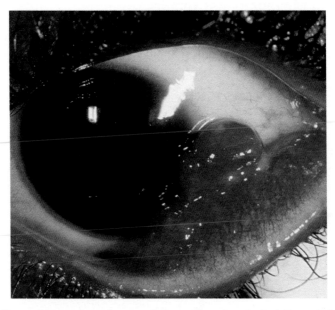

Figure 12-13 Pyogenic granuloma (in association with a chronically inflamed chalazion). *(Reproduced with permission from Mannis MJ, Holland EJ, eds. Cornea. Vol 1. 4th ed. Philadelphia: Elsevier; 2017:326.)*

Subconjunctival granulomas may form around parasitic and mycotic infectious foci. They have also occurred with connective tissue diseases such as rheumatoid arthritis. Sarcoid nodules appear as tan-yellow elevations that can resemble follicles. *Juvenile xanthogranuloma* is a histiocytic disorder that can present as a conjunctival mass. A *fibrous histiocytoma,* composed of fibroblasts and histiocytes with lipid vacuoles, arises, in rare cases, on the conjunctiva or limbus. *Nodular fasciitis* is a very rare benign tumor of fibrovascular tissue in the eyelid or under the conjunctiva; it may originate at the insertion site of a rectus muscle. *Necrobiotic xanthogranuloma* is a very rare tumor that may affect the anterior orbit and eyelids. The lesion can present as subconjunctival or subdermal nodular fibrovascular tissue. Biopsy is essential to establish the diagnosis because this tumor is often associated with paraproteinemias, multiple myeloma, or lymphoma.

Malignant Tumors

Kaposi sarcoma

Kaposi sarcoma, a malignant neoplasm of vascular endothelium, involves the skin and mucous membranes. Internal organs are occasionally involved as well.

PATHOGENESIS Infection with Kaposi sarcoma–associated herpesvirus/human herpesvirus 8 is responsible for this disease. In young patients, Kaposi sarcoma occurs most often in the setting of AIDS. Organ-transplant recipients and other highly immunosuppressed patients are at higher risk of developing Kaposi sarcoma.

CLINICAL PRESENTATION On the eyelid skin, Kaposi sarcoma presents as a purplish nodule. Orbital involvement may produce eyelid and conjunctival edema. In the conjunctiva, Kaposi sarcoma presents as a reddish, highly vascular subconjunctival lesion that may simulate a subconjunctival hemorrhage. The lesions are most often found in the inferior fornix and may be nodular or diffuse (Fig 12-14). Nodular lesions may be relatively less responsive than diffuse lesions to therapy.

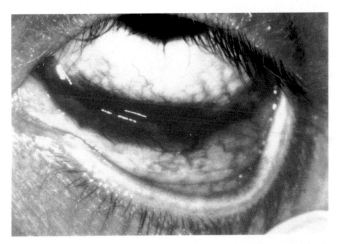

Figure 12-14 Kaposi sarcoma of the conjunctiva. *(Reproduced with permission from Holland GN, Pepose JS, Pettit TH, Gottlieb MS, Yee RD, Foos RY. Acquired immune deficiency syndrome. Ocular manifestations.* Ophthalmology. *1983;90(8):859–873. Photograph courtesy of Gary N. Holland, MD.)*

MANAGEMENT Treatment may not be curative. Options for controlling symptoms include surgical debulking, cryotherapy, and radiotherapy. Local or systemic chemotherapy may be required. Intralesional interferon-α_{2a} has been reported to be effective.

Other malignant tumors

Malignant mesenchymal lesions that infrequently involve the conjunctiva include malignant fibrous histiocytoma, liposarcoma, leiomyosarcoma, and rhabdomyosarcoma.

Lymphatic and Lymphocytic Tumors

Lymphoid tumors of the conjunctiva may be benign, malignant, or indeterminate. Many of these lesions have overlapping clinical and pathologic features. Approximately 20% of patients with a conjunctival lymphoid tumor have detectable extraocular lymphoma.

Lymphatic Malformations: Lymphangiectasia and Lymphangioma

Lymphangiectasia appears in the eye as irregularly dilated lymphatic channels in the bulbar conjunctiva. It may be a developmental anomaly, or it can occur following trauma or inflammation. Anomalous communication with a venule can lead to spontaneous filling of the lymphatic vessels with blood. Lymphangiectasia must be distinguished from ataxia-telangiectasia, an autosomal recessive disease in which the epibulbar and interpalpebral telangiectasia of the arteries lacks an associated lymphatic component.

Lymphangioma is the term applied when the collection of anomalous lymphatic channels has a formed rather than an amorphous appearance. Involvement can be solitary or multifocal. Often, there is a deeper orbital component that can be associated with pain, proptosis, motility problems, and vision loss. Like a capillary hemangioma, a lymphangioma is usually present at birth and may enlarge slowly. Intralesional hemorrhage can produce a "chocolate cyst."

> Jakobiec FA, Werdich XQ, Chodosh J, et al. An analysis of conjunctival and periocular venous malformations: clinicopathologic and immunohistochemical features with a comparison of racemose and cirsoid lesions. *Surv Ophthalmol.* 2014;59(2):236–244.

Lymphoid Hyperplasia

PATHOGENESIS Formerly called *reactive lymphoid hyperplasia*, this benign-appearing accumulation of lymphocytes and other leukocytes may represent a low-grade B-cell lymphoma.

CLINICAL PRESENTATION Lymphoid hyperplasia presents as a minimally elevated, salmon-colored subepithelial tumor with a pebbly appearance corresponding to follicle formation (Fig 12-15); it is clinically indistinguishable from conjunctival lymphoma. The lesion is often moderately or highly vascularized. Primary localized amyloidosis (discussed in Chapter 8) can have a similar appearance. Most patients with lymphoid hyperplasia are older than 40 years, although in rare instances, extranodal lymphoid hyperplasia has occurred in children.

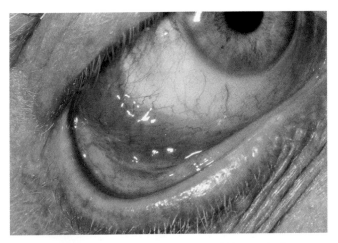

Figure 12-15 Conjunctival lymphoid hyperplasia.

MANAGEMENT Lymphoid hyperplasia may resolve spontaneously, but these lesions have been treated with local excision, topical corticosteroids, or radiation. Biopsy specimens require special handling to complete many of the histochemical and immunologic studies. Fresh tissue is required for immunohistochemistry, flow cytometry, and gene rearrangement studies. Because systemic lymphoma could potentially develop in a patient with an apparently benign polyclonal lymphoid lesion, general medical consultation is advisable.

Lymphoma

A neoplastic lymphoid lesion of the conjunctiva is generally a monoclonal proliferation of B lymphocytes.

PATHOGENESIS A lymphoma can arise in conjunctival lymphoid follicles. Some conjunctival lymphomas are limited to the conjunctiva; others occur in conjunction with systemic malignant lymphoma. The majority of conjunctival lymphomas are monoclonal B-cell mucosa-associated lymphoid tissue (MALT) lymphomas. Conjunctival plasmacytoma, Hodgkin lymphoma, and T-cell lymphomas are less common.

CLINICAL PRESENTATION Conjunctival lymphoma has essentially the same clinical appearance as benign lymphoid hyperplasia. It appears as a salmon-pink, mobile mass on the conjunctiva (Fig 12-16). The lesions are usually unilateral; 20% are bilateral. A diffuse lesion may masquerade as chronic conjunctivitis. An epibulbar mass fixed to the underlying sclera may be a sign of extrascleral extension of uveal lymphoid neoplasia. Most patients with conjunctival lymphoma are either older than 50 years or immunosuppressed.

LABORATORY EVALUATION AND MANAGEMENT Patients with conjunctival lymphoma should be referred to an oncologist for systemic evaluation because underlying systemic lymphoma may be present or may eventually develop in up to 31% of these patients. Unless a tumor is small enough to be removed completely, incisional biopsy is indicated for histologic

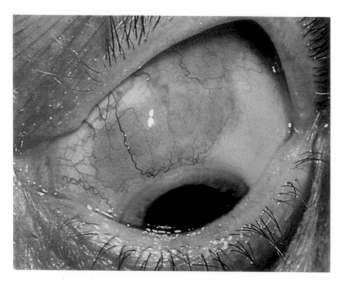

Figure 12-16 Conjunctival lymphoma.

diagnosis. Local external-beam radiation therapy is usually curative for lesions confined to the conjunctiva, but systemic chemotherapy is required for the treatment of systemic lymphoma. More recently described treatments for conjunctival MALT lymphoma include intralesional interferon-α_{2b} and intralesional or systemic rituximab.

Blasi MA, Tiberti AC, Valente P, et al. Intralesional interferon-α for conjunctival mucosa-associated lymphoid tissue lymphoma: long–term results. *Ophthalmology.* 2012;119(3): 494–500.

Raderer M, Kiesewetter B, Ferreri AJ. Clinicopathologic characteristics and treatment of marginal zone lymphoma of mucosa-associated lymphoid tissue (MALT lymphoma). *CA: A Cancer Journal for Clinicians.* 2016;66(2):153–171.

Shields CL, Shields JA, Carvalho C, Rundle P, Smith AF. Conjunctival lymphoid tumors: clinical analysis of 117 cases and relationship to systemic lymphoma. *Ophthalmology.* 2001; 108(5):979–984.

Warner MA, Stagner AM, Jakobiec FA. Subepithelial tumors of the conjunctiva. In: Mannis MJ, Holland EJ, eds. *Cornea.* Vol 1. 4th ed. Philadelphia: Elsevier; 2017:442–465.

Metastatic Tumors

Metastatic tumors to the conjunctiva are much less common than those to the uveal tract and orbit, but such tumors have arisen from cancer of the breast, lung, kidney, and elsewhere, including cutaneous melanoma. Metastatic lesions to the uveal tract, orbit, or paranasal sinuses can extend into the conjunctiva. Metastases or leukemic infiltrates to the limbus or cornea also occur.

CHAPTER 13

Therapeutic Interventions for Ocular Surface Disorders

Highlights

- Leaving bare sclera after pterygium excision is associated with higher morbidity and recurrence rates than covering the defect.
- The recurrence rate after pterygium surgery may be lower with a conjunctival graft than with amniotic membrane.
- Tissue glue can be used effectively to secure a conjunctival graft.
- Lateral tarsorrhaphy is the most underutilized procedure for treatment of problems arising from corneal surface disease.

Introduction

This chapter covers common surgical procedures and other therapeutic interventions used in the management of ocular surface disorders (Table 13-1). More detailed descriptions of these procedures and discussion of alternative surgical techniques can be found in surgical

Table 13-1 Indications for Ocular Surface Reconstruction

Conjunctival Autograft	Limbal Autograft*	Limbal Allograft†	Amniotic‡ or Mucous Membrane Transplantation
Cicatricial strabismus (bilateral)	Chemical injury	Aniridia	Chemical injury§
Fornix reconstruction (unilateral)	Chronic medication toxicity	Atopy	Conjunctival tumor removal
Postexcision of conjunctival tumor	Contact lens keratopathy	Mucous membrane pemphigoid	Fornix reconstruction (bilateral)
Pterygium surgery	Persistent epithelial defect (various etiologies)	Stevens-Johnson syndrome	Immune melts
Symblepharon repair	Limbal depletion after multiple surgeries		Mucous membrane pemphigoid
	Thermal burn		Pterygium surgery
			Stevens-Johnson syndrome

*A limbal autograft from the contralateral eye is preferable only in unilateral cases.
† A limbal allograft from donor tissue is preferable for bilateral disease.
‡ May be used in conjunction with a limbal autograft or allograft.
§ May need fornix reconstruction after cicatricization.

textbooks and other resources (see the references in this chapter). For additional discussion of the entities mentioned in this chapter, refer to the appropriate chapters in this book.

Conjunctival Interventions for Ocular Surface Disorders

Pterygium Excision

A pterygium is a wing-shaped pannus of conjunctiva and fibrovascular tissue on the superficial cornea (see Chapter 6). Indications for pterygium excision include ocular discomfort, decreased vision secondary to scarring or visually significant astigmatism, cosmesis, growth of the pterygium over the cornea toward the visual axis (Fig 13-1), and restricted ocular motility. The goal in pterygium excision is to achieve a clear and topographically smooth ocular surface. After excision, the most commonly used technique for coverage of exposed sclera is an autologous free graft from the same or fellow eye. The procedure is performed on an outpatient basis using topical anesthesia, although in some cases, such as a recurrent pterygium complicated by excessive proliferation of the Tenon layer, peribulbar or retrobulbar anesthesia may be required.

Surgical technique

A traction suture (eg, 6-0 silk or polyglactin on a spatulated needle, placed at the 12-o'clock position, that can be clamped down in various positions to the surgical drape) facilitates maximal exposure of both the pterygium for excision and the superior conjunctival graft site if a conjunctival transplant is planned. A common surgical technique is to remove the pterygium from the cornea by using a flat or angled crescent blade and dissecting a smooth tissue plane toward the limbus, between the pterygium and the underlying corneal tissue (ideally leaving the Bowman layer intact). Although it is preferable to dissect down to bare sclera at the limbus, the surgeon should be careful when dissecting Tenon

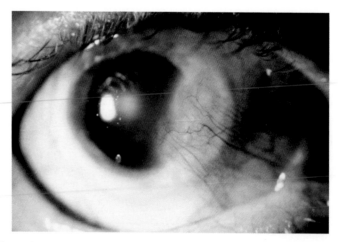

Figure 13-1 Pterygium on the cornea, encroaching on the visual axis. Opacification of the leading edge indicates that the pterygium has been present for some time. *(Courtesy of Woodford S. Van Meter, MD.)*

tissue posteriorly, as doing so can sometimes lead to bleeding and later scarring from inadvertent trauma to subjacent medial rectus muscle tissue and muscle check ligaments.

After excision, light cautery is usually applied to the sclera for hemostasis. It is important to remove as much as possible of the fibrovascular scar tissue in the Tenon layer, down to bare sclera, because residual Tenon tissue is a template for recurrence of the pterygium. If the medial rectus muscle is involved, it should be isolated and carefully freed of all scar tissue. A smooth scleral surface at the site of dissection is a desirable endpoint. Leaving the sclera bare is associated with a higher recurrence rate (32%–88%; Table 13-2). It also increases the occurrence of postoperative pain, perforation, and pyogenic granuloma, as well as corneal complications such as dellen and vascularization. There are many techniques for coverage of bare sclera: a conjunctival flap from contiguous tissue, a free conjunctival graft from the same or fellow eye, application of amniotic membrane using fibrin glue or sutures, and simple limbal epithelial transplantation.

Conjunctival autografting and other techniques for coverage of bare sclera

If there is only a small area of bare sclera after ptyergium excision, many surgeons use a sliding flap technique. This is performed by undermining contiguous conjunctival tissue and rotating it in place without tension. If there is a larger defect, conjunctival autograft transplantation using tissue from the superior bulbar conjunctiva is optimal. With a surgical pen, the area to be harvested is marked 0.5–1.0 mm larger than the size of the defect to account for some later retraction of the graft. It is essential to procure a flap of thin conjunctival tissue with only minimal or no Tenon tissue, which is facilitated by injecting a small amount of anesthetic (lidocaine 1% or 2% without epinephrine) between the conjunctiva and Tenon capsule. The donor material should be oriented in the host bed so that the limbal side of the graft is adjacent to the cornea in the excision site. The superior bulbar donor site under the eyelid can be left bare. Figure 13-2 shows various types of surgical wound closures after pterygium excision. Covering the entire defect decreases postoperative inflammation and speeds reepithelialization of the ocular surface.

Table 13-2 Recurrence Rates of Pterygium With Different Surgical Treatment Options

Surgical Option		Recurrence Rate, %
Bare sclera excision	Isolated	32–88
	With postoperative MMC* eyedrops	0–38
	With intraoperative MMC*	3–38
Amniotic membrane transplantation	Isolated	7–41
	With intraoperative MMC	16
Conjunctival autografting[†]	Isolated	1–39
	With postoperative MMC eyedrops	4–21
	With intraoperative MMC	0–16
	With fibrin glue	0–9
	With suture	9–16
Conjunctival–limbal autografting	Isolated	0–4
	With MMC*	18

MMC = mitomycin C.

*Various concentrations of and regimens for MMC.

[†] Conjunctival autografting refers to a free graft or a rotational or sliding flap.

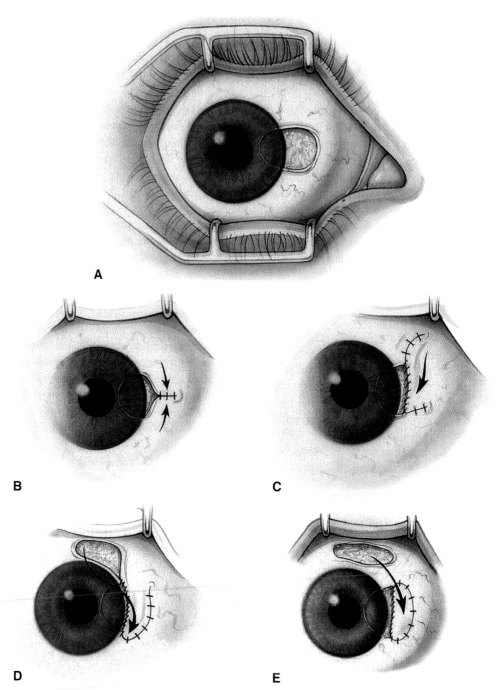

Figure 13-2 Surgical wound closures following pterygium excision. **A,** Bare sclera. **B,** Simple closure with fine, absorbable sutures. **C,** Sliding flap that is closed with interrupted and/or continuous suture. **D,** Rotational flap from the superior bulbar conjunctiva. **E,** Conjunctival autograft that is secured with interrupted and/or continuous sutures. *(Reproduced from Gans LA. Surgical treatment of pterygium. Focal Points: Clinical Modules for Ophthalmologists. San Francisco: American Academy of Ophthalmology; 1996, module 12. Illustration by Christine Gralapp.)*

In the case of either a sliding flap or free graft, the conjunctival tissue is then secured to adjacent conjunctiva (with or without incorporating episclera) with either 8-0 polyglactin (absorbable) sutures or 10-0 nylon (nonabsorbable) sutures, or alternatively with commercially available fibrin glue. Elimination of sutures reduces surgical time and decreases postoperative pain and inflammation.

Fibrin glue (also called fibrin sealant, fibrin tissue adhesive) mimics natural fibrin formation, ultimately resulting in the formation of a fibrin clot. Several fibrin glues have been approved by the US Food and Drug Administration (FDA) and are commercially available. These products include TISSEEL Fibrin Sealant (Baxter Healthcare Corp, Westlake Village, CA), EVICEL Fibrin Sealant (Ethicon Inc, Somerville, NJ), and BioGlue Surgical Adhesive (CryoLife Inc, Kennesaw, GA). Another option is the CryoSeal FS System (ThermoGenesis Corp, Rancho Cordova, CA), which can be used in the automated preparation of fibrin sealant from the patient's own plasma. Currently, use of these products in pterygium surgery is considered off-label. Also, because both pooled human plasma and bovine products are used to obtain some components of these sealants, the clinician should keep in mind the potential for disease transmission with their use.

If the defect created following dissection of the pterygium is considerably larger than what can be covered with an autologous conjunctival graft, then amniotic membrane grafting or simple limbal epithelial transplantation (SLET) are viable options. SLET is a newer technique that optimizes the use of limbal tissue from the healthy fellow eye by combining it with amniotic membrane; see the section Limbal Stem Cell Transplantation, later in the chapter, for a more detailed description.

Although there is evidence that the use of mitomycin C (MMC) with conjunctival grafting reduces the pterygium recurrence rate after surgical excision, further studies are necessary to determine the optimal route of administration and dose, as well as the duration of treatment with MMC and its long-term effects. Any use of topical MMC can be toxic and may cause visually significant complications, such as aseptic scleral necrosis and infectious sclerokeratitis. These complications may occur months or even years after use of the drug. If MMC use is being considered, it is safer to apply this agent intraoperatively than to give it to the patient for postoperative topical application.

Ganelis IB. Pterygium excision with transplantation surgery. In: *Basic Techniques of Ophthalmic Surgery.* 2nd ed. San Francisco: American Academy of Ophthalmology; 2015:101–108.

Hernandez-Bogantes E, Amescua G, Navas A, et al. Minor ipsilateral simple limbal epithelial transplantation (mini-SLET) for pterygium treatment. *Br J Ophthalmol.* 2015;99(7): 1598–1600.

Hirst LW. Pterygium surgery. *Focal Points: Clinical Modules for Ophthalmologists.* San Francisco: American Academy of Ophthalmology; 2009, module 3.

Kheirkhah A, Hashemi H, Adelpour M, Nikdel M, Rajabi MB, Behrouz MJ. Randomized trial of pterygium surgery with mitomycin C application using conjunctival autograft versus conjunctival-limbal autograft. *Ophthalmology.* 2012;119(2):227–232.

Lindquist TP, Lee WB. Amniotic membrane transplantation. In: *Basic Techniques of Ophthalmic Surgery.* 2nd ed. San Francisco: American Academy of Ophthalmology; 2015:109–114.

Long T, Li Z. Bare sclera resection followed by mitomycin C and/or autograft limbus conjunctiva in the surgery for pterygium: a meta-analysis. *Int J Ophthalmol.* 2015;8(5):1067–1073.

Pan HW, Zhong JX, Jing CX. Comparison of fibrin glue versus suture for conjunctival autografting in pterygium surgery: a meta-analysis. *Ophthalmology.* 2011;118(6):1049–1054.

Postoperative care

After pterygium surgery, topical antibiotic drops may be used for 1 week or until reepithelialization occurs, as well as topical steroid drops for approximately 4–6 weeks or as needed until inflammation has subsided. The use of bevacizumab in primary pterygium excision has not been reported to reduce the recurrence rate of this condition.

Complications

Complications of pterygium excision include conjunctival graft edema, corneoscleral dellen, and epithelial cysts. Pyogenic granuloma due to incomplete removal of subconjunctival and Tenon fibrovascular tissue may also occur, as well as chronic nonhealing wounds if exposed sclera remains uncovered by autologous conjunctiva. Diplopia may result from severe scarring around the medial rectus muscle. Postoperative infections are rare, but cases reported in the literature reveal a poor visual outcome; thus, postoperative care should not be taken lightly.

Clearfield E, Muthappan V, Wang X, Kuo IC. Conjunctival autograft for pterygium. *Cochrane Database Syst Rev.* 2016;(2):CD011349.

Kaufman SC, Jacobs DS, Lee WB, Deng SX, Rosenblatt MI, Shtein RM. Options and adjuvants in surgery for pterygium: a report by the American Academy of Ophthalmology. *Ophthalmology.* 2013;120(1):201–208.

Masters JS, Harris DJ Jr. Low recurrence rate of pterygium after excision with conjunctival limbal autograft: a retrospective study with long-term follow-up. *Cornea.* 2015;34(12): 1569–1572.

Autologous Conjunctival Transplantation

Autologous conjunctival transplantation is useful when conjunctival loss is not complicated by extensive damage to the limbal epithelial stem cells. The most common indication for this technique is coverage of bare sclera after pterygium excision (see the section Pterygium Excision, earlier in the chapter). Another indication is a clinically significant pinguecula causing chronic ocular redness and irritation. Conjunctival autografts from the opposite eye have been used to treat fornix foreshortening occurring after localized surgery, such as retinal detachment surgery with a scleral buckle, strabismus surgery, or excision of ocular surface tumors or nevi. Conditions associated with bilateral fornix obliteration (eg, mucous membrane pemphigoid, Stevens-Johnson syndrome) are usually systemic, so uninvolved conjunctiva is not available for grafting. Mucous membrane transplantation may be used in these cases and is discussed later in this chapter.

Conjunctival Flap for Corneal Disease

Indications

A conjunctival flap can be used to cover an unstable or painful corneal surface with a hinged flap of more durable conjunctiva when there is little chance of resolution by normal corneal wound healing. Conjunctival flaps provide a vascularized epithelial cover for the cornea but are not optically clear. Conjunctival flap surgery is performed less frequently now than in the past because of the availability of bandage and scleral contact lenses, commercially available amniotic membrane, use of tarsorrhaphy, and broadened indications for penetrating keratoplasty (PK) and lamellar keratoplasty (see Chapter 15). Nevertheless, the conjunctival flap remains an effective method for managing inflammatory and structural corneal disorders when restoration of vision is not the primary concern. The use of a conjunctival flap is controversial in patients with active microbial keratitis or corneal perforation because residual infectious organisms may proliferate in the avascular corneal stroma beneath the flap. A corneal perforation may continue to leak under the flap.

The principal indications for a conjunctival flap are as follows:

- chronic, sterile, nonhealing epithelial defects (stromal herpes simplex or herpes zoster virus keratitis, chemical and thermal burns, keratoconjunctivitis sicca, post-infectious ulcers, neurotrophic keratopathy)
- closed but unstable corneal wounds
- painful bullous keratopathy in a patient who is not a good candidate for PK
- a phthisical eye being prepared for a prosthetic shell

The disadvantages of conjunctival flap surgery are a reduced view of the anterior chamber and the creation of a potential barrier to drug penetration through the cornea into the anterior chamber. However, a successful conjunctival graft, free of buttonholes, will thin out and if blood vessels regress, may eventually enable usable vision.

Surgical technique

A complete (Gundersen) flap (Figs 13-3, 13-4) is a highly successful technique if the surgeon pays close attention to several fundamental principles for covering the corneal surface with vascularized tissue and keeping this tissue in place:

- complete removal of the corneal epithelium and debridement of necrotic tissue from the cornea
- reinforcement of thin areas with corneal or scleral tissue
- creation of a mobile, thin conjunctival flap that contains minimal Tenon capsule
- absence of any conjunctival buttonholes
- absence of any traction on the flap at its margins, which may lead to flap retraction

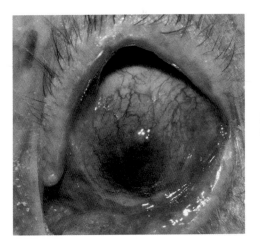

Figure 13-3 Gundersen flap. *(Courtesy of Wood-ford S. Van Meter, MD.)*

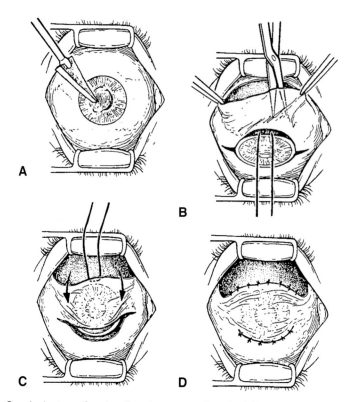

Figure 13-4 Surgical steps for the Gundersen conjunctival flap. **A,** Removal of the corneal epithelium using cellulose sponges. **B,** A 360° peritomy with relaxing incisions, placement of a superior limbal traction suture, a superior forniceal incision, and dissection of a thin flap. **C,** Positioning of the flap. **D,** Suturing of the flap into position with multiple interrupted sutures. *(Reproduced with permission from Mannis MJ. Conjunctival flaps.* Int Ophthalmol Clin. *1988;28(2):165–168.)*

Retrobulbar, peribulbar, or general anesthesia should be used for this procedure. The corneal epithelium and all necrotic tissue are first removed, and the eye is retracted inferiorly with an intracorneal traction suture (6-0 silk) at the superior limbus. Elevation of the flap with subconjunctival injection of lidocaine 1%–2% with epinephrine to separate the conjunctiva from underlying Tenon capsule enhances anesthesia, facilitates dissection, and reduces bleeding. The needle for this injection should not pierce the conjunctiva in the area to be used for the flap.

The dissection may start from either the limbus or the superior fornix. Dissection of conjunctiva from underlying Tenon fascia must be performed carefully to prevent conjunctival perforation, especially in eyes with previous conjunctival surgery. Once the flap has been dissected, a 360° peritomy is performed with relaxing incisions, followed by removal of all remaining limbal and corneal epithelium. Additional undermining of the flap allows it to cover the entire cornea and to rest there without traction. Any residual tension may foster later retraction of the flap. After the flap is positioned over the prepared cornea, it is sutured to the sclera just posterior to the limbus superiorly and inferiorly with 8-0 polyglactin or 10-0 nylon sutures, depending on the surgeon's preference.

Alternatives to the Gundersen flap are smaller or temporary conjunctival flaps (Fig 13-5):

- bipedicle flap
- advancement flap
- single pedicle flap

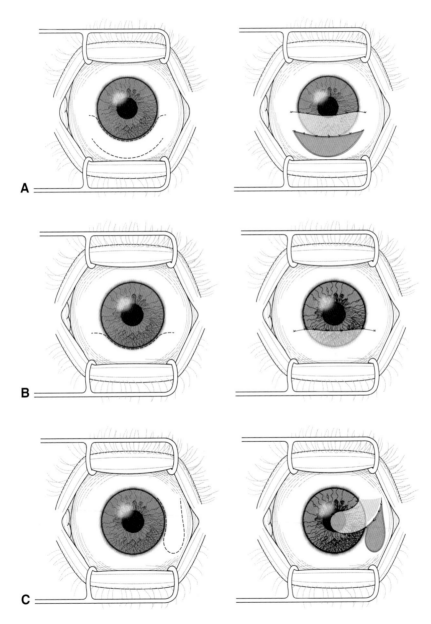

Figure 13-5 **A,** Bipedicle flap. **B,** Advancement flap. **C,** Single pedicle flap. *(Illustration by Mark Miller.)*

These flaps may be used for temporary coverage of small peripheral corneal wounds or areas of ulceration. The advantage is that only small or partial areas of the cornea are covered, so details of the anterior chamber can be visualized, and the patient may regain functional vision. As retraction is a common feature of all of these temporary flaps, the surgeon should take care to minimize tension on any conjunctival flap when it is placed.

> Johnson DA. Gundersen flap. In: *Basic Techniques of Ophthalmic Surgery.* 2nd ed. San Francisco: American Academy of Ophthalmology; 2015:125–130.

Complications

Retraction is the most common complication of conjunctival flaps, occurring in approximately 10% of cases. Other complications include hemorrhage beneath the flap and epithelial cysts. In some cases, inclusion cysts enlarge to the point of requiring excision or marsupialization. Ptosis, usually due to levator dehiscence in elderly patients, may also occur postoperatively and may or may not be related to the flap itself. Unsatisfactory cosmetic appearance can be improved with a painted cosmetic contact lens. Progressive corneal disease under any type of conjunctival flap is a concern in patients with infectious or autoimmune conditions.

Considerations in removal of a flap

If PK or lamellar keratoplasty is to be performed in an eye with a conjunctival flap, the flap may be removed either as a separate procedure or at the time of keratoplasty. Removal of the flap (without keratoplasty) usually does not succeed in restoring vision, as the underlying cornea is almost always opaque from subepithelial scarring and/or thinned. Because the conjunctival flap procedure tends to destroy or displace most limbal stem cells, a limbal autograft or allograft after removal of the flap may be necessary in order to provide a permanent source of normal epithelial cells before an optical corneal transplant is attempted.

> Khodadoust A, Quinter AP. Microsurgical approach to the conjunctival flap. *Arch Ophthalmol.* 2003;121(8):1189–1193.

Conjunctival Biopsy

Indications

A conjunctival biopsy can be helpful in evaluating chronic conjunctivitis and unusual ocular surface diseases, including the following:

- squamous lesions of the conjunctiva (eg, conjunctival intraepithelial neoplasia)
- cicatrizing conjunctivitis
- conjunctival lymphoid tumors
- lichen planus
- pemphigus vulgaris
- graft-vs-host disease
- superior limbic keratoconjunctivitis

Surgical technique

Topical anesthetic eyedrops, as well as a pledget soaked with lidocaine 1% or 2%, are applied to the lesion or biopsy site for approximately 30 seconds. Subconjunctival anesthesia (lidocaine 1% or 2% with epinephrine) may also be used; the advantages of injection of lidocaine for local anesthesia are improved analgesia, blanching of the conjunctival vessels, and reduced bleeding. The surgeon uses forceps and scissors to snip a conjunctival specimen sufficient for histologic examination. For a subepithelial lesion, a wedge or block is excised. Grasping only the edge of the specimen minimizes crushing and preserves tissue integrity. Gentle cauterization can be used to facilitate hemostasis after the specimen has been removed.

Leung TG, Thorne JE. Conjunctival biopsy. In: *Basic Techniques of Ophthalmic Surgery*. 2nd ed. San Francisco: American Academy of Ophthalmology; 2015:121–124.

Tissue processing

The sample is placed in the proper anatomical orientation on a carrier template (eg, filter paper) and inserted into the appropriate fixative, such as 10% neutral-buffered formalin (for histology), 3% glutaraldehyde (for electron microscopy), or Michel or Zeus transport medium (for immunofluorescence microscopy). A preoperative consultation with the pathologist is advised to ensure proper handling and staining of specimens. See BCSC Section 4, *Ophthalmic Pathology and Intraocular Tumors,* for further discussion of tissue processing.

Treatment of Conjunctivochalasis

Conjunctivochalasis is characterized by the presence of redundant conjunctival folds positioned between the globe and the lower eyelid margin (see Chapter 4, Fig 4-4 and discussion of conjunctivochalasis in Chapter 4). Surgical procedures used to treat these redundant folds include superficial cauterization, conjunctival fixation, resection, and amniotic membrane grafting.

Superficial cauterization

A topical anesthetic (eg, proparacaine hydrochloride 0.5%) is administered. The patient is instructed to look upward and remains in this position throughout the procedure. After either topical anesthetic or subconjunctival injection of 0.2 mL of lidocaine 1% with epinephrine is given, the surgeon grasps the redundant conjunctiva 4 mm from the limbus and cauterizes it, starting with low-voltage (power level 0.6) bipolar cauterization and gradually increasing the voltage until the conjunctiva coagulates. Coagulation is considered adequate when the conjunctiva turns white. Coagulation is performed at 5–10 sites in an arc on the inferior bulbar conjunctiva. The slack conjunctiva shrinks and tightens immediately after coagulation.

Nakasato S, Uemoto R, Mizuki N. Thermocautery for inferior conjunctivochalasis. *Cornea.* 2012;31(5):514–519.

Conjunctival fixation (plication)

The lower bulbar conjunctiva is pulled inferiorly, stretched to flatten, and sutured to the inferior sclera with 3 interrupted 6-0 absorbable sutures using episcleral bites inserted 8–10 mm posterior to the limbus. The resulting fold of bulbar conjunctiva must be well below the eyelid margin to prevent the patient from experiencing a foreign-body sensation after the procedure.

Resection

The surgical technique used for resection of the conjunctiva involves a crescent excision of the inferior bulbar conjunctiva 5 mm from the limbus, followed by suture closure. A modified technique to avoid visible scarring or retraction of the inferior conjunctival fornix includes a peritomy made close to the limbus, followed by 2 radial relaxing incisions to excise the redundant conjunctiva. Some surgeons use fibrin glue instead of sutures to close the conjunctival wound.

Amniotic membrane grafting

After excision of the redundant crescent of conjunctiva, an amniotic membrane is fitted to cover the entire defect and placed with the basement membrane surface up to cover the scleral wound. The membrane is secured to the surrounding conjunctival edge with interrupted fine, absorbable, or nylon sutures with episcleral bites. The surgeon must take care to flatten the membrane tightly onto the scleral surface and approximately to or underneath the epithelial edge.

Doss LR, Doss EL, Doss RP. Paste-pinch-cut conjunctivoplasty: subconjunctival fibrin sealant injection in the repair of conjunctivochalasis. *Cornea.* 2012;31(8):959–962.

Meller D, Maskin SL, Pires RT, Tseng SC. Amniotic membrane transplantation for symptomatic conjunctivochalasis refractory to medical treatments. *Cornea.* 2000;19(6):796–803.

Otaka I, Kyu N. A new surgical technique for management of conjunctivochalasis. *Am J Ophthalmol.* 2000;129(3):385–387.

Limbal Stem Cell Transplantation

The peripheral corneal epithelium is derived from stem cells residing in the basal layer of the corneal limbus. However, when the limbal stem cells are not functioning properly, the conjunctival epithelium proliferates over the surface of the cornea. Conjunctival cells do not have the pluripotency of limbal stem cells and cannot differentiate into the corneal phenotype. Replacement of the corneal epithelium by conjunctival epithelium is characterized by abnormal epithelium on the cornea, vascularization, surface irregularity, absence of the limbal palisades of Vogt, and poor epithelial adhesion, a process called *conjunctivalization.*

Minor disturbances to the corneal limbal stem cell function or surface may be reversible with medical therapy using topical corticosteroid drops, topical cyclosporine, oral doxycycline, punctal occlusion, frequent topical lubrication, or a combination of these modalities.

If total loss of limbal stem cells occurs unilaterally, an autograft of limbal epithelium from the fellow eye can repopulate the diseased cornea with normal corneal epithelium (Fig 13-6). In this procedure, the unhealthy corneal epithelium, conjunctiva, and any pannus are removed from within 2 mm of the limbus of the recipient eye, and 2 thin limbal autografts from the fellow eye are then attached to the limbus to facilitate the regeneration and proliferation of corneal epithelial cells.

If total loss of limbal stem cells occurs bilaterally, the patient may receive stem cells from a living related donor (ie, a limbal stem cell allograft) or from an eye bank donor cornea (ie, a keratolimbal allograft). A limbal stem cell allograft may decrease the risk of rejection but requires immunosuppression; it also enables more conjunctiva to be harvested and

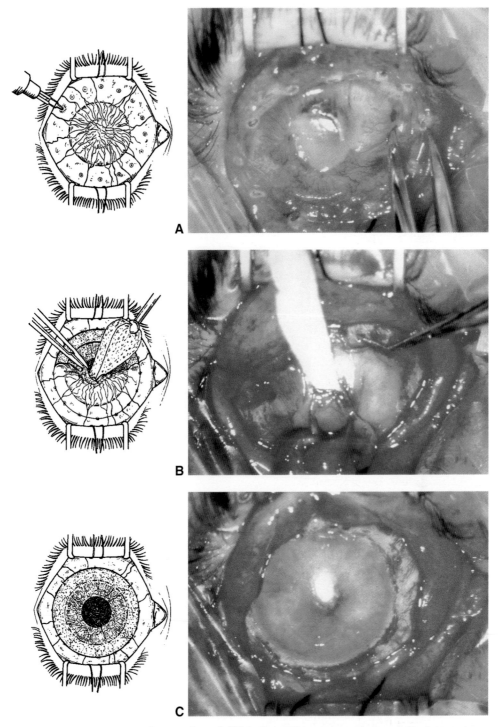

Figure 13-6 Limbal autograft procedure. **A,** With disposable cautery, the area of bulbar conjunctiva to be resected is marked approximately 2 mm posterior to the limbus. **B,** After conjunctival resection, abnormal corneal epithelium and fibrovascular pannus are stripped by blunt dissection using cellulose sponges, metal spatula blades, and/or tissue forceps. **C,** Additional surface polishing smooths the stromal surface and improves visual acuity. *(Continued)*

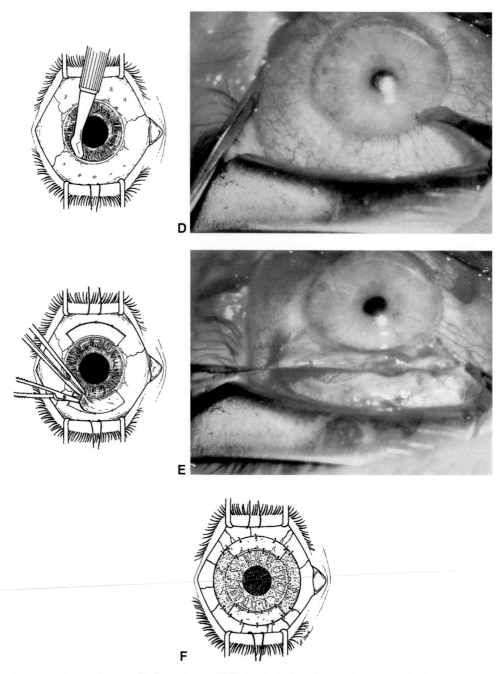

Figure 13-6 *(continued)* **D,** Superior and inferior limbal grafts are delineated in the donor eye with focal applications of cautery approximately 2 mm posterior to the limbus. The initial incision is made superficially within clear cornea using a disposable knife. **E,** The bulbar conjunctival portion of the graft is undermined and thinly dissected from its limbal attachment. **F,** The limbal grafts are transferred to their corresponding sites in the recipient eye and are secured with interrupted sutures, a 10-0 nylon suture at the corneal edge, and an 8-0 polyglactin suture at the conjunctival margin. *(Reproduced from Kenyon KR, Tseng SC. Limbal autograft transplantation for ocular surface disorders. Ophthalmology. 1989;96(5):709–723.)*

transplanted than does a keratolimbal allograft. Although host cells may eventually reject or replace such tissue, good long-term results have been reported using both techniques. Poor epithelial viability and complications from systemic immunosuppression are considerable obstacles to be overcome, but dramatic success has been observed in some cases.

Simple limbal epithelial transplantation (SLET) is a promising new technique for unilateral stem cell injury that obviates the need for intensive systemic immunosuppression, which conventional transplantation requires (see also Pterygium Excision, earlier in the chapter). After the abnormal cornea is denuded of pannus with a superficial keratectomy and covered with amniotic membrane, a small 2×2-mm strip of donor limbal tissue from the healthy fellow eye is divided into 8 or 10 pieces; these are placed evenly over the cornea with fibrin adhesive and then covered with a bandage contact lens.

Cell culture of corneal stem cells has been shown to be an effective source of corneal surface repopulation; however, the long-term survival of these grafts remains uncertain. Epithelial cells present in the oral mucosa and the human umbilical cord are emerging as important sources of cultured stem cells; at present, these approaches remain experimental and are available in few centers worldwide.

Basu S, Sureka SP, Shanbhag SS, Kethiri AR, Singh V, Sangwan VS. Simple limbal epithelial transplantation: long-term clinical outcomes in 125 cases of unilateral chronic ocular surface burns. *Ophthalmology.* 2016;123(5):1000–1010.

Biber JM, Skeens HM, Neff KD, Holland EJ. The Cincinnati procedure: technique and outcomes of combined living-related conjunctival limbal allografts and keratolimbal allografts in severe ocular surface failure. *Cornea.* 2011;30(7):765–771.

Holland EJ, Mogilishetty G, Skeens HM, et al. Systemic immunosuppression in ocular surface stem cell transplantation: results of a 10-year experience. *Cornea.* 2012;31(6):655–661.

Kim BY, Riaz KM, Bakhtiari P, et al. Medically reversible limbal stem cell disease: clinical features and management strategies. *Ophthalmology.* 2014;121(10):2053–2058.

Sangwan VS, Basu S, MacNeil S, Balasubramanian D. Simple limbal epithelial transplantation (SLET): a novel surgical technique for the treatment of unilateral limbal stem cell deficiency. *Br J Ophthalmol.* 2012;96(7):931–934.

Suh LH, Chuck RS. Limbal stem cell transplantation. In: *Basic Techniques of Ophthalmic Surgery.* 2nd ed. San Francisco: American Academy of Ophthalmology; 2015:115–120.

Zhao Y, Ma L. Systematic review and meta-analysis on transplantation of ex vivo cultivated limbal epithelial stem cell on amniotic membrane in limbal stem cell deficiency. *Cornea.* 2015;34(5):592–600.

Mucous Membrane Grafting

In the absence of healthy conjunctiva (eg, in bilateral cicatricial conjunctival disease), mucous membrane may be used to restore the conjunctival surface to a more functional state. The goals of restoration are to create a more normal fornix and to reduce ocular surface inflammation, as well as to minimize corneal damage from the abnormal eyelid–globe relationships (eg, entropion, trichiasis), chronic exposure (lagophthalmos), and direct corneal trauma (palpebral conjunctival keratinization) that usually accompany bilateral cicatricial conjunctival disorders (see Table 13-1). Mucous membrane grafts increase ocular surface wetting by improving eyelid movement and distribution of the tear film over the cornea, thereby reducing exposure and evaporation. These grafts also provide suitable extracellular matrix substrate for epithelial cell migration and adhesion, but they are not effective in replacing normal stem cells.

Mucous membrane grafting has produced good results in inactive cicatricial disorders such as late-stage, nonprogressive Stevens-Johnson syndrome and quiescent mucous membrane pemphigoid (MMP). A combination of limbal allografting, amniotic membrane transplantation, and tarsorrhaphy, followed by the use of serum-derived tears and systemic immunosuppression, allows reconstruction of the ocular surface. Patients with advanced, progressive stage III or IV MMP require advanced immunosuppressive treatment to reduce active inflammation prior to any grafting procedure (see the discussion of MMP in Chapter 11). Keratoprosthesis is another treatment for patients with late-stage cicatricial disease (see Chapter 15).

Multiple surgical techniques for mucosal grafting are available; the reader is encouraged to consult a surgical textbook or video for discussion and illustration of these techniques (see the reference list that follows). Potential complications, regardless of the technique, include buttonholing, graft retraction, trichiasis, surface keratinization of the graft, ptosis, blepharophimosis, depressed eyelid blink, lagophthalmos, submucosal abscess formation, and persistent nonhealing epithelial defects of the cornea.

Black E, Nesi FA, Gladstone G, Levine MR, Clavano CJ, eds. *Smith and Nesi's Oculoplastic and Reconstructive Surgery*. 3rd ed. New York: Springer; 2012.

Chun YS, Park IK, Kim JC. Technique for autologous nasal mucosa transplantation in severe ocular surface disease. *Eur J Ophthalmol*. 2011;21(5):545–551.

Fu Y, Liu J, Tseng SC. Oral mucosal graft to correct lid margin pathologic features in cicatricial ocular surface diseases. *Am J Ophthalmol*. 2011;152(4):600–608.e1.

Liu J, Sheha H, Fu Y, Giegengack M, Tseng SC. Oral mucosal graft with amniotic membrane transplantation for total limbal stem cell deficiency. *Am J Ophthalmol*. 2011;152(5):739–747.

Sant'Anna AE, Hazarbassanov RM, de Freitas D, Gomes JA. Minor salivary glands and labial mucous membrane graft in the treatment of severe symblepharon and dry eye in patients with Stevens-Johnson syndrome. *Br J Ophthalmol*. 2012;96(2):234–239.

Takeda K, Nakamura T, Inatomi T, Sotozono C, Watanabe A, Kinoshita S. Ocular surface reconstruction using the combination of autologous cultivated oral mucosal epithelial transplantation and eyelid surgery for severe ocular surface disease. *Am J Ophthalmol*. 2011;152(2):195–201.

Corneal Interventions for Ocular Surface Disorders

Superficial Keratectomy and Corneal Biopsy

Indications

In superficial keratectomy, the surgeon excises the superficial layers of cornea (epithelium, Bowman layer, or superficial stroma) without replacing the tissue. The primary indications are as follows:

- removal of hyperplastic or necrotic tissue (eg, corneal dermoid, pterygium, Salzmann nodular degeneration, epithelial basement membrane redundancy, degenerative calcification)
- excision of retained foreign material in the cornea

- need for tissue for diagnosis (histology or microbiology)
- excision of scar tissue or superficial corneal dystrophic tissue

If corneal biopsy is performed for histology, preservation of tissue integrity and anatomical orientation is important. A small specimen can be placed on a filter or thin card to maintain the tissue orientation before fixation or cryosection. For microbiology workup, the biopsied specimens can be minced or homogenized before inoculation of the culture media or tissue smear for histochemical staining.

Surgical techniques

Mechanical keratectomy   If the corneal lesion is superficial, it may be possible to scrape or peel it away without sharp dissection. Often, a smooth anatomical tissue plane anterior to the Bowman layer can be achieved with sweeping strokes parallel to the tissue through the use of a metal spatula blade or a cellulose sponge. In some cases, such as in Salzmann nodular degeneration, it is possible to gently peel the abnormal tissue off using a 0.12 forceps. When deeper dissection is required, the surgeon can either mark the area freehand with an adjustable-depth blade or use a trephine. A 2- to 3-mm disposable dermatologic skin punch trephine blade can be used to create a partial-thickness incision, and forceps and scissors are then used to excise a lamellar flap of cornea. The specimen is generally split into 2 pieces, or separate biopsies are taken, so that tissue can be sent for both histologic and microbiologic examination.

Alió JL, Agdeppa MC, Uceda-Montanes A. Femtosecond laser–assisted superficial lamellar keratectomy for the treatment of superficial corneal leukomas. *Cornea.* 2011;30(3):301–307.

Kron-Gray MM, Mian SI. Corneal biopsy. In: *Basic Techniques of Ophthalmic Surgery.* 2nd ed. San Francisco: American Academy of Ophthalmology; 2015:125–135.

Phototherapeutic keratectomy   The excimer laser can be used to remove superficial stromal tissue. However, abnormal tissue, like corneal scars or calcium deposits (as in band keratopathy), may ablate at a different rate than normal tissue, so an uneven surface results even if the original surface was smooth. Manual techniques are more likely to respect the Bowman layer and maintain a smooth ocular surface, as the laser does not respect anatomical planes. Frequent application of viscous liquid to the corneal surface during laser ablation can fill in gaps in the surface and help achieve a smooth surface after ablation. Most patients experience a hyperopic shift after phototherapeutic keratectomy (PTK) from the corneal-flattening effect of the procedure. Nevertheless, PTK is an excellent option in selected patients with superficial (less than 100 µm deep) stromal scarring or dystrophies when manual techniques are not feasible. PTK may postpone or eliminate the need for corneal transplantation. Topical MMC applied to the corneal ablation zone for a brief period following PTK has been shown to decrease postoperative scar formation. Oral vitamin C has been used prophylactically to reduce haze formation in PTK.

Hindman H, MacRae S. Phototherapeutic keratectomy. In: *Basic Techniques of Ophthalmic Surgery.* 2nd ed. San Francisco: American Academy of Ophthalmology; 2015:183–188.

Rapuano CJ. Phototherapeutic keratectomy: who are the best candidates and how do you treat them? *Curr Opin Ophthalmol.* 2010;21(4):280–282.

Shah RA, Wilson SE. Use of mitomycin-C for phototherapeutic keratectomy and photorefractive keratectomy surgery. *Curr Opin Ophthalmol.* 2010;21(4):269–273.

Management of Persistent Corneal Epithelial Defects, Thinning, and Perforation

Patching

Corneal surface disorders such as dellen, rheumatoid melt, and descemetocele can be managed by patching on a short-term basis. A partial tarsorrhaphy can sometimes be very effective and restore some vision to the eye.

Persistent epithelial defects and recurrent erosions of the cornea result from defects in the surface epithelium that fail to heal in a timely fashion (see Chapter 4). Trauma from the eyelids during blinking can retard reepithelialization, and if delayed, reepithelialization is further slowed by chronic changes in the basement membrane and anterior stroma. Patching may be successful over the short term. However, it compromises corneal oxygenation and impairs vision; also, some patients cannot tolerate closure of the eye while it is patched.

Bandage contact lenses

Application of a thin, oxygen-permeable, continuous-wear soft contact lens as a therapeutic bandage can protect loosely adherent remaining or regenerating epithelium from the "windshield-wiper" action of the blinking eyelids. Use of bandage contact lenses has significantly improved and simplified the management of recurrent erosions and persistent epithelial defects. These lenses help reduce stromal leukocyte infiltration and promote regeneration of basement membrane and restoration of tight epithelial–stromal adhesion without compromising corneal oxygenation, patient comfort, or vision.

Careful consideration should be given to the choice of a soft contact lens for patients with severe dry eye. In general, patients with dry eye run a high risk of infection with soft contact lenses; punctal occlusion should be performed in these patients to facilitate lens retention and comfort. Contact lenses with high oxygen transmissibility (eg, hydroxyethyl methacrylate [HEMA]–silicone polymer) are theoretically the most appropriate choice in this setting. Silicone lenses should be replaced every 2–4 weeks or as deposits accumulate on the lens. Frequent lubrication, prophylaxis with antibiotics, and close follow-up are crucial, especially in patients with decreased corneal sensitivity or dry eye. If a conventional soft lens is not tolerated, the use of an acrylic scleral lens may circumvent the problems encountered with a smaller-diameter hydrogel lens.

Continuous wear of a soft lens can relieve the symptoms of painful bullous or filamentary keratopathy. However, long-term use of a bandage contact lens can also lead to hypoxia, corneal pannus, limbal stem cell damage, and vascularization, all of which can compromise the success of future PK for vision rehabilitation.

Tarsorrhaphy should be considered for patients who have contact lens complications or a high risk of infection. The tarsorrhaphy procedure is described later in this chapter.

Treatment of corneal thinning/descemetocele

Corneal thinning may occur secondary to dellen where the tear film is uneven or may result from stromal inflammation and necrosis. In patients with dellen, the epithelium is intact, but there is an area of thinning next to an area of elevated or edematous tissue. In these cases, short-term patching may be sufficient.

In patients with corneal thinning down to the Descemet membrane (descemetocele) that is secondary to stromal infection or inflammation, the condition is much more serious because the epithelium is not intact and the patient is at risk for corneal perforation. The goals of therapy are to treat the inflammation or infectious component and to facilitate reepithelialization, which prevents progression of stromal collagenolysis.

The first order of therapy is to use appropriate antibiotics and anti-inflammatory medications. Topical steroids may reduce inflammation but should be used with caution with aggressive corneal melts. In patients with autoimmune conditions, conjunctival resection in the quadrant of a peripheral melt can be useful. In some cases, cyanoacrylate glue (also called cyanoacrylate adhesive) is helpful. Once the inflammation or infection has been controlled, a bandage lens or tarsorrhaphy may facilitate reepithelialization.

An alternative to using cyanoacrylate for a descemetocele is to use amniotic membrane that has been cut to the shape of the defect and then place a patch into the defect where the near-perforation is located. The patch and smaller amniotic membrane may be held in place with a larger amniotic membrane patch, nylon sutures, and a bandage contact lens, or by means of fibrin glue. With time, scar tissue will reinforce the deficient area and may circumvent the need for a corneal transplant.

Lindquist TP, Lee WB. Amniotic membrane transplantation. In: *Basic Techniques of Ophthalmic Surgery*. 2nd ed. San Francisco: American Academy of Ophthalmology; 2015:109–114.

Treatment of perforation

Some corneal perforations are small and seal spontaneously before ophthalmic examination, with no intraocular damage, prolapse, or adherence. These cases may require only treatment with systemic and/or topical antibiotic therapy, along with close observation. If a corneal wound is leaking but the anterior chamber remains formed, the leakage may be sealed with pharmacologic suppression of aqueous production (topical ocular hypotensive agent or systemic carbonic anhydrase inhibitor), patching, or a bandage contact lens. Generally, if these measures fail to seal the wound within 2 days, cyanoacrylate glue is another option (Fig 13-7). Perforations measuring more than 1–2 mm are usually not amenable to tissue adhesive and require supplemental tissue (Fig 13-8).

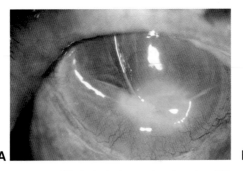 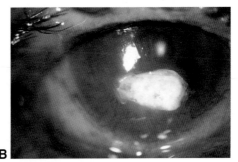

A **B**

Figure 13-7 Clinical photographs showing **(A)** a central corneal melt and **(B)** glue and a contact lens applied to the melt. *(Courtesy of Robert W. Weisenthal, MD.)*

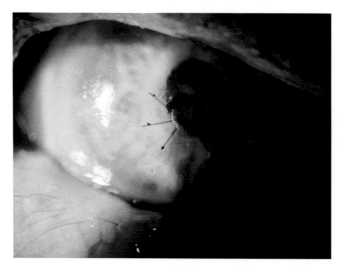

Figure 13-8 Clinical photograph showing a corneal patch graft for a small central perforation unresponsive to gluing. *(Courtesy of Woodford S. Van Meter, MD.)*

Cyanoacrylate glue Although cyanoacrylate glues have not been approved by the FDA for ophthalmic use, they have been utilized effectively and extensively over the past 3 decades to seal impending or small (<2 mm) perforations. Cyanoacrylate glue applied to thinned or ulcerated corneal tissue may prevent further thinning and can prevent leakage through the period of vascularization and repair. The adhesive plug is also thought to retard the entry of inflammatory cells and epithelium into the area, thus decreasing the rate of corneal melting. After the lesion has been sealed, new stromal tissue may be laid down, and accompanying corneal vascularization may help ensure the integrity of the area by providing nutrients and antiproteases.

SURGICAL TECHNIQUE Cyanoacrylate glue can usually be applied on an outpatient basis using topical anesthetics. However, if adherent or prolapsed uvea in the leakage site or a flat chamber is encountered, the procedure may be best performed in the operating room using balanced salt solution and/or viscoelastic to re-form the anterior chamber. An eyelid speculum is necessary to keep the eyelids open and immobilized. Before the adhesive is applied, necrotic tissue and corneal epithelium should be removed from the involved area out to a 2-mm zone. The area should then be dried with a cellulose sponge.

The easiest way to apply glue is under biomicroscopic magnification. A small drop of the fluid adhesive is applied to the corneal wound with the tip of a 30-gauge needle or anterior chamber cannula. The glue does not polymerize on plastic, so an alternative way to apply the adhesive is to spread a small amount on the inside of the sterile plastic wrapping of any medical product that has been cut to a size slightly larger than the perforation. The glue can then be applied to the surface of the cornea in as thin a layer as possible using the plastic handle of a cellulose sponge or the wooden stick of a cotton-tipped applicator. The glue polymerizes completely within 20–60 seconds and usually adheres well to the deepithelialized surface.

The adhesive plug has a rough surface and can be irritating, so a bandage contact lens is necessary to protect the upper tarsal conjunctiva and to prevent the plug from being dislodged by blinking.

Kim HK, Park HS. Fibrin glue–assisted augmented amniotic membrane transplantation for the treatment of large noninfectious corneal perforations. *Cornea.* 2009;28(2):170–176.

Shaw C, Islam MN, Chakroborty S, et al. Tissue adhesive in ophthalmology. *J Indian Med Assoc.* 2010;108(7):460–461.

Suh LH, Akpek EK. Corneal gluing. In: *Basic Techniques of Ophthalmic Surgery.* 2nd ed. San Francisco: American Academy of Ophthalmology; 2015:161–164.

Tattoo for Corneal Scars

Corneal tattooing has been used for centuries to improve the cosmetic appearance of a blind eye with an unsightly leukoma. It has also been used occasionally in seeing eyes to reduce the glare from scars and to eliminate monocular diplopia in patients with large iridectomies, traumatic loss of iris, and congenital iris colobomas (Fig 13-9).

Different techniques may be used to create a tattoo. One involves applying a platinum-ion solution to the cornea. When this solution reacts with a second agent, a black precipitate is formed in the cornea, producing a dark deposit that can simulate a pupil. Another technique involves utilizing the standard methods used in skin tattooing: applying to the cornea a paste of colored pigment, either India ink or a metal oxide, and then using a hypodermic needle or angled blade to drive the pigment into the corneal stroma in the area that needs coverage. Multiple superficial punctures are made until enough pigment has been applied; multiple pigment colors can be used to give a more natural appearance. However, the method is time-consuming and often needs to be repeated if the pigment uptake is inadequate or the pigment migrates. Femtosecond laser–assisted anterior lamellar corneal staining/tattooing in the cosmetic treatment of leukocoria is under investigation.

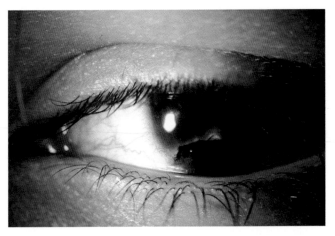

Figure 13-9 Clinical photograph showing a corneal tattoo for a cosmetically displeasing inferior scar in a young woman. *(Courtesy of Robert W. Weisenthal, MD.)*

Kim JH, Lee D, Hahn TW, Choi SK. New surgical strategy for corneal tattooing using a femtosecond laser. *Cornea*. 2009;28(1):80–84.

Rocher N, Hirst L, Renard G, Doat M, Bourges JL, Mancel E. Corneal tattooing: a series of
14 case studies. *J Fr Ophtalmol*. 2008;31(10):968–974.

Tarsorrhaphy

Tarsorrhaphy, the surgical fusion of the upper and lower eyelid margins, is performed to
reduce the exposed surface area of the cornea. It is among the safest, most effective, and
most underutilized procedures for healing difficult-to-treat corneal lesions. Tarsorrhaphy
is most commonly performed to protect the cornea from exposure caused by inadequate
eyelid coverage, as may occur in dellen, neurotrophic cornea, thyroid eye disease, or facial
nerve (cranial nerve VII) dysfunctions such as Bell palsy. It can also be used to aid in the
healing of indolent corneal ulceration, as is sometimes seen with tear film deficiency, herpes simplex or herpes zoster infection, or stem cell dysfunction.

Tarsorrhaphies are classified as lateral (Fig 13-10), medial, or central according to
the position of the adhesion of the palpebral fissure. BCSC Section 7, *Orbit, Eyelids, and
Lacrimal System,* discusses eyelid anatomy and surgical technique for tarsorrhaphy in detail. Because the cosmetic effect of a lateral tarsorrhaphy is significant, patients may be
reluctant to undergo this procedure and should be counseled on its therapeutic benefits.

Tarsorrhaphy may be temporary (Frost suture) or permanent. The Frost suture, a surgical procedure involving use of a transtarsal plate suture to keep the eyelids closed but
entailing no intramarginal adhesion, can be employed to partially occlude the eyelids for
up to 2–3 weeks. If closure of more than 3 weeks is desired or if the length of time is uncertain, then permanent but reversible adhesion is induced by denuding the eyelid margin.
Plastic stints or bolsters can be used to protect the eyelids from tight sutures, allow the
suture tension to close the eyelids the desired amount, and reduce patient discomfort due
to the sutures (see Fig 13-10).

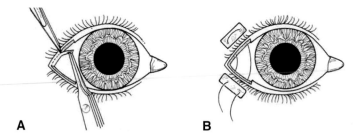

A   **B**

Figure 13-10 Lateral tarsorrhaphy. **A,** A strip of eyelid margin is shaved over the gray line.
B, One or two mattress sutures (double-armed 4-0 polypropylene with cutting needles) are
passed through the upper and lower eyelids to secure the tarsorrhaphy. Sutures are threaded
through bolsters (#40 silicone band) and tied. Each suture end should be placed through the
skin of the upper eyelid approximately 5 mm above the lash line, traverse the upper tarsal
plate, exit through the denuded wound surface of the upper eyelid margin, enter through the
denuded wound surface of the lower eyelid margin, traverse the lower tarsal plate, and exit
through the skin of the lower eyelid approximately 5 mm from the lash line. *(Reproduced with
permission from Hersh PS. Ophthalmic Surgical Procedures. 2nd ed. New York: Thieme Medical Publishers; 2009:253.)*

A tarsorrhaphy can be released under local anesthesia in the office. After infiltration of local anesthetic, a muscle hook is placed under the tissue, and a hemostat is placed (for 5 seconds) across the adhesion to be released. A blade or scissors are used to incise the tarsorrhaphy adhesion parallel to the upper and lower eyelid margins. If the status of the corneal exposure is uncertain, the tarsorrhaphy can be opened in stages, a few millimeters at a time. If the tarsorrhaphy has been performed properly, eyelid margin deformity is minimal.

Alternatives to tarsorrhaphy

Injection of onabotulinumtoxinA into the levator palpebrae superioris muscle to paralyze its function can cause pharmacologic ptosis and, similar to a surgical tarsorrhaphy, can impart a protective effect that lasts up to 6 months. Application of cyanoacrylate adhesive (discussed earlier in this chapter) to the eyelid margins may also enable temporary closure of the eyelids. However, both techniques have endpoints that are out of the control of the treating surgeon.

Tape may also be used to temporarily close the eyelids, but tape rarely lasts longer than 24 hours. Use of moisture-retaining eyewear (also called moisture chamber glasses) is another temporary measure that may be used to minimize desiccation and help protect the ocular surface. These devices are available commercially or may be constructed with plastic wrap and taped over the eyelids.

Reddy UP, Woodward JA. Abobotulinum toxin A (Dysport) and botulinum toxin type A (Botox) for purposeful induction of eyelid ptosis. *Ophthalmic Plast Reconstr Surg.* 2010; 26(6):489–491.

Sonmez B, Ozarslan M, Beden U, Erkan D. Bedside glue blepharorrhaphy for recalcitrant exposure keratopathy in immobilized patients. *Eur J Ophthalmol.* 2008;18(4):529–531.

CHAPTER 14

Clinical Aspects of Toxic and Traumatic Injuries of the Anterior Segment

Highlights

- Chemical solutions in the eye, especially strong alkaline substances, should be irrigated as soon as possible.
- Surgical repair of iridodialysis should be attempted as soon as possible to minimize corectopia from permanent contracture of the radial iris fibers.
- The combination of elevated intraocular pressure, corneal endothelial damage, and blood in the anterior chamber can result in corneal blood staining.
- Prolapsed uveal tissue in penetrating ocular injuries is usually reposited rather than resected unless it is grossly necrotic or contaminated.

Chemical Injuries

Chemical injuries to the external eye can range in severity from mild irritation to complete destruction of the ocular surface and adnexa (eyelids), resulting in corneal opacification, loss of vision, and even loss of the eye. Chemical injuries may occur in the home or workplace. Some of the most severe ocular chemical injuries are caused by strong alkalis (eg, lye) or acids used for assault. Table 14-1 lists some common caustic chemicals that can cause ocular injury.

Whenever possible, the offending chemical agent should be identified. The severity of a chemical injury depends on the pH (acid or alkali), the volume and duration of contact, and the inherent toxicity of the chemical. Frequently, the container of the toxic agent offers instructions for treatment or a phone number to call for detailed assistance.

Alkali Burns

The most severe chemical injuries occur with alkaline (high pH) solutions because they cause saponification of fatty acids in cell membranes and ultimately cellular disruption. Once the surface epithelium is damaged, alkaline solutions readily penetrate the corneal stroma, where they rapidly destroy the proteoglycan ground substance and collagen fibers

Table 14-1 Common Alkalis and Acids Causing Eye Injuries

Substance	Compound	pH*	Use
Alkali	Ammonia (NH₃)	11.60	General-purpose cleaner, fertilizer, refrigerant
	Potassium hydroxide (KOH)	10.98	Caustic potash
	Sodium hydroxide (NaOH): lye, caustic soda	10.98	Drain cleaner, agent in air bag reaction
	Calcium hydroxide (Ca(OH)₂): lime	11.27	Plaster, mortar, cement, whitewash
	Magnesium hydroxide (Mg(OH)₂)	10.40	Fireworks
Acid	Sulfuric acid (H₂SO₄)	2.75	Car battery
	Sulfurous acid (H₂SO₃)	1.60?	Bleach, refrigerant
	Hydrofluoric acid (HF)	3.27	Glass polisher, mineral refiner
	Acetic acid (HAcetate) (CH₃CO₂H or C₂H₄O₂)	3.91	Vinegar, glacial acetic acid
	Hydrochloric acid (HCl)	3.01	Control of pH in swimming pools, pickling of steel

*pH in 1.0 M aqueous.

of the stromal matrix. Strong alkaline substances may also penetrate through the endothelium into the anterior chamber, causing severe tissue damage and intense inflammation.

The visual prognosis is often determined by the extent of ocular surface injury and the effect of skin burns on eyelid function. There are multiple classification and grading schemes for chemical injuries. The Hughes classification scheme (as modified by Thoft) divides chemical injuries of the cornea into 4 categories (Table 14-2) based on clinical findings. The scheme shown in Table 14-3 establishes the grade of injury based on clinical signs, symptoms, and expected outcomes. The most unfavorable visual prognosis is

Table 14-2 Prognostic Features of Chemical Injury of the Eye

Grade of Injury	Clinical Findings	Prognosis
Grade I	Corneal epithelial defect No corneal haze No loss of limbal stem cells	Excellent
Grade II (see Fig 14-1)	Cornea mildly hazy Focal limbal ischemia	Generally good; may have focal vascularization of cornea in area of limbal stem cell loss
Grade III (see Fig 14-2)	Severe corneal haze limits view of anterior segment structures Extensive limbal ischemia with loss of most limbal stem cells	Guarded; cornea must be repopulated with conjunctiva; surgery needed for vision rehabilitation
Grade IV (see Fig 14-3)	Complete loss of corneal and proximal conjunctival epithelium Cornea opaque Complete limbal ischemia and loss of all limbal stem cells	Extremely poor; melting likely; globe salvage may not be possible

Modified from Colby KA. Chemical injuries of the cornea. *Focal Points: Clinical Modules for Ophthalmologists.* San Francisco: American Academy of Ophthalmology; 2010, module 1.

Table 14-3 Classification Scheme for Chemical Injury to the Human Eye Based on Clinical Findings

	Class 0			Class I	Class II	Class III	Class IV
	a	b	c				
Criteria to Be Used in Grading Clinical Cases							
Limbal blood vessel ischemia (circumference affected, %)	No ischemia; no injection present	No ischemia; injection may be present	No ischemia; injection present	<25%	25%–50%	50%–75%	70%–100%
Corneal stroma	Details of iris clearly visible				Opacity causes blurriness of iris details	Pupil is discernible despite opacity	Unable to discern pupil; complete opacity
Corneal epithelium	Appears normal		Punctate damage (expected to clear within 24 hours)	<33% loss in a geographic or punctate pattern	>33% to completely destroyed	Destroyed	
Symptoms	Possible pain, excess tearing		Pain, excess tearing, foreign-body sensation; possibly glare, photophobia, blurred vision	Symptoms include pain and loss of visual acuity (ranging from blurred vision and glare on the low end through complete loss of vision on the high end)			
Expected outcome	No consequence			Recover to full vision	Recover, but there may be some degree of visual impairment	Loss of sight in the eye possible without extensive medical intervention	Loss of globe possible without extensive medical intervention

(Continued)

Table 14-3 *(continued)*

	Class 0			Class I	Class II	Class III	Class IV
	a	b	c				
Additional Criteria Requiring Specialized Equipment and Validation							
Depth of corneal injury	Corneal epithelium				<$\frac{1}{3}$, including epithelium and anterior stroma	>$\frac{1}{3}$, including epithelium and stroma	Entire cornea damaged
Corneal endothelial cell loss (% of total)	None			0%<10%	10%–60%	>40%	100%
Suggested Preventive Measures							
First aid labels	None	Wash/irrigate eye for 2–5 minutes; see an ophthalmologist if symptoms persist for 24 hours*		Wash/irrigate eye for 15–30 minutes; see an ophthalmologist immediately thereafter			
Packaging		Childproof closure				Safety packaging	

*For alkali-containing materials, irrigate for 15–30 minutes and see an ophthalmologist.

Modified with permission from Bagley DM, Casterton PL, Dressler WE, et al. Proposed new classification scheme for chemical injury to the human eye. *Regul Toxicol Pharmacol.* 2006;45(2):206–213.

associated with extensive limbal epithelial damage. The limbus contains corneal epithelial stem cells; damage to this region can lead to disruption in the cells repopulating the corneal epithelium. Blanching occurs when the vascular supply to this critical area is disrupted via death of vascular endothelial cells in the conjunctiva. The resultant limbal and anterior segment ischemia is a poor prognostic feature for eyes thus affected (Figs 14-1 through 14-4). If the conjunctiva recovers, vascularization may occur (Fig 14-5). Repopulation of the corneal surface epithelium with undifferentiated conjunctival cells leads to poor epithelial adhesion and recurrent breakdown, and possibly chronic inflammation if the original trauma is severe. Intraocular chemical penetration may result in cataract formation and secondary glaucoma; the latter is thought to result from damage to the trabecular meshwork, which can affect outflow facility.

Patients with severe alkali burns are fortunate if the conjunctival and corneal surface vascularize and stabilize. Patients with alkali burns may not be candidates for penetrating

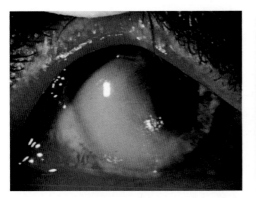

Figure 14-1 Grade II alkali burn, with inferior scleral ischemia (see Table 14-2). *(Courtesy of James J. Reidy, MD.)*

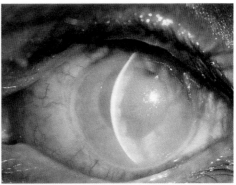

Figure 14-2 Grade III alkali burn with corneal edema and haze (see Table 14-2).

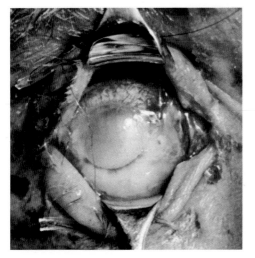

Figure 14-3 Grade IV alkali burn with corneal epithelial loss and stromal necrosis (see Table 14-2). The blue polypropylene sutures are holding the amniotic membrane in place over the cornea. *(Courtesy of James J. Reidy, MD.)*

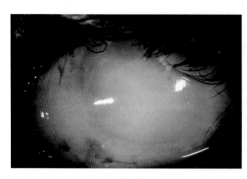

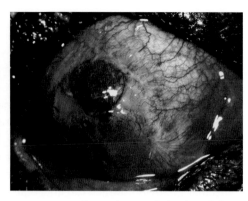

Figure 14-4 Severe alkali burn with opaque cornea and total limbal blanching. *(Courtesy of Woodford S. Van Meter, MD.)*

Figure 14-5 Corneal vascularization following severe alkali burn. *(Courtesy of Woodford S. Van Meter, MD.)*

keratoplasty because the loss of goblet cells impairs graft survival, but they may be candidates for limbal stem cell transplantation followed by keratoplasty or keratoprosthesis. In the most severe cases, phthisis of the globe may occur or, in the absence of vascularization, melting may lead to enucleation.

Bagley DM, Casterton PL, Dressler WE, et al. Proposed new classification scheme for chemical injury to the human eye. *Regul Toxicol Pharmacol.* 2006;45(2):206–213.

Colby KA. Chemical injuries of the cornea. *Focal Points: Clinical Modules for Ophthalmologists.* San Francisco: American Academy of Ophthalmology; 2010, module 1.

Acid Burns

Acid solutions with very low pH tend to cause less severe tissue damage than do alkaline solutions because acids denature and precipitate proteins in the tissues they contact, forming a barrier to penetration. Mild acid burns can cause an epithelial defect (Fig 14-6). Acid burns can cause severe damage to the ocular surface, but compared with alkali burns, there is a lower chance of corneal melting or penetration of the solution into the anterior chamber. The exception to diminished penetration is a hydrofluoric acid burn, which can cause significant anterior segment destruction. Acid burns do not directly cause loss of

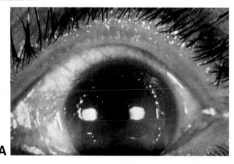

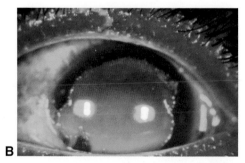

A   B

Figure 14-6 **A,** Mild acid burn with central corneal epithelial defect. **B,** Fluorescein staining showing the outline of the epithelial defect. *(Courtesy of Woodford S. Van Meter, MD.)*

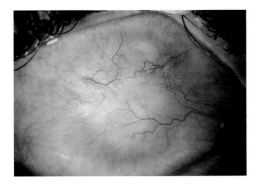

Figure 14-7 Corneal keratinization and opacification following severe acid burn. *(Courtesy of Woodford S. Van Meter, MD.)*

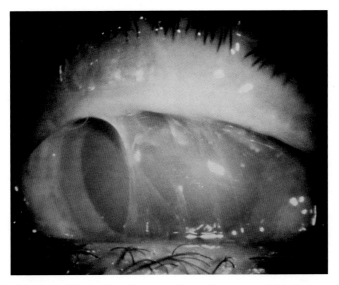

Figure 14-8 Symblepharon formation after a moderately severe acid burn. *(Courtesy of Woodford S. Van Meter, MD.)*

the proteoglycan ground substance in the cornea, although they can incite severe inflammation and damage to the corneal matrix and result in corneal opacification (Fig 14-7) or symblepharon formation (Fig 14-8).

Management of Chemical Injuries

The most important step in the management of chemical injuries is immediate and copious irrigation of the ocular surface with water or balanced saline solution. If these liquids are not available, the clinician may use any other pure, nontoxic solution to rinse the ocular surface and dilute the offending agent. Alkali burns are true emergencies, and irrigation should be initiated at the site of the chemical injury and continued until an ophthalmologist evaluates the patient.

The eyelid can be opened with a retractor or eyelid speculum, and topical anesthetic should be instilled. Irrigation may be accomplished using handheld intravenous tubing, an irrigating eyelid speculum, or a special scleral contact lens that connects to intravenous tubing. Irrigation should continue until the pH of the conjunctival sac normalizes. The conjunctival pH should be checked with a urinary pH strip. If this strip is not available, it is better to overtreat with prolonged periods of irrigation than to assume that the pH has normalized and discontinue treatment too early.

Because prolonged exposure to toxic particles can exacerbate chemical damage to the ocular surface, particulate chemicals should be removed from the ocular surface with cotton-tipped applicators and forceps. Eversion of the upper eyelid should be performed to search for material in the upper fornix (Fig 14-9), and the fornices should be swept with an applicator to ensure that no particulate matter remains in the eye.

Management over the next few days, the *intermediate period,* should aim to decrease inflammation, monitor intraocular pressure (IOP), limit matrix degradation, and promote

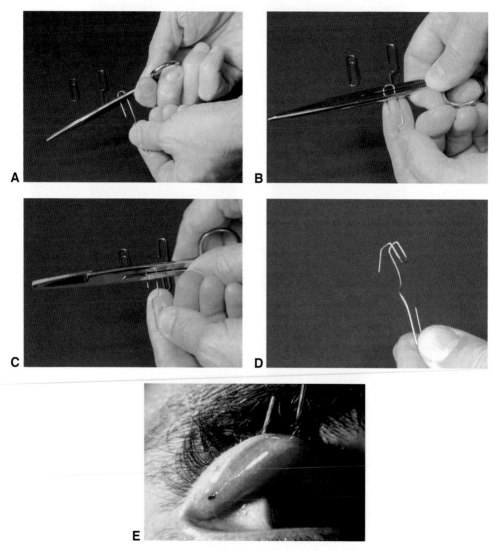

Figure 14-9   A–D, Steps in fashioning an eyelid retractor from a paper clip. **E,** Use of the retractor for double eversion reveals a foreign body on the upper eyelid. *(Courtesy of John E. Sutphin, MD.)*

reepithelialization of the cornea. Many of the following recommendations for management are based on animal models of acute alkaline injury.

An intense polymorphonucleocyte (PMN) infiltration of the corneal stroma can occur following acute alkali burns. PMNs deliver proteolytic enzymes that, in the absence of an intact epithelium, dissolve corneal stromal collagen and ground substance. Corticosteroids are excellent inhibitors of PMN function, and intensive treatment with a topical corticosteroid is recommended for 10–14 days following a chemical injury. Thereafter, the frequency of the corticosteroid drops should be markedly reduced to prevent inhibition of wound healing and exacerbation of stromal melting. Corticosteroids retard epithelial wound healing and increase the risk of secondary infection by inhibiting normal ocular surface immune defense mechanisms, so their adverse effects in the chronic phase probably exceed their beneficial effects.

A deficiency of calcium in the plasma membrane of PMNs inhibits their ability to degranulate. Both tetracycline and citric acid are potent chelators of extracellular calcium. Therefore, oral tetracyclines and topical sodium citrate 10% have theoretical benefits for inhibiting PMN-induced collagenolysis. Topical medroxyprogesterone 1% may be effective in suppressing collagen breakdown and is used at some centers. Use of topical cycloplegics should be initiated and may be continued for patients with discomfort or significant anterior chamber reaction.

In the early stage of a chemical injury, there may be a rise in IOP, which can be controlled by use of oral carbonic anhydrase inhibitors in order to avoid toxicity from topical glaucoma medications. However, if the corneal epithelium is healing normally, topical therapies may be used as well. See BCSC Section 10, *Glaucoma*, for a detailed discussion of medications used to control IOP.

Measures that promote wound healing and inhibit collagenolytic activity prevent stromal ulceration. Severe alkali burns in rabbit eyes reduce aqueous humor ascorbate levels to one-third of normal levels. Reduced aqueous humor ascorbate has been correlated with corneal stromal ulceration and perforation. Systemic administration of ascorbic acid to rabbits with acute corneal alkaline injuries restores the level of aqueous humor ascorbate to normal and significantly reduces the incidence of ulceration. High-dose ascorbic acid is believed to promote collagen synthesis in the alkali-burned eye, given that ascorbic acid is required as a cofactor for collagen synthesis. Currently, there is no widely accepted standard for administration of ascorbic acid after chemical injury, but some recommend that patients take 1–2 g of vitamin C per day. Because this therapy is potentially toxic to the kidneys, ascorbic acid should not be administered to patients with compromised renal function.

Frequent use of nonpreserved topical lubricants helps facilitate epithelial healing in the acute and chronic stages of chemical injury. Necrotic corneal epithelium should be debrided to minimize the release of inflammatory mediators from damaged epithelial cells and to promote reepithelialization. A bandage contact lens may be beneficial for protecting ocular surface epithelium once migration onto the peripheral cornea has begun; however, acute conjunctival swelling and inflammation or late symblepharon formation may prevent retention of the contact lens. A temporary or permanent tarsorrhaphy facilitates reepithelialization due to increased corneal coverage, but as with contact lens use, the drawback is the increased risk of infection in eyes with compromised defense mechanisms. Avascular sclera usually does not epithelialize until revascularization occurs. If scleral melting occurs, a rotational graft of tarsoconjunctival tissue from the adjacent eyelid can be performed to promote revascularization.

Autologous conjunctival or limbal stem cell transplantation using tissue from the patient's uninjured eye may facilitate healing of the corneal epithelial defect. Amniotic membrane may be helpful in suppressing inflammation, promoting reepithelialization, and preventing symblepharon formation; this option should be considered 1–2 weeks after injury. Limbal stem cell transplantation may be performed as soon as 2 weeks after chemical injury if no signs of corneal epithelialization have appeared. However, the prognosis of limbal grafts is better when the eye is not very inflamed; therefore, it is preferable to wait until the acute inflammation has subsided. A new technique known as *simple limbal epithelial transplantation (SLET)* combines limbal stem cell transplantation with use of amniotic membrane (see Chapter 13). If there is damage to the conjunctiva of both eyes, then either amniotic membrane alone or oral mucosal grafts may be necessary.

The long-term prognosis for a corneal transplant is improved if the ocular surface inflammation has resolved either over time (months to years) or after limbal stem cell grafting (ocular surface reconstruction), if necessary. Even when there is no active ocular surface inflammation, stromal vascularization in the host bed is associated with a much higher risk of rejection in these keratoplasty cases. Keratoprosthesis is another surgical option for these patients, but again, the prognosis is best when the inflammation has been brought under control.

Chan CC, Biber JM, Holland EJ. The modified Cincinnati procedure: combined conjunctival limbal autografts and keratolimbal allografts for severe unilateral ocular surface failure. *Cornea.* 2012;31(11):1264–1272.

Tejwani S, Kolari RS, Sangwan VS, Rao GN. Role of amniotic membrane graft for ocular chemical and thermal injuries. *Cornea.* 2007;26(1):21–26.

Vazirani J, Basu S, Sangwan V. Successful simple limbal epithelial transplantation (SLET) in lime injury–induced limbal stem cell deficiency with ocular surface granuloma. *BMJ Case Rep.* 2013;bcr2013009405.

Injuries Caused by Temperature and Radiation

Thermal Burns

Heat

Heat is a primary cause of inflammation and stromal protease expression and can lead to collagen melting if severe. Rapid-reflex eyelid closure, Bell phenomenon, and reflex movement away from the source of intense heat usually limit damage to the globe from flames. Burns from molten metal that stays in contact with the eye are more likely to cause corneal injuries that result in permanent scarring.

Curling irons, cigarettes, and hot liquids splashing into the eye, especially during cooking, are common household causes of corneal burns (Fig 14-10). These burns are usually limited to the epithelium and generally require only a brief period of antibiotic and cycloplegic therapy.

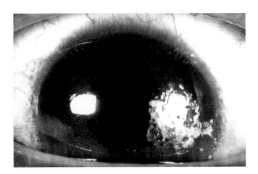

Figure 14-10 Cigarette burn on the cornea. *(Courtesy of Woodford S. Van Meter, MD.)*

Ocular electrical injury may be caused by heat or electric current. Electric current can eventually cause corneal epithelial erosion.

The primary objectives of therapy for burns caused by heat are the following:

- relieve discomfort
- prevent secondary corneal inflammation, ulceration, and perforation from infection or from exposure caused by eyelid damage
- minimize eyelid scarring and resultant malfunction

A cycloplegic agent can help relieve discomfort from ciliary spasm or iridocyclitis. Prophylactic antibiotics (topical and/or systemic) can help prevent infection of burned eyelids and/or reduce the chances of infectious corneal ulceration. Limited debridement of devitalized tissues and granulation tissue, used with full-thickness skin grafts and tarsorrhaphy, helps minimize eyelid scarring and ectropion. Burned ocular tissue can be protected temporarily by covering the eye with a lubricant and a piece of sterile plastic wrap. Topical corticosteroids help suppress any associated iridocyclitis, but they can also inhibit corneal wound healing and must be used with caution and, in general, for short periods.

Freezing

Transient corneal stromal edema induced by cold has been reported in a variety of settings, including prolonged exposure to cold when skiing or mountain climbing. Cold temperatures adversely affect the Na^+,K^+-ATPase pump function of the endothelial cells and render it less effective. Individuals with Raynaud disease and those with cranial nerve V (trigeminal) dysfunction may be especially susceptible. Research suggests that sensory denervation of the eye increases the susceptibility of the endothelium to cold temperatures.

Ultraviolet Radiation

The corneal epithelium is susceptible to injury from ultraviolet (UV) radiation, both naturally occurring and artificial. The most common causes of UV-radiation injury to the eye are unprotected exposure to sunlamps or tanning beds, and arc welding. Prolonged outdoor exposure to reflected sunlight, or *snow blindness,* occurs in skiers and mountain climbers at high elevations, where there is less atmospheric diffraction of UV radiation.

Patients with ocular UV-radiation injuries present with eyelid edema, conjunctival hyperemia, and diffuse punctate keratitis. Treatment consists of patching to minimize discomfort from eyelid movement, use of a topical antibiotic ointment, and cycloplegia.

If discomfort is severe, patients may require oral analgesics. Complete epithelial healing usually occurs within 24–72 hours. Appropriate protection with UV-filtering glasses can prevent most such injuries.

Ionizing Radiation

Exposure to ionizing radiation may occur with UV light, x-rays, gamma rays, medical imaging equipment, nuclear explosions, and radioisotopes. The level of exposure is related to the amount of energy in the ionizing radiation, the type of rays emitted, the duration of exposure, and the patient's proximity to the ionizing source. Tissue destruction may result from direct killing of cells, cellular DNA changes that produce lethal or other mutations, or radiation damage to blood vessels with secondary ischemic necrosis.

Ionizing radiation can damage the conjunctiva, cornea, and occasionally the lacrimal glands. Conjunctival edema occurs acutely, often followed by scarring, shrinkage, loss of tear production, and alterations in conjunctival blood vessels with telangiectasia. Necrosis of the conjunctiva and underlying sclera can occur if radioactive material (or a radiomimetic agent such as mitomycin C) is embedded in the conjunctiva. Punctate corneal epithelial erosions are noted acutely. Explosions involving ionizing radiation may lead to perforation of ocular tissues with immediate radiation necrosis.

The first step in management of acute radiation injury is removal of all foreign bodies. Poor wound healing is a hallmark of ionizing radiation injuries. Late complications are related to decreased tear production, loss of corneal sensation, sloughing of corneal epithelial cells, and failure of the cornea to heal. Secondary microbial keratitis, vascularization, and ocular surface disease can result from dry eyes and compromised epithelial cells. The use of artificial tears or a bandage contact lens may help stabilize the ocular surface in mild cases. More severe cases may require tarsorrhaphy and/or tissue adhesive. If there is recurrent epithelial breakdown despite these measures, significant conjunctival scarring typically precludes the use of a conjunctival flap from that eye. If the fellow eye has not been injured, a contralateral autologous conjunctival flap may be helpful. Alternatively, an amniotic membrane transplant, limbal stem cell transplant, or mucous membrane graft may be employed. The visual prognosis associated with penetrating keratoplasty or limbal stem cell transplantation in these situations is guarded because of the severely compromised ocular surface.

Injuries Caused by Animal and Plant Substances

Insect and Arachnid Injuries

Bee and wasp stings to the cornea and/or conjunctiva cause conjunctival hyperemia and chemosis acutely, sometimes associated with severe pain, corneal edema, and infiltration, with subsequent decreased vision. The significant variability in the acute response is thought to reflect differences in the quantity of the venom injected and whether the reaction to the venom is primarily toxic or immunologic. In rare instances, other sequelae have been documented, including hyphema, lenticular opacities, anterior uveitis, secondary glaucoma, and heterochromia. Initial therapy with cycloplegics and topical (and occasionally systemic) corticosteroids is beneficial. Removal of externalized stingers may be attempted. After the acute episode, retained stingers may remain inert in the cornea for years. Caterpillar and tarantula hairs (urticating hairs) may also become embedded in the cornea and conjunctiva. These hairs are very fine and usually cannot be removed manually. Because of their structure, these urticating hairs tend to migrate more deeply into ocular tissues and elicit a localized granulomatous inflammatory response *(ophthalmia nodosum)*. In these cases, the patient will have an extreme foreign-body sensation until the hairs migrate below the corneal surface. Inflammatory sequelae usually respond to topical corticosteroids.

Mangat SS, Newman B. Tarantula hair keratitis. *N Z Med J.* 2012;125(1364):107–110.

Shrum KR; Robertson DM, Baratz KH, Casperson TJ, Rostvold JA. Keratitis and retinitis secondary to tarantula hair. *Arch Ophthalmol.* 1999;117(8):1096–1097.

Vegetative Injuries

Ocular contact with the milky sap (latex) from a variety of trees can cause toxic reactions manifested by acute keratoconjunctivitis, epithelial defects, and stromal infiltration. The pencil tree and the manchineel tree, widely distributed in tropical regions, are known offenders. Houseplants in the genus *Dieffenbachia* are known to cause keratoconjunctivitis from calcium oxalate crystals in the cornea; crunching the leaves can cause these crystals to shoot into the cornea. The crystals cause a foreign-body sensation and are difficult to see on slit-lamp examination; the diagnosis of *Dieffenbachia* keratitis is made from the history as much as anything else. Corneal foreign bodies from coconut shell, sunflower stalk, and ornamental cactus have also been documented.

Initial management of injuries caused by all such plant materials should include irrigation and removal of foreign bodies when possible and administration of topical cycloplegics with prophylactic antibiotic coverage, as indicated by the clinical situation. Corticosteroids are best avoided, as they suppress immunity to microbes in general and may promote fungal infection specifically, which is of concern in all cases involving vegetable matter because plant sources are common causes of fungal keratitis. Surgical removal of vegetative foreign bodies should be attempted in order to mitigate the inflammatory response or associated secondary microbial infections. If a patient with a severe injury from plant sources fails to improve after supportive therapy, the possibility of bacterial or fungal infection should be considered and appropriate workup (including culturing and/or biopsy) performed. For additional discussion of microbial keratitis, see Chapter 10.

Concussive (Blunt) Trauma

Subconjunctival Hemorrhage

A subconjunctival hemorrhage is blood beneath the conjunctiva, with an alarming bright red appearance against the white sclera below (Fig 14-11). Patients with subconjunctival hemorrhage typically have no history of antecedent trauma. When trauma has occurred,

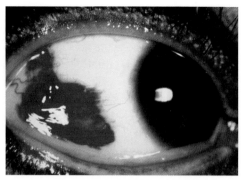

Figure 14-11 Subconjunctival hemorrhage shows prominently against white sclera. *(Courtesy of Woodford S. Van Meter, MD.)*

damage to deeper structures of the eye (ie, eye perforation when there is massive and raised hemorrhage) must be ruled out. Subconjunctival hemorrhage is usually not associated with an underlying systemic disease and rarely has an identifiable cause. Occasionally, a history of vomiting, coughing, or other forms of the Valsalva maneuver can be elicited. Patients may be taking a medication that impedes clotting.

Typically, no therapy is necessary for the hemorrhage, as it usually resolves in 7–12 days, and the patient simply requires reassurance that the condition is not serious. If the hemorrhage elevates the limbal conjunctiva off of the cornea, corneal dellen may occur. Patients should be warned that the hemorrhage can spread around the circumference of the globe before it resolves and that it may change in color from red to yellow during its dissolution.

Repeated episodes of spontaneous subconjunctival hemorrhage may indicate a possible bleeding diathesis (eg, easy bruising, frequent bloody nose), and a careful systemic medical evaluation may be warranted. Recurrent subconjunctival hemorrhages can be seen in association with uncontrolled hypertension; diabetes mellitus; systemic blood disorders; and use of antiplatelet (aspirin), anticoagulant (heparin or warfarin), and thrombolytic (streptokinase) drugs.

Corneal Changes From Blunt Trauma

Blunt trauma to the cornea can result in abrasions, edema, tears in the Descemet membrane (Fig 14-12), and corneoscleral lacerations, usually located at the limbus. Traumatic posterior annular keratopathy or corneal endothelial rings have also been described; these rings are whitish gray and occur directly posterior to the traumatic impact. The endothelial rings appear within several hours of a contusive injury and usually disappear within a few days.

Traumatic Mydriasis and Miosis

Traumatic mydriasis results from iris sphincter tears that can permanently dilate or otherwise alter the shape of the pupil (Fig 14-13). The iris tears may result in a hyphema. The pupil changes are generally permanent; patients should use sunglasses for resultant photophobia, as permanent surgical repair is less effective.

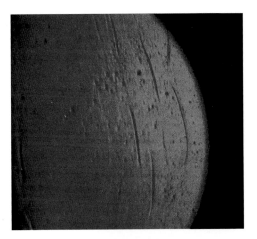

Figure 14-12 Tears in the Descemet membrane due to blunt trauma from forceps delivery. *(Courtesy of Woodford S. Van Meter, MD.)*

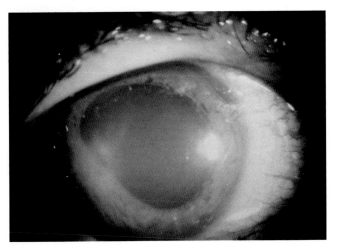

Figure 14-13 Traumatic mydriasis caused by tears in the iris sphincter muscle, resulting from blunt trauma. *(Courtesy of Woodford S. Van Meter, MD.)*

Miosis tends to be associated with anterior chamber inflammation (*traumatic anterior uveitis;* see the following section). Topical corticosteroid drops to reduce inflammation and cycloplegia to prevent formation of posterior synechiae are helpful in controlling symptoms.

Traumatic Anterior Uveitis

The inflammation present in traumatic anterior uveitis is often associated with decreased vision and perilimbal conjunctival hyperemia. Photophobia, tearing, and ocular pain may occur within 24 hours of injury. The anterior chamber reaction can be surprisingly minimal to cause symptoms of pain and photophobia.

Treatment consists of a topical cycloplegic agent to relieve patient discomfort, as well as topical corticosteroid drops if significant inflammation is present. Once the anterior uveitis has diminished, cycloplegia may be discontinued, and topical corticosteroids should be tapered slowly to prevent rebound anterior uveitis. See BCSC Section 9, *Intraocular Inflammation and Uveitis*, for a more detailed discussion of uveitis.

Iridodialysis and Cyclodialysis

Iridodialysis

Blunt trauma may cause *iridodialysis*, or traumatic separation of the iris root from the ciliary body (Fig 14-14). Anterior segment hemorrhage often ensues, and the iridodialysis may not be recognized until the hyphema has cleared. A small iridodialysis requires no treatment. A large iridodialysis may cause polycoria, polyopia, and monocular diplopia, requiring surgical repair (Figs 14-15, 14-16) (see Surgical Management later in the chapter). If possible, the iridodialysis should be repaired within a few weeks of the injury,

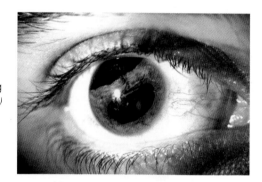

Figure 14-14 Severe iridodialysis resulting from blunt trauma. *(Courtesy of David Rootman, MD.)*

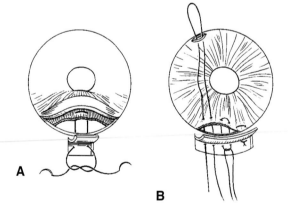

A

B

Figure 14-15 Repair of iridodialysis. **A,** A cataract surgery–type incision is made at the site of iridodialysis or iris disinsertion. A double-armed, 10-0 polypropylene suture is passed through the iris root and out through the angle and is tied on the surface of the globe under a partial-thickness scleral flap. The corneoscleral wound is then closed with 10-0 nylon sutures. **B,** In an alternative technique, multiple 10-0 Prolene sutures on double-armed Drews needles are passed through a paracentesis opposite the site of iris disinsertion to avoid the need to create a large corneoscleral entry wound. *(Reproduced from Hamill MB. Repair of the traumatized anterior segment. Focal Points: Clinical Modules for Ophthalmologists. San Francisco: American Academy of Ophthalmology; 1992, module 1. Illustrations by Christine Gralapp.)*

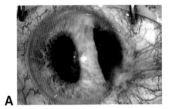 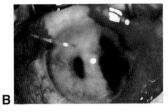 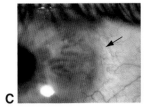

A   B   C

Figure 14-16 Repair of iridodialysis with polypropylene sutures. **A,** Traumatic iridodialysis. **B,** A needle is passed across the anterior chamber through the limbus opposite the dialysis for reattachment. **C,** Normal pupil following suturing of the iridodialysis. The *arrow* points to the polypropylene suture. *(Courtesy of Woodford S. Van Meter, MD.)*

because prolonged contracture of the radial iris fibers may prevent a round pupil after normal iris anatomy is reestablished.

Cyclodialysis

Traumatic cyclodialysis is characterized by separation of the ciliary body from its attachment to the scleral spur, resulting in a cleft. A hyphema may result from the tearing of the tissue. Gonioscopically, this cleft appears as a gap at the posterior edge of the scleral spur from posterior displacement of the ciliary body band. Sclera may be visible through the gap. Ultrasound biomicroscopy can be useful in identifying the location and extent of the cyclodialysis (Fig 14-17). A cyclodialysis cleft can cause increased uveoscleral outflow, leading to chronic hypotony, and macular edema. If treatment with topical cycloplegics does not suffice, closure may be attempted using an argon laser, diathermy, cryotherapy, or direct suturing. If repair is necessary, it should be performed after resolution of the hyphema.

Traumatic Hyphema

Traumatic hyphema occurs most commonly in young men, as this demographic experiences more ocular trauma than any other. Trauma causes posterior displacement of the lens–iris interface with equatorial scleral expansion. The increase in equatorial diameter

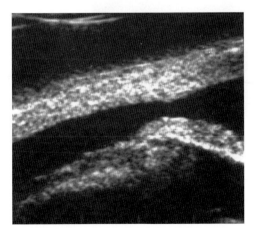

Figure 14-17 Ultrasound biomicroscopy of cyclodialysis. *(Courtesy of David Rootman, MD.)*

stretches the major iris arterial circle, arterial branches of the ciliary body, and/or recurrent choroidal arteries and veins. The hyphema results from injury to the vessels of the peripheral iris, iris sphincter, or anterior ciliary body (Fig 14-18). The bleeding may be so subtle that it can be detected only as a few circulating red blood cells on slit-lamp examination (microscopic hyphema; Fig 14-19), or it may form a clot in the anterior chamber (layered hyphema; Fig 14-20). Alternatively, the bleeding may be severe enough to fill

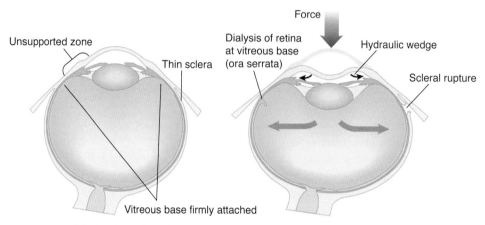

Figure 14-18 Mechanism of hyphema and blunt force injury to the eye. Blunt force applied to the eye displaces the aqueous volume peripherally, causing an increase in hydraulic pressure at the lens, iris root, and trabecular meshwork. If this "wedge of pressure" exceeds the tensile strength of ocular structures, the vessels in the peripheral iris and the anterior ciliary body may rupture, leading to hyphema. The force may cause scleral ruptures, typically at the limbus and posterior to the muscle insertions, where the sclera is thinner and unsupported by the orbital bones. Severe trauma leads to lens subluxation, retinal dialysis, optic nerve avulsion, and/or vitreous hemorrhage. *(Illustration by Cyndie C.H. Wooley.)*

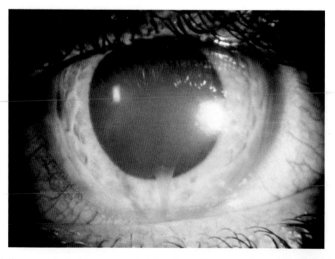

Figure 14-19 Microscopic hyphema with blood on the endothelial surface following blunt trauma. *(Courtesy of Woodford S. Van Meter, MD.)*

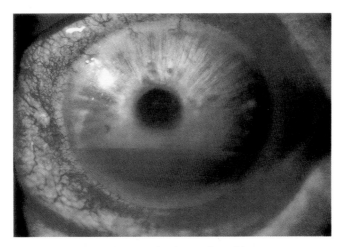

Figure 14-20   Layered hyphema from blunt trauma.

the anterior chamber completely. The prognosis for traumatic hyphema is generally good and is independent of the size of the hyphema, as long as no additional complications are present. Even *total,* or *eight-ball, hyphemas* (Fig 14-21) can resolve without sequelae. Traumatic hyphema is frequently associated with corneal abrasion, anterior uveitis, and mydriasis, as well as with simultaneous injuries to the angle structures, lens, posterior segment, and orbit.

Spontaneous hyphema (ie, a hyphema that occurs without any history of trauma) is much less common and should alert the examiner to the possibility of rubeosis iridis (mainly central retinal vein obstruction and diabetic retinopathy), clotting abnormalities, herpetic disease, or intraocular lens (IOL) problems. Juvenile xanthogranuloma, retino-blastoma, iris vascular hamartomas, and leukemia are associated with spontaneous hyphema in children.

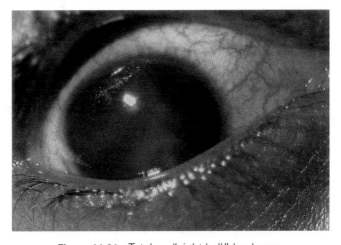

Figure 14-21   Total, or "eight-ball," hyphema.

Rebleeding

The major concern after a traumatic hyphema is rebleeding, which is seen in less than 5% of cases. Rebleeding usually occurs between 3 and 7 days after injury as a result of clot lysis and retraction. A complication associated with rebleeding is elevated IOP (seen in 50% of patients), which can potentially lead to glaucoma and optic atrophy.

The combination of elevated IOP, corneal endothelial damage, and blood in the anterior chamber can result in corneal blood staining (Fig 14-22A). Red blood cells within the anterior chamber release hemoglobin that penetrates the posterior corneal stroma, where it is absorbed by keratocytes. Within the keratocytes, breakdown of the hemoglobin into hemosiderin can result in the death of the keratocytes. It may be difficult to detect when blood is in apposition to the endothelium on slit-lamp examination; however, close observation reveals early blood staining as yellow granular changes and reduced fibrillar definition in the posterior corneal stroma. Blood staining can lead to a reduction in corneal transparency that may be permanent. Histologically, red blood cells and their breakdown products can be seen within the corneal stroma. Corneal blood staining often clears slowly, starting in the periphery (Fig 14-22B).

Medical management of traumatic hyphema

The treatment plan for traumatic hyphema should be directed at minimizing the possibility of secondary hemorrhage, controlling inflammation, and mitigating elevated IOP. It is essential that the patient wear a protective shield over the injured eye; restrict physical activity; elevate the head of the bed; and be observed closely, with daily observation initially. To reduce the risk of rebleeding, nonaspirin analgesics should be used for pain relief; however, even nonsteroidal anti-inflammatory medications can increase the risk of rebleeding. Most patients can be managed on an outpatient basis, but if satisfactory home care and outpatient observation cannot be ensured, admission to the hospital may be required.

Most ophthalmologists administer long-acting topical cycloplegic agents initially to control inflammation and improve patient comfort, facilitate posterior segment evaluation, and eliminate iris movement. Topical corticosteroids are beneficial in controlling anterior chamber inflammation and preventing synechiae formation, and they may play a role in preventing rebleeding. Oral corticosteroids are controversial in the treatment of

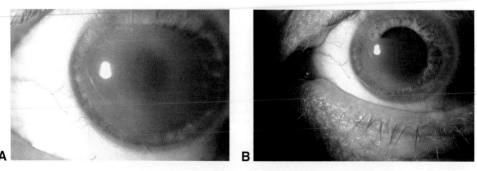

A

B

Figure 14-22 **A,** Dense corneal blood staining after a traumatic hyphema. **B,** Clearing of central corneal blood staining. *(Courtesy of Robert W. Weisenthal, MD.)*

hyphema but may be used to facilitate the resolution of severe inflammation and/or to prevent rebleeding.

Aggressive treatment of elevated IOP is important to reduce the risk of corneal blood staining and optic atrophy. Topical antihypertensive agents (β-blockers and α-agonists) are the mainstay of therapy, although intravenous or oral hyperosmotic agents may occasionally be required. If medical management fails to control IOP, surgical evacuation of the blood may be required in order to reduce the risk of permanent corneal blood staining.

Antifibrinolytic agents (eg, aminocaproic acid, tranexamic acid, prednisone) were previously thought to reduce the incidence of rebleeding, but studies have shown no statistical improvement in visual outcome. Because these agents can have significant adverse effects (eg, nausea, vomiting, postural hypotension, muscle cramps, conjunctival suffusion, nasal stuffiness, headache, rash, pruritus, dyspnea, toxic confusional states, and arrhythmias), they are rarely used today in the treatment of hyphema.

Gharaibeh A, Savage HI, Scherer RW, Goldberg MF, Lindsley K. Medical interventions for traumatic hyphema. *Cochrane Database Syst Rev.* 2013;(12):CD005431.

Surgical intervention in traumatic hyphema

Surgery should be performed at the earliest definitive detection of corneal blood staining. Some authors suggest that surgery is indicated when IOP is higher than 25 mm Hg on average for 5 days with a total hyphema or when IOP is higher than 60 mm Hg for 2 days. Patients with preexisting optic nerve damage or sickle cell hemoglobinopathies may require earlier intervention. Indications for surgical intervention are summarized in Table 14-4.

The simplest way to surgically treat a persistent anterior chamber clot is anterior chamber irrigation with balanced salt solution through a limbal paracentesis. The goal is to remove circulating red blood cells that may obstruct the trabecular meshwork; removal of the entire clot is neither necessary nor wise because of the risk of a secondary hemorrhage. The irrigation procedure can be repeated. If irrigation is not successful, the

---

Table 14-4 Indications for Surgical Intervention in Traumatic Hyphema

To prevent optic atrophy
  IOP averages >60 mm Hg for 2 days
  IOP averages >35 mm Hg for 7 days

To prevent corneal blood staining
  IOP averages >25 mm Hg for 5 days
  Evidence of early corneal blood staining

To prevent peripheral anterior synechiae
  Total hyphema that persists for 5 days
  Any hyphema failing to resolve to a volume of <50% within 8 days

In hyphema patients with sickle cell hemoglobinopathies
  IOP averages ≥25 mm Hg for 24 hours
  IOP has repeated transient elevations to >30 mm Hg for 2–4 days, despite medical intervention

---

IOP = intraocular pressure.

Adapted from Deutsch TA, Goldberg MF. Traumatic hyphema: medical and surgical management. *Focal Points: Clinical Modules for Ophthalmologists.* San Francisco: American Academy of Ophthalmology; 1984, module 5.

irrigation/aspiration handpiece, used in cataract surgery, may be effective. The use of a cutting instrument or intraocular diathermy may be necessary in severe cases. Iris damage, lens injury, endothelial cell trauma, and additional bleeding are potentially serious complications of surgical intervention.

Sickle cell complications

When a traumatic hyphema develops in an African American patient, a sickle cell workup should be performed to investigate the possibility of sickle cell hemoglobinopathy. Patients with sickle cell disease and carriers of the sickle cell trait are predisposed to sickling of red blood cells in the anterior chamber. Because sickle cells have restricted outflow through the trabecular meshwork, they may raise IOP dramatically. In addition, the optic nerve seems to be at greater risk of damage in patients with sickle cell disease, even those with modest IOP elevation, presumably as a result of a decrease in blood flow to the optic nerve.

The clinician must make every effort to control elevated IOP in these patients. Carbonic anhydrase inhibitors and osmotic agents reduce aqueous pH and lead to hemoconcentration, both of which may exacerbate sickling of red blood cells. For this reason, carbonic anhydrase inhibitors should be avoided in sickle cell patients. Surgical intervention is recommended if average IOP remains 25 mm Hg or higher after the first 24 hours or if there are repeated, transient elevations, with IOP higher than 30 mm Hg for 2–4 days, despite medical intervention.

Bansal S, Gunasekeran DV, Ang B, et al. Controversies in the pathophysiology and management of hyphema. *Surv Ophthalmol.* 2015;61(3):297–308.

Campagna JA. Traumatic hyphema: current strategies. *Focal Points: Clinical Modules for Ophthalmologists.* San Francisco: American Academy of Ophthalmology; 2007, module 10.

Penetrating and Perforating Ocular Trauma

It is important to understand the difference between a penetrating wound and a perforating wound for accurate communication and documentation. In a *penetrating* wound, a foreign body passes into an anatomical structure; in a *perforating* wound, a foreign body passes through such a structure. In a penetrating corneal injury, an object enters but does not pass all the way through the cornea, as in the case of a metallic foreign body that enters the corneal stroma but lodges anterior to the Descemet membrane. In a perforating corneal injury, an object passes through the cornea and lodges in the anterior chamber. A perforating corneal foreign-body injury can also be called a *penetrating ocular* foreign-body injury if the foreign body passes through the cornea but does not exit through the globe. In a *perforating ocular* injury, the foreign body enters and exits the globe.

Conjunctival Laceration

When managing conjunctival lacerations associated with trauma, the physician must be certain that the deeper structures of the eye have not been damaged and that no foreign body is present. After a topical anesthetic has been applied, the conjunctival laceration should be explored under slit-lamp examination using sterile forceps or cotton-tipped applicators. If any question remains as to whether the globe has been penetrated, consideration must be given to exploration in the operating room. In general, small linear conjunctival lacerations do not need to be sutured. However, stellate conjunctival lacerations, lacerations with bare sclera exposed, or lacerations with lost or retracted conjunctival tissue will heal faster if sutured closed.

Conjunctival Foreign Body

Foreign bodies on the conjunctival surface are best recognized with slit-lamp examination. Foreign bodies can lodge in the cul-de-sac, or they may be located on the palpebral conjunctival surface of the upper eyelid (Fig 14-23). When a patient reports an ocular foreign-body sensation, topical fluorescein should be instilled to check for the fine, vertical, linear corneal abrasions characteristic of retained foreign bodies on the eyelid margin or superior tarsal plate (Fig 14-24). Foreign matter embedded in tissue can be removed with a sterile, disposable hypodermic needle. Glass particles, cactus spines, and insect hairs are often difficult to see, but a careful search of the cul-de-sac with high magnification aids in identification and removal. These foreign bodies may be removed with fine-tipped jeweler's forceps or a blunt spatula. If a foreign body is suspected but not seen, the cul-de-sac should be irrigated and wiped with a cotton-tipped applicator moistened with topical anesthetic. Double eversion of the eyelid with a Desmarres retractor or a bent paper clip may be necessary to allow the examiner to effectively search the entire arc of the superior cul-de-sac (see Fig 14-9).

If no foreign body is found after a thorough examination, the next step is copious irrigation to cleanse the fornix. This procedure should then be repeated for both the upper and lower eyelids. Gunpowder or carbon fragments, such as those that may be embedded in the conjunctiva by a blast injury, should be removed if possible, but can be well tolerated in the substantia propria.

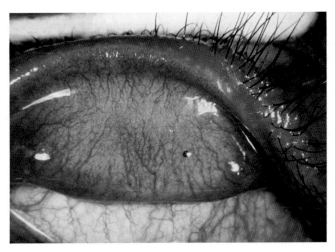

Figure 14-23 Rust foreign body embedded on the superior tarsal plate. *(Courtesy of Woodford S. Van Meter, MD.)*

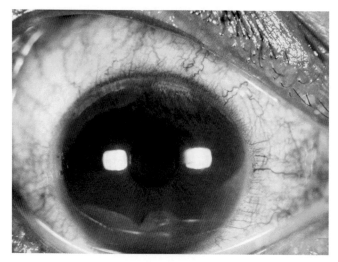

Figure 14-24 Vertical linear abrasions in the superior cornea are suggestive of a foreign body embedded in the superior tarsal conjunctiva. *(Courtesy of Woodford S. Van Meter, MD.)*

Corneal Abrasion

Disruption of the corneal epithelium is usually associated with immediate pain, foreign-body sensation, tearing, and discomfort with blinking. A slit-lamp examination is essential in determining the presence, extent, and depth of the corneal defect. Fluorescein staining of the cornea is very helpful in diagnosing a foreign body. It is important to distinguish between a corneal abrasion, which generally has sharply defined edges and little to no associated inflammation (when seen acutely), and a corneal ulcer, which is characterized by opacification and an inflammation-mediated breakdown of the stromal matrix and possible thinning. Also, it is important to rule out a foreign body as the cause of the abrasion. Occasionally, a patient may not recall a definite history of trauma but still present with signs and symptoms suggestive of a corneal abrasion. An eye with a corneal abrasion from a fingernail, piece of paper, or tree branch is more likely to develop recurrent erosions, the symptoms of which are the same as those of a corneal abrasion and typically occur upon awakening (see Chapter 4 for a discussion of recurrent corneal erosions). Herpes simplex virus keratitis should also be excluded as a possible diagnosis in such cases.

Pressure patching can relieve pain from an abrasion by immobilizing the upper eyelid to prevent rubbing against the corneal defect, although patching is not necessary for most abrasions and some patients may find patches uncomfortable. Topical antibiotic ointment is suggested in either case. Another alternative is a bandage contact lens, which provides pain relief and facilitates reepithelialization. Antibiotic drops rather than ointment should be used with a bandage lens. Topical antibiotic drops are recommended until the epithelium heals. Cycloplegics can help with the ciliary spasm associated with a corneal abrasion. Topical nonsteroidal anti-inflammatory agents have anesthetic properties and may be used for the first 24–48 hours for pain relief in selected patients; however, these agents should be used with caution, as they can cause local toxicity and delay wound healing. Oral pain management for the first 24–48 hours can be helpful for many patients.

Patients with abrasions caused by organic material require close follow-up to monitor for fungal infection. Abrasions caused by vegetable matter such as a fingernail, paper, leaves, or thorns heal more slowly than abrasions caused by inorganic materials such as steel, glass, or plastic.

Patients with contact lens–associated epithelial defects due to excessive wear or an improper fit should not receive a patch or have a therapeutic contact lens applied because of the risk of promoting or worsening a corneal infection. These patients should be treated with topical antibiotic drops or ointment.

Corneal Foreign Body

Small foreign bodies can become embedded in the corneal epithelial surface, as the texture of the cornea is similar to gelatin. Larger foreign bodies can cause a corneal abrasion and then leave the eye. Because of the density of corneal pain fibers in the normal eye, an abrasion and a foreign body feel the same to the patient. Blinking abrades the epithelial defect and exacerbates discomfort. Treatment should mitigate the effect of the upper eyelid on the epithelial defect to minimize discomfort and promote healing.

Corneal foreign bodies are identified most effectively by slit-lamp examination. Before removing a corneal foreign body, the clinician should assess the depth of corneal penetration. Occult intraocular foreign bodies must be ruled out when there is a history of exposure to high-speed metallic foreign bodies, typically from grinding tools and metal-on-metal hammering.

Identifying the composition of a corneal foreign body by either history or examination is important. Vegetable matter, such as leaves, thorns, bark, and dirt, presents an increased risk of fungal keratitis, so corticosteroid drops are contraindicated in patients with these types of foreign bodies, because of the risk of potentiating fungal infection. Contaminated foreign material from a hospital or medical setting may pose a higher risk of bacterial infection.

If glass foreign bodies are present, all exposed fragments should be removed. Fragments deeply embedded in the cornea are often inert and can be left in place (Fig 14-25). Careful gonioscopic evaluation of the anterior chamber is essential to ensure that the iris and the angle are free of any retained glass particles. Glass particles in the anterior chamber are indicative of a perforating ocular injury.

When an iron foreign body has been embedded in the cornea for more than a few hours, an orange-brown "rust ring" results (Fig 14-26). Corneal iron foreign bodies and rust rings can usually be removed at the slit lamp with a disposable (25-gauge or 26-gauge) hypodermic needle, after application of a topical anesthetic. A battery-powered dental burr with a sterile tip may also be utilized; however, the rotating burr can cause excessive tissue disruption and increased scar formation. A foreign body that enters the corneal stroma deep to the Bowman layer always results in some degree of scar formation. When these scars occur in the visual axis, they may result in glare and decreased vision from irregular astigmatism. Optimal management of a corneal foreign body therefore includes

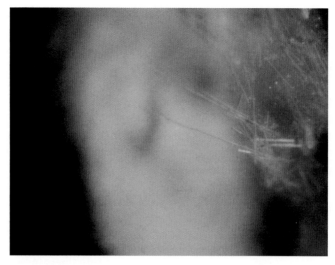

Figure 14-25 Glass or fiberglass foreign bodies (as seen in this photograph) may be well tolerated in the corneal stroma. *(Courtesy of Woodford S. Van Meter, MD.)*

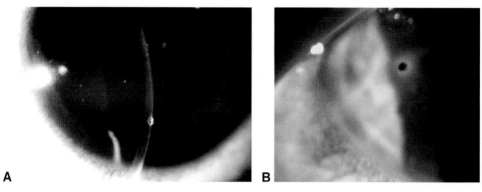

A   B

Figure 14-26 **A,** Orange ring around a rust foreign body present for 24–48 hours. **B,** White infiltrate around an iron foreign body present for 3–5 days. *(Courtesy of Woodford S. Van Meter, MD.)*

minimal disruption of the Bowman layer to avoid further scarring and obstruction of the visual axis.

Therapy following the removal of a corneal foreign body includes the use of topical antibiotics, cycloplegia, and occasionally the application of a firm pressure patch or bandage contact lens to help the healing process. If a pressure patch or bandage contact lens is used, the risk of infection due to the foreign body is increased and the patient should be closely monitored until this risk has passed.

Blast injuries may cause both penetrating and perforating corneal foreign bodies (Fig 14-27). For patients with blast injuries, the clinician should meticulously remove all possible foreign bodies on or near the surface of the cornea to prevent subsequent erosion of the superficial foreign bodies and accompanying discomfort.

Scott R. The injured eye. *Philos Trans R Soc Lond B Biol Sci.* 2011;366(1562):251–260.

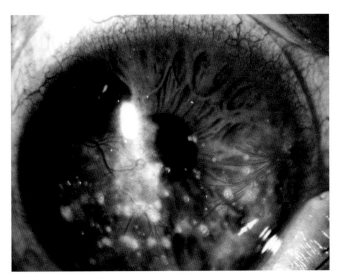

Figure 14-27 Multiple foreign bodies in the cornea following a blast injury. *(Courtesy of Woodford S. Van Meter, MD.)*

Evaluation and Management of Perforating Ocular Trauma

Evaluation

History

If a patient presents with both ocular and systemic trauma, diagnosis and treatment of any life-threatening injury take precedence over evaluation and management of the ophthalmic injury. Once the patient is medically stable, the ophthalmologist should elicit a complete preoperative history. The diagnosis of a traumatic ocular injury may be obvious from casual examination of the eye. However, a thorough history of the nature of the injury should always be obtained and should include questions about the history and details of the injury, such as whether the injury was associated with

- metal-on-metal strike
- high-velocity projectile
- high-energy impact on globe
- sharp injuring object
- lack of eye protection

Examination

Evaluation of a patient with a traumatic ocular injury should include a complete general and ophthalmic examination. As soon as possible, the examiner should determine and record visual acuity, which is the most reliable predictor of final visual outcome in traumatized eyes. Pupillary examination should be performed to detect the presence of an afferent pupillary defect (including a reverse Marcus Gunn response) arising from the possibility of traumatic mydriasis. The examiner should then look for key signs that are suggestive or diagnostic of a penetrating or perforating ocular injury (Table 14-5).

Table 14-5 Signs of Penetrating or Perforating Ocular Trauma

Suggestive	Diagnostic
Deep eyelid laceration	Exposed uvea, vitreous, retina
Orbital chemosis	Positive Seidel test result
Conjunctival laceration/hemorrhage	Visualization of intraocular foreign body
Focal iris–corneal adhesion	Intraocular foreign body seen on x-ray or
Shallow anterior chamber	ultrasonography
Iris defect	
Hypotony	
Lens capsule defect	
Acute lens opacity	
Retinal tear/hemorrhage	

Table 14-6 Ancillary Tests in the Evaluation of Penetrating Ocular Trauma

Useful in many cases (to assess extent of injury and provide needed information for preoperative assessment of patient)
CT scan
Plain-film x-ray (generally not as useful as CT scans)
CBC, differential, platelet level
Electrolyte, blood urea nitrogen, creatinine levels
Test for HIV status, hepatitis

Useful in selected cases
MRI (especially in cases of suspected organic foreign objects in the eye or orbit; this should *never* be used if a metallic foreign object is suspected)
Prothrombin time, partial thromboplastin time, bleeding time
Sickle cell test
Drug and/or ethanol levels

CBC = complete blood count; CT = computed tomography; HIV = human immunodeficiency virus; MRI = magnetic resonance imaging.

If a significant perforating injury is suspected, forced duction testing, gonioscopy, tonometry, and scleral depression should be avoided. Ancillary tests that may be useful in this setting are summarized in Table 14-6. All cases should be managed with safeguards appropriate for patients known to have blood-borne infections.

Nonsurgical Management

Some perforating injuries are so minimal that they seal spontaneously before ophthalmic examination, with no intraocular damage, prolapse, or adherence. These cases may require only systemic and/or topical antibiotic therapy along with close observation. Small, nongaping wounds may be treated as corneal abrasions with patching or a bandage contact lens until the epithelial defect has resolved and the patient is comfortable.

If a corneal wound is leaking (ie, the Seidel test result is positive; see Chapter 2, Fig 2-22) but the anterior chamber remains formed, the clinician can attempt to stop the leak with the following interventions, used in combination or alone: pharmacologic suppression of aqueous production (topical [eg, β-blocker] or systemic), patching, a therapeutic contact lens, or a tissue adhesive. Generally, if these measures fail to seal the wound within 2 days, surgical closure with sutures is recommended. If the corneal wound is leaking in the presence of a very shallow or flat anterior chamber, urgent surgical repair is required.

When a foreign body is present, the management of a corneal perforation poses a special challenge. The Descemet membrane is the strongest structural barrier to perforation of the cornea; foreign bodies may penetrate through the stroma and lodge anterior to the Descemet membrane. It may be difficult to determine whether removal of a deep foreign body will dislodge a self-sealed wound, so judicious decision making is mandatory. If multiple, very small foreign bodies are seen in the deep stroma (as may occur after an explosion) with no resultant inflammation or sign of infection, the patient may be monitored closely, given that aggressive surgical manipulation of the cornea in search of the very last particle may be unnecessary. If anterior chamber extension is present or suspected, the foreign body should be removed in a sterile environment such as an operating room. Overly aggressive attempts to remove deeply embedded foreign bodies at the slit lamp may result in leakage of aqueous humor and collapse of the anterior chamber.

Surgical Management

Preoperative management

If surgical repair is required, the timing of the operation is crucial. Although studies have not documented any disadvantage in delaying the repair of an open globe for up to 36 hours, intervention ideally should occur as soon as possible. Prompt closure of the wound to restore the integrity of the globe helps minimize the risk of additional damage to intraocular contents, inflammation, microbial proliferation, and endophthalmitis.

The following should be done before proceeding to the operating room:

- apply a protective shield
- avoid interventions that require prying open the eyelids
- ensure that the patient has no food or liquids
- prescribe appropriate medications for sedation and pain control
- initiate intravenous antibiotics and antiemetics
- provide tetanus prophylaxis
- seek anesthesia consultation

Injuries associated with soil contamination and/or retained intraocular foreign bodies increase the risk of *Bacillus* endophthalmitis. Because this organism can destroy the eye within 24 hours, intravenous and/or intravitreal therapy with an antibiotic effective against *Bacillus* species may be necessary; fluoroquinolones (eg, levofloxacin, moxifloxacin, or gatifloxacin), clindamycin, or vancomycin should be considered. Surgical repair should be undertaken with minimal delay in cases at risk for contamination with this organism.

Anesthesia

General anesthesia is almost always preferred for repair of an open globe because retrobulbar or peribulbar anesthetic injection increases posterior orbital pressure, which may cause or exacerbate the extrusion of intraocular contents. Local or topical anesthesia may be considered for the repair in rare instances, such as a patient with a small, self-sealing laceration who is at medical risk from general anesthesia. After the surgical repair is complete, a periocular anesthetic injection may be used to control postoperative pain.

Surgical repair considerations

Management of a typical full-thickness corneoscleral laceration with uveal prolapse generally requires surgical repair in the operating room (Fig 14-28). The primary goal of the repair is to restore the integrity of the globe. The secondary goal at the time of the primary repair or during subsequent procedures is to restore vision.

Primary enucleation should be performed only for an injury so devastating that restoration of the anatomy is impossible, when it may spare the patient another procedure. If the prognosis for vision in the injured eye is hopeless and the patient is at risk for sympathetic ophthalmia, enucleation must be considered. In the overwhelming majority of cases, however, the advantages of delaying enucleation for a few days far outweigh any advantage of primary enucleation. This delay (which should not exceed the 12–14 days thought necessary for an injured eye to incite sympathetic ophthalmia) allows for assessment of postoperative visual function, consultation with a vitreoretinal or ophthalmic plastic surgeon, and stabilization of the patient's medical condition. Most importantly, delay in enucleation following attempted repair and subsequent loss of light perception allow the patient time to acknowledge both loss of vision and accompanying disfigurement and to thoughtfully consider the benefits of enucleation in a nonemergency setting.

Agrawal R, Rao G, Naigaonkar R, Ou X, Desai S. Prognostic factors for vision outcome after surgical repair of open globe injuries. *Indian J Ophthalmol.* 2011;59(6):465–470.

Castiblanco CP, Adelman RA. Sympathetic ophthalmia. *Graefes Arch Clin Exp Ophthalmol.* 2009;247(3):289–302.

Galor A, Davis JL, Flynn HW Jr, et al. Sympathetic ophthalmia: incidence of ocular complications and vision loss in the sympathizing eye. *Am J Ophthalmol.* 2009;148(5):704–710.e2.

Repair of a corneoscleral laceration

Repair of a corneoscleral laceration in the operating room should take precedence over non-life-threatening surgical problems elsewhere on the body. Repair of an adnexal injury

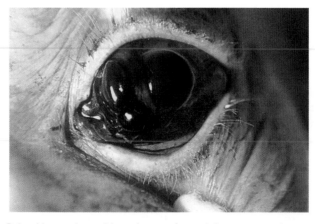

Figure 14-28 Scleral laceration with prolapse of uveal tissue secondary to blunt trauma.

should follow repair of the globe itself because eyelid surgery can put pressure on an open globe, and certain eyelid lacerations may actually improve globe exposure.

The corneal component of the injury is approached first. If vitreous or lens fragments have prolapsed through the wound, the surgeon should cut these fragments flush with the surface of the globe (Fig 14-29), taking care not to exert traction on the vitreous or zonular

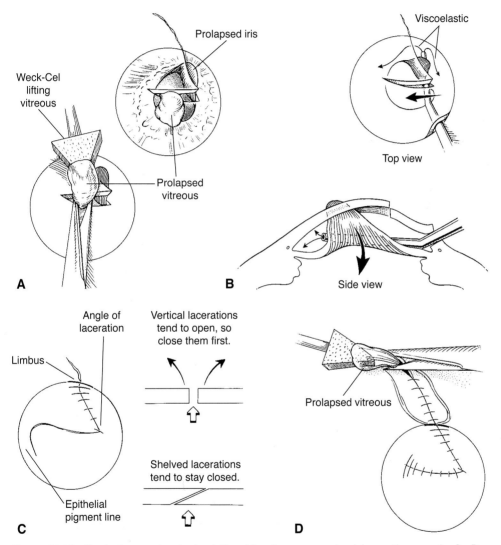

Figure 14-29 Restoring anatomical relationships in corneoscleral laceration repair. **A,** Prolapsed vitreous or lens fragments are excised. **B,** Iris is reposited by means of viscoelastic and a cannula inserted through a separate paracentesis. **C,** Landmarks such as limbus, laceration angles, or epithelial pigment lines are closed. Vertical lacerations are closed first to create a watertight globe more quickly, followed by shelved lacerations. **D,** The scleral part of the wound is exposed, prolapsed vitreous is severed, and the wound is closed from the limbus, working posteriorly. *(Reproduced from Hamill MB. Repair of the traumatized anterior segment. Focal Points: Clinical Modules for Ophthalmologists. San Francisco: American Academy of Ophthalmology; 1992, module 1. Illustrations by Christine Gralapp.)*

fibers. If uvea or retina (seen as translucent, tan tissue with extremely fine vessels) protrudes, the surgeon should reposit it using a gentle sweeping technique through a separate limbal incision, with the assistance of viscoelastic injection to keep the anterior chamber formed. If epithelium has obviously migrated onto a uveal surface or into the wound, an effort should be made to peel the epithelial layer off. Only in cases of frankly necrotic macerated tissue should uveal tissue be excised.

Points at which the laceration crosses landmarks such as the limbus are then closed with 9-0 or 10-0 nylon suture, followed by closure of the remaining corneal components of the laceration. It may be necessary to reposit iris tissue repeatedly after each suture is placed to avoid entrapment of iris in the wound. Despite these efforts, uvea may remain apposed to the posterior corneal surface. Very shallow sutures may be helpful at this stage of closure to avoid impaling the uvea with the suture needle. Then, after the closure is watertight, the uvea can be definitively separated from the cornea with viscoelastic injection, followed by replacement of the shallow sutures with deeper ones of near-full-thickness depth. Suture knots should be buried in the corneal stroma with the knot on the side of firmest tissue support to facilitate eventual removal.

If watertight closure of the wound proves difficult to achieve because of unusual laceration configuration or loss of tissue, X-shaped or purse-string sutures or other customized techniques may suffice. Cyanoacrylate glue or even primary lamellar keratoplasty may be required in extremely difficult cases, but a bandage contact lens over the glue is necessary for comfort. A conjunctival flap should not be used to treat a wound leak.

When the anatomy of the wound allows, specific suturing techniques may be helpful to restore the normal corneal contour. Longer, more widely spaced sutures create flattening in the area of the suture and are therefore placed in the peripheral cornea to re-create the aspheric curvature of the cornea—flatter in the periphery and steeper centrally. Shorter, more closely spaced sutures are then used centrally, when possible, in order to close the wound without excessive central flattening (Fig 14-30). When the sutures are being tied, it is important to have sufficient tension to create a watertight closure but not excessive tightness, which can induce corneal folds, astigmatism, or maceration of the inflamed stromal tissue. The knots should be buried for patient comfort. Very short sutures are harder to remove than longer sutures.

To evaluate the scleral component of the laceration, a gentle peritomy and conjunctival separation are performed to expose the wound. Prolapsed vitreous is excised, and prolapsed nonnecrotic uvea and retina are reposited, as in corneal repair, by use of a spatula or similar instrument (Fig 14-31). The scleral wound is closed with 9-0 nylon or 8-0 silk sutures. Often, resection of Tenon capsule and management of prolapsed tissue must be repeated incrementally after each suture is placed. The McCannel technique is a popular approach for repair of an iris defect (Fig 14-32).

Some posterior wounds may require visualization with a loupe and a headlight if the open globe cannot be rotated enough for visualization under the operating microscope. If the laceration extends under an extraocular muscle, the muscle may be carefully removed at its insertion and then reinserted following repair. The surgeon should exercise extreme care if fixation of an open globe with rectus muscle sutures is necessary for visualization, as is sometimes done in retinal surgery, because doing so would put undue pressure on the eye and could exacerbate the extrusion of intraocular structures. Closure of the laceration

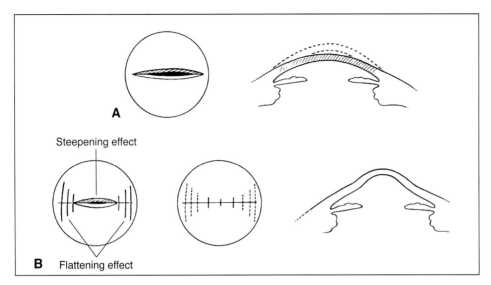

Figure 14-30 Restoring functional architecture in corneal wound closure. **A,** Laceration has a flattening effect on the cornea. **B,** Long, compressive sutures are taken in the periphery to flatten the peripheral cornea and steepen the central cornea. Subsequently, short, minimally compressive sutures are taken in the steepened central cornea to preserve sphericity despite the flattening effect of the sutures. *(Reproduced from Hamill MB. Repair of the traumatized anterior segment.* Focal Points: Clinical Modules for Ophthalmologists. *San Francisco: American Academy of Ophthalmology; 1992, module 1.)*

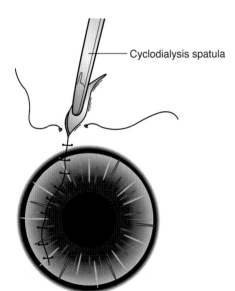

Figure 14-31 The zippering technique of scleral wound closure. Prolapsed uveal tissue is depressed while the scleral wound is progressively closed, moving in an anterior-to-posterior direction. *(Redrawn from Hersh PS, Shingleton BJ, Kenyon KR. Management of corneoscleral lacerations. In: Hersh PS, Shingleton BJ, Kenyon KR, eds.* Eye Trauma. *St Louis: Mosby Year Book; 1991.)*

should continue posteriorly only to the point at which it becomes technically difficult or requires undue pressure on the globe to complete. Very posterior lacerations may be tamponaded effectively by orbital tissue and are best left alone.

Once the globe is watertight, the surgeon must decide whether intraocular surgery (if necessary) should be attempted immediately or postponed. Deciding whether to pursue such intervention at the time of initial repair is a complex process. The expertise of the

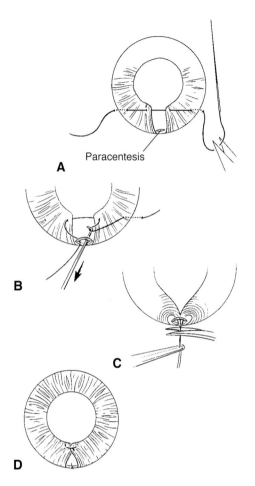

Figure 14-32 The McCannel technique for repairing iris lacerations. With large lacerations, multiple sutures may be used. **A,** A limbal paracentesis is made over the iris discontinuity. A long Drews needle with 10-0 polypropylene is then passed through the peripheral cornea, the edges of the iris, and the peripheral cornea opposite, and the suture is cut. **B,** A Sinskey hook, introduced through the paracentesis and around the suture peripherally, is drawn back out through the paracentesis. **C,** The suture is securely tied. **D,** After the suture is secure, it is cut, and the iris is allowed to retract. *(Reproduced from Hamill MB. Repair of the traumatized anterior segment. Focal Points: Clinical Modules for Ophthalmologists. San Francisco: American Academy of Ophthalmology; 1992, module 1. Illustrations by Christine Gralapp.)*

surgeon; the quality of the facility, technical equipment, and instruments; the adequacy of the view of anterior segment structures; and issues of informed consent should be considered. In general, it is recommended that, if there are concerns regarding any of these parameters, the surgeon complete the closure of the laceration to maintain globe integrity and postpone the secondary procedures until a later date. For example, the average anterior segment surgeon should not attempt automated vitrectomy with retina present in the anterior chamber, and the most expert cataract surgeon might not attempt a lens extraction with limited visualization.

As always, the welfare of the patient determines the proper course. In general, if a foreign body is visible in the anterior segment and can be grasped, it is reasonable to remove it, either through the wound or through a separate limbal incision. Metal fragments are difficult to remove through their entrance wounds because the rough metal edges usually require a surprisingly larger wound for extraction than would appear necessary. If removal of opacified lens material is attempted, it is helpful to know whether the posterior capsule has been violated and lens–vitreous admixture has occurred. The removal of a ruptured lens may be undertaken from a posterior approach with vitrectomy during a second procedure. BCSC Section 11, *Lens and Cataract,* also discusses the issues of cataract surgery and IOL placement following trauma to the eye.

Closure of iris lacerations helps keep the iris in its proper plane, decreasing the formation of anterior or posterior synechiae while reducing glare and polyopia from severe corectopia, but may be difficult to achieve during the primary procedure. Iridodialysis may cause monocular diplopia and an eccentric pupil if left untreated. In the event that corneal opacity prevents safe repair of internal ocular injury, repairs can be performed secondarily.

Subconjunctival injections of antibiotics to cover both gram-positive and gram-negative organisms may be given prophylactically at the conclusion of the repair. Intravitreal antibiotics such as vancomycin 1 mg and ceftazidime 2.25 mg should be considered for contaminated wounds involving the vitreous.

Postoperative management

Postoperatively, therapy is directed at preventing infection, suppressing inflammation, controlling IOP, and relieving pain. Patients may be given intravenous antibiotics (eg, a cephalosporin and an aminoglycoside) for 48 hours or an oral antibiotic such as moxifloxacin (400 mg per day) for 3–5 days. Topical antibiotics are generally instilled 4 times a day for 7 days or until epithelial closure of the ocular surface is complete. Topical corticosteroids may be given 4–8 times a day, depending on the amount of inflammation or the risk of infection. Corticosteroid drops and cycloplegics are slowly tapered as the inflammation subsides. A fibrinous response in the anterior chamber may respond well to a short course of systemic prednisone. IOP should be monitored; low pressure may suggest a wound leak, cyclodialysis, ciliary body shutdown, choroidal effusion, or intraocular hemorrhage. Elevated IOP should be controlled to minimize the risk of optic nerve damage.

Corneal sutures that do not loosen spontaneously are generally left in place for at least 3 months, depending on wound healing and patient age, and then removed incrementally over the next few months. Fibrosis and vascularization are indicators that enough healing has occurred to render suture removal safe. Applying fluorescein at each postoperative visit is mandatory to ensure that suture loosening or erosion through the epithelium has not occurred, as these eroded sutures can induce pain, infection, and inflammation.

Traumatized eyes are at increased risk of choroidal effusion or retinal detachment, so frequent examination of the posterior segment is mandatory. If media opacity precludes an adequate fundus examination, evaluation for an afferent pupillary defect and B-scan ultrasonography are useful in monitoring retinal status.

Refraction and vision correction with contact lenses or glasses can proceed when the ocular surface and media permit. Partial or complete suture removal should be performed when safe to facilitate improvement in vision. Because of the risk of amblyopia in a child or loss of fusion in an adult, vision correction should not be unnecessarily delayed.

For more information on wound repair, see BCSC Section 4, *Ophthalmic Pathology and Intraocular Tumors.*

Macsai MS, Rohr A. Surgical management and rehabilitation of anterior segment trauma. In: Mannis MJ, Holland EJ, eds. *Cornea.* Vol 2. 4th ed. Philadelphia: Elsevier; 2017:1588–1600.

CHAPTER 15

Clinical Approach to Corneal Transplantation

 This chapter includes related videos, which can be accessed by scanning the QR codes provided in the text or going to www.aao.org/bcscvideo_section08.

Highlights

- The trend toward selectively replacing pathologic corneal tissue has led to an increase in lamellar corneal surgery.
- Endothelial keratoplasty (EK) is now the procedure of choice for treating endothelial cell dysfunction. Advantages include preservation of structural integrity, faster visual recovery, and more predictable refractive outcomes.
- Deep anterior lamellar keratoplasty (DALK) preserves the host corneal endothelium, eliminating the risk of endothelial rejection and providing additional structural support in the case of trauma. However, DALK does not reduce postoperative astigmatism or prevent stromal rejection.

Corneal Transplantation

Corneal transplantation refers to surgical replacement of a full-thickness host cornea (penetrating keratoplasty [PK]) or lamellar portion of the host cornea with that of a donor cornea. Ongoing innovations in lamellar transplantation have produced a virtual alphabet soup of nomenclature to describe the various approaches (Table 15-1). If the donor is another person, the tissue is called an *allograft* and the procedure is referred to as *allogeneic transplantation*. If the donor tissue is from the same or fellow eye, it is called an *autograft* and the procedure is referred to as *autologous transplantation* (see the section Corneal Autograft Procedures, later in the chapter).

A 2015 review by Park et al of corneal transplant procedures *(keratoplasty)* performed over the past 10 years in the United States identified several trends. The number of transplants performed annually increased slightly from 2005 to 2014 (but peaked in 2008). However, there has been a dramatic shift in the types of procedures performed.

Table 15-1 Contemporary Keratectomy and Keratoplasty Procedures

Acronym	Procedure
ALK (ALTK)	Anterior lamellar keratoplasty (therapeutic)
DALK	Deep anterior lamellar keratoplasty
DLEK	Deep lamellar endothelial keratoplasty
DMEK	Descemet membrane endothelial keratoplasty
DSEK (DSAEK)	Descemet stripping endothelial keratoplasty (automated)
EK	Endothelial keratoplasty
FALK	Femtosecond anterior lamellar keratoplasty
FLAK	Femtosecond laser–assisted keratoplasty
PKP/PK	Penetrating keratoplasty
PRK	Photorefractive keratectomy
PTK	Phototherapeutic keratectomy
SK	Superficial keratectomy

Modified from American Academy of Ophthalmology Cornea/External Disease Panel. Preferred Practice Pattern Guidelines. *Corneal Edema and Opacification.* San Francisco: American Academy of Ophthalmology; 2013. Available at www.aao.org/ppp.

The percentage of all transplants that were PK procedures decreased from 94.9% in 2005 to 41.5% in 2014. The percentage that were anterior lamellar keratoplasty (ALK) procedures (including DALK) increased slightly, but even by 2014, accounted for only 2.0% of total transplants. Most significantly, the percentage of all transplants that were EK procedures increased from 3.2% in 2005 to 55.9% in 2014; in the latter year, 49.7% were Descemet stripping endothelial keratoplasty (DSEK) and 6.2% were Descemet membrane endothelial keratoplasty (DMEK). The percentage that were keratoprosthesis procedures remained fairly stable at 0.6% of total transplants annually.

Table 15-2 lists the indications for transplantation of corneal tissue from US eye banks for procedures performed in the United States and internationally in 2016. The success of any transplant depends on the availability and quality of corneal tissue. The cornea surgeon is thus indebted to the Eye Bank Association of America and to the outstanding US and international eye banks that provide tissue.

> Park CY, Lee JK, Gore PK, Lim CY, Chuck RS. Keratoplasty in the United States: a 10-year review from 2005 through 2014. *Ophthalmology.* 2015;122(12):2432–2442.

Table 15-2 Indications for Transplant in US and International Eye Banks, 2016

Surgical Diagnosis	Endothelial Cell Failure						Total	
	PK		ALK		EK		Total	
Post–cataract surgery edema	2729	33.0%	—	—	5558	67.0%	8287	
Fuchs dystrophy	1171	6.9%	—	—	15,845	93.1%	17,016	
Other causes of endothelial dysfunction	1035	26.0%	—	—	2882	74.0%	3917	
Subtotal	**4935**	**17.0%**	**0**	**0%**	**24,285**	**83.0%**	**29,220**	
	12.8% of PK				75.4% of EK		40% of grafts	

Table 15-2 *(continued)*

Surgical Diagnosis	Stromal or Full-Thickness (Nonendothelial) Disease						Total	
	PK		ALK		EK		Total	
Keratoconus	5463	88.0%	732	12.0%	—	—	6195	
Other degenerations or dystrophies	1164	93.0%	88	7.0%	—	—	1252	
Post–refractive surgery	70	94.6%	4	5.4%	—	—	74	
Microbial changes	677	95.0%	36	5.0%	—	—	713	
Mechanical or chemical trauma	982	97.0%	31	3.0%	—	—	1013	
Congenital opacities	620	96.1%	25	3.9%	—	—	645	
Pterygium	10	77.0%	3	23.0%	—	—	13	
Noninfectious ulcerative keratitis or perforations	1301	95.5%	62	4.5%	—	—	1363	
Other causes of corneal dysfunction or distortion	2346	92.5%	191	7.5%	—	—	2537	
Subtotal	**12,633**	**91.5%**	**1172**	**8.5%**	**0**	**0%**	**13,805**	
	32.9% of PK		49.1% of ALK				18.9% of grafts	

Surgical Diagnosis	Regraft						Total	
	PK		ALK		EK		Total	
Repeated corneal transplant	4529	61.3%	38	0.5%	2822	38.2%	7389	
	11.8% of PK		1.6% of ALK		8.7% of EK		10.1% of grafts	

Surgical Diagnosis	Unknown/Unspecified						Total	
	PK		ALK		EK		Total	
Unknown, unreported, or unspecified	16,316	72.2%	1176	5.2%	5114	22.6%	22,606	
	42.5% of PK		49.3% of ALK		15.9% of EK		31.0% of grafts	

	PK		ALK		EK		Total	
Total for each procedure	**38,413**	**52.6%**	**2386**	**3.3%**	**32,221**	**44.1%**	**73,020**	

Modified with permission from the Eye Bank Association of America (EBAA). *2016 Eye Banking Statistical Report.* Washington, DC: EBAA; 2017.

Keratoplasty and Eye Banking

Milestones in the History of Keratoplasty and Eye Banks

The first human corneal transplant, for a 45-year-old laborer with an opaque cornea due to a lime burn, was performed by Eduard Zirm in 1906. In 1919, Anton Elschnig performed a partial central corneal penetrating transplant. Vladimir Filatov, his student, was the first to use donor corneas from cadavers. In the 1930s, Ramon Castroviejo developed instruments specially designed for performing corneal transplantation. In 1944, R. Townley Paton established the first eye bank to provide a source of donated human eye tissue for keratoplasty.

In 1961, to establish uniform policies and procedures for corneal transplantation, 10 eye banks formed the Eye Bank Association of America (EBAA). The 2017 EBAA membership currently includes all 69 eye banks in the United States, as well as 13 international eye banks.

Modern Eye Banking and Donor Selection

The EBAA and the US Food and Drug Administration track all donor tissue, monitoring for infection to minimize the chance of transmission. Screening of the donor medical record for potentially transmissible diseases is mandatory and is performed by an eye bank technician. Medical criteria that render a potential donor unsuitable for tissue recovery are listed in Table 15-3, and diseases that can be transmitted from donor corneas are listed in Table 15-4.

The eye bank technician also rigorously inspects the cadaver to rule out signs of high-risk behavior or other possible sources of potentially transmissible infectious diseases. Features like bluish-red cutaneous nodules (Kaposi sarcoma), needle marks, and recent tattoos can make the potential donor ineligible. If the cadaver passes inspection, blood samples are taken to rule out infectious diseases such as hepatitis B, hepatitis C, human immunodeficiency virus (HIV) infection, and syphilis.

Most eye banks accept corneal tissue from donors 2 to 75 years of age, but eye donation at any age is to be encouraged. Donor tissue from a person younger than 2 years is typically not used for transplant because it is extremely steep and flaccid, which makes the tissue difficult to handle and poses challenges in creating a watertight closure and achieving a predictable refractive outcome. The corneas of donors who have undergone cataract surgery are acceptable as long as they exceed the minimum acceptable cell count outlined in the eye bank's policy (typically 2000 cells/mm^2). Corneas with lower endothelial cell counts and clear stroma may be suitable for anterior lamellar procedures. Conversely, corneas with anterior stromal opacities but high cell counts may be used for EK. Patients who have undergone keratorefractive surgery are not suitable donors for PK, but if all other parameters are satisfactory, their corneas may be used for EK. Responsibility for determining whether a donor cornea is suitable for transplantation ultimately rests with the transplant surgeon.

Tissue Processing and Preservation

Originally, donor corneal tissue was preserved within the whole globe, which was refrigerated at 4°C in a glass jar that served as a moisture chamber; this allowed tissue to be used up to 24–48 hours after donation. Extensive research on the importance of the endothelium for corneal allograft survival led to the development of McCarey-Kaufman (MK) medium, which extended the storage time to 4 days. Optisol GS (Bausch + Lomb, Bridgewater, NJ) is the most commonly used intermediate-term storage medium in the United States today, allowing the tissue to be stored for up to 7 days after death and in some circumstances up to 14 days. It contains chondroitin 2.5%, dextran 1%, ascorbic acid, and vitamin B$_{12}$; it also includes gentamicin and streptomycin for broad-spectrum antibacterial coverage (Fig 15-1).

Table 15-3 Medical Criteria Contraindicating Donor-Cornea Use

Death of unknown cause with likelihood of other exclusion criteria
Congenital rubella
Reye syndrome within the past 3 months
Active viral encephalitis of unknown origin or progressive encephalopathy (eg, subacute
    sclerosing panencephalitis, progressive multifocal leukoencephalopathy)
Active bacterial or viral encephalitis
Active bacterial or fungal endocarditis
Suspected rabies virus infection or history of being bitten, within the past 6 months, by an animal
    suspected to be infected with rabies virus
Down syndrome (exclusion criterion for PK or ALK)
Intrinsic eye diseases
    Retinoblastoma
    Malignant tumor of the anterior ocular segment or known adenocarcinoma in the eye (primary
        or metastatic origin)
    Active ocular or intraocular inflammation: conjunctivitis, keratitis, scleritis, anterior uveitis,
        uveitis, vitreitis, choroiditis, or retinitis
    Congenital or acquired disorders of the eye that would preclude a successful outcome for the
        intended use (eg, a central donor corneal scar for an intended PK, keratoconus, or keratoglobus)
Leukemias
Active disseminated lymphomas
High-risk behavior or incarceration in prison
Prior refractive corneal surgery, such as radial keratotomy, PRK, LASIK, and lamellar inserts, with the
    exception that previous laser refractive surgery may not disqualify a donor's tissue for use in EK
Positive test for anti-HIV-1 and anti-HIV-2 (or combination test) and nonreactive for HBsAg and
    anti-HCV antibody
History of Ebola virus disease
History of melanoma with known metastatic disease

Donors for PK
Prior intraocular or anterior segment surgery
    Refractive corneal procedures (radial keratotomy, lamellar inserts)
    Laser photoablation surgery
Pterygium or other disorders involving the optical center of the cornea

Donors for ALK
Criteria are the same as those listed for PK, except that tissue with local eye disease affecting the
    corneal endothelium or previous ocular surgery that does not compromise the corneal stroma
    can be used.

Donors for EK
Criteria are the same as those listed for PK, except that tissue with noninfectious anterior
    pathology that does not affect the posterior stroma and endothelium is acceptable.

HBsAg = hepatitis B surface antigen; HCV = hepatitis C virus; HIV = human immunodeficiency virus;
LASIK = laser in situ keratomileusis.

Information from the Eye Bank Association of America (EBAA). *EBAA Medical Standards, October 2016.*
Washington, DC: EBAA; 2016.

The process of tissue recovery includes slit-lamp evaluation and an endothelial cell count at the eye bank before release for transplantation. The optimal time from death to recovery is less than 12 hours, but recovery is acceptable for up to 24 hours postmortem. After recovery, the donor tissue is stored at 4°C until use. Many eye banks prepare tissue for Descemet stripping automated endothelial keratoplasty (DSAEK) and DMEK once a cornea is deemed suitable for EK.

Table 15-4 Disease Transmission From Corneal Transplantation

Proven disease transmission from corneal transplantation
Rabies
Hepatitis B
Creutzfeldt-Jakob disease (previously diagnosed)
Retinoblastoma
Bacterial or fungal keratitis
Bacterial or fungal endophthalmitis

Potential disease transmission from corneal transplantation*
Human immunodeficiency virus infection
Herpes simplex virus infection
Prion diseases

*Other diseases that contraindicate donor-cornea use and that could be transmitted via corneal transplantation are listed in Table 15-3.

Information from the Eye Bank Association of America (EBAA). *EBAA Medical Standards, October 2016.* Washington, DC: EBAA; 2016.

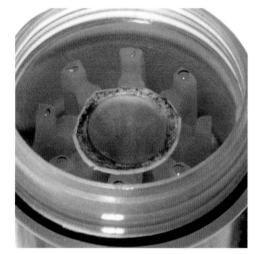

Figure 15-1 Corneal tissue preserved in Optisol GS. *(Courtesy of Woodford S. Van Meter, MD.)*

Most eye banks in Europe incubate donor corneal tissue in organ culture storage at 37°C. Organ culture allows tissue to be stored for up to 35 days but requires a culture at the end of the storage period to confirm sterility before the tissue is used. The organ culture system is more complex, costly, and labor-intensive than intermediate storage at 4°C, but the longer storage time is advantageous in places where the supply of donor corneas is limited.

Results of the Cornea Donor Study (CDS), a landmark study of eye bank–supplied corneal tissue, have greatly helped surgeons analyze and select donor tissue for their patients. The CDS, which completed enrollment in 2002 and conducted follow-up observations through 2012, evaluated the effect of donor age on graft survival in PK patients. Donors were grouped into cohorts age 10–64 years and age 65–75 years. At 5 years, the study showed no difference in the rate of graft survival between the 2 groups. However, at 10 years the rate of graft survival was slightly higher in patients receiving tissue from donors in the younger group than those receiving tissue from donors in the older group.

Eye Bank Association of America (EBAA). *2016 Eye Banking Statistical Report.* Washington, DC: EBAA; 2017.

Glasser DB. Medical standards for eye banking. In: Mannis MJ, Holland EJ, eds. *Cornea.* Vol 1. 4th ed. Philadelphia: Elsevier; 2017:287–297.

Lass JH, Beck RW, Benetz BA, et al; Cornea Donor Study Investigator Group. Baseline factors related to endothelial cell loss following penetrating keratoplasty. *Arch Ophthalmol.* 2011; 129(9):1149–1154.

Malling JV. Eye banking: structure and function. In: Mannis MJ, Holland EJ, eds. *Cornea.* Vol 1. 4th ed. Philadelphia: Elsevier; 2017:283–286.

Sugar A, Gal RL, Kollman C, et al; Writing Committee for the Cornea Donor Study Research Group. Factors associated with corneal graft survival in the Cornea Donor Study. *JAMA Ophthalmol.* 2015;133(3):246–254.

Transplantation for the Treatment of Corneal Disease

Ophthalmologists have many options for surgically treating the wide spectrum of corneal disease. The procedure of choice depends primarily on the depth and extent of corneal pathology (Table 15-5). Discussion of the surgical technique for these procedures is beyond the purview of this book; however, many excellent resources are available for this purpose and are listed in the references provided throughout the chapter. The following section discusses the preoperative evaluation of corneal transplant patients, and the rest of the chapter highlights the postoperative management of these patients in order to help the clinician make appropriate referrals and initiate treatment if necessary.

Gorovoy MS. Advances in lamellar corneal surgery. *Focal Points: Clinical Modules for Ophthalmologists.* San Francisco: American Academy of Ophthalmology; 2008, module 4.

Hausheer JR, ed. *Basic Techniques of Ophthalmic Surgery.* 2nd ed. San Francisco: American Academy of Ophthalmology; 2015.

Mannis MJ, Holland EJ, eds. *Cornea.* Vol 2. 4th ed. Philadelphia: Elsevier; 2017.

Table 15-5 Layer-Based Approach to the Surgical Management of Corneal Opacities and Edema

Layer of Pathology	Representative Disease	ED	SK	PTK	ALK	DALK	EK	PK
Epithelium	Redundant, irregular epithelium	●						
Subepithelial layer	Epithelial (anterior) basement membrane dystrophy	●						
	Salzmann nodular degeneration	●	●					
Bowman layer	Band keratopathy	●	●	●				
	Reis-Bücklers dystrophy		●	●	●			
Anterior–midstroma	Granular corneal dystrophy		●	●	●			●
Midposterior stroma	Scarring				●	●		●
Endothelium							●	●

ED = epithelial debridement; SK = superficial keratectomy.

From American Academy of Ophthalmology Cornea/External Disease Panel. Preferred Practice Pattern Guidelines. *Corneal Edema and Opacification.* San Francisco: American Academy of Ophthalmology; 2013. Available at www.aao.org/ppp.

Preoperative Evaluation and Preparation of the Transplant Patient

A complete ophthalmic evaluation, including a history and examination, is necessary before corneal transplantation. The clinician should obtain a detailed social history to help determine whether the patient or caretakers can adhere to the potentially complex postoperative regimen. A history of amblyopia, macular degeneration, and glaucoma or other optic neuropathy will affect the visual prognosis and the decision to proceed with surgery.

The examination should include simple clinical tests, such as checking for color vision, light projection, and afferent pupillary defect, particularly in patients with media opacity. It is important to recognize that corneal and lens opacities can dramatically constrict visual fields. Overrefraction with a rigid contact lens can aid in determining the cause of decreased vision. Improvement in vision with the contact lens indicates that superficial irregular astigmatism is the cause; in such cases, the patient can be offered treatment with a contact lens. If vision does not improve, corneal opacification is the most likely cause of the reduced vision, necessitating surgical intervention. Optical coherence tomography (OCT) may help detect retinal problems such as macular edema (cystoid or diabetic) and age-related macular degeneration. If the media are completely opaque, standard B-scan ultrasonography is helpful in evaluating the posterior segment.

Prior to any corneal procedure but particularly before PK, DALK, or ALK, it is important to check for reduced corneal sensation. The loss of corneal sensation seen in herpes zoster or simplex disease may complicate the postoperative course because of prolonged epithelial healing. It is also important to diagnose and treat ocular surface problems such as dry eye, blepharitis, and rosacea, as well as eyelid problems such as trichiasis, lagophthalmos, entropion, and ectropion prior to corneal surgery. In older patients, the postoperative course may be more problematic; slower wound healing, decreased corneal sensation, and reduced or incomplete eyelid closure can lead to persistent epithelial defects, infections, and wound dehiscence. Deep corneal vascularization and a history of graft failure increase the risk of rejection in PK and DALK. The presence of an active keratitis or uveitis at the time of surgery is associated with a higher incidence of postoperative complications, such as graft rejection or failure, glaucoma, and cystoid macular edema. Ideally, there should be no ocular inflammation for several months prior to surgery. A history of glaucoma surgery, such as placement of filters or tube shunts, reduces endothelial cell survival and increases the risk of graft failure in EK and PK.

Fortunately, the advent of EK for endothelial dysfunction has minimized the impact of ocular surface disorders on the success of transplantation. The extent of stromal edema can be measured with corneal pachymetry, Scheimpflug imaging, or anterior segment OCT. (See Chapter 2 for more discussion of these tests.) Typically, corneal edema is worse in the morning and improves throughout the day; this fluctuation can be documented through testing in the early morning and in the afternoon. In some patients, extensive guttae alone may cause enough reduction in vision or symptoms of glare to warrant surgery. For further discussion of the evaluation and indications for corneal surgery, see the references that follow.

American Academy of Ophthalmology Cornea/External Disease Panel. Preferred Practice Pattern Guidelines. *Corneal Edema and Opacification.* San Francisco: American Academy of Ophthalmology; 2013. Available at www.aao.org/ppp.

Hannush SB, Riveroll-Hannush L. Preoperative considerations and decision-making in kerato-plasty. In: Mannis MJ, Holland EJ. eds. *Cornea.* Vol 2. 4th ed. Philadelphia: Elsevier; 2017: 1256–1263.

Watanabe S, Oie Y, Fujimoto H, et al. Relationship between corneal guttae and quality of vision in patients with mild Fuchs endothelial corneal dystrophy. *Ophthalmology.* 2015; 122(10):2103–2109.

Penetrating Keratoplasty

The most common indications for PK are combined stromal and endothelial pathology, concomitant intraocular lens (IOL) suturing and anterior segment reconstruction, kera-toconus, and, less frequently, endothelial dysfunction (Fig 15-2). Video 15-1 shows PK performed to treat stromal scarring and endothelial decompensation due to congenital hereditary endothelial dystrophy. Video 15-2 shows PK combined with scleral suture fixa-tion of a posterior chamber IOL using an open-sky approach. To educate the patient about the risks and benefits of transplant surgery, the surgeon must understand potential intra-operative and postoperative complications, as well as postoperative management; these are discussed in the following subsections and summarized in Table 15-6.

 VIDEO 15-1 Penetrating keratoplasty for stromal scarring and endothelial dysfunction in congenital hereditary endothelial dystrophy.
Courtesy of Robert W. Weisenthal, MD.
Access all Section 8 videos at www.aao.org/bcscvideo_section08.

 VIDEO 15-2 PK with scleral-sutured intraocular lens using an open-sky approach.
Courtesy of Robert W. Weisenthal, MD.

Chan CC, Perez MA, Verdier DD, Van Meter WS. Penetrating keratoplasty: the fundamentals. In: Mannis MJ, Holland EJ, eds. *Cornea.* Vol 2. 4th ed. Philadelphia: Elsevier; 2017:1264–1276.

Intraoperative Complications

Complications that can occur during surgery are listed in Table 15-6.

Chen MC, Mannis MJ. Intraoperative complications of penetrating keratoplasty. In: Mannis MJ, Holland EJ, eds. *Cornea.* Vol 2. 4th ed. Philadelphia: Elsevier; 2017:1277–1282.

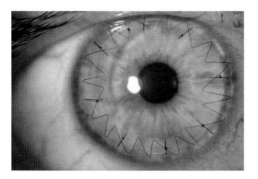

Figure 15-2 Slit-lamp photograph of a full-thickness corneal transplant with interrupted and continuous 10-0 nylon sutures. The inter-rupted sutures can be removed to control astigmatism. *(Courtesy of Robert W. Weisenthal, MD.)*

Table 15-6 Comparison of Procedures for Penetrating and Selective Keratoplasty

	Penetrating Keratoplasty (PK)	Anterior Lamellar Keratoplasty (ALK)	Deep Anterior Lamellar Keratoplasty (DALK)	Endothelial Keratoplasty (DSEK/DMEK)
Indications	Combined stromal or endothelial corneal pathology Keratoconus Concomitant IOL suturing/anterior segment reconstruction Fuchs corneal dystrophy/pseudophakic corneal edema (less frequently) Corneal perforation treated with patch graft, either lamellar or full thickness	Superficial stromal dystrophies and degenerations Salzmann nodular degeneration Scars, trauma, and dermoids Infections Superficial corneal tumors Descemetocele	Keratoconus Infections Corneal stromal dystrophies not involving endothelium Corneal thinning Corneal ectasia secondary to LASIK	Fuchs corneal dystrophy Posterior polymorphous corneal dystrophy Congenital hereditary endothelial dystrophy Pseudophakic corneal edema ICE syndrome Failed corneal graft
Intraoperative complications	Scleral perforation with fixation sutures Expulsive or choroidal hemorrhage Vitreous hemorrhage Damage to lens or iris Irregular trephination Poor graft centration Iris or vitreous incarceration in the wound Torn posterior capsule Damage to donor endothelium Excessive bleeding from the iris or wound edge Retained Descemet membrane	Poor microkeratome dissection for donor tissue Corneal perforation Thin or irregular donor tissue Irregular dissection of host stromal tissue	Corneal perforation requiring transition to PK Difficulty obtaining smooth dissection to Descemet membrane Double (pseudo) anterior chamber or Descemet membrane detachment Placement of an air bubble to tamponade Descemet membrane can cause formation of an anterior subcapsular cataract	Poor microkeratome dissection of donor tissue (DSEK) or inability to harvest Descemet membrane with endothelium (DMEK) Inability to strip host Descemet tissue Improper orientation or loss of donor tissue Excessive manipulation of donor tissue, leading to cell loss and possible graft failure Tearing of donor tissue Retention of viscoelastic

	Penetrating Keratoplasty (PK)	Anterior Lamellar Keratoplasty (ALK)	Deep Anterior Lamellar Keratoplasty (DALK)	Endothelial Keratoplasty (DSEK/DMEK)
Intraoperative complications (cont'd)	Retinal tear or detachment			Vitreous or blood in the interface Choroidal hemorrhage (lower risk than in PK) Hemorrhage leading to blood in the interface
Postoperative complications	Suture-related problems Infectious keratitis Neovascularization Graft rejection Graft failure Wound leak/misalignment Flat chamber Glaucoma Endophthalmitis Cystoid macular edema Elevated IOP Persistent epithelial defect Recurrent primary disease	Suture-related problems Infectious keratitis Neovascularization Graft (stromal) rejection Graft failure Opacification and vascularization of the interface Retained interface debris Microbial infections	Suture-related problems Infectious keratitis Neovascularization Epithelial or stromal allograft rejection Graft failure Opacification and/or vascularization of the interface Inflammatory necrosis of the graft Retained interface debris Microbial infections Visually significant wrinkling of Descemet membrane	Pupillary block glaucoma Dislocation or decentration of lenticule Primary graft failure Epithelial ingrowth Interface opacification Graft rejection (lower risk than after PK) Infection in the interface Cystoid macular edema Reduced endothelial cell survival
Advantages	Full-thickness tissue eliminates interface-related visual problems Ability to treat epithelial, stromal, and endothelial disease and allow anterior segment reconstruction in a single procedure if necessary	Selective removal of pathologic tissue Reduced risk of penetration of anterior chamber More rapid vision rehabilitation Less need for sutures Minimal requirements for donor tissue Reduced incidence of graft rejection	Selective removal of pathologic tissue Reduced risk of penetration of anterior chamber Preservation of globe integrity due to stronger wound than in PK Minimal requirements for donor tissue Early removal of sutures	Rapid vision rehabilitation Preservation of ocular surface Less induced astigmatism Greater accuracy in selection of intraocular lens for triple procedures Stronger wound Reduction in suture-related problems

(Continued)

Table 15-6 *(continued)*

	Penetrating Keratoplasty (PK)	Anterior Lamellar Keratoplasty (ALK)	Deep Anterior Lamellar Keratoplasty (DALK)	Endothelial Keratoplasty (DSEK/DMEK)
Advantages *(cont'd)*		Less risk for patients who adhere poorly to treatment or rub their eyes	Less chance of graft rejection without donor endothelium, allowing more flexibility in dose and duration of postop steroid prophylaxis Less risk for patients who adhere poorly to treatment or rub their eyes	Reduced incidence of graft rejection Smaller incision with preservation of globe integrity
Disadvantages	Difficulty determining anterior corneal curvature, potentially leading to anisometropia Ocular surface disease or neurotrophic cornea leads to prolonged healing or persistent epithelial defect Irregular/significant regular astigmatism	Irregular/significant regular corneal astigmatism Irregular interface Ocular surface disease or neurotrophic cornea leads to prolonged healing or persistent epithelial defect Stromal opacification/ interface debris	Irregular/significant regular corneal astigmatism Irregular interface Ocular surface disease or neurotrophic cornea leads to prolonged healing or persistent epithelial defect Stromal opacification/ interface debris Procedure more technically demanding and time-consuming	Significant stromal haze, subepithelial fibrosis, or epithelial irregularity may require second procedure Reduction in BCVA in DSEK, less so in DMEK Increased risk of primary graft failure during surgical learning curve

BCVA = best-corrected visual acuity; ICE = iridocorneal endothelial; IOP = intraocular pressure.

Postoperative Care and Complications

The long-term success of a PK depends on appropriate postoperative management and conscientious patient adherence. Routine postsurgical care includes short-term use of topical antibiotics and a prolonged, perhaps indefinite, course of topical steroids (prednisolone, difluprednate ophthalmic emulsion 0.05%, fluorometholone 0.25% or 0.1%). (See "Prevention of graft rejection," later in the chapter.) Frequent office visits are necessary to facilitate rapid vision rehabilitation and early recognition of the many complications that can occur after PK. The following sections review some common postsurgical complications.

> Section 3, Penetrating Keratoplasty: Postoperative Management. In: Mannis MJ, Holland EJ, eds. *Cornea.* Vol 2. 4th ed. Philadelphia: Elsevier; 2017:1289–1354.

Primary donor failure (primary endothelial failure)

When a graft is edematous from the first postoperative day and remains so without inflammatory signs, a deficiency of donor endothelium should be suspected (Fig 15-3). Most surgeons allow at least 4 weeks and up to 2 months for spontaneous resolution of edema before considering regrafting. The cause of the donor failure is not always clear and may be related to intraoperative handling of the tissue.

Wound misalignment or leak

The wound is always checked carefully for aqueous leakage at the end of surgery. A Seidel test can be helpful in postoperatively assessing wound integrity, particularly in patients with low intraocular pressure (IOP) and a normal or shallow anterior chamber. Small wound leaks or suture track leaks without iris incarceration often close spontaneously. Patching, therapeutic contact lenses, and use of aqueous suppressants may facilitate a watertight seal. Resuturing is advised for leaks associated with shallow anterior chambers and low pressures lasting longer than 3 days.

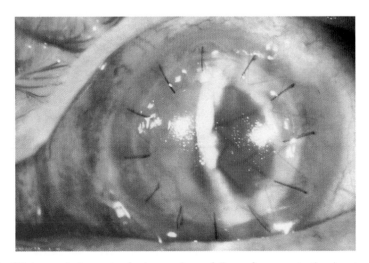

Figure 15-3 Slit-lamp photograph of primary donor failure after penetrating keratoplasty (PK).

Flat chamber or iris incarceration in the wound

If the IOP is low and there is a flat chamber or iris incarceration in the wound, the clinician should return the patient to surgery to reposit the iris, re-form the anterior chamber, and suture the wound. If the problem is not addressed promptly and appropriately, anterior synechiae may form, increasing the risk of graft rejection, glaucoma, or graft failure. Normal or high IOP with a shallow or flat anterior chamber may signify pupillary block or malignant glaucoma (aqueous misdirection). Initially, the surgeon should dilate the pupil to help break the pupillary block; if this is not successful, other measures are required. See BCSC Section 10, *Glaucoma,* for discussion of pupillary block and malignant glaucoma.

Endophthalmitis

After PK, endophthalmitis may arise owing to intraoperative contamination, contamination of the donor corneal button, or postoperative invasion by microorganisms. The incidence of endophthalmitis is considerably higher in PK patients than cataract surgery patients, particularly if the vitreous is invaded or if the donor died of infection. Immunosuppressed patients with moderate to severe eyelid inflammation are also at greater risk for infection. Early recognition and aggressive intervention can save the eye and vision in some cases. Donor rim culture may identify any potential contaminants. See also BCSC Section 9, *Intraocular Inflammation and Uveitis.*

Chen JY, Jones MN, Srinivasan S, Neal TJ, Armitage WJ, Kaye SB; NHSBT Ocular Tissue Advisory Group and Contributing Ophthalmologists (OTAG Audit Study 18). Endophthalmitis after penetrating keratoplasty. *Ophthalmology.* 2015;122(1):25–30.

Persistent epithelial defect

Large epithelial defects are common after PK, but they should heal within 7–14 days. After this time, irreversible scarring and ulceration may occur. Patients who have reduced corneal sensation or decreased blink rate before surgery are at greater risk. Ocular surface disease (eg, dry eye, exposure, rosacea, blepharitis) should be identified and treated. Lubrication, patching, therapeutic contact lenses, punctal occlusion with plugs or cautery, and temporary or permanent lateral tarsorrhaphy may be helpful in difficult cases. (See the discussions of neurotrophic keratopathy and persistent epithelial defects in Chapter 4 and of tarsorrhaphy in Chapter 13.) If these measures are not successful, the diagnosis of herpetic keratitis (Fig 15-4) should be considered even if this was not the underlying reason for the graft. Oral antivirals can be used as a therapeutic trial.

Elevated intraocular pressure

High IOP may occur at any time after PK. Often, the first clinical sign is the loss of folds in the Descemet membrane. IOP elevation early in the postoperative period can be due to pupillary block, malignant glaucoma, hemorrhage or pigment blocking the trabecular meshwork, or an overly tight running suture. Elevated IOP starting a month or more after the procedure may be due to response to steroids such as topical prednisolone or difluprednate ophthalmic emulsion 0.05%. If glaucoma develops, aggressive treatment with

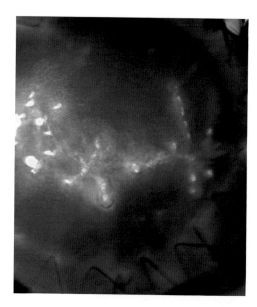

Figure 15-4 Slit-lamp photograph showing recurrence of herpes simplex keratitis in a graft. *(Courtesy of Robert W. Weisenthal, MD.)*

appropriate topical medications, laser surgery, or other surgical intervention is indicated. Though uncommon, epithelial downgrowth or fibrous ingrowth can also cause postoperative pressure elevation. See also BCSC Section 10, *Glaucoma*.

Recurrence of primary disease

Bacterial, fungal, viral, or amebic keratitis can recur in a graft in the early postoperative period. In recurrent infections, medical treatment directed at the causative agent is the initial form of therapy (see Chapters 9 and 10). Epithelial–stromal dystrophies such as granular or lattice dystrophy can superficially recur a year or later after the initial procedure (Fig 15-5). Visually significant lesions can be removed using phototherapeutic keratectomy (PTK); see Chapter 13.

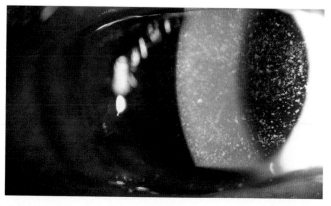

Figure 15-5 Slit-lamp photograph showing recurrence of granular corneal dystrophy after corneal transplantation. *(Courtesy of Robert W. Weisenthal, MD.)*

Suture-related problems

Postoperative problems related to sutures include the following:

- excessive tightness of the sutures, producing an irregular astigmatism or elevated IOP
- loosening (usually as a result of wound contraction, suture breakage, resolution of wound edema, or suture cheese-wiring; Fig 15-6)
- breakage of a continuous suture
- infectious abscesses (usually localized around loose, broken, or exposed sutures; Fig 15-7)
- noninfectious (toxic) suture infiltrates, often multiple and in areas of pannus, or extension of sutures beyond the limbus
- giant papillary conjunctivitis from exposed knots
- vascularization along suture tracks

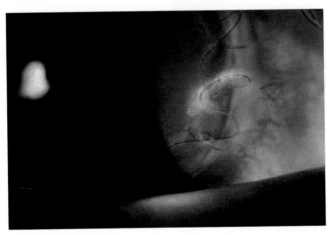

Figure 15-6 Slit-lamp photograph of an eroded continuous suture after PK. *(Courtesy of Robert W. Weisenthal, MD)*

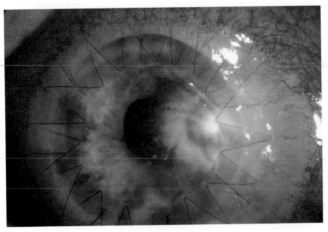

Figure 15-7 Slit-lamp photograph of a suture abscess in a corneal graft. *(Courtesy of Stephen Orlin, MD.)*

Loose or broken sutures do not contribute to wound stability and should be removed as soon as possible. Loose sutures stain with fluorescein because they usually have broken through the corneal epithelium. Totally buried fragments of interrupted sutures may be left. Vascularization along the suture indicates that the wound is adequately healed in the vicinity and that sutures may be removed safely. Vascularized sutures are also prone to loosening and may increase the likelihood of graft rejection. After the sutures are removed, the refractive error or astigmatism may shift dramatically, so the surgeon should see the patient in 3–4 weeks to ensure wound stability and to recheck refraction. The shift may occur even years after surgery.

Microbial keratitis

Long-term use of topical steroids, loss of corneal sensation after transplantation, uneven tear film, and suture exposure or erosion all predispose the patient to infectious keratitis, sometimes caused by unusual organisms. Culture of the infiltrate and the exposed suture is recommended, and initiation of broad-spectrum antibiotic therapy can help avoid graft failure. A peculiar form of keratitis, infectious crystalline keratopathy (Fig 15-8), is occasionally seen in grafts and other immunocompromised corneas. Branching colonies of organisms proliferate in the deep corneal stroma, with minimal or no inflammatory response. Many organisms have been implicated, but viridans streptococci are the most frequent causative organisms.

Late non–immune-mediated endothelial failure

In the absence of acute inflammation or graft rejection, visually significant corneal edema months to years after the procedure may be due to the normal loss of endothelial cells in tissue that had a marginal number of endothelial cells originally. The Cornea Donor Study showed that the 10-year cumulative probability of non–immune-mediated graft failure was higher in patients treated for pseudophakic or aphakic corneal edema than in patients treated for Fuchs endothelial corneal dystrophy. The higher failure rate may be related to the placement of a poorly designed anterior chamber lens or improper placement of the

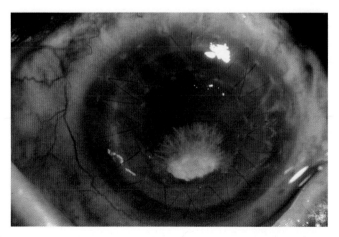

Figure 15-8   Slit-lamp photograph showing infectious crystalline keratopathy after PK. *(Courtesy of Stephen Orlin, MD.)*

lens during previous, complex cataract surgery. Such problems may require an exchange of the IOL at the time of PK. In addition, patients with a prior diagnosis of glaucoma— especially those with a history of glaucoma surgery (particularly tube shunt implantation) and, to a lesser extent, those taking glaucoma medications—face a higher probability of graft failure than do patients who have no history of glaucoma.

Sugar A, Gal RL, Kollman C, et al; Writing Committee for the Cornea Donor Study Research Group. Factors associated with corneal graft survival in the Cornea Donor Study. *JAMA Ophthalmol.* 2015;133(3):246–254.

Graft rejection

Corneal allograft rejection rarely occurs within the first month; however, it may occur many years after PK. Fortunately, most episodes of graft rejection do not cause irreversible graft failure if recognized early and treated aggressively with steroids. Corneal transplant rejection after PK occurs in 4 distinct clinical forms, which may occur either singly or in combination. (See BCSC Section 9, *Intraocular Inflammation and Uveitis*, and Chapter 11 in this volume for further discussion on the immunology of graft rejection.)

Epithelial rejection The immune response may be directed entirely at the donor epithelium (Fig 15-9). Lymphocytes cause an elevated, linear epithelial ridge that advances centripetally. Because host cells replace lost donor epithelium, this form of rejection is problematic only in that it may herald the onset of endothelial rejection. Epithelial rejection occurs in a minority of patients experiencing rejection and is usually seen early in the postoperative period (1–13 months). It may be asymptomatic; however, blurred vision can occur if the epithelial ridge is near the visual axis.

Subepithelial rejection Corneal transplant rejection may also present as subepithelial infiltrates (Fig 15-10). These may be asymptomatic or may cause glare or reduced vision. It is not known whether these lymphocytic cells are directed at donor keratocytes or at donor epithelial cells. In atypical cases, a cellular anterior chamber reaction may accompany this form of rejection. Easily missed on cursory examination, subepithelial infiltrates

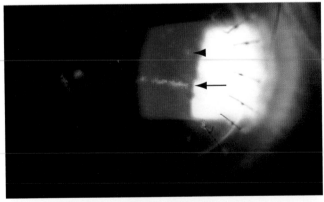

Figure 15-9 Slit-lamp photograph showing an epithelial rejection line *(arrow)* with subepithelial infiltrates *(arrowhead)* after PK. *(Courtesy of Robert W. Weisenthal, MD.)*

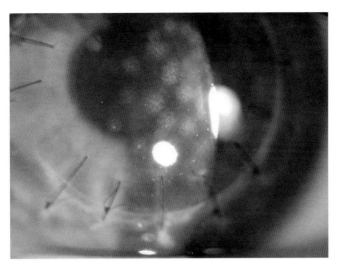

Figure 15-10 Slit-lamp photograph showing corneal graft rejection manifested by subepithelial infiltrates. *(Courtesy of Charles S. Bouchard, MD.)*

can best be seen with broad, tangential illumination. They resemble the infiltrates associated with adenoviral keratoconjunctivitis. Subepithelial graft rejection may completely resolve if treated, but it may presage the more severe endothelial graft rejection.

Stromal rejection Isolated stromal rejection is not common after PK; it is seen more commonly after DALK. It may present as stromal infiltrates, neovascularization, or, typically, noninfiltrative keratolysis within the graft–host interface that does not extend into the peripheral recipient stroma. In severe or prolonged episodes of graft rejection, the stroma can become necrotic.

Endothelial rejection The most common and serious form of graft rejection is endothelial rejection, because loss of a significant number of endothelial cells leads to graft failure. Inflammatory precipitates are seen on the endothelial surface in fine precipitates, in random clumps, or in linear form underlying or in some cases outlining the area of corneal edema (Khodadoust line; Fig 15-11). Inflammatory cells are usually seen in the anterior chamber as well, but anterior uveitis is usually mild. As endothelial function is lost, the corneal stroma thickens with the development of posterior folds, and microcystic or bullous epithelial edema can occur. Patients have symptoms related to inflammation and corneal edema, such as photophobia, redness, irritation, halos around lights, or fogginess of vision.

Treatment Frequent administration of steroid eyedrops is the mainstay of therapy for corneal allograft rejection. Either dexamethasone 0.1% or prednisolone 1% eyedrops are used, as often as every 15 minutes to 2 hours, depending on the severity of the episode. Difluprednate ophthalmic emulsion 0.05% can also be used, in less frequent doses; however, close follow-up to monitor for increased IOP is recommended. Although topical steroid ointment may be used on occasion, the reduced bioavailability of topical ointment is not as effective as frequently applied eyedrops.

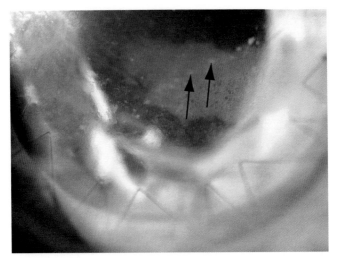

Figure 15-11 Slit-lamp photograph showing corneal endothelial graft rejection with epithelial and stromal edema. Note the Khodadoust line *(arrows)*. *(Courtesy of Robert W. Weisenthal, MD.)*

Steroids may be given by periocular injection (triamcinolone acetonide 0.5 cc of 40 mg/mL or dexamethasone 0.5 cc of 4 mg/mL) for severe rejection episodes or nonadherent patients. Caution is advised in patients who may have steroid-induced elevation of IOP or a history of herpetic keratitis. In particularly fulminant cases, steroids may be administered either orally (80 mg per day, tapered as the graft rejection responds) or intravenously (a one-time dose of 125–500 mg methylprednisolone).

Prevention of graft rejection Surgical techniques that avoid proximity to the peripheral cornea and early attention to loosening sutures and infections will minimize the risk of rejection.

According to a survey of members of the Cornea Society conducted in 2011, prednisolone is the topical steroid of choice for prophylaxis against graft rejection; however, some surgeons prefer dexamethasone instead. In low-risk cases, the dosage is typically 4 times per day for at least 3 months; it is then tapered by 1 drop either each month or every 2 months until it has been reduced to once per day. Notably, 13% of respondents reported using difluprednate in high-risk eyes for the first 6 months. In patients with a steroid response causing ocular hypertension, respondents reported substituting loteprednol etabonate ophthalmic suspension or fluorometholone. The phakic patient may be tapered off steroids or maintained on one of low-concentration to minimize the risk of cataract. The pseudophakic patient is typically kept on a once-daily steroid regimen. Patients using steroids should continue to be followed for IOP elevation, which can occur many months or even years after treatment.

Long-term immunosuppressive agents such as topical cyclosporine have been used to prevent graft rejection, but in general, cyclosporine is not as effective as topical steroids. In high-risk cases, the use of various immunosuppressive agents, including oral cyclosporine, tacrolimus, and mycophenolate mofetil, has been reported, but these medications require very careful follow-up because of their narrow therapeutic index. Topical tacrolimus has also been advocated for use in high-risk patients.

Kharod-Dholakia B, Randleman JB, Bromley JG, Stulting RD. Prevention and treatment of corneal graft rejection: current practice patterns of the Cornea Society (2011). *Cornea.* 2015; 34(6):609–614.

Control of Postoperative Corneal Astigmatism and Refractive Error

A corneal transplant was once considered successful merely if the graft remained clear. Today, success is also measured based on the refractive outcome. Severe astigmatism may be associated with decreased visual acuity, anisometropia, aniseikonia, image distortion, and monocular diplopia, rendering an otherwise clear graft poorly functional. Many methods have been suggested to reduce astigmatism, including

- variation of suture techniques
- intraoperative adjustments with qualitative keratometry
- improvement of trephines and use of new technology, such as the femtosecond laser (femtosecond laser–assisted keratoplasty [FLAK]), to better match donor and host tissue (however, the efficacy of matching the tissue with the femtosecond laser has not been shown to reduce astigmatism in long-term clinical studies)
- selective suture removal or adjustment of the continuous suture using corneal topography and tomography for postoperative management
- incisional or ablative refractive surgery
- secondary intraocular procedures after the graft has stabilized

The primary method of reducing astigmatism postoperatively is to readjust or remove the sutures. However, before suture removal or adjustment is considered, it is essential to ensure that a smooth and regular epithelium is present. Careful attention to the ocular surface and appropriate management of topical therapy expedite reaching this point. If a single continuous suture technique has been used, the surgeon may redistribute the suture tension at 1 month postoperatively, using corneal topography as a guide. Alternatively, if there is a combination of continuous and interrupted sutures, the interrupted sutures can be removed starting at 1 month. If the patient has only interrupted sutures, suture removal should begin at a later stage to avoid wound slippage or dehiscence. Clinicians must be especially careful with older patients placed on long-term topical steroid therapy, as wound healing is often slower in these patients.

Prior to removal of the sutures, the most critical step is to identify the steep axis using corneal topography, photokeratoscopy, or manual keratometry. For example, in Figure 15-12 the simulated keratometry readings from the topographer show a steep axis of 49.93 diopters (D) at 11 and a flat axis of 44.06 D at 101. The photokeratoscopic image shows clear rings that are oval in contour, with the shorter axis horizontally corresponding to the steep axis. The presence of distinct rings demonstrates the smooth surface indicative of regular astigmatism. Rings that are very irregular or indistinct may indicate irregular astigmatism; in such cases, suture removal is not recommended until clear and stable measurements can be obtained. Surface disruption may distort keratoscopic mires, but a drop of a tear supplement can temporarily make the mires more distinct.

Manifest refraction can aid in confirming the steep axis (plus cylinder). The autorefraction in Figure 15-12 is –9.00 +6.75 at 4°. The manifest refraction is –7.00 +5.00 at 4°, resulting in 20/25 acuity; the good visual acuity confirms the presence of regular

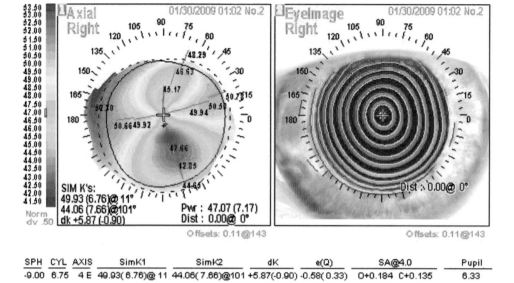

SPH	CYL	AXIS	SimK1	SimK2	dK	e(Q)	SA@4.0	Pupil
-9.00	6.75	4 E	49.93(6.76)@ 11	44.06(7.66)@101	+5.87(-0.90)	-0.58(0.33)	O+0.184 C+0.135	6.33

Figure 15-12 Corneal topography with a Nidek OPD showing astigmatism after corneal transplantation. *(Courtesy of Robert W. Weisenthal, MD.)*

astigmatism. Removing the interrupted sutures on one or both sides of the 4° meridian or adjusting the continuous suture will compensate for the induced astigmatism. After manipulation or removal of the sutures, the patient uses a topical antibiotic for 4 days and returns for a follow-up visit in 1 month for corneal topography and manifest refraction.

If the patient has intolerable anisometropia or significant astigmatism after adjustment or removal of selected sutures, a contact lens can be tried. After removal of all sutures, relaxing incisions—performed with a metal or diamond knife or a femtosecond laser—are effective in treating residual regular astigmatism. The arcuate incisions are placed either in the donor cornea anterior to the graft–host junction or in the graft–host interface at the steep (plus cylinder) meridian. Suture placement at the flat meridian can augment the effect. Laser in situ keratomileusis (LASIK) and photorefractive keratectomy (PRK) have also been used to manage residual anisometropia and astigmatism after transplantation (see BCSC Section 13, *Refractive Surgery*).

If the patient has a visually significant cataract associated with anisometropia following PK, cataract extraction with appropriate IOL power selection will reduce anisometropia. If the patient has visually significant regular, stable astigmatism with a healthy graft endothelium, a toric IOL is also an option. If the patient has intolerable anisometropia with a clear lens, the surgeon may elect to place a phakic IOL or perform a refractive lens exchange.

Risks of surgical intervention include microperforation and macroperforation, infection, rejection, undercorrection or overcorrection, persistent epithelial defects, and production of irregular astigmatism. Any intraocular procedure following corneal transplantation has the potential to damage the endothelial cells and can lead to graft failure.

Lamellar Keratoplasty

With advances in surgical instruments and techniques, cornea surgeons are now able to selectively remove diseased or scarred corneal tissue while preserving healthy tissue. Removal and replacement of select layers of the cornea is called lamellar keratoplasty. The general ophthalmologist should be familiar with the indications and limitations of, and common complications associated with, the various types of lamellar keratoplasty, including ALK, DALK, DSEK, and DMEK (see Table 15-6). DSEK and DMEK are discussed separately later in this chapter.

Anterior Lamellar Keratoplasty

Anterior lamellar keratoplasty is an excellent option for patients with opacities or loss of tissue not involving the full thickness of the cornea. These conditions include corneal thinning (eg, Terrien marginal degeneration, descemetocele formation, pellucid marginal degeneration, keratoconus; Fig 15-13), superficial corneal tumors, and peripheral ulcerative keratitis with significant keratolysis. See Table 15-6 for additional information.

Advantages

Anterior lamellar keratoplasty has many advantages over PK. It eliminates a full-thickness corneal incision into the anterior chamber, thereby avoiding the risks of glaucoma, cataract, retinal detachment, cystoid macular edema, expulsive hemorrhage, and endophthalmitis. Because the endothelium is not transplanted, it also eliminates the risk of endothelial rejection and, consequently, decreases the need for topical steroids.

Disadvantages

Anterior lamellar keratoplasty does not replace damaged endothelium. Also, the procedure is more technically demanding and time-consuming than PK. It may be associated with irregular or significant regular astigmatism, opacification and vascularization of the graft–host interface, and stromal rejection is still possible and may be problematic.

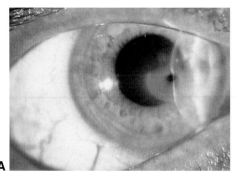 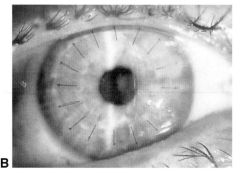

A **B**

Figure 15-13 **A,** Slit-lamp photograph of a descemetocele in a patient with rheumatoid arthritis. **B,** The same patient after lamellar keratoplasty.

Fontana L, Iovieno A. Techniques of anterior lamellar keratoplasty. In: Mannis MJ, Holland EJ, eds. *Cornea*. Vol 2. 4th ed. Philadelphia: Elsevier; 2017:1361–1365.

Gorovoy MS. Advances in lamellar corneal surgery. *Focal Points: Clinical Modules for Ophthalmologists*. San Francisco: American Academy of Ophthalmology; 2008, module 4.

John T, ed. *Surgical Techniques in Anterior and Posterior Lamellar Corneal Surgery*. New Delhi, India: Jaypee Brothers Medical Publishers; 2006.

Deep anterior lamellar keratoplasty

In contrast to ALK, in which the excision of tissue may extend only to the pathology found in the superficial or midstromal tissue, the goal of DALK is to remove the entire stromal layer. DALK has become more popular for the treatment of keratoconus, corneal dystrophies, and corneal scarring. (See Videos 15-3 and 15-4, which demonstrate DALK procedures.) To obtain a visual outcome similar to that achieved with PK, the surgeon must dissect down to or close to the Descemet membrane to create a clear, smooth graft–host interface. There are many techniques for dissecting stromal tissue to expose the Descemet membrane, including the Anwar big-bubble technique (see Videos 15-5 and 15-6 for animations of the big-bubble technique), the Melles technique, and, more recently, the use of the femtosecond laser. As discussion of these techniques is beyond the purview of this chapter, the reader is encouraged to consult the references that follow. Even in experienced hands, it may not always be possible to expose the Descemet membrane using these techniques. In these cases, manual dissection is possible, but it poses a risk of reduced best-corrected visual acuity due to incomplete removal of the host stromal tissue and secondary interface haze. In an OCT study of patients who underwent DALK, 20 μm of residual stromal bed was not visually significant; however, 80 μm of residual tissue caused a reduction in vision.

 VIDEO 15-3 Deep anterior lamellar keratoplasty for keratoconus. *Courtesy of Robert W. Weisenthal, MD.*

 VIDEO 15-4 DALK. *Courtesy of David D. Verdier, MD. Deep anterior lamellar keratoplasty. In:* Copeland and Afshari's Principles and Practice of Cornea. *New Delhi, India: Jaypee Brothers Medical Publishers; 2013.*

 VIDEO 15-5 Formation of the big bubble in DALK. *Courtesy of Dasa Gangadhar, MD.*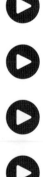

 VIDEO 15-6 Decompression of the big bubble in DALK. *Courtesy of Dasa Gangadhar, MD.*

Anwar M, Teichmann KD. Big-bubble technique to bare Descemet's membrane in anterior lamellar keratoplasty. *J Cataract Refract Surg*. 2002;28(3):398–403.

Ardjomand N, Hau S, McAlister JC, et al. Quality of vision and graft thickness in deep anterior lamellar and penetrating corneal allografts. *Am J Ophthalmol*. 2007;143(2):228–235.

Chen G, Tzekov R, Wensheng L, Jiang F, Mao S, Tong Y. Deep anterior lamellar keratoplasty versus penetrating keratoplasty: a meta-analysis of randomized controlled trials. *Cornea*. 2016;35(2):169–174.

Reinhart WJ, Musch DC, Jacobs DS, Lee WB, Kaufman SC, Shtein RM. Deep anterior lamellar keratoplasty as an alternative to penetrating keratoplasty: a report by the American Academy of Ophthalmology. *Ophthalmology.* 2011;118(1):209–218.

Complications

Complications associated with lamellar keratoplasty

Opacification and vascularization of the interface Meticulous dissection of the lamellar plane during both ALK and DALK is essential to creation of a smooth, clear interface. Irrigation and cleaning of the lamellar bed at the time of surgery reduces the likelihood of postoperative opacification. Retained interface debris, secondary vascularization, microbial infections, or wrinkling of the Descemet membrane can reduce vision or prolong vision rehabilitation. Neovascularization can increase the risk of lipid keratopathy, leading to further corneal opacification.

Allograft rejection Because the corneal endothelium is not transplanted, endothelial rejection cannot take place. Epithelial rejection, subepithelial infiltrates, and stromal rejection can still occur, but they usually respond to corticosteroid therapy. Stromal rejection, characterized by significant haze and deep vascularization, can lead to corneal opacification and is more common after DALK than PK (Fig 15-14).

Complications unique to deep anterior lamellar keratoplasty

Rupture of the Descemet membrane If there is a small rupture, the procedure may still be completed but may result in a Descemet detachment (see the following discussion). If there is a large perforation, conversion to PK may be necessary.

Double anterior chamber or Descemet detachment Descemet detachment or double (pseudo) anterior chambers can occur because of fluid in the interface, which results from a host perforation or retained viscoelastic material. Injection of air into the anterior chamber can help with reattachment; however, it may also reduce the endothelial cell count and lead to the development of an anterior subcapsular cataract.

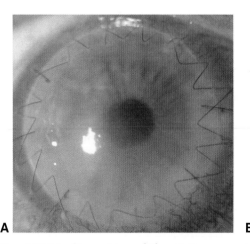
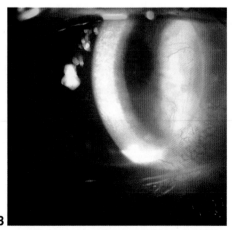

A   **B**

Figure 15-14 Stromal haze **(A)** and deep vascularization **(B)** following deep anterior lamellar keratoplasty. *(Courtesy of Robert W. Weisenthal, MD.)*

Postoperative complications common to lamellar and penetrating keratoplasty

Complications common to lamellar and penetrating keratoplasty include prolonged healing due to ocular surface disease, suture erosion and abscess, infectious keratitis, neovascularization, graft rejection, and graft failure.

Endothelial Keratoplasty

In 1998, Gerrit Melles introduced the concept of lamellar surgery for endothelial dysfunction through a procedure called deep lamellar endothelial keratoplasty (DLEK). Because the manual dissection (of the host and donor corneal tissue) in DLEK was technically challenging, this technique was not widely adopted by cornea surgeons. Melles modified the technique to include stripping of the host Descemet membrane and endothelium (descemetorrhexis) and insertion of a hand-dissected posterior lamellar donor button, which was positioned against the host with an air bubble in the anterior chamber; the revised technique was coined Descemet stripping endothelial keratoplasty (DSEK). Mark Gorovoy later automated the lamellar dissection of the donor tissue by using a microkeratome, giving rise to the procedure he called Descemet stripping automated endothelial keratoplasty (DSAEK). Over time, the term DSEK has been adopted for these automated procedures as well; in this book, the term DSEK is similarly used.

Melles further modified the DSEK procedure by using only donor Descemet membrane and endothelium in a procedure termed Descemet membrane endothelial keratoplasty (DMEK). Further innovations to the technique used to insert and unscroll the tissue, the adoption of an "S" stamp for graft orientation, and the use of SF_6 gas to extend the duration of the gas bubble have significantly reduced the incidence of postoperative complications and increased the use and success of DMEK. In addition, the availability of eye bank–prepared tissue for DSEK and DMEK has increased the safety and popularity of both procedures.

EK is now the preferred technique for treatment of patients with corneal endothelial dysfunction, and it has been adopted for use in pediatric patients with congenital or early corneal edema (see the discussion of pediatric keratoplasty later in the chapter). Due to the success of, and rapid rehabilitation observed with, EK, the indications for this procedure have expanded to include patients with visually significant cornea guttae in the absence of stromal edema. Table 15-7 shows the increased use of DSEK and DMEK in the United States since 2013. Comparisons of PK and endothelial surgery are provided in Tables 15-6 and 15-8. Videos 15-7 through 15-10 show the DSEK and DMEK procedures.

Table 15-7 Statistics for DSEK and DMEK Procedures Performed in the United States, 2013–2016

	2016	%	2015	%	2014	%	2013	%
Total EK procedures	28,327		27,208		25,965		24,987	
DSAEK	21,868	77.0	22,514	83.0	23,100	89.0	23,465	91.0
DMEK	6459	23.0	4694	17.0	2865	11.0	1522	9.3

Modified with permission from the Eye Bank Association of America (EBAA). *2016 Eye Banking Statistical Report.* Washington, DC: EBAA; 2017.

Table 15-8 Comparison of Short-Term Results for Different Surgical Techniques for Corneal Edema (Fuchs Dystrophy and PBK)

	PK	DLEK	DSAEK	DMEK
Dislocation rate	0.0%	6.6%	14.5%	5.0%–62.0%*
Wound dehiscence	1.3%–5.8%			
Donor failure within 60 days	0.3%	3.3%	0%–29.0%; mean 5.0%	2.2%–8.0%
Rejection rate at:				
1 year	17.0%	3.4%	2.0%–9.0%	0.7%–3.0%
2 years	9.7%–13.0%	5.5%	12.0%–14.0%	
5 years	22.2%		22.0% (2.0%)	
Graft failure rate at 5 years	5.0% for Fuchs/ 27.0% for PBK	27.5%	5.0% for Fuchs/ 24.0% for PBK	NA
BSCVA:				
% 20/40 or better at 1 year	65.0%–84.0% with selective suture removal	40.0%–44.1%	38.0%–90.0%	94.0% at 6 months 97.0% 20/30 or better at 1 year
% 20/20 or better				39.0%–47.0%
Time to BCVA	6–12 months with selective suture removal	NA	NA	⅔ stable by 3 months
Mean keratometric cylinder:				
Sutures out	4.40±2.80 D	1.50±1.20 D		
at 2 years	3.70±3.20 D	0.40–0.60 D induced; mean 0.10 D	0.40–0.60 D induced; mean 0.10 D	+0.40 D hyperopic shift; no change
With sutures in at 1 year	2.50 D			
Mean spherical equivalent change	2.80±2.10 D	0.90±0.70 D	+1.10 D induced hyperopia	+0.24 to +0.32 D
Endothelial cell loss at:				
1 year	9.0%–19.0% Fuchs[†] 34.0% Fuchs/PBK	43.0%–57.9%	37.0%	32.0±20.0%, 34.0%, 36.0%
2 years	27.0%–42.0% Fuchs, 54.0% Fuchs/PBK	57.0%	44.0%	
5 years	69.0%–75.0% Fuchs, 61.0% Fuchs/PBK	62.0% at 4 years	53.0%	

BSCVA = best spectacle-corrected visual acuity; BCVA = best-corrected visual acuity; D = diopter; DSAEK = Descemet stripping automated endothelial keratoplasty; NA = data not available; PBK = pseudophakic bullous keratopathy.

*Includes only dislocations that influenced the result; edge dislocation or tag not counted. If all dislocations are counted, then 8.0%–24.0%.

[†] Range: 2 donor age groups.

Modified from American Academy of Ophthalmology Cornea/External Disease Panel. Preferred Practice Pattern Guidelines. *Corneal Edema and Opacification.* San Francisco: American Academy of Ophthalmology; 2013. Available at www.aao.org/ppp.

VIDEO 15-7 Descemet stripping endothelial keratoplasty.
Courtesy of Robert W. Weisenthal, MD.

 VIDEO 15-8 DSEK combined with phacoemulsification and IOL implantation.
Courtesy of Robert W. Weisenthal, MD.

 VIDEO 15-9 Descemet membrane endothelial keratoplasty.
Courtesy of Robert W. Weisenthal, MD.

 VIDEO 15-10 DMEK combined with phacoemulsification and IOL implantation.
Courtesy of Robert W. Weisenthal, MD.

Lee WB, Jacobs DS, Musch DC, Kaufman SC, Reinhart WJ, Shtein RM. Descemet's stripping endothelial keratoplasty: safety and outcomes: a report by the American Academy of Ophthalmology. *Ophthalmology.* 2009;116 (9):1818–1830.

Section 6, Endothelial Keratoplasty. In: Mannis MJ, Holland EJ, eds. *Cornea.* Vol 2. 4th ed. Philadelphia: Elsevier; 2017:1427–1508.

Terry MA, Straiko MD, Veldman PB, et al. Standardized DMEK technique: reducing complications using prestripped tissue, novel glass injector, and sulfur hexafluoride (SF6) gas. *Cornea.* 2015;34(8):845–852.

Waggoner M, Cohen AW. Descemet stripping automated endothelial keratoplasty (DSAEK) and Descemet membrane endothelial keratoplasty (DMEK). In: *Basic Techniques of Ophthalmic Surgery.* 2nd ed. San Francisco: American Academy of Ophthalmology; 2015:145–152.

Advantages

Because the donor tissue is inserted through a small corneal or scleral incision in EK procedures (compared with the large full-thickness central corneal incision used in other keratoplasty procedures), the structural integrity of the eye is preserved, and any subsequent trauma to the eye will result in less damage (Fig 15-15). Other advantages include reduced incidence of graft rejection, reduction in suture-related problems, less induced astigmatism with greater accuracy in IOL power calculations, and more rapid vision rehabilitation (due to preservation of the ocular surface and the rapid return of endothelial function).

Disadvantages

The main disadvantages of EK include the potential for wasting donor tissue (due to poor harvesting, which is minimized with eye bank–prepared tissue), increased risk of primary graft failure during surgical learning curve, and the need for additional surgical interventions postoperatively (re-injection of air, or *rebubbling*). Reduced postoperative visual acuity is another potential drawback and is discussed separately in the following subsection.

Potential for reduced postoperative visual acuity

Coexisting corneal pathology such as basement membrane changes or subepithelial fibrosis may cause surface irregularity that limits vision after DSEK or DMEK. In some

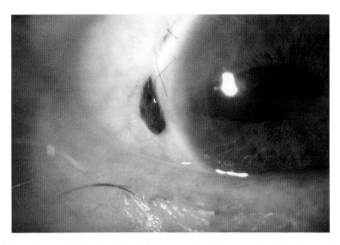

Figure 15-15 Iris prolapse following blunt trauma after Descemet stripping endothelial kerato-plasty (DSEK). *(Courtesy of Robert W. Weisenthal, MD.)*

cases, debridement or superficial keratectomy may be necessary. Another possible cause of decreased vision after EK is light scattering due to preexisting long-standing corneal edema. An evaluation of patients with Fuchs corneal dystrophy who underwent DSEK revealed that the corneal light scattering associated with anterior stromal haze improved significantly after surgery but was still increased compared with that in a normal cornea 24 months after the procedure.

A review of the literature on DSEK outcomes found that the average best-corrected Snellen visual acuity (BCSVA) ranged from 20/34 to 20/66. Also, an American Academy of Ophthalmology (AAO) *Preferred Practice Pattern* guideline reported that in a review of studies, a best spectacle-corrected visual acuity of 20/40 or better was achieved at 1 year in 38%–90% of patients after DSEK compared with 97% of patients after DMEK; further, 39%–47% of patients had 20/20 vision after DMEK (see Table 15-8). A number of studies have compared DMEK and DSEK, and all concluded that DMEK provided more rapid recovery of visual acuity and a better final visual outcome. The difference in visual outcome between DSEK and DMEK may be related to the alteration of the posterior corneal curvature that occurs with DSEK. This alteration is due to the unevenness and thickness of the donor tissue and the irregularity of the interface between the donor stromal tissue and the host Descemet membrane. This is in contrast to the nearly normal anatomical restoration of the cornea achieved with DMEK, which is due to the extremely thin graft tissue used and the exceedingly smooth interface created between the host Descemet membrane and transplanted Descemet membrane and endothelium in DMEK.

Nevertheless, for many surgeons, DSEK is still the procedure of choice for routine EK, because manipulation and placement of tissue are easier with this technique. DSEK is particularly useful in patients with disorganized anterior segments, those with sutured posterior chamber or anterior chamber IOLs, and in patients who have undergone tube shunt implantation or other glaucoma procedures. In an effort to improve the visual outcome after DSEK, some surgeons advocate using thinner donor grafts (between 90 and 120 µm), a variation called *ultrathin DSEK*. However, Wacker et al, in a meta-analysis of

23 series, found that there may be a weak correlation but overall insufficient evidence to conclude that graft thickness is clinically important with respect to BCVA after DSEK. These same investigators have also shown that visual acuity after DSEK continues to improve over a 5-year period, with more than half of the patients seeing better than 20/25 at 5 years, which they believe was a result of ongoing remodeling of the cornea reducing corneal haze and aberrations.

American Academy of Ophthalmology Cornea/External Disease Panel. Preferred Practice Pattern Guidelines. *Corneal Edema and Opacification*. San Francisco: American Academy of Ophthalmology; 2013. Available at www.aao.org/ppp.

Baratz KH, McLaren JW, Maguire LJ, Patel SV. Corneal haze determined by confocal microscopy 2 years after Descemet stripping with endothelial keratoplasty for Fuchs corneal dystrophy. *Arch Ophthalmol*. 2012;130(7):868–874.

Dickman MM, Kruit PJ, Remeijer L, et al. A randomized multicenter clinical trial of ultrathin Descemet stripping automated endothelial keratoplasty (DSAEK) versus DSAEK. *Ophthalmology*. 2016;123(11):2276–2284.

Hamzaoglu EC, Straiko MD, Mayko ZM, Sáles CS, Terry MA. The first 100 eyes of standardized Descemet stripping automated endothelial keratoplasty versus standardized Descemet membrane endothelial keratoplasty. *Ophthalmology*. 2015;122(11):2193–2199.

Roberts HW, Mukherjee A, Aichner H, Rajan MS. Visual outcomes and graft thickness in microthin DSAEK—one year results. *Cornea*. 2015;34(11):1345–1350.

Rudolph M, Laaser K, Bachmann BO, Cursiefen C, Epstein D, Kruse FE. Corneal higher-order aberrations after Descemet's membrane endothelial keratoplasty. *Ophthalmology*. 2012; 119(3):528–539.

Tourtas T, Laaser K, Bachmann BO, Cursiefen C, Kruse FE. Descemet membrane endothelial keratoplasty versus Descemet stripping automated endothelial keratoplasty. *Am J Ophthalmol*. 2012;153(6):1082–1090.

Wacker K, Baratz KH, Maguire LJ, McLaren JW, Patel SV. Descemet stripping endothelial keratoplasty for Fuchs' corneal endothelial dystrophy: five-year results of a prospective study. *Ophthalmology*. 2016;123(1):154–160.

Wacker K, Bourne WM, Patel SV. Effect of graft thickness on visual acuity after Descemet stripping endothelial keratoplasty: a systematic review and meta-analysis. *Am J Ophthalmol*. 2016;163:18–28.

Intraoperative Complications

Complications that can occur during DSEK or DMEK include improper orientation during placement of the donor tissue; excessive manipulation of the donor tissue, leading to cell loss and possible graft failure; tearing of the donor tissue; retention of viscoelastic; and vitreous or blood in the interface (Fig 15-16). See Table 15-6 for additional intraoperative complications in EK.

Postoperative Care and Complications

Dislocation or decentration of the donor graft

In DSEK and DMEK, the donor tissue should be well centered over the pupil, without fluid in the interface. To promote tissue adherence over the ensuing days, 40%–60% of the air bubble injected intraoperatively should remain after DSEK on postoperative day 1 (Fig 15-17),

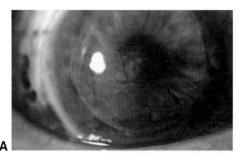
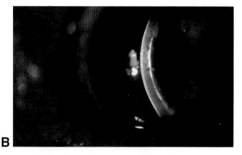

A   **B**

Figure 15-16   A, Hemorrhage in the interface after DSEK. **B,** Slit-lamp photograph showing blood in the interface. *(Courtesy of Robert W. Weisenthal, MD.)*

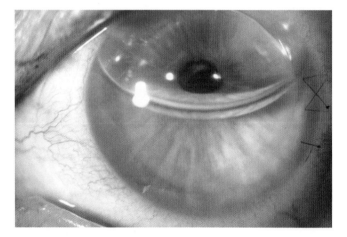

Figure 15-17   Residual air bubble following DSEK (postoperative day 1). *(Courtesy of Robert W. Weisenthal, MD.)*

and 80% of the gas (SF_6) or air bubble should remain after DMEK on day 1 (Fig 15-18). The air bubble resorbs within 2–3 days, and SF_6 resorbs within 4–6 days after DMEK. The rate of dislocation of donor tissue decreases for both DSEK and DMEK as surgeon experience increases. See Table 15-8 for dislocation rates for DSAEK and DMEK.

DSEK   Dislocation or decentration of the donor graft (Fig 15-19) typically occurs within the first 24 hours after DSEK. A soft eye due to a preexisting tube shunt or uncontrolled release of the air increases the likelihood of a decentered or dislocated graft. Retained viscoelastic or the presence of vitreous in the interface may prevent proper adherence of the graft. If the graft remains attached on postoperative day 1, subsequent dislocation is unlikely, although inadvertent trauma or eye rubbing during the first week may displace the donor tissue. Wearing glasses or a shield to protect the eye is recommended, along with exercising caution during instillation of eyedrops.

It is still not clear how long the air bubble should be retained after DSEK, as some surgeons remove the air completely on the day of surgery without an increased incidence of tissue dislocation. This raises the possibility that long-term retention of an air bubble is not necessary for graft adherence in DSEK.

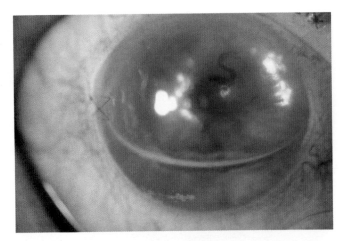

Figure 15-18 Residual air bubble after Descemet membrane endothelial keratoplasty (DMEK) (postoperative day 1). The S stamp is shown for orientation. *(Courtesy of Robert W. Weisenthal, MD.)*

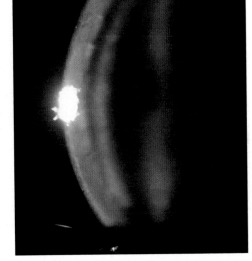

Figure 15-19 Slit-lamp photograph of a detached donor corneal button following DSEK. *(Courtesy of Robert W. Weisenthal, MD.)*

DMEK The donor tissue is more delicate, and as a result, peripheral or central detachments are much more common in DMEK than in DSEK (Fig 15-20). Anterior segment OCT allows visualization of the area of detachment (Fig 15-21). Peripheral detachments not involving the visual axis can be observed over several weeks to ensure there is no progression. They usually seal without adverse impact.

If the graft detachment extends into the visual axis or is greater than one-third of the graft area, the surgeon may consider additional injection of air (rebubbling) to tamponade the graft against the host. Initially, rebubbling was not advised because of reports of extensive, visually significant detachments resolving spontaneously. Yet longer-term follow-up of these cases has been instructive. Baydoun et al reported that, in patients with clinically significant graft detachments managed without rebubbling, there was a significant

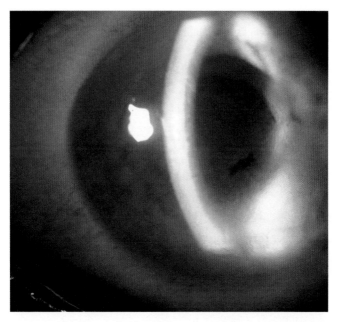

Figure 15-20 Slit-lamp photograph of a peripheral detachment following DMEK. *(Courtesy of Robert W. Weisenthal, MD.)*

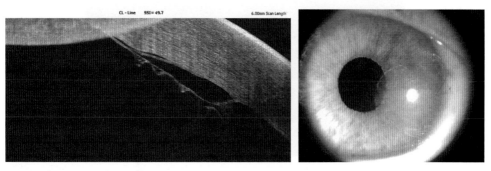

Figure 15-21 Anterior segment optical coherence tomography images of a peripheral detachment following DMEK. *(Courtesy of Robert W. Weisenthal, MD.)*

reduction in endothelial cell counts at 5-year follow-up, which led to a higher rate of late graft failure. In some cases, permanent stromal haze developed secondary to chronic corneal edema, worsening the visual outcome after repeated DMEK. Thus, early rebubbling seems to be the best course in these cases. If rebubbling is necessary, it can be performed in the office or surgery center.

In the event that the graft is attached but the cornea still has visually significant edema after 1–2 months, repeated surgery is indicated prior to the development of chronic corneal edema, which can lead to bullous keratopathy, epithelial breakdown, and possible secondary infection. Repeated EK, either DMEK or DSEK, before the development of permanent corneal changes has a good visual prognosis, similar to that of the original procedure.

Baydoun L, Ham L, Borderie V, et al. Endothelial survival after Descemet membrane endothelial keratoplasty. Effect of surgical indication and graft adherence status. *JAMA Ophthalmol.* 2015;133(1):1277–1285.

Baydoun L, van Dijk K, Dapena I, et al. Repeat Descemet membrane endothelial keratoplasty after complicated primary Descemet membrane endothelial keratoplasty. *Ophthalmology.* 2015;122(1):8–16.

Dirisamer M, van Dijk K, Dapena I, et al. Prevention and management of graft detachment in Descemet membrane endothelial keratoplasty. *Arch Ophthalmol.* 2012;130(3):280–291.

Lehman RE, Copeland LA, Stock EM, Fulcher SF. Graft detachment rate in DSEK/DSAEK after same-day complete air removal. *Cornea.* 2015;34(11):1358–1361.

Price FW Jr, Price MO. To intervene or not to intervene: that is the question. *Ophthalmology.* 2015;122(1):6–7.

Pupillary block

Anterior pupillary block or iris bombé may occur if the anterior chamber bubble migrates posteriorly, preventing aqueous flow through the pupil; Figures 15-22 and 15-23 show such a block after DSEK and DMEK, respectively. The resultant acute rise in IOP produces

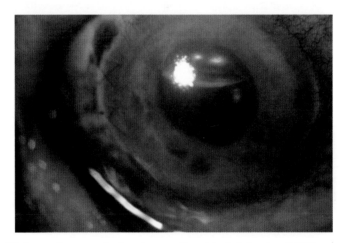

Figure 15-22 Slit-lamp photograph showing pupillary block following DSEK. *(Courtesy of Robert W. Weisenthal, MD.)*

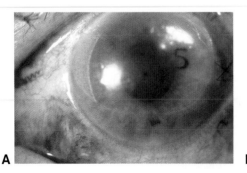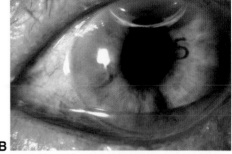

A **B**

Figure 15-23 **A,** Slit-lamp photograph of pupillary block following DMEK. **B,** The same patient after the release of air, leading to resolution of the block. *(Courtesy of Robert W. Weisenthal, MD.)*

pain and can exacerbate preexisting optic nerve damage. Pupillary block may also lead to iridocorneal adhesion, damaging the graft and increasing the risk of rejection. Pupil dilation and supine positioning may relieve the pupil block; if this fails, some air should be removed. An inferior iridectomy performed prior to or at the time of the surgery reduces the likelihood of this scenario.

Epithelial ingrowth

Epithelial ingrowth following DSEK can be seen as a gray-white deposit within the graft–host interface (Fig 15-24). It typically remains stable and is asymptomatic unless it occurs in the visual axis. The source of epithelium may be either the host or the donor. Host epithelium can be pushed into the eye through the main wound, side ports, or venting incisions used to drain interface fluid. It can also enter the eye through a fistulous track. Loose donor epithelium may enter the eye if adherent to the donor corneal button because of eccentric trephination beyond the microkeratome excision. In rare cases, epithelial ingrowth leads to graft failure that is missed on clinical examination but recognized on histologic examination of the tissue after removal. In a large series of cases, the majority of patients with epithelial ingrowth were simply observed and continued to see well without further intervention. In the atypical cases that resulted in graft failure, a second DSEK or PK produced a good outcome without recurrent ingrowth. This is in contrast to the progressive and devastating course of intraocular epithelial downgrowth associated with intracapsular cataract extraction or full-thickness PK. Epithelial ingrowth has not been described in DMEK.

Dalal RR, Raber I, Dunn SP, et al. Epithelial ingrowth following endothelial keratoplasty. *Cornea.* 2016;35(4):465–470.

Suh LH, Shousha MA, Ventura RU, et al. Epithelial ingrowth after Descemet stripping automated endothelial keratoplasty: description of cases and assessment with anterior segment optical coherence tomography. *Cornea.* 2011;30(5):528–534.

Other interface pathology

Infections can occur in the graft–host interface by several means: pathogens passing through venting incisions, contaminated donor tissue, or bacteria from the ocular surface dragged into the eye during insertion.

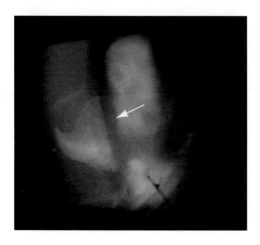

Figure 15-24 Slit-lamp photograph of epithelial ingrowth *(arrow)* in the interface after DSEK. *(Courtesy of Robert W. Weisenthal, MD.)*

In a recent review by the EBAA, 0.7% of donor rim cultures were positive for fungi, and infections developed in 17.1% of corneas with positive fungal rim culture results. The incidence of postoperative fungal infections is significantly higher for EK than PK. These infections have occurred primarily in eyes that have undergone DSEK, but there are case reports of infections after DMEK as well. It is possible that these infections are related to the tissue warming that occurs during preparation of donor tissue for EK.

Interface opacification may occur because of retention of fibers, incomplete removal of the Descemet membrane, and persistence of interface fluid. *Textural interface opacity* describes a recently reported finding that results from retained viscoelastic or from the shearing of stromal fibrils during an irregular microkeratome donor preparation. The opacity has 2 forms: elongated (a lacy honeycomb pattern of deposits with intervening clear zones) (Fig 15-25) and punctate (small, discrete deposits). Textural interface opacity may be associated with reduced vision, but it typically improves or disappears completely over many months. There have been no reports of interface problems after DMEK.

Aldave A. The utility of donor corneal rim culture: a report of the EBAA Medical Advisory Board Subcommittee on fungal infection following corneal transplantation. *Subspecialty Day Program: Cornea.* Las Vegas: American Academy of Ophthalmology; 2015.

Vira S, Shih CY, Ragusa N, et al. Textural interface opacity after Descemet stripping automated endothelial keratoplasty: a report of 30 cases and possible etiology. *Cornea.* 2013; 32(5):e54–59.

Progression of cataracts

DSEK performed in a phakic eye may induce cataract progression, particularly in patients with narrow anterior chambers (<3.0 mm); therefore, DSEK with cataract extraction has been recommended in patients older than 50 years or in the presence of mild to moderate cataract. In a large series of patients with Fuchs dystrophy, DSEK combined with cataract extraction did not increase the risk of graft dislocation, endothelial cell loss, or other complications. There has not been a similar study in patients after DMEK, but many surgeons routinely combine DMEK with cataract surgery.

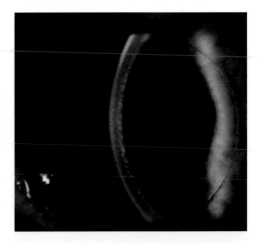

Figure 15-25 Slit-lamp photograph of textural interface opacity after DSEK. *(Courtesy of Jeffrey Goshe, MD.)*

Terry MA, Shamie N, Chen ES, et al. Endothelial keratoplasty for Fuchs' dystrophy with cataract: complications and clinical results with the new triple procedure. *Ophthalmology.* 2009;116(4):631–639.

Tsui JY, Goins KM, Sutphin JE, Wagoner MD. Phakic Descemet stripping automated endothelial keratoplasty: prevalence and prognostic impact of postoperative cataracts. *Cornea.* 2011;30(3):291–295.

Primary graft failure

In published reports, the primary graft failure rates for DSEK and DMEK range from 2.2% to 8.0%, with a mean of 5.0% for DSEK (see Table 15-8); higher rates are associated with less experienced surgeons. The lower rates probably reflect better surgical technique, which results in less tissue manipulation and a lower rate of graft dislocations and thus less endothelial trauma.

Graft rejection

The incidence of corneal graft rejection following DSEK seems to be lower than that after PK; in several long-term studies, the incidence was between 0% and 10% in the first year, increasing slightly at 2 years. In a paper by Wu et al, the incidence of graft rejection in DSEK was reported to be 22% at 5 years, although this result may be skewed, as these investigators routinely discontinued steroids, in some cases at 4 months postoperatively and typically at 1 year. In contrast, in a study by Ratanasit and Gorovoy, where all patients were maintained on topical steroids indefinitely, the rejection rate was 2% after 5 years in 51 eyes. Several studies on graft rejection after DSEK suggest that long-term prophylaxis with a steroid once daily, regardless of the strength of the steroid, is important in reducing the incidence of graft rejection.

For DSEK patients, topical steroids such as prednisolone acetate (1%) 4 times a day are prescribed initially and then tapered over time to once per day at 1 year. A patient who is pseudophakic and not at risk of IOP elevation can continue to use a topical steroid once daily indefinitely, but periodic IOP measurement is recommended. If the patient is a steroid responder, loteprednol etabonate or fluorometholone may be substituted.

The clinical presentation of graft rejection in DSEK patients differs from that in PK patients. The classic endothelial rejection line of PK is not seen; instead, multiple keratic precipitates scattered across the cornea are typically noted (Fig 15-26).

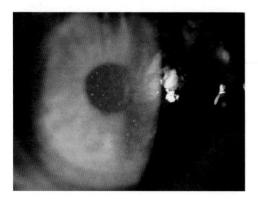

Figure 15-26 Slit-lamp photograph showing endothelial graft rejection after DSEK, characterized by scattered keratic precipitates without an endothelial rejection line. *(Courtesy of Robert W. Weisenthal, MD.)*

The rate of graft rejection after DMEK seems to be even lower than that after DSEK (eg, less than 1%). Further, the medication regimen after DMEK offers more flexibility in terms of dosage, strength, and tapering of the topical steroids. In a randomized prospective study, prednisolone acetate 1% was used for only 1 month following DMEK, after which loteprednol etabonate 0.5% gel was used without increased incidence of graft rejection. The authors of that study report that the incidence of graft rejection was 0% for patients who continued using topical steroids through the second year but increased to 6% in the second year in patients who stopped the steroids after 1 year. The graft rejections experienced were mild and asymptomatic, and all but one reversed with resumption of steroid therapy.

Anshu A, Price MO, Price FW Jr. Risk of corneal transplant rejection significantly reduced with Descemet's membrane endothelial keratoplasty. *Ophthalmology.* 2012;119(3):536–540.

Dapena I, Ham L, Netuková M, van der Wees J, Melles GR. Incidence of early allograft rejection after Descemet membrane endothelial keratoplasty. *Cornea.* 2011;30(12):1341–1345.

Price MO, Feng MT, Scanameo A, Price FW Jr. Loteprednol etabonate 0.5% gel vs prednisolone acetate 1% solution after Descemet membrane endothelial keratoplasty: prospective randomized trial. *Cornea.* 2015;34(8):853–858.

Price MO, Scanameo A, Feng MT, Price FW Jr. Descemet's membrane endothelial keratoplasty: risk of immunologic rejection episodes after discontinuing topical corticosteroids. *Ophthalmology.* 2016;123(6):1232–1236.

Ratanasit A, Gorovoy MS. Long-term results of Descemet stripping automated endothelial keratoplasty. *Cornea.* 2011;30(12):1414–1418.

Wu EI, Ritterband DC, Yu G, Shields RA, Seedor JA. Graft rejection following Descemet stripping automated endothelial keratoplasty: features, risk factors, and outcomes. *Am J Ophthalmol.* 2012;153(5):949–957.

Endothelial cell loss

Several maneuvers potentially contribute to early endothelial cell loss in EK patients, including the manipulation of tissue entailed in the preparation of donor tissue, placement and orientation of the tissue within the anterior chamber, primary injection of air to facilitate graft adherence, and rebubbling and tissue manipulation to treat dislocated grafts. Endothelial cell loss at 1 year for both DSEK and DMEK is reported to be approximately 32%–37%. In a follow-up study of 95 eyes by Price and colleagues, the median endothelial cell loss was 53% at 5 years and 71% at 10 years, which compares favorably to results for PK in the Cornea Donor Study, which showed a mean cell loss of 70% at 5 years and 76% at 10 years. Long-term viability of the endothelial cells is influenced by ocular comorbidity such as previous filtering surgery and, in particular, tube shunts. Long-term prospective trials on DMEK and DSEK are necessary to better understand the clinical biology of the corneal endothelium and the impact of endothelial cell loss on graft viability.

Li JY, Terry MA, Goshe J, Shamie N, Davis-Boozer D. Graft rejection after Descemet's stripping automated endothelial keratoplasty: graft survival and endothelial cell loss. *Ophthalmology.* 2012;119(1):90–94.

Ni N, Sperling BJ, Dai Y, Hannush SB. Outcomes after Descemet stripping automated endothelial keratoplasty in patients with glaucoma drainage devices. *Cornea.* 2015;34(8): 870–875.

Price FW Jr, Feng MT, Price MO. Evolution of endothelial keratoplasty: where are we headed? *Cornea.* 2015;34(Suppl 10):S41–S47.

Price MO, Calhoun P, Kollman C, Price FW Jr, Lass JH. Descemet stripping endothelial keratoplasty: ten-year endothelial cell loss compared with penetrating keratoplasty. *Ophthalmology.* 2016;123(7):1421–1427.

Price MO, Fairchild KM, Price DA, Price FW Jr. Descemet's stripping endothelial keratoplasty: five-year graft survival and endothelial cell loss. *Ophthalmology.* 2011;118(4):725–729.

Ratanasit A, Gorovoy MS. Long-term results of Descemet stripping automated endothelial keratoplasty. *Cornea.* 2011;30(12):1414–1418.

Sugar A. The importance of corneal endothelial cell survival after endothelial keratoplasty. *JAMA Ophthalmol.* 2015;133(11):1285–1286.

Novel Methods for Treatment of Endothelial Dysfunction

A number of case reports have described extensive, visually significant graft detachments; nonadherent, "free-floating," grafts; and even an upside-down graft after DMEK in which the cornea cleared without additional intervention. The restoration of corneal clarity in these cases was thought to result from endothelial migration either from the peripheral cornea or from the free-floating donor tissue. After this experience, Dirisamer et al performed descemetorrhexis with implantation of a free-floating donor graft of Descemet membrane and endothelial cells, a technique called *Descemet membrane endothelial transfer (DMET).* In their study of 12 patients (7 patients with Fuchs endothelial corneal dystrophy [FECD] and 5 with pseudophakic bullous keratopathy [PBK]), all of the patients with FECD had clear corneas of normal thickness after 6 months; however, the patients with PBK did not improve and required further surgery. The authors suggested that descemetorrhexis in the patients with FECD, removing the thickened Descemet membrane characteristic of FECD, allowed the migration of endothelial cells from either the host or donor endothelial cells. In contrast, the corneal edema did not resolve in PBK because there was endothelial depletion in the host cornea.

Subsequently, other investigators attempted a standard descemetorrhexis of 8.0–8.5 mm without placement of donor tissue in patients with FECD. The results of this technique have been mixed, with some surgeons abandoning the procedure and some investigators continuing to look for ways to modify it for a more consistent and successful outcome. In one study of 13 eyes, the investigators opted to decrease the size of the central descemetorrhexis to 4 mm. Corneal edema was present in all 13 eyes in the immediate postoperative period. Four eyes were classified as fast responders, with resolution of the corneal edema occurring at 1 month, and 4 eyes were considered typical responders, with corneal clearing at 3 months. Two eyes were slow responders, with partial corneal clearing, and 3 eyes required EK. In the future, a pharmacologic approach such as the use of Rho-associated kinase inhibitors to induce host endothelial proliferation or endothelial cell culture using reprogrammed adult stem cells from the patient may improve the success of this descemetorrhexis without the use of donor tissue.

In an effort to expand the pool of donor tissue, a new technique has been introduced in which a single donor corneal button is divided into 2 segments for transplantation in 2 different patients. This technique, referred to as *hemi-DMEK,* may not be adopted in the

United States because of regulatory, billing, and liability challenges, but it may be more acceptable in areas where there are donor shortages.

Arbelaez JG, Price MO, Price FW Jr. Long-term follow-up and complications of stripping Descemet membrane without placement of graft in eyes with Fuchs endothelial dystrophy. *Cornea.* 2014;33(12):1295–1299.

Borkar DS, Veldman P, Colby KA. Treatment of Fuchs endothelial dystrophy by Descemet stripping without endothelial keratoplasty. *Cornea.* 2016;35(10):1267–1273.

Dirisamer M, Ham L, Dapena I, van Dijk K, Melles GR. Descemet membrane endothelial transfer: "free-floating" donor Descemet implantation as a potential alternative to "kerato-plasty." *Cornea.* 2012;31(2):194–197.

Dirisamer M, Yeh RY, van Dijk K, Ham L, Dapena I, Melles GR. Recipient endothelium may relate to corneal clearance in Descemet membrane endothelial transfer. *Am J Ophthalmol.* 2012;154(2):290–296.

Koenig SB. Planned descemetorhexis without endothelial keratoplasty in eyes with Fuchs corneal endothelial dystrophy. *Cornea.* 2015;34(9):1149–1151.

Lam FC, Baydoun L, Satué M, Dirisamer M, Ham L, Melles GR. One-year outcome of hemi-Descemet membrane endothelial keratoplasty. *Graefes Arch Clin Exp Ophthalmol.* 2015; 253(11):1955–1958.

Pediatric Corneal Transplantation

Increased understanding of the special problems associated with pediatric grafts, advances in preoperative diagnostic techniques and in surgical methods, and improved postoperative management have enhanced the visual prognosis for children who have undergone corneal transplantation. Further, improvements in pediatric anesthesia and the recognition that development of amblyopia is a major impediment to useful vision have led to earlier surgical intervention. The success rate of pediatric corneal transplantation depends on the extent of coexisting ocular abnormalities. For example, one of the most common indications for pediatric keratoplasty is Peters anomaly. For type I disease, in which there is a central corneal opacity and a normal anterior segment, the survival rate for a clear graft was 83%–90% in 1 large series (mean follow-up time of 78 months), depending on the age of the patient at the time of surgery. By contrast, in another large series of patients with either type I or type II Peters anomaly, the outcomes were significantly worse: only 56% of grafts remained clear at 6 months; 44%, at 3 years. This was attributed to the inclusion of patients with type II disease, in which the anterior segment findings are more severe and characteristically include adhesions among the cornea, iris, and lens; corneal neovascularization; glaucoma; cataract; and corneal staphyloma. Therefore, more extensive surgery was required, and not surprisingly, the survival rate of the graft decreased.

Critical to a successful outcome is the family's (or caregiver's) dedication to following a rigorous postoperative regimen, which includes repeated examinations under anesthesia and adherence to the medication regimen. Postoperative glaucoma, strabismus, self-induced trauma, and immune rejection are common. As part of obtaining informed consent from the family, the physician must discuss the many difficult issues associated with the surgery, including the complicated postoperative course, loss of time from work (with associated loss of income), the extensive ongoing care required for the child, disruption of home life, and less time to devote to other dependents.

Corneal grafting in children younger than 2 years is associated with rapid neovascularization, especially along the sutures. As the wound heals, erosions may occur along the sutures, leading to eye rubbing, epithelial defects, mucus accumulation, and possible infection. Suture erosion has been reported to occur as early as 2 weeks postoperatively in infants and necessitates urgent and frequent examination under anesthesia in the operating room to evaluate the transplant and remove sutures until all have been removed. In addition, early fitting with a contact lens (as early as the time of PK) and ocular occlusive therapy are necessary to stem development of amblyopia in children with monocular aphakia.

Surgeons have become aware of DALK as an option for certain pediatric patients with stromal scarring without any other corneal pathology. For disease that is primarily endothelial, such as congenital hereditary endothelial dystrophy, EK has been reported to provide good outcomes, as observed in a small series of 8 patients (15 eyes).

Busin M, Beltz J, Scorcia V. Descemet-stripping automated endothelial keratoplasty for congenital hereditary endothelial dystrophy. *Arch Ophthalmol.* 2011;129(9):1140–1146.

Nischal KK. Pediatric keratoplasty. In: Mannis MJ, Holland EJ, eds. *Cornea.* Vol 2. 4th ed. Philadelphia: Elsevier; 2017:1382–1398.

Rao KV, Fernandes M, Gangopadhyay N, Vemuganti GK, Krishnaiah S, Sangwan VS. Outcome of penetrating keratoplasty for Peters anomaly. *Cornea.* 2008;27(7):749–753.

Zaidman GW, Flanagan JK, Furey CC. Long-term visual prognosis in children after corneal transplant surgery for Peters anomaly type I. *Am J Ophthalmol.* 2007;144(1):104–108.

Corneal Autograft Procedures

The greatest advantage of a corneal autograft is the elimination of allograft rejection. Cases with clinical circumstances appropriate for autograft are uncommon, but an astute ophthalmologist who recognizes the potential for a successful autograft procedure can spare the patient the risks associated with long-term topical steroid use and the need for lifelong vigilance against rejection.

A *rotational* autograft can be used to reposition a localized corneal scar that involves the pupillary axis. By making an eccentric trephination and rotating the host corneal button before resuturing, the surgeon can place a paracentral zone of clear cornea in the pupillary axis. The procedure is particularly useful in children, in whom the prognosis for PK is poorer, and in areas with tissue scarcity. It is important that the graft–host junction not be too close to the visual axis, because image distortion and irregular astigmatism could result.

A *contralateral* autograft is reserved for patients who have a corneal opacity in one eye with a favorable visual prognosis, and a clear cornea in the opposite eye with coexisting severe dysfunction of the afferent system (eg, retinal detachment, severe amblyopia). The clear cornea is transplanted to the first eye; then, it is replaced with either the diseased cornea from the first eye or an allograft. If an eye with a clear cornea is to be enucleated or eviscerated, the cornea can be used as a donor for keratoplasty in the fellow eye. Such simultaneous bilateral transplant surgery carries the risk of bilateral endophthalmitis.

Keratoprosthesis

In some patients, corneal transplantation is associated with an extremely guarded prognosis because of a history of multiple graft failures or associated ocular surface disease (eg, chronic bilateral inflammation from Stevens-Johnson syndrome or mucous membrane pemphigoid). These patients may be good candidates for a synthetic keratoprosthesis. Claes Dohlman, a pioneer in the development of the keratoprosthesis, divides these high-risk patients into 2 groups: those with a good blink reflex and adequate tear function and those with significant conjunctival scarring, dry eye, and exposure. In the first group of patients, the Boston keratoprosthesis type I (KPro; Massachusetts Eye and Ear Infirmary, Boston) works well (Fig 15-27). For patients with end-stage dry eye, the Boston KPro type II is an option. Other types of keratoprostheses for these high-risk patients are more popular in Europe and include the TKPro, which uses tibia bone tissue, and the osteo-odonto-keratoprosthesis, which uses dentine and alveolar bone tissue.

Some surgeons have expanded the indications to include the treatment of ocular trauma, advanced quiescent herpetic disease, aniridia, and congenital corneal opacification.

The prognosis for keratoprosthesis implantation has improved dramatically because of innovations in the design of keratoprostheses and improvements in postoperative management. The use of a soft contact lens and long-term prophylactic antibiotics has reduced the incidence of infection and necrosis around the keratoprosthesis. A review of the literature on the Boston keratoprosthesis, the results of which were published in a report by AAO, revealed that a BCSVA of 20/200 or better occurred in 45%–89% of eyes, and a BCSVA of 20/40 or better occurred in 11%–39% of eyes after implantation of the Boston KPro. In a large, multicenter study of 300 eyes followed for 17.1±14.8 months after implantation of the Boston KPro, there was significant improvement in vision, although only 6% of eyes had visual acuity of 20/60 or better. The retention rate with the Boston KPro type I ranged from 65% to 100%. Loss of vision resulted from corneal melts due to exposure keratopathy, endophthalmitis, infectious keratitis, or corneal ulceration. The most common complications following keratoprosthesis implantation were persistent epithelial

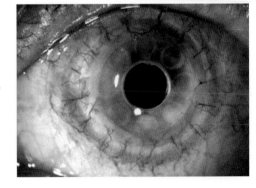

Figure 15-27 Boston keratoprosthesis type I. *(Courtesy of James J. Reidy, MD.)*

Table 15-9 Complications of Keratoprosthesis

Complication	Incidence
Glaucoma	Preexisting in 72.0%–86.0%
Retroprosthetic membrane formation	25.0%–55.0%
Persistent epithelial defects	38.0%
Stromal necrosis	16.0%
Endophthalmitis	12.5%
Cystoid macular edema	8.7%
Infectious keratitis	8.0%
Extrusion of implant	0%–12.5%

Reproduced from American Academy of Ophthalmology Cornea/External Disease Panel. Preferred Practice Pattern Guidelines. *Corneal Edema and Opacification.* San Francisco: American Academy of Ophthalmology; 2013. Available at www.aao.org/ppp.

defects, retroprosthetic membrane formation, stromal necrosis, and elevated IOP, often associated with glaucoma (Table 15-9).

Chang HY, Luo ZK, Chodosh J, Dohlman CH, Colby KA. Primary implantation of type I Boston keratoprosthesis in nonautoimmune corneal disease. *Cornea.* 2015;34(3):264–270.

Lee WB, Shtein RM, Kaufman SC, Deng SX, Rosenblatt MI. Boston keratoprosthesis: outcomes and complications: a report by the American Academy of Ophthalmology. *Ophthalmology.* 2015;122(7):1504–1511.

Part XII, Keratoprosthesis. In: Mannis MJ, Holland EJ, eds. *Cornea.* Vol 2. 4th ed. Philadelphia: Elsevier; 2017:1635–1667.

Rudnisky CJ, Belin MW, Guo R, Ciolino JB; Boston Type 1 Keratoprosthesis Study Group. Visual acuity outcomes of the Boston keratoprosthesis type 1: multicenter study results. *Am J Ophthalmol.* 2016;162:89–98.

Sayegh RR, Afshari NA, Chang HP, Lou ZK, Chodosh J. An overview of keratoprosthesis. *Focal Points: Clinical Modules for Ophthalmologists.* San Francisco: American Academy of Ophthalmology; 2014, module 6.

Basic Texts

External Disease and Cornea

Albert DM, Miller JW, Azar DT, Blodi BA, eds. *Albert & Jakobiec's Principles and Practice of Ophthalmology.* 3rd ed. 4 vols. Philadelphia: Saunders; 2008.

Arffa RC, Grayson M, eds. *Grayson's Diseases of the Cornea.* 4th ed. St Louis: Mosby; 1997.

Brightbill FS, McDonnell PJ, McGhee CN, Farjo AA, Serdarevic O. *Corneal Surgery: Theory, Technique and Tissue.* 4th ed. Philadelphia: Mosby; 2009.

Copeland RA Jr, Afshari NA, eds. *Copeland and Afshari's Principles and Practice of Cornea.* New Delhi, India: Jaypee Brothers; 2013.

Feder RS, ed. *The LASIK Handbook: A Case-based Approach.* 2nd ed. Philadelphia: Lippincott Williams & Wilkins; 2013.

Jorgensen JH, Pfaller MA, Carroll KC, Funke G, Landry ML, Richter SS, Warnock DW, eds. *Manual of Clinical Microbiology.* 11th ed. 2 vols. Washington, DC: ASM Press; 2015.

Krachmer JH, Palay DA. *Cornea Atlas.* 2nd ed. St Louis: Mosby; 2006.

Laver NV, Specht CS, eds. *The Infected Eye: Clinical Practice and Pathological Principles.* Cham, Switzerland: Springer International Publishing; 2016.

Levin LA, Nilsson SFE, Ver Hoeve J, Wu SM, Alm A, Kaufman PL, eds. *Adler's Physiology of the Eye.* 11th ed. Philadelphia: Saunders; 2011.

Mannis MJ, Holland EJ, eds. *Cornea.* 4th ed. 2 vols. Philadelphia: Elsevier; 2017.

Seal DV, Pleyer U. *Ocular Infection.* 2nd ed. New York: Informa Healthcare; 2007.

Spalton DJ, Hitchings RA, Hunter P. *Atlas of Clinical Ophthalmology.* 3rd ed. Oxford: Elsevier/Mosby; 2005.

Related Academy Materials

The American Academy of Ophthalmology is dedicated to providing a wealth of high-quality clinical education resources for ophthalmologists.

Print Publications and Electronic Products

For a complete listing of Academy products related to topics covered in this BCSC Section, visit our online store at https://store.aao.org/clinical-education/topic/cornea-external-disease.html. Or call Customer Service at 866.561.8558 (toll free, US only) or +1 415.561.8540, Monday through Friday, between 8:00 AM and 5:00 PM (PST).

Online Resources

Visit the Ophthalmic News and Education (ONE®) Network at aao.org/onenetwork to find relevant videos, online courses, journal articles, practice guidelines, self-assessment quizzes, images, and more. The ONE Network is a free Academy-member benefit.

Access free, trusted articles and content with the Academy's collaborative online encyclopedia, EyeWiki, at aao.org/eyewiki.

Requesting Continuing Medical Education Credit

The American Academy of Ophthalmology is accredited by the Accreditation Council for Continuing Medical Education (ACCME) to provide continuing medical education for physicians.

The American Academy of Ophthalmology designates this enduring material for a maximum of 15 *AMA PRA Category 1 Credits™*. Physicians should claim only the credit commensurate with the extent of their participation in the activity.

To claim *AMA PRA Category 1 Credits™* upon completion of this activity, learners must demonstrate appropriate knowledge and participation in the activity by taking the posttest for Section 8 and achieving a score of 80% or higher.

This Section of the BCSC has been approved by the American Board of Ophthalmology as a Maintenance of Certification Part II self-assessment and CME activity.

To take the posttest and request CME credit online:

1. Go to www.aao.org/cme-central and log in.
2. Click on "Claim CME Credit and View My CME Transcript" and then "Report AAO Credits."
3. Select the appropriate media type and then the Academy activity. You will be directed to the posttest.
4. Once you have passed the test with a score of 80% or higher, you will be directed to your transcript. *If you are not an Academy member, you will be able to print out a certificate of participation once you have passed the test.*

CME expiration date: June 1, 2020. *AMA PRA Category 1 Credits™* may be claimed only once between June 1, 2017, and the expiration date.

For assistance, contact the Academy's Customer Service department at 866.561.8558 (US only) or + 1 415.561.8540 between 8:00 am and 5:00 pm (PST), Monday through Friday, or send an e-mail to customer_service@aao.org.

Study Questions

Please note that these questions are *not* part of your CME reporting process. They are provided here for your own educational use and identification of any professional practice gaps. The required CME posttest is available online (see "Requesting CME Credit"). Following the questions are a blank answer sheet and answers with discussions. Although a concerted effort has been made to avoid ambiguity and redundancy in these questions, the authors recognize that differences of opinion may occur regarding the "best" answer. The discussions are provided to demonstrate the rationale used to derive the answer. They may also be helpful in confirming that your approach to the problem was correct or, if necessary, in fixing the principle in your memory. The Section 8 faculty thanks the Self-Assessment Committee for providing these self-assessment questions.

1. A 19-year-old woman with a known history of anorexia nervosa presents with symptoms of severe dry eye. On examination, there is wrinkling of the conjunctiva, heavy staining with lissamine green, and beading of tears along the conjunctival surface. A deficiency in what component of the tear film is responsible for these findings?

   a. mucin

   b. immunoglobulin E

   c. lipid

   d. lactoferrin

2. What can contribute to increased hydration or edema of the corneal stroma?

   a. hypertonic drops

   b. Salzmann nodular degeneration

   c. hypotony

   d. topical ofloxacin

3. What would the clinician expect to see on Placido disk–based topography in a patient with epithelial basement membrane dystrophy?

   a. distortion of mires

   b. inferior steepening in a "crab-claw" configuration

   c. symmetric bow-tie pattern

   d. central flattening

4. What corneal finding would display negative staining with fluorescein?

   a. dendrite

   b. corneal abrasion

   c. dellen

   d. maps

5. A 62-year-old man with a known history of rosacea presents with ocular symptoms of bilateral redness and irritation. Examination shows thickened meibomian secretions, eyelid margin telangiectasia, and marginal keratitis. Past medical history is also significant for atrial fibrillation, for which he takes warfarin, and 2 myocardial infarctions. What oral medication would pose the least risk for adverse reaction in this patient?

   a. minocycline

   b. erythromycin

   c. doxycycline

   d. azithromycin

6. A 61-year-old woman is referred by a glaucoma specialist for management of dry eye. Visual acuity is 20/60 in both eyes, with diffuse punctate staining and whorled epithelium. The Schirmer test result is normal, and tear breakup time is greater than 10 seconds. She has been using generic artificial tears 4 times daily in addition to latanoprost and timolol in both eyes. What would be the most effective first step in treatment?

   a. increasing the frequency of artificial tear use

   b. bilateral occlusion of the lower puncta

   c. topical steroid use

   d. providing preservative-free alternatives for all drops

7. A 19-year-old man presents with chronic symptoms of irritation and redness bilaterally. On examination, an extra row of eyelashes emerging from the ducts of the meibomian glands is noted. The patient's father has been examined, and the same findings have been noted. What is the diagnosis?

   a. blepharophimosis

   b. trichiasis

   c. distichiasis

   d. epiblepharon

8. A 56-year-old man presents with decreased vision. The examination reveals a markedly enlarged corneal diameter and visually significant cataract; results of the dilated examination are normal for both eyes. Preoperative measurements for cataract surgery show normal axial length, with white-to-white measurements of 14.5 mm in both eyes. During cataract surgery, the patient is at increased risk for what complication?

   a. choroidal effusion

   b. bleeding

   c. zonular instability

   d. malignant glaucoma

9. A finding of posterior embryotoxon on examination is most commonly associated with what condition?

   a. Axenfeld-Rieger syndrome

   b. Peters anomaly

   c. congenital aniridia

   d. normal eyes

10. Congenital syphilis was recently diagnosed in a child, who was then referred for ocular examination. What corneal finding would be consistent with this diagnosis?

    a. stromal vascularization

    b. pseudodendrites

    c. phlyctenules

    d. enlarged corneal nerves

11. While receiving treatment for a corneal abrasion, a patient presents with a chalky white plaque covering the extent of the abrasion and obscuring the visual axis. What is the most likely medication being used?

    a. ciprofloxacin

    b. neomycin-polymyxin-dexamethasone

    c. polytrim-sulfamethoxazole

    d. gentamicin

12. Band keratopathy may occur in patients with renal failure because of elevated levels of what serum electrolyte?

    a. sodium

    b. potassium

    c. phosphate

    d. chloride

13. What is the primary mechanism of vision loss in patients with Terrien marginal degeneration?

    a. corneal opacification

    b. amblyopia

    c. astigmatism

    d. spontaneous corneal rupture

14. Acute corneal hydrops in the setting of keratoconus is characterized by what histologic appearance?

    a. disruption of the Descemet membrane

    b. fragmentation of the Bowman layer

    c. iron deposition in the basal epithelium

    d. focal thinning of corneal stroma and the overlying epithelium

15. For patients with Hurler syndrome, corneal clouding is the result of a deficiency of what cellular structure?

    a. mitochondrion

    b. lysosome

    c. cell membrane

    d. endoplasmic reticulum

16. For an infant with corneal cystinosis, systemic monitoring for what complication is necessary?

    a. renal failure

    b. cardiomyopathy

    c. hepatosplenomegaly

    d. pulmonary fibrosis

17. A 45-year-old patient presents with a 2-year history of dry eye symptoms and bilateral recurrent corneal ulceration. In addition to a severely dry ocular surface, a foamy, superficial, triangular plaque located on the temporal bulbar conjunctiva of both eyes is noted during clinical examination. What past surgical history should be solicited?

    a. renal transplantation

    b. aortic aneurysm repair

    c. bowel resection

    d. pituitary tumor excision

18. What physical property of adenovirus makes it resistant to routine disinfection precautions (eg, swabbing a tonometer tip with ethyl alcohol)?

    a. absence of a viral envelope

    b. presence of a double-stranded DNA genome

    c. ability to form dormant cysts

    d. absence of glycoproteins in the capsid

19. What is the primary role of oral antiviral therapy in the treatment of interstitial keratitis caused by herpes simplex virus (HSV)?

    a. prevention of epithelial keratitis

    b. prevention of endotheliitis

    c. prevention of neovascularization

    d. prevention of lipid keratopathy

20. For immunocompetent adults receiving the varicella-zoster vaccine, the incidence of zoster is reduced by approximately what percentage?

    a. 30%

    b. 50%

    c. 70%

    d. 90%

21. A 35-year-old patient presents with chronic unilateral follicular conjunctivitis. Slit-lamp examination is remarkable for an ipsilateral eyelid nodule with central umbilication. What would biopsy of the eyelid lesion most likely reveal?

    a. eosinophilic intracytoplasmic inclusions within epidermal cells surrounding a necrotic core

    b. vacuolization of keratinocyte cytoplasm with multinucleated cells and nuclear inclusions

    c. histiocytes with foamy, lipid-laden cytoplasm surrounding blood vessels

    d. hyperkeratosis and acanthosis with a papillary growth pattern

22. A patient presents with a 1-day history of severe, copious conjunctival discharge. No corneal ulceration is present. Gram stain is significant for numerous neutrophils with gram-negative intracellular diplococci. What is the most appropriate treatment?

    a. intramuscular ceftriaxone

    b. intravenous penicillin G

    c. oral azithromycin

    d. topical gentamicin ointment

23. A 50-year-old man born in rural Pakistan presents for evaluation of a 10-year history of chronic decreased vision. Examination reveals bilateral corneal pannus originating superiorly, corneal vascularization, and extensive trichiasis. Both superior tarsi demonstrate stellate scarring. The Schirmer test result is 1 mm bilaterally. The inferior fornix is relatively unaffected. What is the most likely etiology of his vision loss?

    a. autoimmune disease

    b. bacterial infection

    c. viral infection

    d. toxic injury

24. What antifungal agent is indicated as first-line treatment of superficial keratitis caused by *Fusarium* species?

    a. amphotericin B

    b. fluconazole

    c. natamycin

    d. voriconazole

25. A 25-year-old contact lens wearer presents for evaluation of 4 weeks of severe ocular pain (right eye) and photophobia. The slit-lamp examination is notable for diffuse limbal injection, a 3-mm epithelial defect, and an amorphous stromal infiltrate. An adjacent corneal nerve exhibits a dense white-blood-cell reaction following the length of the nerve. What is the most likely etiology?

    a. bacterial

    b. viral

    c. fungal

    d. protozoal

26. What offending agent is most likely to be associated with contact dermatoblepharitis?

    a. topical medication

    b. *Demodex*

    c. pollen

    d. *Staphylococcus*

27. What is the most appropriate long-term treatment of atopic dermatitis and associated atopic keratoconjunctivitis uncontrolled by topical therapies?

    a. oral corticosteroids

    b. oral tacrolimus

    c. oral hydroxychloroquine

    d. oral doxycycline

28. What would be a reasonable treatment regimen for ocular surface squamous neoplasia?

    a. topical interferon-α_{2b} 1 million IU/mL 4 times daily for 3–4 months

    b. topical 5-fluorouracil 1% 4 times daily for 3–4 months

    c. topical mitomycin C (MMC) 1% 4 times daily for 3–4 months

    d. subconjunctival interferon-α_{2b} (3 million IU in 0.5 mL) daily for 3–4 months

29. An optical coherence tomography image depicts a conjunctival subepithelial lesion with cysts. What is the most likely diagnosis?

    a. nevus

    b. melanoma

    c. primary acquired melanosis (PAM)

    d. complexion-associated melanosis (CAM)

30. After surgical removal of a pterygium, what is the best approach to minimize the risk of recurrence and avoid any late-term complications?

    a. conjunctival autograft

    b. amniotic membrane transplant

    c. MMC injection

    d. bevacizumab injection

31. What is the best surgical option in a patient with a 360° conjunctivalization of the cornea after a unilateral chemical burn?

    a. simple limbal epithelial transplantation (SLET)

    b. penetrating keratoplasty (PK)

    c. allogeneic limbal stem cell transplantation

    d. keratoprosthesis

32. What factor exacerbates corneal blood staining from a traumatic hyphema?

    a. shallow anterior chamber

    b. heavily pigmented iris

    c. high intraocular pressure

    d. persistent epithelial defect

33. What is the best management when uveal prolapse occurs during an acute open-globe repair?

    a. reposit tissue

    b. resect tissue

    c. interpolate tissue

    d. enucleate

34. What is the next step in the management of a chemical injury to the ocular surface after initial irrigation fails to normalize the pH?

    a. Perform anterior chamber paracentesis and washout.

    b. Sweep the fornices for retained chemical particles.

    c. Change to speculum or contact lens irrigation system.

    d. Add topical corticosteroids.

35. By what mechanism does the *Dieffenbachia* plant cause keratoconjunctivitis?

    a. type I hypersensitivity

    b. type IV hypersensitivity

    c. calcium oxalate deposition

    d. immune complex deposition

36. Why is tissue from donors younger than 2 years generally not used in corneal transplantation?

    a. The tissue is steep and flaccid.

    b. There are ethical concerns about using tissue from infants and very young children.

    c. The corneal endothelial cells are not sufficiently developed.

    d. The corneal stroma is too thin.

37. What is the most common organism involved in infectious crystalline keratopathy following keratectomy?

    a. *Streptococcus*

    b. *Staphylococcus*

    c. *Candida*

    d. *Nocardia*

Answer Sheet for Section 8
Study Questions

Question	Answer	Question	Answer
1	a b c d	20	a b c d
2	a b c d	21	a b c d
3	a b c d	22	a b c d
4	a b c d	23	a b c d
5	a b c d	24	a b c d
6	a b c d	25	a b c d
7	a b c d	26	a b c d
8	a b c d	27	a b c d
9	a b c d	28	a b c d
10	a b c d	29	a b c d
11	a b c d	30	a b c d
12	a b c d	31	a b c d
13	a b c d	32	a b c d
14	a b c d	33	a b c d
15	a b c d	34	a b c d
16	a b c d	35	a b c d
17	a b c d	36	a b c d
18	a b c d	37	a b c d
19	a b c d		

Answers

1. **a.** Findings from the examination are suggestive of conjunctival xerosis (abnormal dryness of the conjunctiva), which is due to vitamin A deficiency and is associated with deficiency in the mucin component of the tear film caused by degeneration of the goblet cells. Mucin is produced by the goblet cells within the conjunctiva. Lipid, another component of the tear film, is produced by the meibomian glands. A reduced level of lactoferrin, a protein found in tears, can be a marker for dry eye. Immunoglobulin E levels in tears are elevated in allergic conjunctivitis.

2. **c.** Many factors contribute to hydration of the cornea. There is a natural tendency of the cornea to swell as the negatively charged glycosaminoglycans in the stroma repel each other (swelling pressure). Conversely, intraocular pressure has a compressive force on the cornea. In cases of hypotony, the compressive force is reduced, leading to increased corneal hydration and, in some cases, detectable corneal edema. Hypertonic drops draw fluid out of the cornea by creating an osmotic gradient. Salzmann nodular degeneration and topical ofloxacin have no effect on hydration of the corneal stroma.

3. **a.** Placido disk topography is based on the principle of reflecting images of concentric rings or mires off the corneal surface. In areas where the tear film or corneal surface is irregular, such as in epithelial basement membrane dystrophy, the mires are distorted. Reflected images are captured and analyzed by computer software, which can translate them into color topography maps. Color-coded maps help accentuate normal and pathologic patterns. Regular astigmatism is characterized by a symmetric bow-tie pattern oriented on the steep axis. Inferior steepening in a "crab-claw" configuration is classic for pellucid marginal degeneration. Central flattening is suggestive of a previous myopic ablation.

4. **d.** Punctate and macroulcerative epithelial defects stain with fluorescein (positive staining); the staining appears bright green when illuminated with a cobalt-blue filter. Dendrites and corneal abrasions display positive fluorescein staining. Dellen display either positive fluorescein staining or pooling of the dye. Fluorescein can also be used to distinguish lesions that project through the tear film. These lesions are described as having negative staining because they take on a darker appearance when contrasted with the surrounding fluorescein in the tear film. Maps seen in epithelial basement membrane dystrophy display negative staining with fluorescein when viewed with a cobalt-blue filter.

5. **b.** Tetracyclines such as minocycline and doxycycline are commonly used to treat rosacea and meibomian gland dysfunction, but prescribers must be aware of the potential adverse effects of these drugs, which include photosensitization, gastrointestinal upset, and oral or vaginal candidiasis (with long-term use). Tetracyclines are contraindicated in children younger than 8 years (because of the potential for discoloration of developing teeth) and in women who are pregnant or breastfeeding. Also, tetracyclines can reduce the effectiveness of oral contraceptives. In patients taking warfarin, such as the one described in the question, tetracyclines can potentiate anticoagulant effects and should be avoided if possible. Azithromycin is an alternative oral treatment, but the US Food and Drug Administration has issued a warning that this medication may be hazardous to patients with cardiovascular problems because it has the potential to cause irregularities in heart rhythm. Erythromycin is another alternative oral treatment; the risk of adverse reactions in this case would be lowest with this drug.

6. **d.** This patient has bilateral punctate staining with whorled epithelium in the absence of aqueous tear deficiency and evaporative dry eye. These clinical findings, along with her use of multiple eyedrops, are suggestive of toxic keratitis; benzalkonium chloride, the preservative found in most eyedrops, is a common offender. Switching to preservative-free alternatives is likely to improve the ocular surface. Adding topical steroids, increasing the frequency of generic artificial tears (which generally contain preservatives), or performing punctal occlusion would all increase exposure to preservatives and could worsen the condition.

7. **c.** Distichiasis is a condition in which an extra row of eyelashes emerges from the ducts of the meibomian glands. It can be congenital (often autosomal dominant) or acquired. Trichiasis is an acquired condition in which eyelashes emerge from their normal origin and curve inward toward the cornea. Epiblepharon is a condition in which the pretarsal muscle and skin of the eyelid ride above the eyelid margin to form a horizontal fold of tissue. Blepharophimosis is a horizontal shortening of the palpebral fissure.

8. **c.** Megalocornea is a condition with bilateral, nonprogressive corneal enlargement that usually shows X-linked inheritance. In this condition, the cornea is histologically normal, but its diameter is greater than 13 mm. Megalocornea is associated with zonular instability; thus, there are additional risks for these eyes during cataract surgery. Megalocornea is not associated with an increased risk of bleeding or malignant glaucoma. Nanophthalmic eyes are associated with an increased risk of choroidal effusion during cataract surgery.

9. **d.** Posterior embryotoxon is a thickened and anteriorly displaced Schwalbe line that can be seen by external examination. Although it is a known characteristic of Axenfeld-Rieger syndrome, most cases of posterior embryotoxon are seen in normal eyes. Peters anomaly is a congenital condition characterized by a paracentral corneal opacity with absence of underlying Descemet membrane and corneal endothelium. Congenital aniridia is incomplete formation of the iris and is associated with corneal pannus, glaucoma, cataracts, and foveal and optic nerve hypoplasia. Posterior embryotoxon is not associated with Peters anomaly or congenital aniridia.

10. **a.** In children with untreated congenital syphilis, the onset of interstitial keratitis is usually between 6 and 12 years of age. The keratitis initially presents as progressive corneal edema, followed by abnormal vascularization in the deep stroma, adjacent to the Descemet membrane. Pseudodendrites are seen in herpes zoster keratitis. Enlarged corneal nerves can be seen in *Acanthamoeba* keratitis and a variety of inherited diseases. Phlyctenules are nodular lesions that can be seen along the corneal limbus in cases of staphylococcal hypersensitivity.

11. **a.** Use of topical fluoroquinolones, especially ciprofloxacin, may result in chalky white deposits that adhere to corneal epithelial defects. A major factor in drug deposition is pH-dependent solubility of the drug. Also, patients with dry eye using eyedrops more frequently and for a prolonged period are prone to drug precipitation. Corneal deposits are more common in the interpalpebral region because of ultraviolet radiation–induced corneal damage and because of the maximum accumulation of topical ophthalmic medications in this part of the eye. These cases can be managed conservatively, avoiding debridement; deposits resolve after discontinuation of the medication.

12. **c.** Band keratopathy refers to the characteristic appearance of calcium hydroxyapatite deposited in a horizontal "band" across the cornea. The keratopathy commonly occurs in the presence of elevated levels of serum calcium (eg, due to hyperparathyroidism, vitamin D

toxicity, sarcoidosis), although elevated levels of serum phosphate also drive the precipitation of calcium hydroxyapatite, even in the setting of normal calcium levels. This may occur in patients with renal failure, particularly if they are not receiving appropriate treatment to lower serum phosphate concentrations. It is for this reason that the laboratory workup for unexplained band keratopathy should include calcium and phosphate tests.

13. **c.** Patients with Terrien marginal degeneration typically present in the fourth or fifth decade of life with decreased vision due to high against-the-rule, oblique, or irregular astigmatism. Hard contact lens fitting may be challenging because of severe inferior peripheral ectasia in these patients. Amblyopia is rarely, if ever, present, because the degeneration occurs later in life. Corneal opacification secondary to lipid keratopathy typically develops superiorly and may progress circumferentially, but it rarely causes vision loss due to opacification of the visual axis. Although progressive peripheral corneal thinning may occur (leading to increased risk of traumatic rupture), spontaneous corneal perforation is rare.

14. **a.** Acute corneal hydrops develops when a rupture (typically spontaneous) of the Descemet membrane occurs and aqueous rapidly saturates the stromal collagen, producing profound edema. Fragmentation of the Bowman layer, iron deposition in the basal epithelium, and focal corneal thinning are also features of keratoconus but not specific to corneal hydrops.

15. **b.** Hurler syndrome is a type of systemic mucopolysaccharidosis, a condition in which glycosaminoglycans cannot be completely metabolized because of defects in lysosomal enzymes. Mutations in the genes that synthesize the lysosomal enzymes are responsible for more than 30 different human genetic diseases. These conditions are known collectively as lysosomal storage diseases. The incompletely degraded by-products accumulate in cells, causing alterations in cellular function and properties. Excessive accumulation of glycosaminoglycans in the cornea results in progressive corneal clouding, which may recur despite penetrating keratoplasty (PK).

16. **a.** Nephropathy is most common in the infantile form of cystinosis (and least common in the adult-onset form). Corneal symptoms are often present by 2 years of age and manifest as photophobia. Renal damage is the major medical morbidity and may lead to kidney failure by 10 years of age. Corneal symptoms are managed with topical application of cysteamine. Oral administration of cysteamine may be beneficial for posterior segment manifestations (retinopathy, optic neuropathy).

17. **c.** The clinical scenario is suggestive of ocular surface disease due to chronic vitamin A deficiency. The bulbar conjunctival lesions described are known as Bitôt spots, which consist of keratinized epithelium, cellular debris, and *Corynebacterium xerosis*. More common in developing countries, vitamin A deficiency is uncommon in the United States in the absence of a specific risk factor. Possible risk factors that should be solicited during the history include unusually restrictive diets, alcoholism, or any chronic cause of lipid malabsorption (including bowel resection, as well as diseases such as cystic fibrosis). A history of renal transplantation is relevant for patients presenting with band keratopathy. Aortic aneurysm repair may suggest a diagnosis of Marfan syndrome. Because of their proximity to the optic chiasm, pituitary tumors are most relevant to visual field defects.

18. **a.** Adenoviruses (as well as many other viruses responsible for infectious outbreaks) do not have a viral envelope, in contrast to herpes simplex virus (HSV), human immunodeficiency virus (HIV), and influenza virus. Viral envelopes are composed primarily of lipids and proteins, which render them more susceptible to heat, acids, and drying. Alcohol swabbing is

sufficient to inactivate enveloped viruses. Adenoviruses, however, are surrounded only by a capsid of primarily glycoproteins, which are intrinsically more resistant to these same environmental stressors. For this reason, alcohol swabbing of a reusable tonometer tip is insufficient to prevent inoculation of subsequent patients in the setting of adenoviral exposure. Diluted bleach cleaning solution or disposable tonometer tips are necessary. Both HSV and adenovirus are characterized by a double-stranded DNA genome. *Acanthamoeba*, not adenovirus, is capable of prolonging survival by encysting itself in a dormant form.

19. **a.** The mainstay of treatment for HSV interstitial keratitis is topical corticosteroids. This condition is believed to be primarily inflammatory rather than actively infectious in origin. Topical or systemic antiviral coverage is indicated with the use of topical steroids to prevent severe epithelial keratitis should the patient shed HSV while using corticosteroid drops, and it is generally continued until the patient has completely stopped the corticosteroids or is using less than 1 drop of prednisolone 1% per day. Endotheliitis is a less common manifestation of HSV keratitis, and the benefit of antiviral prophylaxis is unclear. Neovascularization and lipid keratopathy are controlled primarily by limiting inflammation through the use of topical corticosteroids.

20. **b.** A study of more than 38,000 adults aged 60 years or older showed a 50% reduction in new cases of zoster and a 66% reduction in postherpetic neuralgia. Of note, the immunity may last only about 5 years, and younger adults may benefit more than older adults.

21. **a.** Chronic follicular conjunctivitis with an umbilicated eyelid nodule should raise suspicion for molluscum contagiosum. The classic histologic appearance of a molluscum lesion is a cup-shaped nodule with central necrosis, surrounded by epidermal cells with large eosinophilic intracytoplasmic inclusions (Henderson-Patterson bodies). Vacuolized cytoplasm with multinucleated cells is typical of a herpetic vesicle. Foamy histiocytes surrounding blood vessels describes xanthelasma. Hyperkeratosis and acanthosis with a papillary growth pattern are typical of *verruca vulgaris*, caused by human papillomavirus.

22. **a.** Hyperacute conjunctivitis with gram-negative intracellular (or extracellular) diplococci is diagnostic of gonococcal conjunctivitis caused by *Neisseria gonorrhoeae*. If corneal ulceration is present, the patient should be admitted to the hospital to receive intravenous ceftriaxone. In the absence of corneal involvement, outpatient therapy with intramuscular ceftriaxone 1 g and close observation is appropriate. Intravenous penicillin G is indicated for treatment of neurosyphilis. Oral azithromycin is indicated for the treatment of chlamydial conjunctivitis. Topical gentamicin ointment may be used as an adjunctive treatment for gonococcal conjunctivitis, but the mainstay of treatment is systemic ceftriaxone.

23. **b.** Taking into account the patient's age, clinical features, and country of origin, the most likely diagnosis is trachoma. Trachoma is caused by the bacterium *Chlamydia trachomatis* (serotypes A–C) and is the leading cause of preventable blindness worldwide. Although major efforts have been undertaken to decrease the incidence of trachoma, it remains endemic in the Middle East, Africa, and parts of Asia. The distinctive features are conjunctival and corneal scarring (predominantly superiorly, although severe cases may be diffuse), bandlike or stellate tarsal scarring (also typically superiorly), trichiasis, and aqueous tear deficiency. Entropion and tear duct obstruction are also common. The ocular manifestations of autoimmune disease (eg, Sjögren syndrome, mucous membrane pemphigoid) can be similar, but the superior predilection, place of birth, and relatively young age favor the diagnosis of trachoma. Cicatrizing changes from severe viral conjunctivitis (adenoviral, HSV, etc) are possible but still less likely. Toxic injuries (eg, from alkaline substances) tend to affect the inferior ocular surface in excess of the superior surface.

24. **c.** Natamycin is generally considered first-line therapy for most cases of fungal keratitis due to infection with filamentous fungi (eg, *Fusarium* species). Amphotericin B is preferred for treatment of yeast keratitis (eg, *Candida*). Voriconazole is efficacious against a variety of fungal infections, but it was shown to be inferior to natamycin in a prospective, randomized clinical trial. Fluconazole has largely been replaced by newer azoles (voriconazole, posaconazole) because of their improved ocular penetration with systemic administration. Of note, ocular penetration through intact corneal epithelium is poor for many antifungal agents, including natamycin; for deep lesions, serial epithelial debridement may be indicated to enhance tissue penetration.

25. **d.** A chronic corneal ulcer in the setting of contact lens wear may be caused by a variety of pathogens. In this case, the presence of radial perineuritis should raise suspicion for keratitis caused by *Acanthamoeba* (a protozoa) species. Although radial perineuritis has been reported rarely in other infections (HSV, *Pseudomonas*), the clinical description, chronicity, and history of contact lens wear should elevate *Acanthamoeba* keratitis to the top of the differential diagnosis. Fungal infections in contact lens wearers may present insidiously or acutely, but radial perineuritis is not typical.

26. **a.** Topical medications, such as dorzolamide, are most likely to cause contact dermatoblepharitis. Medications, cosmetics, and chemicals can trigger a local allergic reaction. Type I (immediate hypersensitivity) reactions, which are immunoglobulin E mediated, typically occur within minutes after exposure to an allergen. A type IV (delayed) hypersensitivity reaction, which is T-cell mediated, usually begins 24–72 hours following instillation of a topical agent. Environmental allergens such as pollen and mold are associated with various ophthalmic manifestations (vernal conjunctivitis, seasonal allergic conjunctivitis) but do not typically cause a contact dermatoblepharitis. *Staphylococcus* hypersensitivity can also have a variety of ocular manifestations, such as marginal keratitis, but its presentation is not typically similar to that of dermatoblepharitis. *Demodex* has been implicated in cases of chronic blepharitis but has not been associated with contact dermatoblepharitis.

27. **b.** Atopic dermatitis is a chronic condition in genetically susceptible individuals that usually begins in infancy or childhood and may or may not involve the external eye. It involves a type IV hypersensitivity reaction, increased immunoglobulin E hypersensitivity, increased histamine released from mast cells and basophils, and impaired cell-mediated immunity. Treatment includes identifying and minimizing allergens in the environment and in foods. Moisturizing lotions and petrolatum gels can be useful for skin hydration. Acute lesions can be controlled with a topical corticosteroid cream or ointment (eg, clobetasone butyrate 0.05%), but to avoid skin thinning and ocular complications of steroids, long-term use of such medications is strongly discouraged. Both topical and oral T-cell inhibitors (eg, tacrolimus) have been found effective and have fewer adverse effects than corticosteroids, so they are preferred in patients with chronic and severe disease. Oral antipruritic agents such as antihistamines and mast-cell stabilizers can alleviate itching but may exacerbate dry eye with their anticholinergic activity. Oral doxycycline and hydroxychloroquine are not used in the treatment of atopic dermatitis or atopic keratoconjunctivitis.

28. **a.** Several topical therapies can be used to treat ocular surface squamous neoplasia. Topical interferon-α_{2b} (IFN-α_{2b}) 1 million IU/mL is typically given 4 times daily until clinical resolution occurs, usually within 2 to 4 months. Several additional months of treatment may be beneficial; recent evidence indicates that residual tumor may be present for up to

3 months following clinical resolution. Subconjunctival/perilesional IFN-α_{2b} (3 million IU in 0.5 mL) can be given weekly in addition to, or as an alternative to, topical drops, especially if patient adherence is an issue. Subconjunctival IFN-α_{2b} is associated with flulike symptoms in 10% of patients. Mitomycin C (MMC) can be used for a shorter duration—typically weeks rather than months—but may have greater adverse effects, including surface toxicity and potential stem cell deficiency. Topical MMC 0.02% or 0.04% is typically administered 4 times daily for 1 week, followed by a 1-week structured treatment interruption (drug holiday), for a maximum of 3 or 4 treatment cycles. Topical 5-fluorouracil 1% may be given 4 times daily for 1 month, with at least several months off if repeated; alternatively, it may be given 4 times daily for 1 week, followed by a 3-week structured treatment interruption, until resolution, for a maximum of 3 cycles.

29. **a.** Nevocellular nevi of the conjunctiva consist of nests or more diffuse infiltrations of benign melanocytes. They arise during childhood and adolescence. Conjunctival nevi are classified as junctional (confined to the epithelial–stromal junction); subepithelial, or stromal (confined to the stroma); or compound (combined junctional and stromal components). Nevi near the limbus are usually almost flat, whereas nevi appearing elsewhere on the bulbar conjunctiva tend to be elevated. Pigmentation of conjunctival nevi is variable. Small epithelial inclusion cysts occur within about half of all conjunctival nevi, particularly the compound or subepithelial varieties. The other pigmented lesions listed do not typically contain cysts.

30. **a.** Several studies have demonstrated that the risk of recurrence after pterygium excision is lower if a conjunctival autograft, rather than an amniotic membrane transplant, is used. However, if the defect created following dissection of the pterygium is considerably larger than what can be covered with an autologous conjunctival graft, an amniotic membrane graft or simple limbal epithelial transplantation (SLET) are viable options to cover the entire area of resection. Covering the entire defect decreases postoperative inflammation and speeds reepithelialization of the ocular surface. Although there is evidence that the use of MMC with conjunctival autografting reduces the pterygium recurrence rate after surgical excision, further studies are necessary to determine the optimal route of administration and dose for MMC, as well as the duration of treatment with MMC and its long-term effects. Any use of topical MMC can be toxic and may cause visually significant complications, such as aseptic scleral necrosis and infectious sclerokeratitis. These complications may occur months, or even years, after use of the drug. The use of bevacizumab in primary pterygium excision apparently has no effect on the recurrence rate of this condition.

31. **a.** If total loss of limbal stem cells occurs unilaterally, an autograft of limbal epithelium from the fellow eye can repopulate the diseased cornea with normal corneal epithelium. The SLET technique is one in which minimal tissue is harvested from the donor eye to reduce the risk of damage to the ocular surface of the healthy eye. If total loss of limbal stem cells occurs bilaterally, options include harvesting stem cells from a living related donor (limbal stem cell allograft) or from an eye bank donor cornea (keratolimbal allograft). Cell culture (ex vivo expansion) of corneal stem cells has been shown to be an effective source for corneal surface repopulation; however, this technique remains experimental and is not available in the United States. Allogeneic limbal stem cell transplantation requires systemic immunosuppression as part of the postoperative regimen and is not needed when the unaffected eye can serve as a donor. Keratoprosthesis can be used in cases of limbal stem cell deficiency, but given its risks (glaucoma, endophthalmitis), this surgery is not

the first-line choice for the clinical scenario described. PK is not the appropriate surgery to perform in eyes with significant limbal stem cell deficiency.

32. **c.** The combination of elevated intraocular pressure, corneal endothelial damage, and blood in the anterior chamber can result in corneal blood staining. Red blood cells within the anterior chamber release hemoglobin; the hemoglobin penetrates the posterior corneal stroma, where it is absorbed by keratocytes. Hemoglobin is broken down into hemosiderin within the keratocytes, which can result in keratocyte death. It may be difficult to detect when blood is in apposition to the endothelium on slit-lamp examination; however, with close observation, early blood staining is seen by yellow granular changes and reduced fibrillar definition in the posterior corneal stroma. Blood staining can lead to a reduction in corneal transparency that may be permanent. Histologically, red blood cells and their breakdown products can be seen within the corneal stroma. Corneal blood staining often slowly clears, starting in the periphery.

33. **a.** If uvea or retina (seen as translucent, tan tissue with extremely fine vessels) protrudes, the surgeon can reposit it using a gentle sweeping technique through a separate limbal incision, with the assistance of viscoelastic injection to keep the anterior chamber formed. Only in cases of frankly necrotic macerated or contaminated tissue should prolapsed uveal tissue be excised. Primary enucleation should be performed only for an injury so devastating that restoration of the anatomy is impossible, when it may spare the patient another procedure. Interpolated conjunctival pedicle flaps have been used in the treatment of exposed glaucoma tube shunts and scleral melts, but this would not be appropriate handling of the tissue in an open-globe injury.

34. **b.** The most important step in the management of chemical injuries is immediate and copious irrigation of the ocular surface with water or balanced saline solution. Irrigation should continue until the pH of the conjunctival sac normalizes. The conjunctival pH should be checked with a urinary pH strip. If this strip is not available, it is better to overtreat with prolonged periods of irrigation than to assume that the pH has normalized and discontinue treatment too early. Because prolonged exposure to toxic particles can exacerbate chemical damage to the ocular surface, particulate chemicals should be removed from the ocular surface with cotton-tipped applicators and forceps. Eversion of the upper eyelid should be performed to search for material in the upper fornix, and the fornices should be swept with an applicator to ensure that no particulate matter remains in the eye. Topical corticosteroids are useful in treating inflammation in the acute postinjury period but are not used to neutralize the ocular surface initially.

35. **c.** Houseplants in the genus *Dieffenbachia* are known to cause keratoconjunctivitis, which occurs after deposition of calcium oxalate crystals in the cornea; when the plant leaves are crunched, these crystals can shoot into the cornea. The crystals cause a foreign-body sensation and are difficult to see on slit-lamp examination; the diagnosis of *Dieffenbachia* keratitis is made from the history as much as anything else. Ocular contact with the milky sap from a variety of trees can cause toxic reactions manifested by acute keratoconjunctivitis, epithelial defects, and stromal infiltration. The pencil tree and the manchineel tree, widely distributed in tropical regions, are known offenders.

36. **a.** Most eye banks accept corneal tissue from donors 2 to 75 years of age. Tissue from donors younger than 2 years is typically not used because it is extremely steep and flaccid. This makes the tissue difficult to handle and poses challenges for the surgeon in creating a watertight closure and achieving a predictable outcome.

37. **a.** The long-term use of topical corticosteroids, loss of corneal sensation after transplantation, uneven tear film, and suture exposure or erosion all predispose the patient to infectious keratitis, sometimes caused by unusual organisms. Culture of the infiltrate and the exposed suture is recommended, and initiation of broad-spectrum antibiotic therapy can help avoid graft failure. A peculiar form of keratitis, infectious crystalline keratopathy, is occasionally seen in grafts and other immunocompromised corneas. Branching colonies of organisms proliferate in the deep corneal stroma with minimal or no inflammatory response. Many organisms have been implicated, but *Streptococcus viridans* is seen most frequently.

Index

(*f* = figure; *t* = table)

Autografts/autologous transplantation
conjunctival, 351*t*, 353–355, 353*t*, 354*f*, 356
for chemical injuries, 384
indications for, 351*t*, 353
for limbal stem cell deficiency, 94
in pterygium surgery, 353–355, 353*t*, 354*f*
recurrence rate and, 353*t*
after tumor removal surgery, 329
conjunctival-limbal, in pterygium surgery,
recurrence rate and, 353*t*
corneal, 411, 451–452. *See also* Keratoplasty
limbal, 351*t*, 362–365, 363–364*f*. *See also* Limbal
transplantation
indications for, 351*t*
Autoimmune diseases
Cogan syndrome as, 309, 310
conjunctivitis caused by, cicatricial conjunctivitis
differentiated from, 301*t*
Mooren ulcer as, 314
mucous membrane pemphigoid as, 299, 301–302
peripheral ulcerative keratitis as, 51*f*, 311–313,
311*t*, 312*f*
scleritis in, 319, 323
Autologous serum drops
for dry eye, 61*t*, 63
for neurotrophic keratopathy/persistent corneal
epithelial defects, 81, 224
for superior limbic keratoconjunctivitis, 84
Autologous transplantation. *See* Autografts/autologous
transplantation
Autonomic pathways, in tear secretion, 5, 5*f*
Avellino (granular type 2) corneal dystrophy, 135*t*,
136*t*, 145*t*, 148–149, 149*f*
amyloid deposits in, 148, 186*t*
Avulavirus, 240*t*
Axenfeld anomaly/syndrome, 102. *See also* Axenfeld-
Rieger syndrome
Axenfeld-Rieger syndrome, 97*t*, 102, 103*f*
posterior embryotoxon in, 97*t*, 102
Axial curvature/axial curvature map, 28, 29*f*. *See also*
Cornea, topography of
Azelaic acid, for rosacea, 71
Azithromycin
for chlamydial conjunctivitis, 263
for meibomian gland dysfunction, 68, 68–69
for rosacea, 71
for trachoma, 262

B-cell lymphomas, conjunctival/ocular surface, 348,
349–350, 350*f*
B cells (B lymphocytes), monoclonal proliferation of,
crystalline corneal deposits and, 198, 198*f*
Bacilli (bacteria), 243
Bacillus, 244*t*, 247
cereus, 247
as normal flora, 206*t*
ocular infection caused by, 247
after ocular trauma, 247, 403
Bacteria, 208*t*, 243, 243–249, 244*t*. *See also specific
organism or type of infection*
classification of, 243–244, 244*t*

conjunctivitis caused by, 208*t*, 255–265
in children, 243, 255–256
classification of, 257*t*
in neonates, 257*t*, 263–265
corneal infection caused by, 208*t*, 267–273, 268*f*,
269*t*, 270*t*, 273*f*
corneal opacity and, 16*f*
eyelid margin and conjunctival infection caused by,
255–256
keratitis caused by, 208*t*, 267–273, 268*f*, 269*t*, 270*t*,
273*f*. *See also* Keratitis, bacterial
contact lens wear and, 266–267, 268, 269, 269*t*
as normal flora, 205, 206*t*
ocular infection caused by, 208*t*, 243, 243–249, 244*t*
invasion and, 207
specimen collection/isolation techniques for
diagnosis of, 209*t*, 211
scleritis caused by, 282–283, 283*f*
Bacterial cell wall, 243–244
Bacteriology, 208*t*, 243–249, 244*t*. *See also* Bacteria
Band keratopathy/calcific band keratopathy, 111,
117–120, 119*f*, 201
in aqueous tear deficiency, 56
gelatinous droplike corneal dystrophy and, 141, 141*f*
in gout, 119, 188
parathyroid disorders and, 201
Bandage contact lenses, 368
for chemical injuries, 383
contraindications to, in exposure keratopathy, 80
for corneal abrasion, 398
for dry eye, 61*t*, 63, 368
for graft-vs-host disease, 304, 305*f*
for penetrating and perforating ocular trauma, 402
for peripheral ulcerative keratitis, 313
for recurrent corneal erosions, 87, 368
for superior limbic keratoconjunctivitis, 84
for Thygeson superficial punctate keratitis, 307
Bare sclera, wound closure after pterygium excision
and, 351, 353–355, 353*t*, 354*f*
recurrence rate and, 353*t*
Bartonella (bartonellosis)
cat-scratch disease caused by, 248, 265–266
henselae, 244*t*, 248, 265, 266
Basement membrane, corneal, 9. *See also* Descemet
membrane/layer
Basement membrane dystrophy, epithelial (EBMD/
map-dot-fingerprint/Cogan microcystic/anterior
basement membrane), 135–138, 135*t*, 136*t*,
137*f*, 138*f*
recurrent corneal erosion and, 86, 87, 133, 138
Basement membrane zone (BMZ), in mucous
membrane pemphigoid, 301–302, 301*f*
Basic secretion test, 38
BCSVA. *See* Best-corrected visual acuity/best-
corrected Snellen visual acuity
Bee stings, ocular injury caused by, 386–387
Bence Jones protein, corneal deposition of, 198
Benign hereditary intraepithelial dyskeratosis, 332*t*
Benign lymphoid folliculosis, 48, 49*f*
Benign monoclonal gammopathy, crystalline corneal
deposits in, 198

Lipoproteins
corneal arcus and, 120, 121, 179
corneal changes in disorders of metabolism of, 179–181, 180f
Lisch epithelial corneal dystrophy (LECD), 135t, 136t, 140, 140f
Lissamine green, 37, 38f
in tear film/dry eye evaluation, 37, 56
Listeria monocytogenes, invasive capability of, 207
LK (lamellar keratoplasty). *See* Keratoplasty, lamellar
Loa loa (loiasis), 253, 282, 282f
Local anesthesia, for penetrating and perforating trauma repair, 403–404
Lodoxamide, for hay fever conjunctivitis, 289
Long ciliary nerve, lacrimal functional unit innervated by, 5f
Louis-Bar syndrome (ataxia-telangiectasia), 115t, 346
Low-coherence interferometry, 21
Low-density-lipoprotein (LDL) cholesterol, corneal arcus and, 121, 179
Lowe disease/syndrome (oculocerebrorenal syndrome), congenital corneal keloids in, 107, 125
Lubricants
for chemical injuries, 383
for conjunctivochalasis, 86
for dellen, 79, 92
for graft-vs-host disease, 304
for neurotrophic keratopathy/persistent corneal epithelial defects, 81, 224, 230
for peripheral ulcerative keratitis, 312–313
for recurrent corneal erosions, 87
for Stevens-Johnson syndrome (Stevens-Johnson syndrome/toxic epidermal necrolysis overlap and toxic epidermal necrolysis), 297, 298
for thermal injuries, 385
LUM (lumican) gene
in cornea plana, 100
in posterior amorphous corneal dystrophy, 136t
Lumican, 9. *See also LUM* (lumican) gene
Lye, ocular injury caused by, 376t
Lyme disease/Lyme borreliosis, 249
Lymph node biopsy, in conjunctival/ocular surface melanoma, 344
Lymphadenopathy, in ocular surface neoplasia, 328
Lymphangiectasia, conjunctival/ocular surface, 348
Lymphangiogenesis, in corneal transplant rejection, 317
Lymphangioma, conjunctival/ocular surface, 348
Lymphatic malformations, conjunctival/ocular surface, 348
Lymphatic/lymphocytic/lymphoid tumors, conjunctival/ocular surface, 348–350, 349f, 350f
Lymphogranuloma venereum, 260
Lymphoid folliculosis, benign, 48, 49f
Lymphoid hyperplasia (reactive lymphoid hyperplasia) of conjunctiva/ocular surface, 327, 348–349, 349f
lymphoma and, 327, 348, 349
Lymphoid tissues
immunoregulation in, 12–13f

mucosa-associated (MALT), of conjunctiva (conjunctiva-associated/CALT), 7
lymphoma arising in, 349–350, 350f
Lymphomas, conjunctival/ocular surface, 349–350, 350f
lymphoid hyperplasia and, 327, 348, 349
Lysosomal acid hydrolase, in mucolipidoses, 178
Lysosomal storage disorders, 174–179. *See also* Mucopolysaccharidoses
corneal changes in, 174–179, 175t, 176f, 177f
Lysyl hydroxylase, in Ehlers-Danlos syndrome, 193

M proteins, plasma cell overproduction of, 198
Macroglobulinemia, Waldenström, crystalline corneal deposits in, 198, 199f
Macrophage colony-stimulating factor, in mucous membrane pemphigoid, 299
Macular dystrophies, corneal (MCD), 135t, 136t, 145t, 149–151, 150f
Macule, of eyelid, 45t
Madarosis, in staphylococcal blepharitis, 74
Magnesium hydroxide (Mg[OH]₂), ocular injury caused by, 376t
Malassezia furfur
as normal flora, 206t
ocular infection caused by, 255
Malignant glaucoma, after penetrating keratoplasty, 424
Malignant melanoma. *See* Melanoma
Malnutrition, corneal changes in, 196–197, 197f
MALT. *See* Mucosa-associated lymphoid tissue
Mandibulofacial dysostosis (Treacher Collins syndrome), 192t
Manifest refraction, after penetrating keratoplasty, 431–432, 432f
Mannose-induced protein (MIP-133), *Acanthamoeba* keratitis and, 276
α-Mannosidase, in mannosidosis, 179
Mannosidosis, 179
Map-dot-fingerprint dystrophy. *See* Basement membrane dystrophy
Map lines, in epithelial basement membrane dystrophy, 137, 137f
Marcus Gunn pupil (relative afferent pupillary defect/RAPD), in ocular trauma, 401
Marfan syndrome, 192t, 193–194, 193f
corneal changes in, 192t, 193f, 194
megalocornea and, 96t, 194
Marginal arterial arcades, eyelids supplied by, 4f
Marginal corneal (catarrhal) infiltrates, 310–311
staphylococcal blepharitis/blepharoconjunctivitis and, 74, 74f
Marginal degeneration
pellucid (PMD), 16f, 168–169, 168f, 169f, 170f
corneal topography in evaluation of, 31, 33f, 169, 170f
Terrien, 122–124, 123f
Marginal keratitis
Fuchs superficial, 123
in rosacea, 70, 70f
Maroteaux-Lamy syndrome (MPS VI), 175t